The Human
Immunodeficiency
Virus

The Human Immunodeficiency Virus

BIOLOGY,
IMMUNOLOGY,
AND THERAPY

EMILIO A. EMINI,
EDITOR

PRINCETON UNIVERSITY PRESS
PRINCETON AND OXFORD

Copyright © 2002 by Princeton University Press

Published by Princeton University Press, 41 William Street, Princeton, New Jersey 08540

In the United Kingdom: Princeton University Press, 3 Market Place,
Woodstock, Oxfordshire OX20 1SY

All Rights Reserved

Library of Congress Control Number:
2001096473

ISBN 0-691-00454-4

British Library Cataloging-in-Publication Data is available

This book has been composed in Palatino by Princeton Editorial Associates, Inc.,
Scottsdale, Arizona

Printed on acid-free paper. ∞

www.pup.princeton.edu

Printed in the United States of America

10 9 8 7 6 5 4 3 2 1

CONTENTS

PREFACE

A quarter of a century has elapsed since the clinical recognition of the acquired immunodeficiency syndrome (AIDS) epidemic, and it has been almost two decades since the human immunodeficiency virus type 1 (HIV-1) was recognized as the infectious cause of the disease. The battle against the epidemic during these years has been characterized by noted scientific achievement as well as failure. The tools of modern molecular biology and biochemistry have permitted an extraordinary understanding of the virus and its pathogenesis with a speed and depth never before attained for any human pathogen. This understanding led to the development of therapeutic agents that, for many infected individuals, resulted in a substantial slowing of the disease process, thereby forestalling the development of serious clinical disease. However, the failure of our understanding and technology is reflected by our inability to cure the infected patient of this affliction permanently. Similarly, the epidemic has been characterized by triumphs and failures of social policies. On the one hand, these resulted in a substantial diminishing of the spread of the infection in certain human populations. Yet they have not prevented an explosive increase in the worldwide incidence of HIV-1 infection and have failed to provide the medical infrastructure necessary to deliver those therapeutic options that are available to all who could benefit from their use.

This monograph takes stock of our understanding, and lack of understanding, as we begin the third decade of our collective struggle against HIV-1 disease. In many respects, this decade may prove to be the most critical. At the end of 1999, the United Nations Program on HIV/AIDS (UN-AIDS) issued the "Report on the Global HIV/AIDS Epidemic," which detailed the extraordinary extent of the epidemic around the world. It is estimated that approximately 35 million humans are living with the infection. In 1999 alone, there were about 5.4 million new infections and 2.8 million deaths associated with the later stages of the disease. This statistic makes HIV-1 the single largest infectious disease cause of human death, surpassing both tuberculosis and malaria. In some sub-Saharan African countries, HIV-1 is so prevalent that the infection afflicts one of every four adults. In addition, many parts of the world are epidemiologically primed to experience an explosive spread of the infection, even though the current incidence may still seem to be low.

Each of the chapters in this book is designed to be as complete as possible and may be read independently of the remaining chapters if desired. It is hoped that, taken together, the chapters present a complete picture of the challenges that lie ahead. Following a brief but necessary introduction to the virus (Chapter 1), the chapters of the therapeutic intervention section detail the molecular aspects of those viral targets against which anti-HIV-1 chemotherapeutic agents are or may be directed. A description of the existing chemotherapies is given in those chapters (Chapters 3–5) that deal with the targets of these therapies (the viral reverse transcriptase and protease enzymes). A prevalent theme throughout these discussions is the development of viral resistance to these agents, which reflects the extraordinary genetic versatility of HIV-1. For this reason, the section begins with a description of the virus's genetics, particularly as it relates to resistance development (Chapter 2). It is the spreading incidence of resistant HIV-1 variants in treated infected individuals and populations that drives the current search for novel chemotherapeutic targets and interventions. These could potentially include novel agents against both the reverse transcriptase and protease as well as agents against novel targets such as the viral integrase enzyme (Chapter 6), the virus-host cell receptor interaction (Chapter 7), and the viral regulatory and accessory functions (Chapters 8 and 9). The final chapter (Chapter 10) of the section details how the currently available therapeutic agents are used for the treatment of the infected patient and describes both the promise and shortcomings of these therapies.

In the end, our ability to contain the worldwide epidemic will have to rely on prevention, either through social programs or through the development of a vaccine. Chapter 11 speaks to those social programs that have been effective in controlling the epidemiological spread of the infection and that today still serve as the best means of mitigating the epidemic. Finally, the eventual solution will likely rest with a vaccine, and the monograph's final two chapters (Chapters 12 and 13) speak to the considerable scientific challenges currently facing HIV-1 vaccine researchers, as well as their hope.

It is my sincere wish that, in another decade's time, we will look back and be able to chronicle the defeat of the HIV-1 epidemic. While this is almost certainly a naive wish, it is nonetheless one that can and should be made.

I thank all the contributors, laboratory and social scientists and physicians, who took valuable time from their ongoing studies of HIV-1 and AIDS to contribute their knowledge and understanding to this volume. The book reflects their years of collective dedication to the diverse aspects of AIDS research. I am especially grateful to Dolores Wilson, who coordinated the final preparation and compilation of the manuscripts.

CONTRIBUTORS

JON P. ANDERSON   *Department of Pathology, Health Sciences Center, University of Washington, Seattle, Washington, USA*

JAN BALZARINI   *Rega Institute for Medical Research, Leuven, Belgium*

ELANA CHERRY   *McGill University AIDS Centre, Montreal, Quebec, Canada*

TOM COATES   *AIDS Research Institute, University of California, San Francisco, California, USA*

CHRIS COLLINS   *Progressive Health Partners, San Francisco, California, USA*

JON H. CONDRA   *Department of Virus and Cell Biology, Merck Research Laboratories, West Point, Pennsylvania, USA*

MARK B. FEINBERG   *Department of Medicine and Department of Microbiology and Immunology, Emory University School of Medicine, Atlanta, Georgia, USA*

RICHARD B. GAYNOR   *Department of Medicine, University of Texas Southwestern Medical Center, Dallas, Texas, USA*

MATTHIAS GÖTTE   *McGill University AIDS Centre, Montreal, Quebec, Canada*

DARIA J. HAZUDA   *Department of Biological Chemistry, Merck Research Laboratories, West Point, Pennsylvania, USA*

SPYROS A. KALAMS   *Partners AIDS Research Center, Charlestown, Massachusetts, USA*

NATHANIEL R. LANDAU *The Salk Institute for Biological Studies, La Jolla, California, USA*

GERALD H. LEARN *Department of Microbiology, Health Sciences Center, University of Washington, Seattle, Washington, USA*

NORMAN L. LETVIN *Harvard Medical School, Beth Israel Deaconess Medical Center, Boston, Massachusetts, USA*

JAMES I. MULLINS *Department of Microbiology, Health Sciences Center, University of Washington, Seattle, Washington, USA*

WILLSCOTT E. NAUGLER *Department of Infectious Diseases, Division of Virology, Children's Hospital and Medical Center, Seattle, Washington, USA*

DAVID NICKLE *Department of Microbiology, Health Sciences Center, University of Washington, Seattle, Washington, USA*

MATTHEW RAIN *Department of Microbiology, Health Sciences Center, University of Washington, Seattle, Washington, USA*

ALLEN G. RODRIGO *School of Biological Sciences, University of Auckland, Auckland, New Zealand*

DANIEL SHRINER *Department of Microbiology, Health Sciences Center, University of Washington, Seattle, Washington, USA*

SHALOM SPIRA *McGill University AIDS Centre, Montreal, Quebec, Canada*

MARIO STEVENSON *University of Massachusetts Medical School, Worcester, Massachusetts, USA*

TODD SUMMERS *Progressive Health Partners, Washington, D.C., USA*

CATHERINE ULICH *University of Massachusetts Medical School, Worcester, Massachusetts, USA*

JOSEPH P. VACCA *Department of Medicinal Chemistry, Merck Research Laboratories, West Point, Pennsylvania, USA*

MARK A. WAINBERG *McGill University AIDS Centre, Montreal, Quebec, Canada*

BRUCE D. WALKER *Partners AIDS Research Center, Charlestown, Massachusetts, USA*

YANG WANG *Department of Microbiology, Health Sciences Center, University of Washington, Seattle, Washington, USA*

The Structure and Biology of HIV-1: Introduction

1

ELANA CHERRY
MARK A. WAINBERG

Retroviruses

Retroviruses comprise a large and diverse family of enveloped RNA viruses. The retroviral replicative strategy characteristically involves reverse transcription of genomic RNA into linear double-stranded (ds) DNA and the subsequent integration of this DNA into the genome of the cell (206, 286).

Retroviruses are divided into two broad categories, simple and complex, based on considerations of genomic organization, mRNA splicing mechanisms, and temporal regulation of gene expression (51, 298). All retroviruses contain three major coding domains, *gag, pol,* and *env,* which encode the structural, replicative, and envelope proteins, respectively. Simple retroviruses usually contain only these three genes, whereas complex retroviruses also encode additional regulatory proteins derived from multiply spliced messages (298). This alternative splicing mechanism is not observed in simple retroviruses, which express only unspliced and singly spliced viral mRNA transcripts. Because complex retroviruses encode regulatory proteins, their gene expression can be divided into two temporal phases, an early, regulatory phase and a late, structural phase. Simple retroviruses have not been shown to display this pattern of regulation of gene expression (51).

Retroviruses are classified into seven genera according to evolutionary sequence homology (278). Five of the genera belong to the group formerly known as the oncoviruses because of their oncogenic potential: avian sarcoma and leukosis viruses (ASLV), mammalian B-type viruses, murine leukemia–related viruses, human T-cell leukemia–bovine leukemia viruses (HTLV-BLV), and D-type viruses (286). Examples of each are Rous sarcoma virus (RSV), mouse mammary tumor virus (MMTV), Moloney murine leukemia virus (Mo-MuLV), human T-cell leukemia virus (HTLV), and

Mason-Pfizer monkey virus (MPMV), respectively. The remaining two genera are the lentiviruses and the spumaviruses. Members of the former include the human immunodeficiency viruses (HIV-1 and HIV-2), simian immunodeficiency virus (SIV), feline immunodeficiency virus (FIV), equine infectious anemia virus (EIAV), and ovine maedi-visna virus (MVV). An example of spumaviruses is human foamy virus (HFV). All oncogenic viral groups except the HTLV-BLV genus are simple retroviruses; HTLV-BLV and the lentiviruses and spumaviruses are complex (286).

Oncoviruses occur in all classes of vertebrates, are highly pathogenic, and usually cause malignancies. For example, human T-cell leukemia virus type I (HTLV-1) can result in adult T-cell leukemia (298). The lentiviruses are "slow" viruses that cause slow progressive degenerative diseases in many vertebrates. This is a consequence of the viral-mediated killing or impairing of specific cells and tissues and frequently results in immunologic dysfunction and neurological disorders (168, 298). Spumaviruses are less well understood; they are not known to be pathogenic in vivo, despite the fact that in vitro they are highly cytopathic, forming large, vacuolated syncytia with a "foamy" appearance (298). The virion morphology of ASLV, murine leukemia–related viruses, HTLV-BLV, and lentiviruses is termed C-type. These viral particles have a centrally localized spherical or conical core, and viral assembly occurs at the cytoplasmic side of the plasma membrane during budding. B-type particles contain eccentric, spherical cores that are initially formed in the cytoplasm, prior to migration toward the plasma membrane. This type of morphogenesis has been observed in mammalian B-type viruses, D-type viruses, and spumaviruses. Particles of A-type morphology assemble within the cytoplasm or at the endoplasmic reticulum (ER) membrane. Such particles are immature and not infectious and are most probably aberrant forms of other retroviruses.

HIV-1 Viral Dynamics and AIDS Pathogenesis

HIV-1 was first isolated from a patient in 1983 and was subsequently recognized as the causative agent of acquired immunodeficiency syndrome (AIDS) (12, 95, 191, 231, 278).

HIV-1 infection is a dynamic process characterized by continual new rounds of viral infection and replication in susceptible cells (125, 295). This process is ongoing throughout the course of HIV disease, even during the prolonged asymptomatic phase between primary infection and the development of AIDS. There is high turnover of virus in the blood and of virus-infected cells; the total number of virions produced, released into the extracellular fluid, and cleared is at least 10^{10} particles per day. Furthermore, there is rapid turnover of productively infected cells, whereby approximately 10^9 new cells are infected per day (33, 125, 227, 295).

Primary HIV-1 infection is characterized by extremely high levels of plasma virus. Values in excess of 10^6 copies of RNA/ml are commonly seen

(81, 227). As the viral-specific immune response of the host develops, plasma virus levels fall to lower steady-state values. These vary in different individuals and are predictive of the rate of disease progression (195). In untreated asymptomatic patients, the plasma HIV-1 RNA levels are typically in the range of 10^3–10^6 copies/ml (81).

HIV-1 principally infects activated CD4$^+$ T lymphocytes and terminally differentiated cells of the monocyte-macrophage lineage (71, 134, 185, 193). Progressive depletion of T lymphocytes is the defining feature of the immunodeficiency. In addition, infection of cells in the central nervous system, such as brain macrophages and microglial cells, may be responsible for AIDS dementia and other neurological diseases (136, 207). Infection of dendritic and Langerhans cells of the macrophage lineage is important for viral transmission. These cells play a central role in the presentation of antigens to CD4$^+$ T lymphocytes, and thus infected macrophages likely transmit the infection to T cells during antigen presentation (266, 316, 322).

The major sites of virus replication occur in the peripheral lymphoid organs, such as the lymph nodes and the spleen, as well as in the mucosal lymphoid tissue (70, 85, 214, 215). It is estimated that at least 99% of the plasma virus is produced by recently infected short-lived CD4$^+$ T lymphocytes in the peripheral lymphoid tissues (33, 42, 81, 125, 227, 295). Long-lived infected cells such as macrophages and latently infected T cells make only a minor contribution to plasma viremia in untreated patients (33, 42, 125, 227, 295).

Despite the great deal of progress that has been made in understanding HIV-1 and AIDS, critical aspects of disease pathogenesis remain to be elucidated. Primarily, it is still unclear how HIV-1 infection induces CD4$^+$ T-lymphocyte depletion, the central pathophysiologic feature of the disease. Numerous mechanisms have been proposed, including (i) direct killing of HIV-1-infected CD4$^+$ T lymphocytes; (ii) indirect effects on uninfected CD4$^+$ and CD8$^+$ T cells; (iii) failure of T-cell regeneration; (iv) disruption of the lymphoid tissue architecture; and (v) multiple viral and host factors (77, 81, 121, 124, 125, 194, 215, 227, 295). Second, knowledge concerning the dominant host immunologic factors involved in controlling disease progression remains imperfect. Disease progression occurs despite a vigorous HIV-specific immune response consisting of cellular (including both cytotoxic CD8$^+$ T-lymphocyte [CTL] and CD4$^+$ helper T-cell response) and humoral mechanisms that effectively contain viral replication for a time (77, 81, 211, 245).

The HIV-1 Genome and Viral Proteins

The Virion

The HIV-1 virion is illustrated schematically in Fig. 1.1. The viral envelope is formed by a cell-derived lipid bilayer into which the viral glycosylated envelope (Env) proteins have been inserted. These spiked projections con-

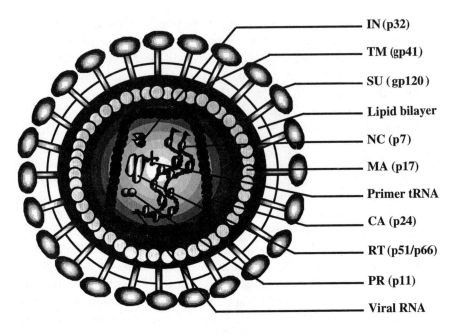

IN (p32)
TM (gp41)
SU (gp120)
Lipid bilayer
NC (p7)
MA (p17)
Primer tRNA
CA (p24)
RT (p51/p66)
PR (p11)
Viral RNA

FIGURE 1.1
Schematic representation of the HIV-1 virion

sist of the transmembrane (TM, gp41) and the surface (SU, gp120) components linked together noncovalently by disulfide bonds. The viral structural proteins are referred to as Gag proteins: in mature particles, the matrix protein (MA, p17) is located under the lipid bilayer, lining the inner surface of the membrane; the capsid protein (CA, p24) forms the conical capsid shell that encases the genomic RNA and the nucleocapsid protein (NC, p7), which together form part of the ribonucleoprotein (RNP) core. Associated with the NC and RNA within the virion are the viral-specific enzymes, reverse transcriptase (RT), protease (PR), and integrase (IN), all of which are essential for virus replication (101, 119).

Genetic Organization of HIV-1

Figure 1.2 is a schematic description of the HIV-1 genome and the known functions of its gene products. The genome consists of two functionally active RNA molecules, each of which is 9.2 kb in length, single-stranded (ss), nonsegmented, and of positive polarity (231). Typical of all retroviruses, HIV-1 initially synthesizes the structural proteins and enzymes in the form of large precursor polyproteins, which are cleaved by the viral PR to yield mature proteins. The HIV-1 genome consists of the three major retroviral genes, *gag, pol,* and *env,* as well as six auxiliary genes, *tat, rev, nef, vif, vpr,* and *vpu* (50).

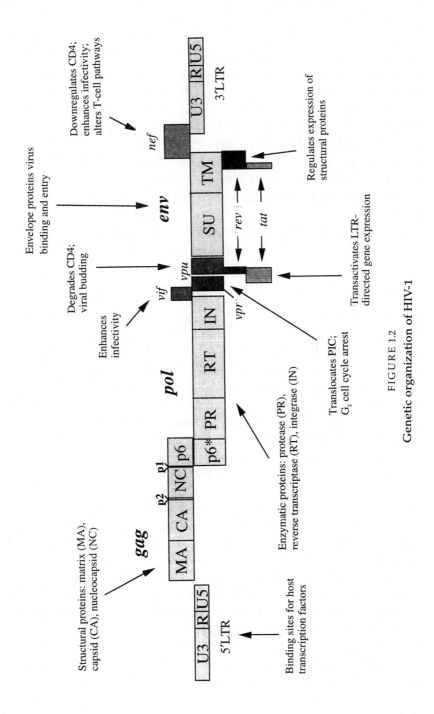

FIGURE 1.2

Genetic organization of HIV-1

HIV-1 also contains a large array of *cis*-acting elements that direct the host cell machinery to mediate viral gene expression from the integrated proviral DNA. Most of these elements reside in the long terminal repeats (LTRs) that are located at each end of the provirus and are divided into three functionally distinct regions known as U3, R, and U5. The U3 region that is found upstream of the transcription start site contains most of the transcription control elements, including the promoter, multiple enhancer sequences, and modulatory regions. RNA synthesis is initiated within the 5' LTR, at the junction between the U3 and R regions. The 3' LTR contains control elements involved in posttranscriptional processing of the 3' end of the RNA product, such as a poly-A tail addition. The R and U5 regions form part of the 5' untranslated leader region, which contains multiple sequences critical for numerous aspects of viral replication. For example, the leader region contains the transactivation region (TAR) element, the primer binding site (PBS), the dimerization initiation signal (DIS), the packaging signal (Ψ), and the major splice donor (SD) site (151, 236).

The gag Gene Products

The *gag* gene encodes the Pr55^{gag} (Gag) polyprotein precursor. During virus maturation, it is cleaved by the viral PR into several smaller polypeptides to yield the viral structural proteins, which play critical roles in the virus life cycle. The final products are (i) MA (p17), which is located at the amino-terminus of Gag and is essential for intracellular transport and membrane association of precursor proteins during viral assembly; (ii) CA (p24), which is derived from the central region of Gag and forms the viral core shell in mature particles; and (iii) NC (p15), which is located at the carboxy-terminus of Gag and is further processed into four smaller fragments, p2, p7 (NC), p1, and p6 (122, 141, 257, 285, 307).

The Gag Precursor Protein. Gag is the only viral protein essential for virus assembly; it is sufficient to direct the production and release of viruslike particles in the absence of any other viral protein, including the *env* gene product (100, 102, 143, 239, 260, 263, 304). Moreover, as the "assembly machine," Gag plays a critical role in orchestrating the assembly process. It contains within its structure all the functional elements required for (i) targeting and binding Gag and Gag-Pol to the plasma membrane; (ii) establishing intermolecular interactions between Gag precursors as well as between Gag and Gag-Pol polyproteins in the immature particle; (iii) envelopment and release of the particle; and (iv) directing the incorporation of the viral genome and of other molecules such as cyclophilin A (CypA) and Vpr (48).

MA. The MA (p17) lies immediately underneath the viral membrane and forms the viral matrix (101). It is *N*-myristylated and is responsible for targeting the Gag precursors to the plasma membrane, as well as facilitating their association with the membrane. These functions are accomplished via the membrane-binding (or M) domain that is located at its amino-terminus (15, 48, 75, 268, 291, 321). Mutations within MA have been shown to have severe effects on stable membrane binding, precursor transport, and particle assembly (88, 268, 291, 292). The efficient incorporation of the envelope glycoproteins into virions is also dependent on the integrity of the MA domain (66, 312). In addition, as part of the viral preintegration complex (PIC), MA is critical for translocating the complex to the nucleus (28, 29, 94, 120, 289). Finally, the MA has also been implicated in an early step in the virus life cycle prior to the completion of reverse transcription (32, 149, 216, 238).

CA. CA (p24) is a hydrophobic protein that forms a bullet-shaped core that encases the NC complex in the mature virion (119). CA plays essential roles early and late in infection. Its C-terminal segment contains a highly conserved sequence, termed the major homology region (MHR), that is essential for virion assembly and release (64, 189, 192, 288, 317). This region is required for Gag oligomerization as well as for CA dimerization (96, 317). Moreover, part of this domain is thought to represent the minimal Gag region capable of particle assembly and release (292). In contrast, the N-terminal region of CA appears to be dispensable for particle assembly but is required for formation of the mature core that is critical for viral infectivity (64, 239, 291).

NC. The mature NC (p7) is a small, basic protein containing two zinc fingers of a characteristic C-C-H-C motif that are associated with nucleic acid–binding proteins (17, 257, 267, 307). NC is essential for virus infectivity and has numerous vital functions in the virus life cycle. These include (i) mediating Gag interactions—via the interaction (or I) domain—that are critical for the formation of mature, infectious cores (15, 40, 48, 65, 88, 102, 111, 189, 213, 239, 304, 319); (ii) promoting dimerization and maturation of viral RNA (20, 55, 80, 89, 90, 256, 257, 311); (iii) facilitating the selective encapsidation of genomic RNA via interaction with the Ψ packaging site (20, 53, 54, 58, 107, 108, 138, 147, 171, 213, 230, 318); (iv) promoting primer tRNA positioning and annealing to the PBS (11, 60, 196, 232); (v) unwinding tRNA molecules; (vi) stimulating reverse transcription by promoting the formation of a tripartite complex composed of the RNA template, primer tRNA, and RT (11, 196, 232) and by stimulating strand transfer (5, 55, 311); and (vii) interacting with the Vpr protein (169).

p6. p6 (or p6^{gag}) is a peptide derived by the 3' region of the Gag precursor and is not present in Gag-Pol because of the ribosomal frameshifting event that occurs upstream (123, 285). In the virion, it is thought to be located between the core and envelope regions (126). The role of p6 in the HIV-1 life cycle is not fully understood, but it seemingly has numerous functions. First, it contains the L (or late) domain that is required for efficient budding by facilitating the release of assembled viral particles from the cell surface (48, 102, 109, 131, 253, 314). Since p6 serves as a negative regulator of PR activity, its role in particle morphogenesis is observed particularly in the presence of PR (131). However, accumulating data suggest that the p6 domain may not be absolutely required for particle assembly and release (138, 268, 292, 314). Second, p6 appears to be critical for the incorporation of Vpr into particles (154, 178, 179, 222). Third, this domain has recently been shown to play an important role in incorporating or retaining Pol proteins in the assembling virus particles when PR is activated during budding (313). Fourth, p6 was found to be critical for determining HIV-1 particle size (98). Finally, some nuclear targeting function was found to be directly or indirectly associated with this domain (40).

p2 and p1. Proteolytic processing of Gag also generates two small peptides, termed spacer peptides 1 and 2 (p1 and p2), which are located between NC and p6 and between CA and NC, respectively (122, 123, 198). Although they are poorly conserved in sequence and length, they are conserved in location within Gag precursors of primate lentiviruses, suggesting an important role in the retroviral life cycle (123). In fact, p2 functions transiently during sequential precursor processing, playing a critical role in regulating the ordered particle assembly and core formation that are crucial for normal virus maturation and infectivity (1, 111, 156, 228, 239). Deletion or alteration of p2 processing had drastic effects on internal core structure, resulting in aberrant virion morphology and loss of infectivity (111, 142, 156, 228, 239). It is thought that p2 regulates the sequential processing of Gag by serving as a negative regulator of cleavage at the CA-p2 site. In this way, it modulates the rate of processing and therefore regulates core formation (228). In addition, a novel function for p2 has recently been suggested in which it acts as a spherical shape determinant of the Gag particle during assembly and maturation (99). Although the function of p1 is unclear, this domain appears to play a role in RNA encapsidation specificity (318).

The pol Gene Products

The *pol* gene encodes the viral enzymes essential for replication, that is, PR (p11), RT (p51/p66), and IN (p32), positioned in that order from the 5′ end of *pol* (105, 285). PR is a homodimeric protein that is responsible for the proteolytic processing and subsequent processing and subsequent maturation of viral proteins (113, 203, 241). The heterodimeric protein RT converts viral genomic RNA into ds DNA via reverse transcription (104, 297). The IN protein catalyzes integration of ds viral DNA into the host chromosome (28, 29).

The Gag-Pol Polyprotein Precursor. The translational reading frame of the *pol* gene is in a −1 position from *gag*, and its expression occurs via a ribosomal frameshift to produce Pr160$^{gag-pol}$ polyproteins (Gag-Pol) (61, 135, 305). The frequency of the shift is about 5%, and therefore the relative abundance of the Gag and Gag-Pol precursor proteins is about 20:1, respectively (61, 135, 305). Encoded in the region between the frameshift site and PR itself is an additional peptide, the transframe region, designated p6* or p6^{pol}. This region has not been ascribed a specific function, but it seems to play an important role in regulating PR activity (113, 221).

The Gag-Pol precursor is incorporated into virus particles and is essential for infectivity (197, 217, 231). It plays a central role in the HIV-1 life cycle, not only because of the structural and enzymatic proteins generated by its cleavage but also because it is a determinant of the subsequent stability of the released virus particles (219). The Gag portion of Gag-Pol is essential for targeting the latter polyprotein into the virion, via multiple interactions between common regions of Gag and Gag-Pol (48, 130, 133, 137, 299, 304). Furthermore, the balance between the levels of Gag and Gag-Pol is critical in influencing the subsequent formation of virus particles (78, 235). In contrast to Gag, the exclusive expression of Gag-Pol does not result in the release of viruslike particles (197, 217, 260). This is due, in part, to the intracellular activation of the viral PR resulting in the premature processing of Gag-Pol.

PR. As with other retroviral proteinases, HIV-1 PR is absolutely required for virion maturation and is therefore essential for viral infectivity (153, 226). Its inactivation, either by a single point mutation in the catalytic active site (Asp-25) or by mutational amino acid insertions within PR, has drastic effects on the assembly, stability, and infectivity of the released virus particles (111, 219, 225, 226).

HIV-1 PR is a member of the aspartic family of PRs, containing the characteristic and conserved amino acid triplet Asp-Thr-Gly (DTG) in its catalytic active site (175, 212, 223). Mutagenic studies have shown the importance of the aspartyl (D25) and other conserved residues for activity (153, 165, 174, 175, 254). The active PR is an obligatory dimeric enzyme, consisting of two 11-kDa monomers that associate symmetrically to form the substrate binding cleft, each monomer contributing one catalytic aspartyl residue to the active site of the enzyme (103, 145, 160, 199, 200, 205, 208, 223, 294, 306). The two monomers are held together as a dimer by the amino- and carboxy-termini of PR, which form a four-stranded antiparallel β-sheet (293, 306). Disruption of these interactions in the dimer interface—for example, by truncation due to self-digestion (244) or by competition by peptides (10, 320)—leads to loss of enzymatic activity.

Reverse Transcriptase. RT is essential for viral replication, being responsible for the conversion of ss viral genomic RNA into ds DNA by a process termed reverse transcription (104, 297). Functional RT molecules are heterodimers consisting of two polypeptides, p66 and p51, which exist in approximately equal proportions in HIV-1 virions (37, 62, 170, 177). Although the two subunits share a common amino-terminus, p51 is produced by proteolytic cleavage of p66 by PR near the carboxy-terminus (62, 170). In the heterodimer, p66 is the subunit with RT activity, while its C-terminal peptide (p15) exhibits RNase H activity (117, 128, 176, 177, 272, 277). RT has at least three enzymatic functions: RNA-dependent DNA polymerase activity (RDDP), DNA-dependent DNA polymerase activity (DDDP), and RNase H activity (105).

IN. IN is a 32-kDa protein derived from the carboxy-terminus of the Gag-Pol polyprotein by proteolytic cleavage during virus maturation. It is responsible for the processing and joining reactions that insert viral DNA into the host genome in a process termed integration, which are essential steps in the virus replication cycle (28, 29, 146). IN functions as a multimer whose enzymatic activities require the presence of a divalent metal ion (13). Integration is both site-specific, involving U3 and U5 terminal sequences of the viral LTR, and nonspecific with respect to the target site in host DNA (146). Although IN is the only protein required for integration in vitro, additional viral and host proteins participate during integration in vivo (76). Initially, it was believed that the only function of IN was to mediate the integration of viral DNA. However, the structure of viral particles produced by some IN-defective HIV-1 mutants is aberrant, suggesting that IN could play a role in virion assembly and maturation (72, 259).

The env *Gene Products*

The *env* gene is translated from a spliced RNA into the precursor gp160, which then enters the secretory pathway of the host cell (86). During the process of transportation to the plasma membrane, the site at which the envelope glycoproteins become incorporated into virions, gp160 undergoes maturation to a bipartite complex composed of the N-terminal, external subunit (gp120, SU), and the TM C-terminal protein (gp41, TM). In addition to this proteolytic cleavage by cellular enzymes, the glycoproteins undergo subsequent modifications such as extensive glycosylation, disulfide bond formation, and interactions with chaperon proteins that facilitate proper folding (68, 69, 116). This results in the formation of a noncovalently associated trimeric complex in the virion membrane (68, 116, 158, 178, 296, 309). The gp120 subunits are responsible for virus adsorption to receptors on host cells (193), while gp41 anchors the complex in the viral membrane and mediates cell fusion (93, 155).

Accessory Proteins

In addition to Gag, Pol, and Env present in all retroviruses, HIV-1 also encodes six accessory proteins, Tat, Rev, Nef, Vpr, Vif, and Vpu (118). These can be classified into two groups based on the temporal regulation of their expression. The Rev-independent proteins are produced at early times after infection and include Tat, Rev, and Nef; the expressions of Vif, Vpr, and Vpu are Rev-dependent and thus occur late in the viral life cycle (51). Tat and Rev are absolutely required for virus growth. Tat is essential early in replication with a primary role in transcriptional activation of the viral promoter, and Rev acts later to ensure the switch from the early, regulatory phase to the late, structural phase of viral gene expression (202, 284). Although early evidence had suggested that Nef, Vif, Vpr, and Vpu were dispensable for virus growth in many in vitro systems, recent studies have shown that they fulfill several critical functions in vivo, particularly with respect to viral replication and pathogenesis (202, 284).

Tat. Tat is a small protein encoded by a spliced mRNA derived from two exons within the central region and *env* gene of the genome (9, 265). Primarily located in the nucleus and nucleolus of infected cells, Tat is a potent transactivator that enhances LTR-driven transcription of viral genes by 10- to 1,000-fold (151, 161, 255). Tat binds to a stable stem-loop structure located at the 5′ end of all RNAs, termed TAR. Both Tat and TAR are essential for HIV-1 replication, and mutations that disrupt their interaction eliminate virus production (52, 151, 255). Binding of Tat to TAR RNA is thought to position Tat in proximity to the RNA start site, allowing its transcriptional activation domains to interact with the cellular transcription apparatus (151). Tat activation of viral gene expression is believed to result from two modes of action. First, it increases the processivity of RNA polymerase II, thereby enhancing the efficiency of elongation of TAR-containing full-length RNA transcripts. Second, the frequency of RNA initiation is increased by Tat (52, 151, 161).

Rev. Rev is an essential viral protein encoded by a small, multiply spliced mRNA synthesized at early times after infection. It is located in the nucleus and nucleolus of infected cells (51). Rev acts posttranscriptionally, playing a critical role in regulating the temporal expression of viral proteins by driving translocation of singly spliced and unspliced RNA out of the nucleus to the cytoplasm (50, 114, 115, 188, 265). In the absence of Rev, only very low levels of full-length RNAs and singly spliced mRNAs are found in the cytoplasm. However, when a threshold level of Rev is produced, unspliced and singly spliced RNAs begin to accumulate in the cytoplasm. This allows the switch from the early, regulatory phase of viral gene expression to the late phase, in which productive infection occurs.

Rev functions through binding to a highly structured segment of HIV-1 RNA located within the *env* gene called the Rev response element (RRE) (115, 188). The RRE is present in all RNAs that are dependent on Rev for their cytoplasmic expression; conversely, it is spliced out of Rev-independent RNAs.

There are a few possible models of Rev action. First, evidence strongly suggests that the primary effect of Rev is in directly mediating the nuclear export of RRE-containing RNAs through interaction with a general nuclear export pathway (82, 188, 300). Second, Rev has also been proposed to inhibit complete splicing of HIV-1 RNAs. This results in the generation of a pool of unspliced and singly spliced RNAs that are now available for nuclear export (38). Finally, it has been suggested that Rev may enhance the translation of unspliced and singly spliced RNAs in the cytoplasm (8). Taken together, it appears that Rev may have effects on several levels of RNA processing and function, acting as a "chaperon" through various stages of RNA transport.

Nef. Encoded only by primate lentiviruses, Nef is produced at all stages of viral gene expression and is packaged in virions in low amounts. Nef is necessary for high levels of viral replication and disease progression of SIV in vivo, as well as for induction of AIDS (56, 148, 152). Although the mechanism of action of Nef in pathogenesis is unclear, it is thought to result from the protein's capacity to alter several cellular functions. First, Nef downregulates the surface expression of CD4 (2, 97) and major histocompatibility complex class I molecules (MHC-I) (164, 253). This is a consequence of Nef triggering their rapid endocytosis and lysosomal degradation and results in the inhibition of CTL-mediated lysis of HIV-1 infected cells (46). Second, virion-associated Nef enhances viral infectivity by promoting early events after virus entry such as uncoating of the core and stimulation of proviral DNA synthesis (3, 27, 201, 270). In addition, Nef has been reported to alter T-cell activation pathways and increase viral transcription in vitro, but the relevance of these findings to HIV-1 pathogenesis in vivo has yet to be determined (52, 202, 284).

Vpr. Vpr is a nuclear protein expressed from a singly spliced mRNA. It is incorporated into budding virus particles in high amounts by a specific mechanism, that is, by association with the p6 domain of Gag (44, 154, 179, 222). Its presence in mature virions is related to its two principal functions. First, Vpr mediates the active transport of the PIC to the nucleus of nondividing cells, independent of MA's role in the same process (120). The second function of Vpr is to arrest dividing cells in the G_2 phase of the cell cycle, by inhibiting cyclin-dependent kinase p34[cdc2] activity (14, 139, 242). Cell-cycle arrest has several important consequences, such as (i) maximizing virus production by delaying cells at the point of the cell cycle where the viral LTR is most active, before the infected cell is eliminated by the host immune response (71, 106); (ii) upregulating viral gene expression (44, 106, 310); (iii) preventing persistent infection in vitro (242); (iv) causing terminal differentiation of some cells (167); and (v) inducing HIV-mediated cell killing in vitro that may be associated with CD4[+] T-cell depletion during disease progression in vivo (275, 310). Thus, in vivo, it appears that the cytostatic Vpr-mediated G_2 arrest plays a pivotal role in viral replication by providing the virus with a selective advantage, namely, maximizing virus production and perhaps mediating CD4[+] T-cell depletion (106, 275, 310). Furthermore, recent evidence suggests that Vpr molecules present in both infectious and noninfectious viral particles are equally capable of arresting CD4[+] T cells and may therefore contribute to immune dysfunction in vivo (229).

Vif. Vif is a cytoplasmic protein that is produced from a singly spliced mRNA late in infection. It plays an important role in conferring infectivity on progeny virions, rendering them competent for the early steps of infection (92, 290). This effect is probably indirect, because only trace amounts are found in virions (31, 173). Moreover, the requirement for Vif is strictly cell dependent and is determined solely by producer and not target cells (247). Several mechanisms for Vif's role in early events have been proposed, each relating to infectivity enhancement and virion association. First, Vif ensures the proper packing of the nucleoprotein core (127). Second, it facilitates the transport of virions through the microfilament network that connects the outer cell membrane to the nuclear membrane (144). Third, it stabilizes newly synthesized DNA intermediates (261). Vif may also play a role in provirus formation; this function is believed to be required during virus formation rather than during infection (202).

Vpu. Vpu is an integral membrane protein that is produced late in the replication cycle from a singly spliced bicistronic mRNA that also contains the *env* open reading frame. Two biological functions have been identified for Vpu. First, Vpu interacts with the cytoplasmic domain of ER-retained CD4 molecules that are complexed with gp160 and triggers their accelerated degradation (23, 190, 302). This not only enhances the intracellular transport and maturation of Env, which is predicted to increase the infectivity of virions, but also reduces the density of CD4 at the cell surface. This may preclude superinfection and hence the premature destruction of the infected cell (202). Second, Vpu stimulates the release of virions from the surface of infected cells (110, 150). Although the mechanism for the release is unknown, it is thought to result from the ability of Vpu to form ion channels in the cell membrane (74, 159, 252).

The Replication Cycle of HIV-1

An overview of the HIV-1 replication cycle is illustrated schematically in Fig. 1.3.

Virus Entry and Cellular Tropism

The process of HIV-1 infection begins with the virus binding to a susceptible target cell. Cellular entry requires binding of the viral gp120 envelope glycoprotein both to the CD4 cell surface receptor (185, 273) and to one of the seven TM G-protein-coupled chemokine receptors (GPCR) recently discovered to act as coreceptors and that play an important role in viral tropism (4, 59, 67, 79). Most viruses that are able to infect cultured T-cell lines are termed T-tropic, or X4, viruses. These are syncytium inducing (SI), are frequently found in late-stage HIV disease, and utilize the chemokine receptor CXCR4. The majority of macrophage-tropic (M-tropic, or R5) viruses are non–syncytium inducing (NSI) in T-cell lines, are found throughout disease, and utilize CCR5 (4, 21, 41, 59, 63, 67, 79, 172). Although other members of the GPCR family are involved in entry for various viral strains, CCR5 and/or CXCR4 remain the receptors used by all known strains of HIV-1 (41, 63, 172). The natural ligands for these chemokine receptors (SDF-1 for CXCR4; RANTES, MIP-1α, and MIP-1β for CCR5) inhibit the infection of the particular HIV-1 variants that utilize these molecules for entry (22, 43, 209, 237, 249).

T-tropic HIV-1 isolates can infect both resting and activated CD4+ T cells, but replication does not occur in the former because of a block at a postentry level (29, 30). Similarly, these viruses can enter macrophages efficiently by using CD4 and CXCR4 as coreceptors; however, replication is restricted at the level of nuclear import of viral DNA (251). M-tropic HIV-1 isolates can infect activated CD4+ T cells but do not easily infect resting T cells because of the low expression of CCR5; productive infection of recently infected resting CD4+ T cells requires antigen-driven activation (29, 30, 269, 315).

The primary viral determinant of cellular tropism is the third variable (V3) loop of Env gp120 (41, 134). CD4 binding to gp120 induces conformational changes in the gp120 glycoprotein, exposing or creating high affinity binding sites for chemokine receptors on the V3 loop (158, 240, 308, 309). Subsequently, gp120 interacts with either CXCR4 or CCR5 (283, 308). Importantly, the affinity of gp120 for CCR5 is greatly enhanced in the presence of CD4, emphasizing that CD4 not only provides a docking surface for gp120 but also promotes exposure of a domain that interacts with chemokine receptors (283, 308). The binding site for CCR5 on gp120 has been mapped to a fragment that contains the CD4 binding site and over-

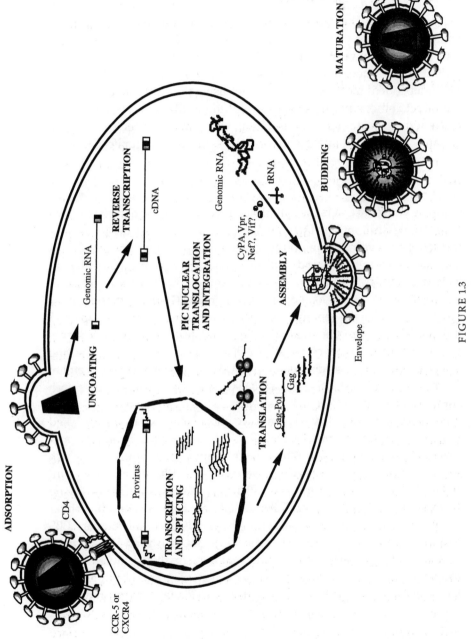

FIGURE 1.3

Schematic representation of the HIV-1 life cycle

lapping determinants within the V3 loop (308); the binding site of gp120 for CXCR4 is thought to lie within the highly conserved stem of the V1/V2 structure near the base of the V3 loop and in other regions folded into proximity (158, 240, 309).

Chemokine-receptor binding is believed to trigger additional conformational changes that lead to the exposure of the fusogenic peptide at the amino-terminus of the gp41 glycoprotein (158). This in turn modifies gp41 into its fusion-active state, whereby it inserts into the target membrane (158, 198). Subsequently, the viral and plasma membranes fuse via a direct, pH-independent mechanism, thereby releasing the viral core particle into the target cell cytoplasm to initiate replication (273). Furthermore, it is thought that, in addition to their roles in viral entry, the chemokine receptors may be involved in postentry activities during virus replication (34).

Reverse Transcription

Once the viral core enters the cytoplasm, reverse transcription converts viral genomic RNA into ds DNA (104, 297). The current model for reverse transcription involves numerous steps and is depicted in Fig. 1.4.

RT initiates minus-strand DNA synthesis by elongating a partially unwound primer tRNA that is hybridized to the PBS in genomic RNA. In HIV-1, tRNA^{Lys3} serves as the replication primer (166). Synthesis continues to the 5′ end of the genome, generating minus-strand strong-stop DNA [(−)ssDNA]. As RT reaches the end of the template, its RNase H activity degrades the RNA strand of the RNA/DNA duplex. This allows the first strand transfer to proceed whereby (−)ssDNA is tranferred to the 3′ end of the genome, guided by the repeat (R) sequences of the LTRs present on both ends of the RNA (129, 184, 224). Minus-strand DNA synthesis then resumes and is completed by RT, again accompanied by RNase H–mediated degradation of the template strand. Template digestion is incomplete and results in the generation of RNase H–resistant oligoribonucleotides rich in purines, called the polypurine tract (PPT) (35). Plus-strand DNA synthesis is initiated primarily at the PPT and then proceeds by copying minus-strand DNA to its 5′ end (39, 234). RNase H removal of the primer tRNA facilitates the second strand transfer, in which complementary PBS segments in the plus-strand DNA and in the minus-strand DNA anneal (129, 224). The plus- and minus-strand syntheses are then completed, with each strand serving as a template for the other (132). This generates a linear ds DNA duplex, containing a duplicated LTR at either end (105, 279).

Proviral DNA Nuclear Localization and Integration

Following reverse transcription, the newly synthesized ds DNA is contained within a PIC, whose other components include RT, IN, NC, MA, and

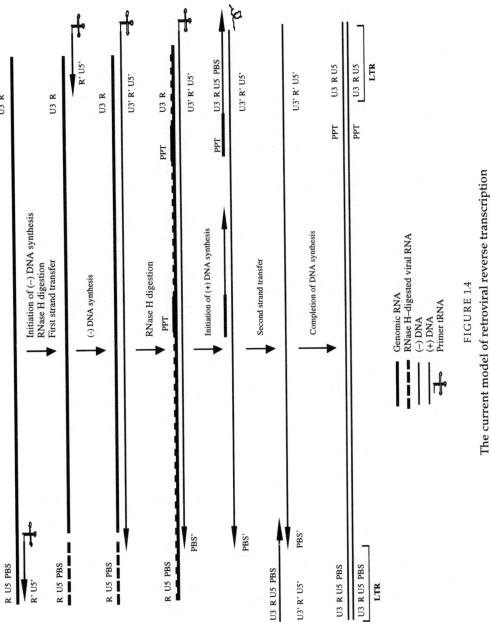

FIGURE 1.4

The current model of retroviral reverse transcription

Vpr (28, 76, 94). Entry of the PIC into the nucleus is an essential step in retrovirus replication and is required for subsequent integration of the viral DNA genome into host DNA and thus for virus production (28). The oncoviruses are dependent on cell proliferation for their replication, because breakdown of the nuclear envelope at mitosis allows the PIC to interact with the host cell chromosomes. In contrast, HIV-1 and other lentiviruses have evolved specific mechanisms for PIC nuclear import that are independent of nuclear membrane breakdown, so that replication can occur in nondividing cells. Consequently, HIV-1 can infect terminally differentiated and nondividing cells such as macrophages and dendritic cells, a property important for viral dissemination and transmission (28, 29, 202). Factors involved in HIV-1 PIC translocation include Vpr and MA, which independently, yet partially redundantly, permit the import of the viral PIC through the nuclear pore via distinct nuclear localization sequences (NLS) (94, 120, 290, 310).

Once inside the nucleus, the viral DNA, which is a blunt-ended linear molecule whose termini correspond to the boundaries of the LTRs, is integrated into the host chromosome at nonspecific target sites by the viral enzyme IN (28, 29). The first step (3′ processing) is IN-dependent cleavage of two nucleotides from the 3′ end of each strand of viral DNA; this occurs in the cytoplasm prior to nuclear entry of the PIC (246). The next step (joining or DNA strand transfer) is a concerted cleavage and ligation reaction, in which a staggered cut is generated in the target DNA by nucleophilic attack involving the hydroxyl group present at the recessed 3′ ends of the viral DNA. This is followed by linkage of the viral DNA to the 5′ ends of the target DNA at the cleavage site (73, 157, 233, 258). The resulting gaps in the target DNA are repaired, likely by host enzymes, to create short direct repeats flanking the provirus, a hallmark of all retroviral integration reactions (146, 157).

Expression of the Viral Genome

Once integrated into the chromosome, HIV-1 utilizes the host cellular machinery for transcription and translation of its genome, in addition to the virally encoded Tat protein (50, 119). Host RNA polymerase II is responsible for synthesis of the primary RNA transcripts, which serve either as mRNA for translation into viral proteins or as viral genomic RNA that will be incorporated into progeny virions during assembly. The rate of initiation of viral transcription depends on cellular transcription factors, particularly in the early stages of viral gene expression prior to the production of Tat. Cellular activation and proliferation signals cause the binding of transcription factors to the LTR and result in increased rates of transcription (50, 151). The efficient transcription of the viral genome requires a series of complex mechanisms involving the viral regulatory proteins Tat and

Rev, as well as cellular transcription factors such as NF-κB, NFAT-1, AP-1, and Sp1 (151).

Following the synthesis of full-length RNA transcripts, a complex array of alternatively spliced mRNAs are produced. The differential expression of distinct species of viral mRNAs is controlled by the HIV-1 Rev protein (52). The level of Rev present in an infected cell determines the proportion of the unspliced, singly spliced, and multiply spliced RNAs that are produced. This in turn regulates the switch from the early phase of viral gene expression to the late phase, in which productive infection occurs (52). Because Rev, Tat, and Nef are encoded by fully spliced nRNAs, these gene products are expressed and function shortly after infection and are therefore referred to as early gene products. In contrast, the Gag, Pol, Env, Vif, Vpr, and Vpu proteins, as well as full-length genomic RNA, are all dependent on Rev for the nucleocytoplasmic transport of their cognate mRNAs and are therefore expressed with delayed kinetics; they are referred to as the late proteins (50, 52, 114, 115, 188, 265).

Viral Packaging, Assembly, and Budding

HIV-1, like other lentiviruses and C-type oncoviruses, assembles at the plasma membrane of the infected cells (286). The formation of retroviral particles is a self-assembly process requiring only the expression of the Gag precursor polyprotein. Gag is responsible for orchestrating the assembly process, as well as recruiting viral proteins, viral genomic RNA, and host cell–derived elements into virus particles (48, 102, 119, 181, 239, 312). However, it is unclear whether the self-assembly of Gag polyprotein monomers is initiated in the cytoplasm or only after association of the molecules with the lipid bilayer (206).

Assembly is thought to begin with the association of genomic RNA with the Gag and Gag-Pol precursor proteins. Efficient encapsidation of the viral genome requires the presence of *cis*-acting packaging sequences, termed ι(psi), located upstream of Gag in the full-length viral genomic RNA (171, 182). Sequences in the NC domain of Gag are necessary for specific genomic RNA recognition and packaging, particularly the zinc finger motifs and the flanking basic residues (20, 53, 54, 58, 147, 171, 182, 213, 230).

The Gag-Pol precursor is incorporated into virions via association with Gag, presumably through interactions between the Gag domains of the two polyproteins (48, 133, 218, 264, 271, 304). Although multiple regions throughout Gag are important in Gag interactions, such as numerous domains within MA, CA, NC, and p2 (40, 213, 239, 319), the critical determinants within Gag-Pol that mediate its entry into virions have been mapped to the MHR and the adjacent C-terminal sequences of CA (130, 189, 218, 239, 264, 271). In addition, the RT and IN regions of Gag-Pol may also play roles in Gag-Pol incorporation by facilitating dimerization of the polyprotein precursors (6, 7, 26, 72).

Membrane targeting and binding of the precursors involve the N-myristic acid that has been cotranslationally added to the amino-terminal glycine residues of MA on both Gag and Gag-Pol, as well as a cluster of basic amino acids near the N-terminus of MA. The myristate moiety is thought to provide a hydrophobic anchor in the membrane while the basic charges mediate electrostatic interactions that stabilize the association (25, 111, 217, 268, 321). In addition, it has recently been suggested that the interaction of the membrane-binding domain of Gag with the plasma membrane is facilitated by the interaction (or I) domain within NC (250). Myristylation of Gag is required for assembly and particle formation (40, 102, 111, 218, 264). In contrast, myristylation of Gag-Pol is not necessary for Gag-Pol assembly into virions; rather, the unmyristylated Gag-Pol polyprotein is recruited via interactions with Gag (25, 111, 218, 264).

Budding is initiated following the association of genomic RNA/polyprotein complexes with the Env glycoproteins at the cell membrane (11, 19, 110, 162, 186, 204, 248). The envelope proteins are incorporated into the virion through interactions with MA (69, 87, 163, 312). The efficient release of virus particles is dependent on a sequence element named the L (or late) domain, located within the C-terminal p6 sequence of Gag (48, 109, 303).

Other Proteins Incorporated into the Virion. During virus assembly, additional molecules, that is, other virus-encoded proteins as well as cellular proteins and nucleic acids, are incorporated into virions while budding from infected cells. Although the mechanism by which some host-derived proteins, such as MHC class I and class II, HLA-DR, β_2-microglobulin, and intercellular adhesion molecule 1 (ICAM-1), are packaged is not clear, it does appear that these host-derived proteins may have functional roles in the virus life cycle (281). Other proteins and RNA molecules, which are critical for virus replication and infectivity, are incorporated into budding virions via specific mechanisms.

The Vpr protein is found in large quantities in virions (44) and is recruited through interactions with the p6 domain of Gag (154, 179, 222). Some controversy remains regarding the presence of Nef and Vif in mature particles, primarily because the amounts of these proteins are low and the mechanisms for their encapsidation are unclear; nevertheless, data supporting their presence are becoming stronger (202, 284). Virion-associated Nef has been shown to enhance the infectivity of the incoming virus, most likely by promoting uncoating of the core and stimulating reverse transcription (3, 27, 201, 270). Although Vif has been identified as a component of the virion that also enhances infectivity (31, 173), recent data suggest that the packaging of Vif is neither specific nor necessary for its function (262).

The incorporation of the host cell chaperon CypA into HIV-1 virions is mediated by a specific interaction with the CA domain of Gag (45, 84, 181, 280). CypA is required for the formation of fully infectious virus particles (24, 83, 84). It is thought that CypA binding to CA induces the correct Gag structure for proper assembly and processing and, after virus entry, facilitates destabilization of the viral core and thereby permits the initiation of reverse transcription (24, 83, 180, 276).

In addition, viral particles contain numerous cellular RNA species, including primer tRNA^{Lys3}, which is selectively packaged into the virus via specific RT sequences within Gag-Pol (186, 187).

Maturation

Newly released viral particles are immature, containing uncleaved precursor proteins that form a spherical protein shell closely apposed to the lipid membrane, as well as an electron-lucent core (91, 100, 126, 206). They are rendered mature and therefore infectious by a process termed maturation. This involves precursor protein processing whereby Gag cleavage induces a dramatic reorganization of the internal viral structure associated with condensation of the core, yielding morphologically mature viruses (287). Processing and maturation are not required for particle assembly or release but are essential for viral infectivity (153, 226).

Virion maturation involves cleavage of Gag by the virally encoded PR, which is brought into the virion as a component of Gag-Pol (49, 111, 153). Either at the membrane of infected cells or shortly after virion release, PR activity is initiated by what is believed to be an autocatalytic process (140, 241). PR activation occurs only after dimerization of Gag-Pol polyproteins at the time of virion assembly (57, 183). The active dimeric PR then processes the polyprotein precursors into functional protein components. This causes the internal structure of the particle to rearrange and to condense into an electron-dense core, generating mature, infectious viral particles (48, 61, 212, 241, 287). Furthermore, PR activity in precursor processing is also important for maximizing the efficiency with which virions are released from the surface of infected cells (140).

Accurate and complete processing of the Gag precursor by PR is essential for the formation of infectious, morphologically mature virions (140, 142). Maturation and core condensation constitute a sequential process that is regulated by the rate of cleavage at individual sites within Gag. Three determinants are likely to control the ordered proteolytic processing: (i) the sequence of the processing site; (ii) the structural context of the processing site; and (iii) the accessibility of the site to PR (220, 228). The initial cleavage occurs at the carboxy-terminus of p2 and separates an N-terminal MC-CA-p2 intermediate and a C-terminal NC-p1-p6 intermediate (16, 47, 112, 198, 282). This rapid cleavage between CA and NC releases the RNA-binding NC protein and leads to condensation of the ribonucleo-protein (RNP) core (301). Subsequent cleavates separating MA from CA-p2 and NC-p1 from p6 occur at an approximately 10-fold lower rate (228). The release of MA from CA, which allows CA to separate from the membrane, plays a pivotal role in core condensation; inhibition of processing at this site leads to noninfectious particles with abnormal morphologies (111, 142, 156, 220, 239, 287). The final cleavage in the processing cascade releases p2 from the carboxy-terminus of CA. This late event is slow and is thought to be mediated by cleavage at the p2-NC site, which reduces the efficiency of cleavage at the upstream CA-p2 site (228). In fact, C-terminally extended CA species have been observed in virions or viruslike particles with reduced PR activity (197, 243). This final CA cleavage is not needed for condensation of the RNP core but is essential for condensation of the capsid shell and is believed to stabilize the viral core into its mature conformation (1, 301).

Implicit in the morphological change precipitated by the cleavage of Gag during virion maturation is the condensation of RNA. The genomic RNA dimer is initially encapsidated in an extended conformation and later adopts a condensed structure (54, 90, 287). This maturation requires the activity of PR, since it is the mature NC that induces the conformational changes that stabilize the RNA dimer (18, 54, 80, 89, 90, 101, 210, 274, 287). Some Gag cleavages are dependent on the presence of RNA, and thus it is thought that events other than proteolysis, in particular NC-RNA interactions, may be critical for proper morphological maturation (20, 256, 257). Moreover, it has been proposed that genomic RNA acts as a scaffold, organizing the assembly process for condensation of a dense, infectious particle (48, 91, 138).

REFERENCES

1. Accola, M. A., S. Hoglund, and H. G. Gottlinger. 1998. A putative α-helical structure which overlaps the capsid-p2 boundary in the human immunodeficiency type 1 Gag precursor is critical for viral particle assembly. J. Virol. 72:2072–2078.

2. Aiken, C., J. Konner, N. R. Landau, M. E. Lenburg, and D. Trono. 1994. Nef induces CD4 endocytosis: requirement for a critical dileucine motif in the membrane-proximal CD4 cytoplasmic domain. Cell 76:853–864.

3. Aiken, C., and D. Trono. 1995. Nef stimulates human immunodeficiency virus type 1 proviral DNA synthesis. J. Virol. 69:5048–5056.

4. Alkhatib, G., C. Combadiere, C. C. Broder, Y. Feng, P. E. Kenedy, P. M. Murphy, and E. A. Berger. 1996. CC CKR5: a RANTES, MIP-1α, and MIP-1β receptor as a fusion cofactor for macrophage-tropic HIV-1. Science 272:1955–1962.

5. Allain, B., M. Lapadat-Tapolsky, C. Berlioz, and J.-L. Darlix. 1994. Transactivation of the minus strand DNA transfer by nucleocapsid protein during reverse transcription of the retroviral genome. EMBO J. 13:2464–2472.

6. Ansari-Lari, M. A., L. A. Donehower, and R. A. Gibbs. 1996. Analysis of human immunodeficiency type 1 integrase mutants. Virology 70:3870–3875.

7. Ansari-Lari, M. A., and R. A. Gibbs. 1996. Expression of human immunodeficiency virus type 1 reverse transcriptase in *trans* during virion release and after infection. J. Virol. 70:3870–3875.

8. Arrigo, S. J., and I. S. Chen. 1991. Rev is necessary for translation but not cytoplasmic accumulation of HIV-1 *vif, vpr,* and *env/vpu* 2 RNAs. Genes Dev. 5:808–819.

9. Arya, S. K., C. Guo, S. J. Josephs, and F. Wong-Staal. 1985. *Trans*-Activator gene of human T-lymphotropic virus type III (HTLV-III). Science 229:69–73.

10. Babe, L. M., J. Rose, and C. S. Craik. 1992. Synthetic "interface" peptides alter dimeric assembly of the HIV 1 and 2 proteases. Protein Sci. 1:1244–1253.

11. Barat, C., O. Schatz, S. H. J. LeGrace, and J.-L. Darlix. 1993. Analysis of the interactions of HIV-1 replication primer tRNA(Lys,3) with nucleocapsid protein and reverse transcriptase. J. Mol. Biol. 231:185–190.

12. Barre-Sinoussi, F., J. C. Cherman, R. Rey, M. T. Nugeryte, S. Chamaret, J. Gruest, C. Dauget, C. Axler-Blin, F. Vezinet-Brun, C. Rouzioux, W. Rosenbaum, and L. Montagnier. 1983. Isolation of a T-lymphotropic retrovirus from a patient at risk for acquired immune deficiency syndrome (AIDS). Science 220:868–871.

13. Barsov, E. V., W. E. Huber, J. Marcotrigiano, P. K. Clark, A. D. Clark, E. Arnold, and S. H. Hughes. 1996. Inhibition of human immunodeficiency virus type 1 integrase by the Fab fragment of a specific monoclonal antibody suggests that different multimerization states are required for different enzymatic functions. J. Virol. 70:4484–4494.

14. Bartz, S. R., M. E. Rogel, and M. Emerman. 1996. Human immunodeficiency virus type 1 cell cycle control: Vpr is cytostatic and mediates G2 accumulation by a mechanism which differs from DNA damage checkpoint control. J. Virol. 70:2324–2331.

15. Bennett, R. P., T. D. Nelle, and J. W. Wills. 1993. Functional chimeras of the Rous sarcoma virus and human immunodeficiency virus Gag proteins. J. Virol. 67:6487–6498.

16. Bennett, R. P., S. Rhee, R. C. Craven, E. Hunter, and J. W. Wills. 1991. Amino acids encoded downstream of Gag are not required by Rous sarcoma virus protease during Gag-mediated assembly. J. Virol. 65:272–280.

17. Berg, J. 1986. Potential metal-binding domains in nucleic acid binding proteins. Science 25:485–487.

18. Berkowitz, R., J. Fisher, and S. P. Goff. 1996. RNA packaging. Curr. Top. Microbiol. Immunol. 214:177–218.

19. Berkowitz, R. D., and S. P. Goff. 1993. Point mutations in Moloney murine leukemia virus envelope protein: effects on infectivity, virion association and superinfection-resistance. Virology 196:748–757.

20. Berkowitz, R. D., A. Ohagen, S. Hoglund, and S. P. Goff. 1995. Retroviral nucleocapsid domains mediate the specific recognition of genomic viral RNAs by chimeric Gag polyproteins during RNA packaging *in vivo*. J. Virol. 69:6445–6456.

21. Berson, J. F., D. Long, G. J. Doranz, J. Rucker, F. R. Jirik, and R. W. Doms. 1996. A seven-transmembrane domain receptor involved in fusion and entry of

T-cell-tropic human immunodeficiency virus type 1 strains. J. Virol. 70: 6288–6295.

22. Bleul, C. C., M. Farzan, H. Choe, C. Parolin, I. Clark-Lewis, J. Sodroski, and T. A. Springer. 1996. The lymphocyte chemoattractant SDF-1 is a ligand for LESTR/fusin and blocks HIV-1 entry. Nature 382:829–832.

23. Bour, S., U. Schubert, and K. Strebel. 1995. The human immunodeficiency virus type 1 Vpu protein specifically binds to the cytoplasmic domain of CD4: implications for the mechanism of degradation. J. Virol. 69:1510–1520.

24. Braaten, D., E. K. Franke, and J. Luban. 1996. Cyclophilin A is required for an early step in the life cycle of human immunodeficiency virus type 1 before the initiation of reverse transcription. J. Virol. 70:3551–3560.

25. Bryant, M., and L. Ratner. 1990. Myristylation-dependent replication and assembly of human immunodeficiency virus 1. Proc. Natl. Acad. Sci. USA 87:523–527.

26. Bukovsky, A., and H. Gottlinger. 1996. Lack of integrase can markedly affect human immunodeficiency virus type 1 particle production in the presence of an active viral protease. J. Virol. 70:6820–6825.

27. Bukovsky, A. A., T. Dorfman, A. Weimann, and H. G. Gottlinger. 1997. Nef association with human immunodeficiency virus type 1 virions and cleavage by the viral protease. J. Virol. 71:1013–1018.

28. Bukrinsky, M. I., S. Haggerty, M. P. Dempsey, N. Sharova, A. Adzhubel, L. Spitz, D. Goldfarb, M. Emerman, and M. Stevenson. 1993. A nuclear localization signal-1 matrix that governs infection of non-dividing cells. Nature 365:666–669.

29. Bukrinsky, M. I., N. Sharova, M. P. Dempsey, T. L. Stanwick, A. G. Bukrinskaya, S. Haggerty, and M. Stevenson. 1992. Active nuclear import of HIV-1 preintegration complexes. Proc. Natl. Acad. Sci. USA 98:6580–6584.

30. Bukrinsky, M. I., T. L. Stanwick, M. P. Dempsey, and M. Stevenson. 1991. Quiescent T lymphocytes as inducible virus reservoir in HIV-1 infection. Science 254:423–427.

31. Camaur, D., and D. Trono. 1996. Characterization of human immunodeficiency virus type 1 Vif particle incorporation. J. Virol. 70:6106–6111.

32. Casella, C. R., L. J. Raffini, and A. T. Panganiban. 1997. Pleiotropic mutations in the HIV-1 matrix protein that affect diverse steps in replication. Virology 228:294–306.

33. Cavert, W., D. W. Notermans, K. Staskus, S. W. Wietgrefe, M. Zupancic, K. Gebhard, K. Henry, S.-C. Zhang, R. Mills, H. McDade, C. M. Schuwirth, J. Goudsmit, S. A. Danner, and A. T. Haase. 1997. Kinetics of response in lymphoid tissue to antiretroviral therapy of HIV-1 infection. Science 276:690–694.

34. Chackerian, B., E. M. Long, P. A. Luciw, and J. Overbaugh. 1997. Human immunodeficiency virus type 1 coreceptors participate in postentry stages in the virus replication cycle and function in simian immunodeficiency virus infection. J. Virol. 71:3932–3939.

35. Champoux, J. J. 1993. Roles of ribonuclease H in reverse transcription, p. 103–117. In A. M. Skalka and S. P. Goff (ed.), Reverse transcriptase. Cold Spring Harbor Laboratory Press, Cold Spring Harbor, N.Y.

36. Chan, D. C., and P. S. Kim. 1998. HIV entry and its inhibition. Cell 93:681–684.

37. Chandra, A., T. Gerber, and P. Chandra. 1986. Biochemical heterogeneity of reverse transcriptase purified from the AIDS virus, HTLV-III. FEBS Lett. 197:84–88.
38. Chang, D. D., and P. A. Sharp. 1989. Regulation by HIV Rev depends upon recognition of splice sites. Cell 59:769–795.
39. Charneau, P., and F. Clavel. 1991. A single-stranded gap in human immunodeficiency virus unintegrated linear DNA defined by a central copy of the polypurine tract. J. Virol. 65:2415–2421.
40. Chazal, N., C. Carriere, B. Gay, and P. Boulanger. 1994. Phenotypic characterization of insertion mutants of the human immunodeficiency virus type 1 Gag precursor expressed in recombinant baculovirus-infected cells. J. Virol. 68:111–122.
41. Choe, H., M. Farzan, Y. Sun, N. Sullivan, B. Rollins, P. D. Ponath, L. Wu, C. R. Mackay, G. LaRosa, W. Newman, N. Gerard, C. Gerard, and J. Sodroski. 1996. The β-chemokine receptors CCR3 and CCR5 facilitate infection by primary HIV-1 isolates. Cell 85:1135–1148.
42. Chun, T.-W., L. Carruth, D. Finzi, X. Shen, J. A. DiGiuseppe, H. Taylor, M. Hermankova, K. Chadwick, J. Margolick, T. C. Quinn, Y.-H. Kuo, R. Brookmeyer, M. A. Zeiger, P. Barditch-Crovo, and R. F. Silicano. 1997. Quantification of latent tissue reservoirs and total body viral load in HIV-1 infection. Nature 387:183–188.
43. Cocchi, F., A. DeVico, A., Garzino-Demo, S. Arya, R. Gallo, and P. Lusso. 1995. Identification of RANTES, MIP-1α, and MIP-1β as the major HIV-1 suppressive factors produced by CD8+ T cells. Science 270:1811–1815.
44. Cohen, E. A., G. Dehni, J. G. Sodroski, and W. A. Haseltine. 1990. Human immunodeficiency virus Vpr product is a virion-associated regulatory protein. J. Virol. 64:3097–3099.
45. Colgan, J., H. E. H. Yuan, E. K. Franke, and J. Luban. 1996. Binding of the human immunodeficiency virus type 1 Gag polyprotein to cyclophilin A is mediated by the central region of capsid and requires Gag dimerization. J. Virol. 70:4299–4310.
46. Collins, K. L., B. K. Chen, S. A. Kalams, and B. D. Walker. 1998. HIV-1 Nef protein protects infected primary cells against killing by cytotoxic T lymphocytes. Nature 391:397–401.
47. Craven, R. C., A. E. Leure-duPree, C. R. Erdie, C. B. Wilson, and J. W. Wills. 1993. Necessity of the spacer peptide between CA and NC in the Rous sarcoma virus Gag protein. J. Virol. 67:6246–6252.
48. Craven, R. C., and L. J. Parent. 1996. Dynamic interactions of the Gag polyprotein. Curr. Top. Microbiol. Immunol. 214:65–94.
49. Crawford, S., and S. P. Goff. 1985. A deletion mutant in the 5′ part of the *pol* gene of Moloney murine leukemia virus blocks proteolytic processing of the *gag* and *pol* polyproteins. J. Virol. 53:899–907.
50. Cullen, B. R. 1991. Regulation of HIV-1 gene expression. FASEB J. 5:2361–2368.
51. Cullen, B. R. 1992. Mechanism of action of regulatory proteins encoded by complex retroviruses. Microbiol. Rev. 56:375–394.
52. Cullen, B. R. 1998. HIV-1 auxiliary proteins: making connections in a dying cell. Cell 93:685–692.

53. Dannull, J., A. Surovoy, G. Jung, and K. Moelling. 1994. Specific binding of HIV-1 nucleocapsid protein to PSI RNA *in vitro* requires N-terminal zinc finger and flanking basic amino acid residues. EMBO J. 13:1525–1533.

54. Darlix, J.-L., M. Lapadat-Tapolsky, H. DeRocquigny, and B. P. Roques. 1995. First glimpses at structure-function relationships of the nucleocapsid protein of retroviruses. J. Mol. Biol. 254:523–537.

55. Darlix, J.-L., A. Vincent, C. Gabus, H. DeRocquigny, and B. Roques. 1993. Trans-activation of the 5' to 3' viral DNA strand transfer by nucleocapsid protein during reverse transcription of HIV-1 RNA. Life Sciences 316:763–771.

56. Deacon, N. J., A. Tsykin, A. Solomon, K. Smith, M. Ludford-Menting, D. J. Hooker, D. A. McPhee, A. L. Greenway, A. Ellett, C. Chatfield, V. A. Lawson, S. Crowe, A. Maerz, S. Sonza, J. Learmont, J. S. Sullivan, A. Cunningham, D. Dwyer, D. Dowton, and J. Mills. 1995. Genomic structure of an attenuated quasi species of HIV-1 from a blood transfusion donor and recipients. Science 270:988–991.

57. Debouck, C., I. C. Deckman, S. K. Grant, R. J. Craig, and M. L. Moore. 1990. The HIV-1 aspartyl protease: maturation and substrate specificity, p. 9–17. *In* L. H. Pearl (ed.), Retroviral proteases: control of maturation and morphogenesis. Stockton Press, New York.

58. DeGuzman, R. N., Z. R. Wu, C. C. Stalling, L. Pappalardo, P. N. Borer, and M. F. Summers. 1998. Structure of the HIV-1 nucleocapsid protein bound to the SL3 Ψ-RNA recognition element. Science 279:384–388.

59. Deng, H., R. Liu, W. Ellmeier, S. Choe, D. Unutmaz, M. Burkhart, P. DiMarzio, R. Sutton, C. M. Hill, C. B. Davis, S. C. Peiper, T. J. Schall, D. R. Littman, and N. R. Landau. 1996. Identification of a major coreceptor for primary isolates of HIV-1. Nature 381:661–666.

60. DeRocquigny, H., C. Gabes, A. Vincent, M. G. Formie-Zaluski, B. Roques, and J.-L. Darlix. 1992. Viral RNA annealing activities of human immunodeficiency virus type 1 nucleocapsid protein requires only peptide domains outside of the zinc fingers. Proc. Natl. Acad. Sci. USA 89:6472–6476.

61. Dickson, C., R. Eisenman, H. Fan, E. Hunter, and N. Teich. 1984. Protein biosynthesis and assembly, p. 513–640. *In* R. Weiss, N. Teich, H. Varmus, and J. Coffin (ed.), RNA tumor viruses. Cold Spring Harbor Laboratory Press, Cold Spring Harbor, N.Y.

62. DiMarzo-Veronese, F., T. D. Copeland, A. L. DeVico, R. Rahman, S. Oroszlan, R. C. Gallo, and M. G. Samgadharan. 1986. Characterization of highly immunogenic p66/p51 as reverse transcriptase of HTLV-III/LAV. Science 231:1289–1291.

63. Doranz, B. J., J. Rucker, Y. Yi, R. J. Smyth, M. Samson, S. C. Peiper, M. Parmentier, R. G. Collman, and R. W. Doms. 1996. A dual-tropic primary HIV-1 isolate that uses fusin and the β-chemokine receptors CKR-5, CKR-3, and CKR-2b as fusion cofactors. Cell 85:1149–1158.

64. Dorfman, T., A. Bukovsky, A. Ohagen, S. Hoglund, and H. G. Gottlinger. 1994. Functional domains of the capsid protein of human immunodeficiency virus type 1. J. Virol. 68:8180–8187.

65. Dorfman, T., J. Luban, S. P. Goff, W. Haseltine, and H. G. Gottlinger. 1993. Mapping of functionally important residues of a cysteine-histidine box in

the human immunodeficiency virus type 1 nucleocapsid protein. J. Virol. 67: 6159–6169.

66. Dorfman, T., F. Mammano, W. A. Haseltine, and H. G. Gottlinger. 1994. Role of the matrix protein in the virion association of the human immunodeficiency virus type 1 envelope glycoprotein. J. Virol. 68:1689–1696.

67. Dragic, T., V. Litwin, G. P. Allaway, S. R. Martin, Y. Huang, K. A. Nagashima, C. Cayanan, P. J. Maddon, R. A. Koup, J. P. Moore, and W. A. Paxton. 1996. HIV-1 entry into CD4+ cells is mediated by the chemokine receptor CC-CKR5. Nature 381:667–673.

68. Earl, P. L., B. Moss, and R. W. Doms. 1991. Folding, interaction with GRP78-BiP, assembly and transport of human immunodeficiency virus type 1 envelope protein. J. Virol. 65:2047–2055.

69. Einfeld, D. 1996. Maturation and assembly of retroviral glycoproteins. Curr. Top. Microbiol. Immunol. 214:133–176.

70. Embretson, J., M. Zupancic, J. L. Ribas, A. Burke, P. Racz, K. Tenner-Racz, and A. T. Haase. 1993. Massive covert infection of helper T lymphocytes and macrophages by HIV during the incubation period of AIDS. Nature 362: 359–362.

71. Emerman, M. 1996. HIV-1, Vpr and the cell cycle. Curr. Biol. 6:1096–1103.

72. Engelman, A., G. Englund, J. M. Orenstein, M. A. Martin, and R. Craigie. 1995. Multiple effects of mutations in human immunodeficiency virus type 1 integrase on viral replication. J. Virol. 69:2729–2736.

73. Engelman, A., K. Mizuuchi, and R. Craigie. 1991. HIV-1 DNA integration: mechanism of viral DNA cleavage and strand transfer. Cell 67:1211–1221.

74. Ewart, G. D., T. Sutherland, P. W. Gage, and G. B. Cox. 1996. The Vpu protein of human immunodeficiency virus type 1 forms cation-selective ion channels. J. Virol. 70:7108–7115.

75. Facke, M., A. Janetzko, R. L. Shoeman, and H.-G. Krausslich. 1993. A large deletion in the matrix domain of the human immunodeficiency virus *gag* gene redirects virus particle assembly from the plasma membrane to the endoplasmic reticulum. J. Virol. 67:4972–4980.

76. Farnet, C. M., and W. A. Haseltine. 1991. Determination of viral proteins present in the human immunodeficiency virus type 1 preintegration complex. J. Virol. 65:1910–1915.

77. Fauci, A. S. 1996. Host factors and the pathogenesis of HIV-induced disease. Nature 384:529–534.

78. Felsenstein, K. M., and S. P. Goff. 1988. Expression of the Gag-Pol fusion protein of Moloney murine leukemia virus without Gag protein does not induce virion formation or proteolytic processing. J. Virol. 62:2179–2182.

79. Feng, Y., C. C. Broder, P. R. E. Kennedy, and E. A. Berger. 1996. HIV-1 entry cofactor: functional cDNA cloning of a seven-transmembrane, G protein-coupled receptor. Science 272:872–877.

80. Feng, Y.-X., T. D. Copeland, L. E. Henderson, R. J. Gorelick, W. J. Bosche, J. G. Levin, and A. Rein. 1996. HIV-1 nucleocapsid protein induces "maturation" of dimeric retroviral RNA *in vitro.* Proc. Natl. Acad. Sci. USA 93:7577–7581.

81. Finzi, D., and R. F. Silicano. 1998. Viral dynamics in HIV-1 infection. Cell 93:665–671.

82. Fischer, U., J. Huber, W. C. Boelens, I. W. Mattaj, and R. Luhrmann. 1995. The HIV-1 activation domain is a nuclear export signal that accesses an export pathway used by specific cellular RNAs. Cell 82:475–483.

83. Franke, E. K., and J. Luban. 1996. Inhibition of HIV-1 replication by cyclosporine A or related compounds correlates with the ability to disrupt the Gag-cyclophilin A interaction. Virology 222:279–282.

84. Franke, E. K., H. E. H. Yuan, and J. Luban. 1994. Specific incorporation of cyclophilin A into HIV-1 virions. Nature 372:359–362.

85. Frankel, S. S., B. M. Wenig, A. P. Burke, P. Mannan, L. D. R. Thompson, S. L. Abbondanzo, A. M. Nelson, M. Pope, and R. M. Steinman. 1996. Replication of HIV-1 in dendritic cell-derived syncytia at the mucosal surface of the adenoid. Science 272:115–117.

86. Freed, E. O., and M. A. Martin. 1995. The role of human immunodeficiency virus type 1 envelope glycoproteins in virus infection. J. Biol. Chem. 270: 23883–23886.

87. Freed, E. O., and M. A. Martin. 1996. Domains of the human immunodeficiency virus type 1 matrix and gp41 cytoplasmic tail required for envelope incorporation into virions. J. Virol. 70:341–351.

88. Freed, E. O., J. M. Orenstein, A. J. Buckler-White, and M. A. Martin. 1994. Single amino changes in the human immunodeficiency virus type 1 matrix protein block virus particle production. J. Virol. 68:5311–5320.

89. Fu, W., R. J. Gorelick, and A. Rein. 1994. Characterization of human immunodeficiency virus type 1 dimeric RNA from wild-type and protease-deficient virions. J. Virol. 68:5013–5018.

90. Fu, W., and A. Rein. 1993. Maturation of dimeric RNA of Moloney murine leukemia virus. J. Virol. 67:5443–5449.

91. Fuller, S. D., T. Wilk, B. E. Gowen, H.-G. Krausslich, and V. M. Vogt. 1997. Cryo-electron microscopy reveals ordered domains in the immature HIV particle. Curr. Biol. 7:729–738.

92. Gabuzda, D. H., K. Lawrence, E. Langhoff, E. Terwilliger, T. Dorfman, and W. A. Haseltine. 1992. Role of *vif* in replication of human immunodeficiency virus type 1 in CD4+ lymphocytes. J. Virol. 66:6489–6495.

93. Gallaher, W. R., J. M. Ball, R. F. Garry, M. C. Griffin, and R. C. Montelaro. 1989. A general model for the transmembrane proteins of HIV and other retroviruses. AIDS Res. Hum. Retroviruses 5:431–440.

94. Gallay, P., S. Swingler, C. Aiken, and D. Trono. 1995. HIV-1 infection of nondividing cells: C-terminal tyrosine phosphorylation of the viral matrix protein is a key regulator. Cell 80:379–388.

95. Gallo, R. C., S. Z. Salahuddin, M. Popovic, G. M. Shearer, M. Kaplan, B. F. Haynes, T. J. Palker, R. Redfield, J. Oleske, B. Safai, G. White, P. Foster, and P. D. Markham. 1984. Frequent detection and isolation of cytophatic retrovirus (HTLV-III) from patients with AIDS and at risk for AIDS. Science 224:500–503.

96. Gamble, T. R., S. Yoo, F. F. Vajdos, U. K. Von Schwedler, J. P. McCutcheon, W. I. Sundquist, and C. P. Hill. 1997. Structure of the carboxy-terminal dimerization domain of the HIV-1 capsid protein. Science 273:849–853.

97. Garcia, J. V., and A. D. Miller. 1991. Serine phosphorylation-independent downregulation of cell-surface CD4 by *nef.* Nature 350:508–511.

98. Garnier, L., L. Ratner, B. Rovinski, S.-X. Cao, and J. W. Wills. 1998. Particle size determinants in the human immunodeficiency virus type 1 Gag protein. J. Virol. 72:4667–4677.

99. Gay, B., J. Tournier, N. Chazal, C. Carriere, and P. Boulanger. 1998. Morphologic determinants of HIV-1 Gag particles assembled in baculovirus-infected cells. Virology 247:160–169.

100. Gelderbloom, H. R. 1991. Assembly and morphology of HIV: potential effect of structure on viral function. AIDS 5:617–638.

101. Gelderbloom, H. R., E. H. S. Hausmann, M. Ozel, G. Pauli, and M. A. Koch. 1987. Fine structure of human immunodeficiency virus (HIV) and immunolocalization of structural proteins. Virology 156:171–176.

102. Gheysen, D., E. Jacobs, F. DeForesta, C. Thiriart, M. Francotte, D. Thines, and M. DeWilde. 1989. Assembly and release of HIV-1 precursor Pr55^{gag} virus-like particles from recombinant baculovirus-infected insect cells. Cell 59:103–112.

103. Giam, C.-Z., and I. Boros. 1988. *In vivo* and *in vitro* autoprocessing of human immunodeficiency virus protease expressed in *Escherichia coli*. J. Biol. Chem. 263:14617–14620.

104. Gilboa, E., S. W. Mitra, S. P. Goff, and D. Baltimore. 1979. A detailed model of reverse transcription and tests for crucial aspects. Cell 18:93–100.

105. Goff, S. P. 1990. Retroviral reverse transcriptase: synthesis, structure, and function. J. Acquired Immune Defic. Syndr. 3:817–831.

106. Goh, W. C., M. E. Rogel, C. M. Kinsey, S. F. Michael, P. N. Fultz, M. A. Nowak, B. H. Hahn, and M. Emerman. 1998. HIV-1 Vpr increases viral expression by manipulating the cell cycle: a mechanism for selection of Vpr *in vivo*. Nature Med. 4:65–71.

107. Gorelick, R. J., L. E. Henderson, J. P. Hanser, and A. Rein. 1988. Point mutants of the Moloney murine leukemia virus that fail to package viral RNA: evidence for specific RNA recognition by a "zinc finger-like" protein sequence. Proc. Natl. Acad. Sci. USA 85:8420–8424.

108. Gorelick, R. J., S. M. Nigida, J. R. Bess, L. O. Arthur, L. E. Henderson, and A. Rein. 1990. Noninfectious human immunodeficiency virus type 1 mutants deficient in genomic RNA. J. Virol. 64:3207–3211.

109. Gottlinger, H., T. Dorfman, J. Sodroski, and W. Haseltine. 1991. Effect of mutations affecting the p6 Gag protein on human immunodeficiency viral particle release. Proc. Natl. Acad. Sci. USA 88:3195–3199.

110. Gottlinger, H. G., T. Dorfman, E. A. Cohen, and W. A. Haseltine. 1993. Vpu protein of human immunodeficiency virus type 1 enhances the release of capsids produced by *gag* gene constructs of widely divergent retroviruses. Proc. Natl. Acad. Sci. USA 90:7381–7385.

111. Gottlinger, H. G., J. G. Sodroski, and W. A. Haseltine. 1989. Role of capsid precursor processing and myristylation in morphogenesis and infectivity of human immunodeficiency virus type 1. Proc. Natl. Acad. Sci. USA 86:5781–5785.

112. Gowda, S. D., B. S. Stein, and E. G. Engelman. 1989. Identification of protein intermediates in the processing of the p55 HIV-1 *gag* precursor in cells infected with recombinant vaccinia virus. J. Biol. Chem. 264:8459–8462.

113. Graves, M. C., J. J. Lim, E. P. Heimer, and R. A. Kramer. 1988. An 11-kDa form of human immunodeficiency virus protease expressed in *Escherichia coli* is sufficient for enzymatic activity. Proc. Natl. Acad. Sci. USA 85:2449–2453.

114. Greene, W. C. 1991. The molecular biology of human immunodeficiency virus type 1 infection. N. Engl. J. Med. 324:308–317.

115. Hadzopolou-Cladares, M., B. K. Felber, C. Cladaros, A. Athanassopoulos, A. Tse, and G. N. Pavlikis. 1989. The Rev (*trs/art*) protein of human immunodeficiency virus type 1 affects viral mRNA and protein expression via a *cis*-acting sequence in the *env* region. J. Virol. 63:1265–1274.

116. Hallenberger, S., V. Bosch, H. Angliker, E. Shaw, H.-D. Klenk, and W. Garten. 1993. Inhibition of furin-mediated cleavage activation of HIV-1 glycoprotein gp160. Nature 360:358–362.

117. Hansen, J., T. Schulze, W. Mellert, and K. Moelling. 1988. Identification and characterization of HIV-specific RNaseH by monoclonal antibody. EMBO J. 7:239–243.

118. Haseltine, W. A. 1988. Replication and pathology of the AIDS virus. J. Acquired Immune Defic. Syndr. 1:217–240.

119. Haseltine, W. A. 1991. Molecular biology of human immunodeficiency virus type 1. FASEB J. 5:2349–2360.

120. Heinzinger, N., M. Bukrinsky, S. Haggerty, A. Ragland, V. Kewal-Ramini, M. Lee, H. Gendelman, M. Stevenson, and M. Emerman. 1994. The HIV-1 Vpr protein influences nuclear targeting of viral nucleic acids in non-dividing cells. Proc. Natl. Acad. Sci. USA 91:7311–7315.

121. Hellerstein, M. K., and J. M. McCune. 1997. T cell turnover in HIV-1 disease. Immunity 7:583–589.

122. Henderson, L. E., M. A. Bowers, R. C. Sowder, S. A. Serabyn, D. G. Johnson, J. W. Bess, L. O. Arthur, D. K. Bryant, and C. Finselan. 1992. Gag proteins of the highly replicative LM strain of human immunodeficiency virus type 1: post-translational modifications, proteolytic processing and complete amino acid sequences. J. Virol. 66:1856–1865.

123. Henderson, L. E., T. D. Copeland, R. C. Sowder, A. M. Schultz, and S. Oroszian. 1988. Analysis of proteins and peptides purified from sucrose gradient bonded HTLV-III, p. 135–147. *In* D. Bolognesi (ed.), Human retroviruses, cancer, and AIDS: approaches to prevention and therapy. Alan R. Liss, Inc., New York.

124. Herbein, G., U. Mahlknecht, F. Batliwalla, G. Gregersen, T. Pappas, J. Butler, W. A. O'Brien, and E. Verdin. 1998. Apostosis of CD8+ T cells is mediated by macrophages through interaction of HIV gp120 with chemokine receptor CXCR4. Nature 395:189–194.

125. Ho, D. D., A. U. Neumann, A. S. Perelson, W. Chen, J. M. Leonard, and M. Markowitz. 1995. Rapid turnover of plasma virions and CD4 lymphocytes in HIV-1 infection. Nature 373:123–126.

126. Hoglund, S., L.-G. Ofverstedt, A. Nilsson, P. Lundquist, H. Gelderblom, M. Ozel, and U. Skoglund. 1992. Spatial visualization of the maturing HIV-1 core and its linkage to the envelope. AIDS Res. Hum. Retroviruses 8:1–17.

127. Hoglund, S., A. Ohagen, K. Lawrence, and D. Gabuzda. 1994. Role of *vif* during packing of the core of HIV-1. Virology 201:349–355.

128. Hostomska, Z., D. A. Matthews, J. F. Davies II, B. R. Nodes, and Z. Hostomsky. 1991. Proteolytic release and crystallization of the RNaseH domain of human immunodeficiency virus type 1 reverse transcriptase. J. Biol. Chem. 266: 14697–14702.

129. Hu, W.-S., and H. M. Temin. 1990. Retroviral recombination and reverse transcription. Science 250:1227–1233.

130. Huang, M., and M. A. Martin. 1997. Incorporation of Pr160$^{gag-pol}$ into virus particles requires the presence of both the major homology region and adjacent C-terminal capsid sequences within the Gag-Pol polyprotein. J. Virol. 71:4472–4478.

131. Huang, M., J. M. Orenstein, M. A. Martin, and E. O. Freed. 1995. p6^{gag} is required for particle production from full-length human immunodeficiency virus type 1 molecular clones expressing protease. J. Virol. 69:6810–6818.

132. Huber, H. E., J. M. McCoy, J. S. Seehra, and C. C. Richardson. 1989. Human immunodeficiency virus 1 reverse transcriptase: template binding, processivity, strand displacement synthesis and template switching. J. Biol. Chem. 264:4669–4678.

133. Hunter, E. 1994. Macromolecular interactions in the assembly of HIV-1 and other retroviruses. Semin. Virol. 5:71–83.

134. Hwang, S. S., T. J. Boyle, H. K. Lyerly, and B. R. Cullen. 1991. Identification of the envelope V3 loop as the primary determinant of cell tropism in HIV-1. Science 253:71–74.

135. Jacks, T., M. D. Power, F. R. Masiarz, P. A. Luciw, P. J. Barr, and H. E. Varmus. 1988. Characterization of ribosomal frameshifting in HIV-1 *gag-pol* expression. Nature 331:280–283.

136. Johnson, R. T. 1995. The pathogenesis of HIV infections of the brain. Curr. Top. Microbiol. Immunol. 202:3–10.

137. Jones, T. A., G. Blaug, M. Hansen, and E. Barklis. 1990. Assembly of gag-beta-galactosidase proteins into retrovirus particles. J. Virol. 64:2265–2279.

138. Jowett, J., D. Hockley, M. V. Nermut, and I. M. Jones. 1992. Distinct signals of human immunodeficiency virus type 1 Pr55 necessary for RNA binding and particle formation. J. Gen. Virol. 73:3079–3086.

139. Jowett, J. B., V. Planelles, B. Poon, N. P. Shah, M. L. Chen, and I. S. Chen. 1995. The human immunodeficiency virus type 1 *vpr* gene arrests infected T cells in the G_2 + M phase of the cell cycle. J. Virol. 69:6304–6313.

140. Kaplan, A. H., M. Manchester, and R. Swanstrom. 1994. The activity of the protease of human immunodeficiency virus type 1 is initiated at the membrane of infected cells before the release of viral proteins and is required for release to occur with maximum efficiency. J. Virol. 68:6782–6786.

141. Kaplan, A. H., and R. Swanstrom. 1991. HIV-1 Gag proteins are processed in two cellular compartments. Proc. Natl. Acad. Sci. USA 88:4528–4532.

142. Kaplan, A. H., J. A. Zack, M. Knigge, D. Paul, D. J. Kempf, D. W. Norbeck, and R. Swanstrom. 1993. Partial inhibition of the human immunodeficiency virus type 1 protease results in aberrant virus assembly and the formation of noninfectious particles. J. Virol. 67:4050–4055.

143. Karacostas, V., K. Nagashima, M. A. Gonda, and B. Moss. 1989. Human immunodeficiency virus-like particles produced by a vaccinia virus expression vector. Proc. Natl. Acad. Sci. USA 86:8964–8967.

144. Karczewski, M. K., and K. Strebel. 1996. Cytoskeleton association and virion incorporation of the human immunodeficiency virus type 1 Vif protein. J. Virol. 70:494–507.

145. Katoh, I., Y. Ikawa, and Y. Yoshinaka. 1989. Retrovirus protease characterized as a dimeric aspartic protease. J. Virol. 63:2226–2232.

146. Katz, R. A., and A. M. Skalka. 1994. The retroviral enzymes. Annu. Rev. Biochem. 63:133–173.

147. Kaye, J. F., and M. L. Lever. 1996. Trans-acting proteins involved in RNA encapsidation and viral assembly in human immunodeficiency virus type 1. J. Virol. 70:880–886.

148. Kestler, H. W., D. J. Dingler, K. Mori, D. L. Panicali, P. K. Sehgal, M. D. Daniel, and R. C. Desrosiers. 1991. Importance of the *nef* gene for maintenance of high virus loads and for development of AIDS. Cell 65:651–652.

149. Kiernan, R. E., A. Ono, G. Englund, and E. O. Freed. 1998. Role of matrix in an early postentry step in the human immunodeficiency type 1 life cycle. J. Virol. 72:4116–4126.

150. Klimkait, T., K. Strebel, M. D. Hoggan, M. A. Martin, and J. M. Orenstein. 1990. The human immunodeficiency virus type 1-specific protein Vpu is required for efficient virus maturation and release. J. Virol. 64:621–629.

151. Kingsman, S. M., and A. J. Kingsman. 1996. The regulation of human immunodeficiency virus type 1 gene expression. Eur. J. Biochem. 240:491–507.

152. Kirchhoff, F., T. C. Greenough, D. B. Brettler, J. L. Sullivan, and R. C. Desrosiers. 1995. Absence of intact *nef* sequences in a long-term survivor with nonprogressive HIV-1 infection. N. Engl. J. Med. 332:228–232.

153. Kohl, N. E., E. A. Emini, W. A. Schleif, L. J. Davis, J. C. Heimbach, R. A. F. Dixon, E. M. Scolnick, and I. S. Sigal. 1988. Active human immunodeficiency virus protease is required for viral infectivity. Proc. Natl. Acad. Sci. USA 85:4686–4690.

154. Kondo, E., F. Mammano, E. A. Cohen, and H. G. Gottlinger. 1995. The p6^{gag} domain of human immunodeficiency virus type 1 is sufficient for the incorporation of Vpr into heterologous viral particles. J. Virol. 69:2759–2764.

155. Kowalski, M., J. Potz, L. Bsiripour, T. Dorfman, W. C. Goh, E. Terwilliger, A. Dayton, C. Rosen, W. Haseltine, and J. Sodroski. 1987. Functional regions of the envelope glycoprotein of human immunodeficiency virus type 1. Science 237:1351–1355.

156. Krausslich, H.-G., M. Facke, A.-M. Heuser, J. Knovalinka, and H. Zentgra. 1995. The spacer peptide between human immunodeficiency virus capsid and nucleocapsid proteins is essential for ordered assembly and viral infectivity. J. Virol. 69:3407–3419.

157. Kulkosky, J., and A. M. Skalka. 1994. Molecular mechanism of retroviral DNA integration. Pharmocol. Ther. 61:185–203.

158. Kwong, P. D., R. Wyatt, J. Robinson, R. W. Sweets, J. Sodroski, and W. A. Hendrickson. 1998. Structure of an HIV gp120 envelope glycoprotein in complex with the CD4 receptor and a neutralizing human antibody. Nature 393:648–659.

159. Lamb, R. A., and L. H. Pinto. 1997. Do Vpu and Vpr of human immunodeficiency virus type 1 and NB of influenza B virus have ion channel activities in the viral life cycles? Virology 229:1–11.

160. Lappatto, R., T. Blundell, A. Hemmings, J. Overington, A. Wilderspin, S. Wood, R. Merson, P. J. Whittle, D. E. Danley, K. F. Geoghegan, S. J. Hawrylik,

S. E. Lee, K. G. Scheld, and P. M. Hobart. 1989. X-ray analysis of HIV-1 proteinase at 2.7 Å resolution confirms structural homology among retroviral enzymes. Nature 342:299–302.

161. Laspia, M. F., A. P. Rice, and M. B. Matthews. 1989. HIV-1 Tat protein increases transcriptional activation and stabilizes elongation. Cell 59:283–292.

162. Lavallee, C., X. J. Yao, A. Ladha, H. G. Gottlinger, W. A. Haseltine, and E. A. Cohen. 1994. Requirement of Pr55^{gag} precursors for incorporation of the Vpr product into human immunodeficiency virus type 1 particles. J. Virol. 68: 1926–1934.

163. Lee, Y.-M., X.-B. Tang, L. M. Cimakasky, J. E. K. Hildreth, and X.-F. Yu. 1997. Mutations in the matrix protein of human immunodeficiency virus type 1 inhibit surface expression and virion incorporation of viral envelope glycoproteins in CD4+ T lymphocytes. J. Virol. 71:1443–1452.

164. LeGall, S., L. Erdtmann, S. Benichou, C. Berlioz-Torrent, L. Liu, R. Benarous, J.-M. Heard, and O. Schwartz. 1998. Nef interacts with the μ subunit of clatherin adaptor complexes and reveals a cryptic sorting signal in MHC I molecules. Immunity 8:483–495.

165. LeGrice, S. F. J., J. Mills, and J. Mous. 1988. Active site mutagenesis of the AIDS virus protease and its alleviation by *trans* complementation. EMBO J. 7:2547–2553.

166. Leis, J., A. Aiyar, and D. Cobrinik. 1993. Regulation of initiation of reverse transcription of retroviruses, p. 33–48. *In* A. M. Skalka and S. P. Goff (ed.), Reverse transcriptase. Cold Spring Harbor Laboratory Press, Cold Spring Harbor, N.Y.

167. Levy, D. N., L. E. Fernandes, W. V. Williams, and D. B. Weiner. 1993. Induction of cell differentiation by human immunodeficiency virus 1 *vpr*. Cell 72:541–550.

168. Levy, J. A. 1988. HIV and the pathogenesis of AIDS. JAMA 261:2887–3006.

169. Li, M., A. G. Garcia, U. Bhattacharyya, P. Mascagni, B. M. Austen, and M. M. Roberts. 1996. The Vpr protein of human immunodeficiency virus type 1 binds to nucleocapsid protein p7 *in vitro*. Biochem. Biophys. Res. Commun. 218:352–355.

170. Lightfoote, M. M., J. E. Coligan, T. M. Folks, A. S. Fauci, M. A. Martin, and S. Venkatesan. 1986. Structural characterization of reverse transcriptase and endonuclease polypeptides of the acquired immunodeficiency syndrome retrovirus. J. Virol. 60:771–775.

171. Linial, M. L., and A. D. Miller. 1990. Retroviral RNA packaging: sequence requirements and implications. Curr. Top. Microbiol. Immunol. 157:125–152.

172. Littman, D. R. 1998. Chemokine receptors: keys to AIDS pathogenesis? Cell 93:677–680.

173. Liu, H., X. Wu, M. Newman, G. M. Shaw, B. H. Hahn, and J. C. Kappes. 1995. The Vif protein of human and simian immunodeficiency viruses is packaged into virions and associates with viral core structures. J. Virol. 69:7630–7638.

174. Loeb, D. D., C. A. Hutchison III, M. H. Edgell, W. G. Farmerie, and R. Swanstrom. 1989. Mutational analysis of human immunodeficiency virus type 1 protease suggests functional homology with aspartic proteinases. J. Virol. 63:111–121.

175. Loeb, D. D., R. Swanstrom, L. Everitt, M. Manchester, S. E. Stamper, and C. A. Hutchison III. 1989. Complete mutagenesis of the HIV-1 protease. Nature 340:397–400.

176. Lori, F., A. I. Scovassi, D. Zella, G. Achilli, E. Cattaneo, C. Casoli, and U. Bertazzoni. 1988. Enzymatically active forms of reverse transcriptase of the human immunodeficiency virus. AIDS Res. Hum. Retroviruses 5:393–398.

177. Lowe, D. M., A. Aitken, C. Bradley, G. K. Darby, B. A. Larder, K. L. Powell, D. J. M. Purifoy, M. Tistale, and D. K. Stammers. 1988. HIV-1 reverse transcriptase: crystallization and analysis of domain structure by limited proteolysis. Biochemistry 27:8884–8889.

178. Lu, Y.-L., R. P. Bennett, J. W. Wills, R. Gorelick, and L. Ratner. 1995. A leucine triplet repeat sequence $(LXX)_4$ in p6^{gag} is important for Vpr incorporation into human immunodeficiency virus type 1 particles. J. Virol. 69:6873–6879.

179. Lu, Y.-L., P. Spearman, and L. Ratner. 1993. Human immunodeficiency virus type 1 viral protein R localizes in infected cells and virions. J. Virol. 67:6542–6550.

180. Luban, J. 1996. Absconding with the chaperone: essential cyclophilin-Gag interaction in HIV-1 virions. Cell 87:1157–1159.

181. Luban, J., K. L. Bossolt, E. K. Franke, G. V. Kalpana, and S. P. Goff. 1993. Human immunodeficiency virus type 1 Gag protein binds to cyclophilins A and B. Cell 73:1067–1078.

182. Luban, J., and S. P. Goff. 1991. Binding of human immunodeficiency virus type 1 (HIV-1) RNA to recombinant HIV-1 Gag polyprotein. J. Virol. 65:3203–3212.

183. Luftig, R., I. Kazuyoshi, M. Bu, and P. Clakins. 1990. Terminal stages of retrovirus morphogenesis in retroviral protease, p. 141–148. In L. H. Pearl (ed.), Control of maturation and morphogenesis. Macmillan, London.

184. Luo, G. X., and J. Taylor. 1990. Template switching by reverse transcriptase during DNA synthesis. J. Virol. 64:4321–4328.

185. Maddon, P. J., A. J. Dalgleish, J. S. McDougal, P. R. Clapham, R. A. Weiss, and R. Axel. 1986. The T4 gene encodes the AIDS virus receptor and is expressed in the immune system and the brain. Cell 47:333–348.

186. Mak, J., M. Jiang, M. A. Wainberg, M. L. Hammerskjold, D. Rekosh, and L. Kleiman. 1994. Role of Pr160$^{gag-pol}$ in mediating the selective incorporation of tRNA(Lys) into human immunodeficiency virus type 1 particles. J. Virol. 68:2065–2072.

187. Mak, J., A. Khorchid, Q. Cao, Y. Huang, I. Lowy, M. A. Parniak, V. R. Prasad, M. A. Wainberg, and L. Kleiman. 1997. Effects of mutations in Pr160$^{gag-pol}$ upon tRNA^{Lys3} and Pr160$^{gag-pol}$ incorporation into HIV-1. J. Mol. Biol. 265:419–431.

188. Malim, M. H., J. Hauber, S.-Y. Le, J. V. Maizel, and B. R. Cullen. 1989. The HIV-1 Rev *trans*-activator acts through a structural target sequence to activate nuclear export of unspliced viral mRNA. Nature 338:254–257.

189. Mammano, F., A. Ohagen, S. Hoglund, and H. G. Gottlinger. 1994. Role of the major homology region of human immunodeficiency virus type 1 in virion morphogenesis. J. Virol. 68:4927–4936.

190. Margottin, F., S. P. Bour, H. Durand, L. Selig, S. Benichou, V. Richard, T. Thomas, K. Strebel, and R. Benarous. 1998. A novel human WD protein,

h-αTrCP, that interacts with HIV-1 Vpu connects CD4 to the ER degradation pathway through an F-box motif. Mol. Cell 1:565–574.

191. Mathews, R. E. F. 1982. Classification and nomenclature of viruses, IVth report of the International Committee on Taxonomy of Viruses. Karger, Basel.

192. McDermott, J., L. Farrell, R. Ross, and E. Barklis. 1996. Structural analysis of human immunodeficiency virus type 1 Gag protein interactions, using cysteine-specific reagents. J. Virol. 70:5106–5114.

193. McDougal, J. J., M. S. Kenedy, J. M. Seigh, S. P. Cort, A. Mawla, and J. K. A. Nicholson. 1986. Binding of HTLV-III/LAV to T4+ cells by a complex of the 110K viral protein and the T4 molecule. Science 231:382–385.

194. McMichael, A. 1998. T cell responses and viral escape. Cell 93:673–676.

195. Mellors, J. W., C. W. Rinaldo, Jr., P. Gupta, R. M. White, J. A. Todd, and L. A. Kingsley. 1996. Prognosis in HIV-1 infection predicted by the quantity of virus in plasma. Science 272:1167–1170.

196. Mely, Y., H. DeRocquigny, M. Sorinas-Jimeno, G. Keith, B. P. Roques, R. Marquet, and D. Gerard. 1995. Binding of the HIV-1 nucleocapsid protein to the primer tRNA(3Lys), *in vitro*, is essentially not specific. J. Biol. Chem. 270: 1650–1656.

197. Mergener, K., M. Facke, R. Welker, V. Brinkmann, H. R. Gelderblom, and H.-G. Krausslich. 1992. Analysis of HIV particle formation using transient expression of subviral constructs in mammalian cells. Virology 186:25–39.

198. Mervis, R. J., N. Ahmad, E. P. Lillehoj, M. G. Raum, F. H. R. Salazar, H. W. Chan, and S. Venkatesan. 1988. The *gag* gene products of human immunodeficiency virus type 1: alignment within the *gag* open reading frame, identification of posttranslational modifications, and evidence for alternative *gag* precursors. J. Virol. 62:3993–4002.

199. Miller, M., M. Jaskolski, J. K. M. Rao, J. Leis, and A. Wlodawer. 1989. Crystal structure of a retroviral protease proves relationship to aspartic protease family. Nature 337:576–579.

200. Miller, M., B. K. Sathyanarayana, M. V. Toth, G. R. Marshall, L. Clawson, L. Selk, J. Schneider, S. B. H. Kent, and A. Wlodawer. 1989. Structure of complex of synthetic HIV-1 protease with a substrate-based inhibitor at 2.3Å resolution. Science 246:1149–1152.

201. Miller, M. D., M. T. Warmerdam, I. Gaston, W. C. Green, and M. B. Feinberg. 1994. The human immunodeficiency virus-1 *nef* gene product: a positive factor for viral infection and replication in primary lymphocytes and macrophages. J. Exp. Med. 179:101–113.

202. Miller, R. H., and N. Sarver. 1997. HIV accessory proteins as therapeutic targets. Nature Med. 3:389–394.

203. Mous, J., E. P. Heimer, and S. F. J. LeGrice. 1988. Processing protease and reverse transcriptase from human immunodeficiency virus type 1 polyprotein in *Escherichia coli*. J. Virol. 62:1433–1436.

204. Murphy, J. E., and S. P. Goff. 1989. Construction and analysis of deletion mutations in the U5 region of Moloney murine leukemia virus: effects on RNA packaging and reverse transcription. J. Virol. 63:319–327.

205. Navia, M. A., P. M. D. Fitzgerald, B. M. McKeever, C.-T. Leu, J. C. Heimbach, W. K. Herber, I. S. Sigal, P. L. Darke, and J. P. Springer. 1989. Three-dimensional

structure of aspartyl protease from human immunodeficiency virus HIV-1. Nature 337:615–620.

206. Nermut, M. V., and D. J. Hockley. 1996. Comparative morphology and structural classification of retroviruses. Curr. Top. Microbiol. Immunol. 214: 1–24.

207. Nottet, H. S., and H. E. Gendelman. 1995. Unraveling the neuroimmune mechanisms for the HIV-1-associated cognitive/motor complex. Immunol. Today 16:441–448.

208. Nutt, R. F., S. F. Brady, P. L. Darke, T. M. Ciccarone, E. M. Nutt, J. A. Rodkey, C. D. Bennett, L. H. Waxman, and I. S. Sigal. 1988. Chemical synthesis and enzymatic activity of a 99-residue peptide with a sequence proposed for the human immunodeficiency virus protease. Proc. Natl. Acad. Sci. USA 85: 7129–7133.

209. Oberlin, E., A. Amara, F. Bachelerie, C. Bessia, J.-L. Virelizier, F. Arenzana-Seisdedos, O. Schwartz, J.-M. Heard, I. Clark-Lewis, D. F. Legier, M. Loetscher, M. Baggiolini, and B. Moser. 1996. The CXC chemokine SDF-1 is the ligand for LESTER/fusin and prevents infection by T-cell-line-adapted HIV-1. Nature 382:833–835.

210. Oertle, S., and P.-F. Spahr. 1990. Role of Gag polyprotein precursor in packaging and maturation of Rous sarcoma virus genomic RNA. J. Virol. 64: 5757–5763.

211. Ogg, G. S., X. Jin, S. Bonhoeffer, P. R. Dunbar, M. A. Nowak, S. Monard, J. P. Segal, Y. Cao, S. L. Rowland-Jones, V. Cerundolo, A. Hurley, M. Markowitz, D. D. Ho, D. F. Nixon, and A. J. McMichael. 1998. Quantitation of HIV-1-specific cytotoxic T lymphocytes and plasma load of viral RNA. Science 279:2103–2106.

212. Oroszlan, S., and R. B. Luftig. 1990. Retroviral proteinases. Curr. Top. Microbiol. Immunol. 157:153–185.

213. Ottman, M., C. Gabus, and J.-L. Darlix. 1995. The central globular domain of the nucleocapsid protein of human immunodeficiency virus type 1 is critical for virion structure and infectivity. J. Virol. 69:1778–1784.

214. Panteleo, G., C. Graziosi, L. Butini, P. A. Pizzo, S. M. Schnittman, D. P. Kotler, and A. S. Fauci. 1991. Lymphoid organs function as major reservoirs for human immunodeficiency virus. Proc. Natl. Acad. Sci. USA 88:9838–9842.

215. Panteleo, G., C. Graziosi, J. F. Demarest, L. Butini, M. Montroni, C. H. Fox, J. M. Orenstein, D. P. Kotler, and A. S. Fauci. 1993. HIV infection is active and progressive in lymphoid tissue during the clinically latent stage of disease. Nature 362:355–358.

216. Parent, L. J., C. B. Wilson, M. D. Resh, and J. W. Wills. 1996. Evidence for a second function of the MA sequence in the Rous sarcoma virus Gag protein. J. Virol. 70:1016–1026.

217. Park, J., and C. D. Morrow. 1991. Overexpression of the *gag-pol* precursor from human immunodeficiency virus type 1 proviral genomes results in efficient proteolytic processing in the absence of virion production. J. Virol. 65: 5111–5117.

218. Park, J., and C. D. Morrow. 1992. The nonmyristylated Pr160$^{gag-pol}$ polyprotein of human immunodeficiency virus type 1 interacts with Pr55^{gag} and is incorporated into virus-like particles. J. Virol. 66:6304–6313.

219. Park, J., and C. D. Morrow. 1993. Mutations in the protease gene of human immunodeficiency virus type 1 affect release and stability of virus particles. Virology 194:843–850.

220. Partin, K., H.-G. Krausslich, L. Ehrlich, E. Wimmer, and C. Carter. 1990. Mutational analysis of a native substrate of the human immunodeficiency virus type 1 proteinase. J. Virol. 64:3938–3947.

221. Partin, K., G. Zybarth, G. Ehrlich, L. Decrombrugghe, E. Wimmer, and C. Carter. 1991. Deletion of sequences upstream of the proteinase improves the proteolytic processing of human immunodeficiency virus type 1. Proc. Natl. Acad. Sci. USA 88:4776–4780.

222. Paxton, W., R. I. Connor, and N. R. Landau. 1993. Incorporation of Vpr into human immunodeficiency virus type 1 virions: requirement for the p6 region of *gag* and mutational analysis. J. Virol. 67:7229–7237.

223. Pearl, L. H., and W. R. Taylor. 1987. A structural model for the retroviral proteases. Nature 329:351–354.

224. Peliska, J. A., and S. J. Benkovic. 1992. Mechanism of DNA strand transfer reactions catalyzed by HIV-1 reverse transcriptase. Science 258:1112–1118.

225. Peng, C., N. T. Chang, and T. W. Chang. 1991. Identification and characterization of human immunodeficiency virus type 1 *gag-pol* fusion protein in transfected mammalian cells. J. Virol. 65:2751–2756.

226. Peng, C., B. K. Ho, T. W. Chang, and N. T. Chang. 1989. Role of human immunodeficiency virus type 1-specific protease in core protein maturation and viral infectivity. J. Virol. 63:2550–2556.

227. Perelson, A. S., A. U. Neumann, M. Markowitz, J. M. Leonard, and D. D. Ho. 1996. HIV-1 dynamics *in vivo*: virion clearance rate, infected cell life-span, viral generation time. Science 271:1582–1586.

228. Pettit, S. C., M. D. Moody, R. S. Wehbie, A. H. Kaplan, P. V. Nantermet, C. A. Klein, and R. Swanstrom. 1994. The p2 domain of human immunodeficiency virus type 1 Gag regulates sequential proteolytic processing and is required to produce fully infectious virus. J. Virol. 68:8017–8027.

229. Poon, B., K. Grovit-Ferbas, S. A. Stewart, and I. S.Y. Chen. 1998. Cell cycle arrest by Vpr in HIV-1 virions and insensitivity to antiretroviral agents. Science 281:266–269.

230. Poon, D. T., J. Wu, and A. Aldovini. 1996. Charged amino acid residues of human immunodeficiency virus type 1 nucleocapsid p7 protein involved in RNA packaging and infectivity. J. Virol. 70:6607–6616.

231. Popovic, M., M. G. Sarngadharan, E. Read, and R. C. Gallo. 1984. Detection, isolation, and continuous production of cytopathic retroviruses (HTLV-III) from patients with AIDS and pre-AIDS. Science 224:497–500.

232. Prats, A.-C., L. Sarih, C. Gabus, S. Litvak, G. Keith, and J.-L. Darlix. 1988. Small finger protein of avian and murine retroviruses has nucleic acid annealing activity and positions the replication primer tRNA onto genomic RNA. EMBO J. 7:1777–1783.

233. Pryciak, P. M., and H. E. Varmus. 1992. Nucleosomes, DNA-binding proteins, and DNA sequence modulate retroviral integration target site selection. Cell 69:769–780.

234. Pullen, K. A., and J. J. Champoux. 1990. Plus-strand origin for human immunodeficiency virus type 1: implications for integration. J. Virol. 64:6274–6277.

235. Quillent, C., A. M. Borman, S. Paulous, C. Dauguet, and F. Clavel. 1996. Extensive regions of *pol* are required for efficient human immunodeficiency virus polyprotein processing and particle formation. Virology 219:28–36.

236. Rabson, A. B., and J. W. Wills. 1997. Synthesis and processing of viral RNA, p. 205–262. *In* J. M. Coffin, S. H. Hughes, and H. E. Varmus (ed.), Retroviruses. Cold Spring Harbor Laboratory Press, Cold Spring Harbor, N.Y.

237. Rapport, C. J., J. Gosling, V. L. Schweickart, P. W. Gray, and I. F. Charo. 1996. Molecular cloning and functional characterization of a novel human CC chemokine receptor (CCR5) for RANTES, MIP-1α, and MIP-1β. J. Biol. Chem. 271:17161–17166.

238. Reicin, A. S., A. Ohagen, L. Yin, S. Hoglund, and S. P. Goff. 1996. The role of Gag in human immunodeficiency virus type 1 virion morphogenesis and early steps of the viral life cycle. J. Virol. 70:8645–8652.

239. Reicin, A. S., S. Paik, R. D. Berkowitz, J. Luban, I. Lowy, and S. P. Goff. 1995. Linker insertion mutations in the human immunodeficiency virus type 1 *gag* gene: effects on virion particle assembly, release, and infectivity. J. Virol. 69:642–650.

240. Rizzuto, C. D., R. Wyatt, N. Hernandez-Ramos, Y. Sun, P. D. Kwong, W. A. Hendrickson, and J. Sodroski. 1998. A conserved HIV gp120 glycoprotein structure involved in chemokine receptor binding. Science 280: 1949–1953.

241. Roberts, M. M., and S. Oroszlan. 1990. The action of retroviral protease in various phases of virus replication, p. 131–139. *In* L. H. Pearl (ed.), Retroviral proteases: control of maturation and morphogenesis. Stockton Press, New York.

242. Rogel, M. E., L. I. Wu, and M. Emerman. 1995. The human immunodeficiency virus type 1 *vpr* gene prevents cell proliferation during chronic infection. J. Virol. 69:882–888.

243. Rose, J. R., L. M. Babe, and C. S. Craik. 1995. Defining the level of human immunodeficiency virus type 1 (HIV-1) protease activity required for HIV-1 particle maturation and infectivity. J. Virol. 69:2751–2758.

244. Rose, J. R., R. Salto, and C. S. Craik. 1993. Regulation of autoproteolysis of the HIV-1 and HIV-2 proteases with engineered amino acid substitutions. J. Biol. Chem. 268:11939–11945.

245. Rosenberg, E. S., J. M. Billingsley, A. M. Caliendo, S. L. Boswell, P. E. Sax, S. A. Kalams, and B. D. Walker. 1997. Vigorous HIV-1-specific CD4+ T cell responses associated with control of viremia. Science 278:1447–1450.

246. Roth, M. J., P. L. Schwartzberg, and S. P. Goff. 1989. Structure of the termini of DNA intermediates in the integration of retroviral DNA: dependence on IN function and terminal DNA sequence. Cell 58:47–54.

247. Saikai, H., R. Shibata, J.-I. Sakuragi, S. Sakuragi, M. Kawanura, and A. Adachi. 1993. Cell-dependant requirement of human immunodeficiency virus type 1 Vif protein for maturation of virus particles. J. Virol. 67:1663–1666.

248. Sakaguchi, K., N. Zambrano, E. T. Baldwin, B. A. Shapiro, J. W. Erickson, J. G. Omichinski, G. M. Clore, J. W. Gronenbon, and E. Appella. 1993. Identification of a binding site for human immunodeficiency virus type 1 nucleocapsid protein. Proc. Natl. Acad. Sci. USA 90:5219–5223.

249. Sampson, M., O. Labbe, C. Mollereau, G. Vassart, and M. Parmentier. 1996. Molecular cloning and functional expression of a new CC-chemokine receptor gene. Biochemistry 35:3362–3367.

250. Sandefur, S., V. Varthakavi, and P. Spearman. 1998. The I domain is required for efficient plasma membrane binding of human immunodeficiency virus type 1 Pr55^{Gag}. J. Virol. 72:2723–2732.

251. Schmidtmayerova, H., M. Alfano, G. Nuovo, and M. Bukrinsky. 1998. Human immunodeficiency virus type 1 T-lymphotropic strains enter macrophages via a CD4- and CXCR4-mediated pathway: replication is restricted at a postentry level. J. Virol. 72:4633–4642.

252. Schubert, U., A. V. Ferrer-Montiel, M. Oblatt-Montal, P. Henklein, K. Strebel, and M. Montal. 1996. Identification of an ion channel activity of the Vpu transmembrane domain and its involvement in the regulation of virus release from HIV-1 infected cells. FEBS Lett. 398:12–18.

253. Schwartz, O., V. Marechal, S. Le Gall, F. Lemonnier, and J.-M. Heard. 1996. Endocytosis of major histocompatibility complex class I molecules is induced by HIV-1 Nef protein. Nature Med. 2:338–342.

254. Seelmeier, S., H. Schmidt, V. Turk, and K. von der Helm. 1988. Human immunodeficiency virus has an aspartic-type protease that can be inhibited by pepstatin A. Proc. Natl. Acad. Sci. USA 85:6612–6616.

255. Sharp, P. A., and R. A. Marciniak. 1989. HIV TAR: an RNA enhancer? Cell 59:229–230.

256. Sheng, N., S. C. Pettit, R. J. Tritch, D. H. Ozturk, M. M. Rayner, R. Swanstrom, and S. Erickson-Viitanen. 1997. Determinants of the human immunodeficiency virus type 1 p15NC-RNA interaction that affect enhanced cleavage by the viral protease. J. Virol. 71:5723–5732.

257. Sheng, S., and S. Erickson-Viitanen. 1994. Cleavage of p15 *in vitro* by human immunodeficiency virus type 1 protease is RNA dependant. J. Virol. 68: 6207–6214.

258. Sherman, P. A., M. L. Dickson, and J. A. Fyfe. 1992. Human immunodeficiency virus type 1 integration protein: DNA sequence requirements for cleaving and joining reactions. J. Virol. 66:3593–3601.

259. Shin, C.-G., B. Taddeo, W. A. Haseltine, and C. M. Farnet. 1994. Genetic analysis of the human immunodeficiency virus type 1 integrase protein. J. Virol. 68:1633–1642.

260. Shioda, T., and H. Shibuta. 1990. Production of human immunodeficiency virus (HIV)-like particles from cells infected with recombinant vaccinia viruses carrying the *gag* gene of HIV. Virology 175:139–148.

261. Simon, J. H. M., and M. H. Malim. 1996. The human immunodeficiency virus type 1 Vif protein modulates the postpenetration stability of viral nucleoprotein complexes. J. Virol. 70:5297–5305.

262. Simon, J. H. M., D. L. Miller, R. A. M. Fouchier, and M. H. Malim. 1998. Virion incorporation of human immunodeficiency virus type-1 Vif is determined by intracellular expression level and may not be necessary for function. Virology 248:182–187.

263. Smith, A. J., M.-I. Cho, M.-L. Hammerskjold, and D. Rekosh. 1990. Human immunodeficiency virus type 1 Pr55^{gag} and Pr160$^{gag-pol}$ expressed from a

simian virus 40 late replacement vector are efficiently processed and assembled into virus-like particles. J. Virol. 64:2743–2750.

264. Smith, A. J., N. Srinivasakumar, M.-L. Hammerskjold, and D. Rekosh. 1993. Requirements for incorporation of Pr160$^{gag-pol}$ from human immunodeficiency virus type 1 into virus-like particles. J. Virol. 67:2266–2275.

265. Sodroski, J., R. Patarca, C. Rosen, F. Wong-Staal, and W. Haseltine. 1985. Location of the *trans*-activating region on the genome of human T-cell lymphotropic virus type III. Science 229:74–77.

266. Sotoramirez, L. E., B. Renjifo, M. F. McLane, R. Marlink, C. Ohara, R. Sutthent, C. Wasi, P. Vithayasai, V. Vithayasai, and C. Apichartpiyakul. 1996. HIV-1 Langerhans cell tropism associated with heterosexual transmission of HIV. Science 271:1291–1293.

267. South, T. L., B. Kim, D. R. Hare, and M. F. Summers. 1990. Zinc fingers and molecular recognition. Biochem. Pharmacol. 40:123–129.

268. Spearman, P., J.-J. Wang, N. V. Heydon, and L. Ratner. 1994. Identification of human immunodeficiency virus type 1 Gag protein domains essential to membrane binding and particle assembly. J. Virol. 68:3232–3242.

269. Spina, C. A., J. C. Guatelli and D. D. Richman. 1995. Establishment of a stable, inducible form of human immunodeficiency virus type 1 DNA in quiescent CD4 lymphocytes in vitro. J. Virol. 69:2977–2988.

270. Spina, C. A., T. J. Kwoh, M. Y. Chowers, J. C. Guatelli, and D. D. Richman. 1994. The importance of *nef* in the induction of human immunodeficiency virus type 1 replication from primary quiescent CD4 lymphocytes. J. Exp. Med. 179:115–123.

271. Srinivasakumar, N., M.-L. Hammerskjold, and D. Rekosh. 1995. Characterization of deletion mutants in the capsid region of human immunodeficiency virus type 1 that affect particle formation and Gag-Pol precursor incorporation. J. Virol. 69:6106–6114.

272. Starnes, M. C., W. Gao, R. Y. C. Ting, and Y.-C. Chang. 1988. Enzyme activity gel analysis of human immunodeficiency virus reverse transcriptase. J. Biol. Chem. 263:52–54.

273. Stein, B. S., S. D. Gowda, J. D. Lifson, R. C. Penhallow, K. G. Bensch, and E. G. Engelman. 1987. pH-independent HIV entry into CD4-positive T cells via virus envelope fusion to the plasma membrane. Cell 49:659–668.

274. Stewart, L., G. Schatz, and V. M. Vogt. 1990. Properties of avian retrovirus particles defective in viral protease. J. Virol. 64:5076–5092.

275. Stewart, S. A., B. Poon, J. B. M. Jowett, and I. S. Chen. 1997. Human immunodeficiency virus type 1 Vpr induces apoptosis following cell cycle arrest. J. Virol. 71:4331–4338.

276. Streblow, D. N., M. Kitabwalla, M. Malkovsky, and C. D. Pauza. 1998. Cyclophilin A modulates processing of human immunodeficiency virus type 1 p55^{Gag}: mechanism for antiviral effects of cyclosporin A. Virology 245: 197–202.

277. Tanese, N., V. R. Prasad, and S. P. Goff. 1988. Structural requirements for bacterial expression of stable, enzymatically active fusion proteins containing human immunodeficiency virus reverse transcriptase. DNA 7:407–416.

278. Teich, N. 1985. Taxonomy of retroviruses, p. 1–16. *In* R. A. Weiss, N. Teich, H.

Varmus, and J. Coffin (ed.), RNA tumor viruses. Cold Spring Harbor Laboratory Press, Cold Spring Harbor, N.Y.

279. Telesnitsky, A., and S. P. Goff. 1997. Reverse transcription and the generation of retroviral DNA, p. 121–160. *In* J. M. Coffin, S. H. Hughes, and H. E. Varmus (ed.), Retroviruses. Cold Spring Harbor Laboratory Press, Cold Spring Harbor, N.Y.

280. Thali, M., A. Bukovski, E. Kondo, B. Rosenwirth, C. T. Walsh, J. Sodroski, and H. G. Gottlinger. 1994. Functional association of cyclophilin A with HIV-1 virions. Nature 372:363–365.

281. Tremblay, M. J., J.-F. Fortin, and R. Cantin. 1998. The acquisition of host-encoded proteins by nascent HIV-1. Immunol. Today 19:346–351.

282. Tritch, R. J., Y.-S. Cheng, F. H. Yin, and S. Erickson-Viitanen. 1991. Mutagenesis of protease cleavage sites in the human immunodeficiency virus type 1 Gag polyprotein. J. Virol. 65:922–930.

283. Trkola, A., T. Dragic, J. Arthos, J. M. Binley, W. C. Olson, C. Chen-Meyer, J. Robinson, P. J. Maddon, and J. P. Moore. 1996. CD4-dependent, antibody-sensitive interactions between HIV-1 and its co-receptor CCR-5. Nature 384:184–187.

284. Trono, D. 1995. HIV accessory proteins: leading roles for the supporting cast. Cell 82:189–192.

285. Veronese, F. D., R. Rahman, T. D. Copeland, S. Oroszlan, and R. C. Gallo. 1987. Immunological and clinical analysis of p6, the carboxy-terminal fragment of HIV p15. AIDS Res. Hum. Retroviruses 3:253–264.

286. Vogt, P. K. 1997. Historical introduction to the general properties of retroviruses, p. 1–27. *In* J. M. Coffin, S. H. Hughes, and H. E. Varmus (ed.), Retroviruses. Cold Spring Harbor Laboratory Press, Cold Spring Harbor, N.Y.

287. Vogt, V. M. 1996. Proteolytic processing and particle maturation. Curr. Top. Microbiol. Immunol. 214:95–132.

288. Von Poblotzki, A., R. Wanger, M. Neidrig, G. Wanner, H. Wolf, and S. Modrow. 1993. Identification of a region in the Pr55gag polyprotein essential for HIV-1 particle formation. Virology 193:981–985.

289. Von Schwedler, U., R. S. Kornbluth, and D. Trono. 1994. The nuclear localization signal of the matrix protein of HIV-1 allows the establishment of infection in macrophages and quiescent T lymphocytes. Proc. Natl. Acad. Sci. USA 91:6992–6996.

290. Von Schwedler, U., J. Song, C. Aiken, and D. Trono. 1993. Vif is crucial for human immunodeficiency virus type 1 proviral DNA synthesis in infected cells. J. Virol. 67:4945–4955.

291. Wang, C.-T., and E. Barklis. 1993. Assembly, processing, and infectivity of human immunodeficiency virus type 1 Gag mutants. J. Virol. 67:4264–4273.

292. Wang, C.-T., H. Y. Lai, and J.-J. Li. 1998. Analysis of minimal human immunodeficiency type 1 *gag* coding sequences capable of virus-like particle assembly and release. J. Virol. 72:7950–7959.

293. Weber, I. T. 1990. Comparison of the crystal structures and intersubunit interactions of human immunodeficiency and Rous sarcoma virus proteases. J. Biol. Chem. 265:10492–10496.

294. Weber, I. T., M. Miller, M. Jaskolski, J. Leis, A. M. Skalka, and A. Wlodawer.

1989. Molecular modeling of the HIV-1 protease and its substrate binding site. Science 243:928–931.

295. Wei, X., S. K. Ghosh, M. E. Taylor, V. A. Johnson, E. A. Emini, P. Deutsch, J. D. Lifson, S. Bonhoeffer, M. A. Norwak, B. H. Hahn, M. S. Saag, and G. M. Shaw. 1995. Viral dynamics in human immunodeficiency virus type 1 infection. Nature 373:117–122.

296. Weiss, C. D., J. A. Levy, and J. M. White. 1990. Oligomeric organization of gp120 on infectious human immunodeficiency type 1 particles. J. Virol. 64:5674–5677.

297. Weiss, R., N. Teich, H. Varmus, and J. Coffin. 1984. RNA tumor viruses. Cold Spring Harbor Laboratory Press, Cold Spring Harbor, N.Y.

298. Weiss, R. A. 1996. Retrovirus classification and cell interactions. J. Antimicrob. Chemother. 37(Suppl. B):1–11.

299. Weldon, R. A., C. R. Erdie, M. G. Oliver, and J. W. Wills. 1990. Incorporation of chimeric Gag protein into retroviral particles. J. Virol. 64:4169–4179.

300. Wen, W., J. L. Meinkoth, R. Y. Tsien, and S. S. Taylor. 1995. Identification of a signal for rapid export of proteins from the nucleus. Cell 82:463–473.

301. Wiegers, K., G. Rutter, H. Kottler, U. Tessmer, H. Hohenberg, and H.-G. Krausslich. 1998. Sequential steps in human immunodeficiency virus particle maturation revealed by alterations of individual Gag polyprotein cleavage sites. J. Virol. 72:2846–2854.

302. Willey, R. L., F. Maldrelli, M. A. Martin, and K. Strebel. 1992. Human immunodeficiency virus type 1 Vpu protein induces rapid degradation of CD4. J. Virol. 66:7193–7200.

303. Wills, J. W., C. E. Cameron, C. B. Wilson, Y. Xiang, R. P. Bennett, and J. Leis. 1994. An assembly domain of the Rous sarcoma virus Gag protein required late in budding. J. Virol. 68:6605–6618.

304. Wills, J. W., and R. C. Craven. 1991. Form, function, and use of retroviral Gag proteins. AIDS 5:639–654.

305. Wilson, W., M. Braddock, S. E. Adams, P. D. Rathjen, S. M. Kingsman, and A. J. Kingsman. 1988. HIV expression strategies: ribosomal frameshifting is directed by short sequence in both mammalian and yeast systems. Cell 55:1159–1169.

306. Wlodawer, A., M. Miller, M. Jaskolski, B. K. Sathyanarayana, E. Baldwin, I. T. Weber, L. M. Selk, L. Clawson, J. Schneider, and S. B. H. Kent. 1989. Conserved folding in retroviral proteases: crystal structure of a synthetic HIV-1 protease. Science 245:616–621.

307. Wondrak, E. M., J. M. Louis, H. DeRocquigny, J. C. Chermann, and B. P. Roques. 1993. The Gag precursor contains a specific HIV-1 protease cleavage site between the NC (p7) and p1 proteins. FEBS Lett. 333:21–24.

308. Wu, L., N. P. Gerard, R. Wyatt, H. Choe, C. Parolin, N. Ruffing, A. Borsetti, A. A. Cardoso, E. Desjardin, W. Newman, C. Gerard, and J. Sodroski. 1996. CD4-induced interaction of primary HIV-1 gp120 glycoproteins with the chemokine receptor CCR-5. Nature 384:179–183.

309. Wyatt, R., P. D. Kwong, E. Desjardins, R. W. Sweet, J. Robinson, W. A. Hendrickson, and J. G. Sodroski. 1998. The antigenic structure of the HIV gp120 envelope glycoprotein. Nature 393:705–711.

310. Yao, X.-J., A. J. Mouland, R. A. Subbramanian, J. Forget, N. Rougeau, D. Bergeron, and E. A. Cohen. 1998. Vpr stimulates viral expression and induces cell killing in human immunodeficiency virus type 1-infected dividing Jurkat T cells. J. Virol. 72:4686–4693.

311. You, J. C., and C. S. McHenry. 1994. Human immunodeficiency virus type 1 nucleocapsid protein accelerates strand transfer of the terminally redundant sequences involved in reverse transcription. J. Biol. Chem. 269:31491–31495.

312. Yu, X., X. Yuan, Z. Matsuda, T. H. Lee, and M. Essex. 1992. The matrix protein of human immunodeficiency virus type 1 is required for incorporation of viral envelope protein into mature virions. J. Virol. 66:4966–4971.

313. Yu, X.-F., L. Dawson, C.-J. Tian, C. Flexner, and M. Dettenhofer. 1998. Mutations of the human immunodeficiency virus type 1 p6^{gag} domain result in reduced retention of Pol proteins during assembly. J. Virol. 72:3412–3417.

314. Yu, X.-F., Z. Matsuda, Q.-C. Yu, T. H. Lee, and M. Essex. 1995. Role of the C-terminus Gag protein in human immunodeficiency virus type 1 assembly and maturation. J. Gen. Virol. 76:3171–3179.

315. Zack, J. A., S. J. Arrigo, S. R. Weitsman, A. S. Go, A. Haislip, and I. S. Y. Chen. 1990. HIV-1 entry into quiescent primary lymphocytes: molecular analysis reveals a labile, latent viral structure. Cell 61:213–222.

316. Zhang, L. Q., P. Mackenzie, A. Cleland, E. C. Holmes, A. J. Brown, and P. Simmonds. 1993. Selection for specific sequences in the external envelope protein of human immunodeficiency virus type 1 upon primary infection. J. Virol. 67:3345–3356.

317. Zhang, W.-H., D. J. Hockley, M. V. Nermut, Y. Morikawa, and I. M. Jones. 1996. Gag-Gag interactions in the C-terminal domain of human immunodeficiency virus type 1 p24 capsid antigen are essential for Gag particle assembly. J. Gen. Virol. 77:743–751.

318. Zhang, Y., and E. Barklis. 1995. Nucleocapsid protein effects on the specificity of retrovirus RNA encapsidation. J. Virol. 69:5716–5722.

319. Zhang, Y., H. Qian, Z. Love, and E. Barklis. 1998. Analysis of the assembly function of the human immunodeficiency virus type 1 Gag protein nucleocapsid domain. J. Virol. 72:1782–1789.

320. Zhang, Z. Y., R. A. Poorman, L. L. Maggiora, R. L. Heinrikson, and F. J. Kezdy. 1991. Dissociative inhibition of dimeric enzymes, kinetic characterization of the inhibition of HIV-1 protease by its COOH-terminal tetrapeptide. J. Biol. Chem. 266:15591–15594.

321. Zhou, W., L. J. Parent, J. W. Wills, and M. D. Resh. 1994. Identification of membrane-binding domain within the amino-terminal region of human immunodeficiency virus type 1 Gag protein which interacts with acidic phospholipids. J. Virol. 68:2556–2569.

322. Zhu, T., H. Mo, N. Wang, D. S. Man, Y. Cao, R. A. Koup, and D. D. Ho. 1993. Genotypic and phenotypic characterization of HIV-1 patients with primary infection. Science 261:1179–1181.

2

JON P. ANDERSON
MATTHEW RAIN
DANIEL SHRINER
ALLEN G. RODRIGO
YANG WANG
DAVID NICKLE
GERALD H. LEARN
WILLSCOTT E. NAUGLER
JAMES I. MULLINS

The Genetics of HIV-1

Features and Products of the HIV-1 Genome

The genome of HIV contains many features common to all other retroviruses (45). For instance, retroviruses contain an enzyme, reverse transcriptase (RT), that has the ability to transcribe viral genomic RNA into a double-stranded, linear DNA molecule, which in turn is integrated into the host genome through the action of the virally encoded integrase (IN) to produce the DNA provirus (96). Additionally, all retroviruses are pseudodiploid: they consist of two single-stranded, sense-strand RNA molecules.[1] Retrovirus genomes characteristically contain group-specific antigen (*gag*), polymerase (*pol*), and envelope (*env*) genes that encode the structural proteins used to replicate within a host cell (Fig. 2.1) (374).

Gag

During transcription of the proviral DNA template, multicistronic (encoding several gene products) messenger RNA (mRNA) molecules are produced. The *gag* gene product, the Gag protein precursor (Pr55), is cleaved into the matrix (MA), capsid (CA), nucleocapsid (NC), and p6 proteins as well as two small peptides (Fig. 2.1). These proteins form the core of the viral particle and function to package the genomic viral RNA into the virion. In mature viral particles, the MA protein is localized between the virion CA and the viral envelope. The N-terminal region of the MA protein is necessary for targeting Pr55 to the cell membrane, associating it with the inner side of the lipid envelope (348), while the C-terminal region of MA is involved in the transport of the preintegration complex[2] to the nucleus (24). Single amino acid substitutions, located at specific sites across several different domains of MA, can greatly reduce the efficiency of virion pro-

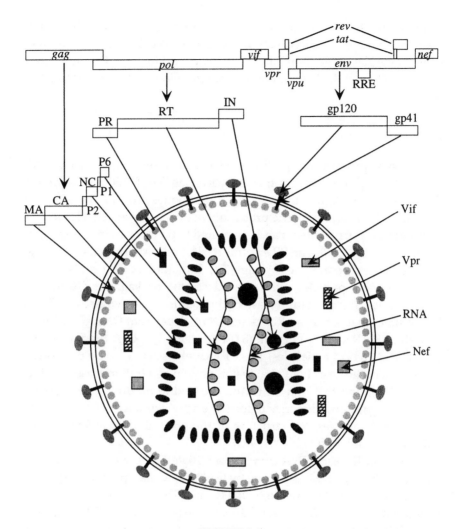

FIGURE 2.1

Virion structure of HIV-1

The genomic organization of HIV-1 is shown with viral genes labeled. The *gag*, *pol*, and *env* genes are subdivided into multiple gene products. Each of the gene products is indicated on the schematic of the HIV-1 virus particle.

duction (108). The CA protein forms the capsid shell within the viral particle (116). It contains a domain required for efficient viral replication that contains several amino acids that are absolutely invariant in all primate lentiviruses. Amino acid changes within the CA protein can block viral replication, reduce viral particle formation, and affect the assembly of the viral core (86, 224, 235, 384). The NC protein binds genomic viral RNA within the capsid and catalyzes the formation of a dimer of the two genomic RNA molecules (66). The NC protein is rich in basic residues that favor binding to nucleic acids and contains two copies of a zinc-finger domain that bind to unspliced viral RNA at psi sites (62, 131). Disruption of either of the zinc-finger domains results in the production of noninfectious viral particles, while their deletion eliminates viral particle formation (87, 348).

Pol

The *pol* gene products are produced following a low-frequency (~5%) ribosomal frameshifting event that creates a Gag/Pol Pr160 fusion protein that contains, in addition to Pr55, the viral enzymes protease (PR), RT, and IN (Fig. 2.1). PR is an aspartic protease that, when dimerized, cleaves the Gag and Gag-Pol precursors and is required to produce an infectious viral particle[3] (57, 197, 260). The PR enzyme itself is released from the Pr160 aggregate by an autocatalytic cleavage (71). Inhibition of PR results in noninfectious viral particles, with the successful packaging of Gag and Gag/Pol, but unsuccessful release of the mature proteins. Active RT is a heterodimer that acts as an RNA- and DNA-dependent DNA polymerase as well as an RNase H enzyme (84) that degrades RNA present within RNA/DNA hybrid molecules. The RT enzyme is activated by proteolytic processing of the Gag/Pol Pr160 fusion protein by viral protease, producing a p66 subunit that may be further cleaved to produce a p51 subunit (378). These subunits dimerize to form the active viral RT heterodimer. As in other polymerases, the structure of the p66 subunit contains finger, palm, and thumb domains (351, 373).

The viral RT uses RNA primers to initiate DNA synthesis. The first strand of DNA synthesis is primed by tRNA^{Lys}, while a polypurine tract of viral RNA that is not degraded by the RNase H activity primes the second strand synthesis (Fig. 2.2). Several drugs have been developed to target the viral RT. Nucleoside analogs (e.g., AZT, ddI, ddC, d4T, 3TC) that either lack a 3′–hydroxyl group or have it replaced with another group have been used to inhibit the elongation of the DNA strand. Non-nucleoside analogs have also been developed to interact with the catalytic site of the HIV RT. The IN enzyme integrates the proviral DNA into the genomic DNA of the host cell. Once integrated, the virus utilizes the host's cellular machinery to produce viral RNA and proteins that assemble into virions, which in turn are capable of infecting new cells (25). IN removes a dinucleotide region from the ends of the linear HIV DNA strand, randomly cleaves the host's cellular DNA, and joins the viral DNA to the host's chromosomal DNA.

Env

The *env* gene produces a glycoprotein, gp160, that is cleaved by a host protease, furin (148, 262), into the two Env proteins, SU and TM (also known respectively as gp120 and gp41), that remain associated as gp160 trimers

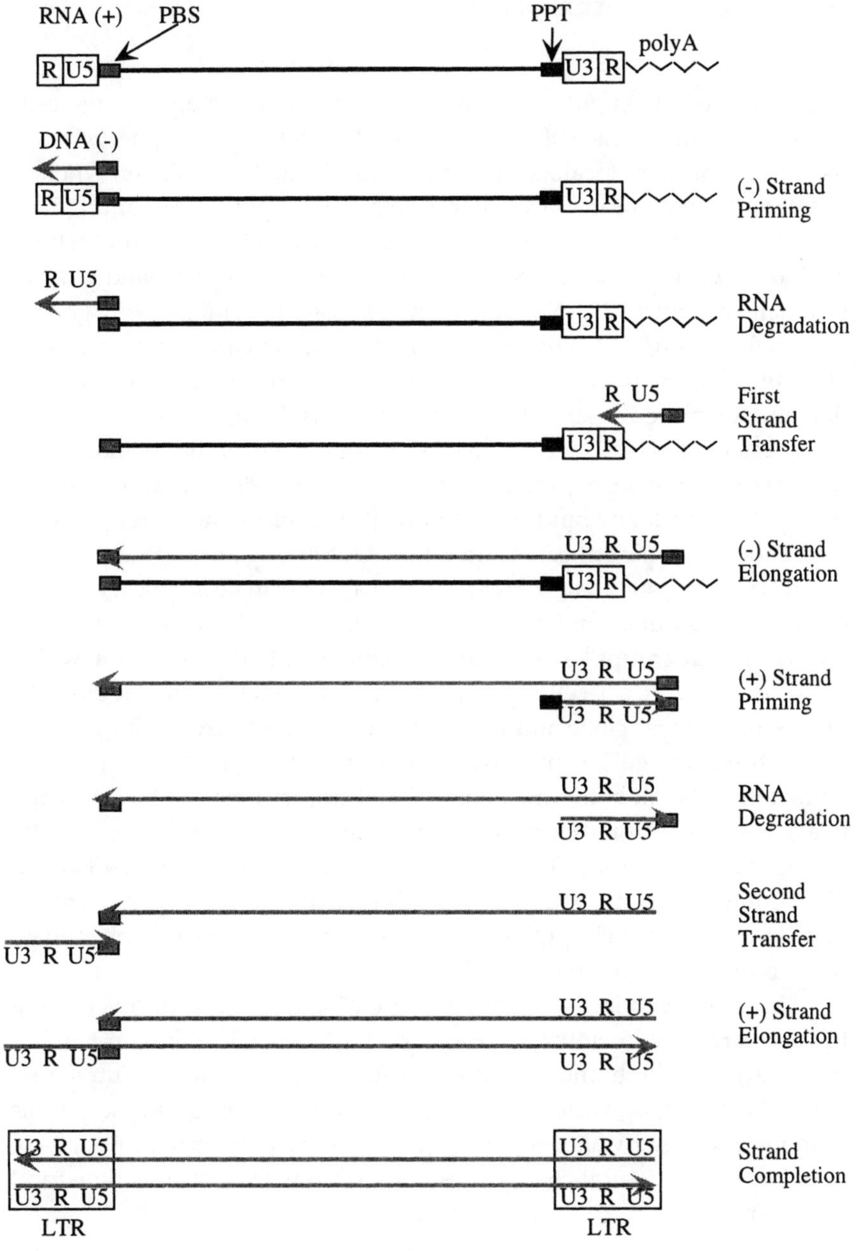

FIGURE 2.2

Reverse transcription mechanism

Viral RNA is shown as a black line, and DNA is shown as a gray line. The synthesis of the first strand of HIV-1 DNA is primed by tRNA^{Lys} binding to the primer binding site (PBS). RNase H activity degrades the RNA in the DNA/RNA hybrid, allowing the newly transcribed DNA to act as a primer for further transcription. The DNA hybridizes to the RNA R region, allowing for DNA extension. Again RNA in the DNA/RNA hybrid is degraded except for a polypurine tract (PPT), which is used as a primer for synthesis of the plus-strand DNA. The end result of reverse transcription is a double-stranded DNA copy that is longer than the single-stranded RNA genome template. The additional length arises from the synthesis of long terminal repeats (LTR) derived from sequences repeated at both ends of the RNA (R) as well as sequences derived from elements unique to the 5′ end of the RNA (U5) and the 3′ end of the RNA (U3).

at the surface of the lipid bilayer membrane of productively infected cells as well as on the surface of virions released from these cells (Fig. 2.1). SU, the surface protein, localizes to the exterior of the lipid bilayer, whereas TM, the transmembrane protein, transverses the lipid bilayer and tethers SU through noncovalent interactions. SU is involved in several functions vital to the virus including receptor recognition, cell tropism, and viral attachment and entry (26, 181, 198). There is substantial and growing genetic divergence among HIV Env sequences. Much of the variation is located in SU in five discrete hypervariable regions (V1 to V5). Between each of these domains are more conserved "constant" regions (C1 to C4). Viral entry requires interaction of SU with both CD4 and members of the chemokine receptor family that are expressed in the host cell (60, 99). Mutational analysis of SU and antibody binding experiments that block the binding of CD4 have shown that the critical residues for CD4 binding are located throughout SU (204, 279, 405). The V3 region of SU appears to be a critical locus for determining cellular tropism (i.e., the cell types that HIV can attach to and infect). Several groups have produced recombinant HIV-1 clones in which the V3 region from a T-cell-tropic virus was replaced by the V3 region of a macrophage-tropic clone and vice versa. In such cases, exchanging the V3 region has reversed the phenotype of several different clones; the phenomenon works in both directions: a T-cell-tropic clone can be converted to a macrophage-tropic clone by V3 exchange and vice versa (40, 43, 349). Further studies on the V3 region have identified two positions (306 and 320, counted from the beginning of SU) that can confer a change from a non-syncytium-inducing (NSI) to a syncytium-inducing (SI) phenotype when positively charged (105, 107).

TM is involved in the postreceptor binding cascade of events leading to virus-target cell membrane fusion and viral entry. The Env protein is a major target of the humoral immune response system, with neutralizing antibodies targeting various epitopes of gp120. The virus can escape this immune response by altering the gp120 region by point mutations, glycosylation, and structural changes resulting from insertions, deletions, and recombination.

The Auxiliary Genes of HIV-1

HIV-1 is a member of the lentivirus subgroup of retroviruses (41). Animal lentiviruses, such as HIV, simian immunodeficiency virus (SIV), feline immunodeficiency virus (FIV), and bovine immunodeficiency virus (BIV), primarily infect cells of the immune system including macrophages and T lymphocytes (146, 221). Animals infected by a lentivirus often experience immunodeficiency, neurodegeneration, wasting disorders, and death (146). In contrast to "simple" onco-retroviruses, which contain the three retroviral-defining proteins Gag, Pol, and Env, the "complex" lenti-retroviruses encode a complex set of regulatory and accessory gene products. The essential regulators of gene expression in HIV-1 include the transcriptional regulator Tat and the posttranscriptional regulator Rev. HIV-1 also contains several accessory proteins that remain conserved in vivo but are often found to be nonessential in vitro. These accessory proteins of HIV-1 include the so-called negative factor (Nef), viral protein R (Vpr), viral protein U (Vpu), and viral infectivity factor (Vif). Although these proteins vary in their importance to virus growth in culture systems, considering the high degree of conservation of all the corresponding reading frames, it seems highly likely that all are critical to appropriate virus replication and spread in vivo. Indeed, several studies support the idea that mutations in these genes that result in attenuated or defective viruses correlate with delayed disease progression (27, 69, 167, 189, 193, 213, 243, 259, 317). These observations spurred the hope of creating a live attenuated vaccine strain containing multiple deletions (80, 126), although recent findings cast considerable doubt on this approach (see below). Recent studies have revealed intriguing new functions of these viral proteins, suggesting a variety of roles in AIDS pathogenesis, while also elucidating new features of host cell biology.

Tat. Tat is one of two auxiliary proteins essential for virus growth in all cell systems evaluated and one of three "early" viral proteins, expressed before substantial amounts of the viral structural proteins are produced. Tat is translated from two coding exons derived from a spliced mRNA (Fig. 2.1). The first encodes a cysteine-rich N-terminal activation domain and an RNA binding domain responsible for nuclear localization and binding to the transactivation response element (TAR) of the LTR. The activation domain contains the amino acid motif (RKGLGI), which is conserved in HIV-1, HIV-2, and SIV Tat proteins. The RNA binding domain contains the highly basic amino acid motif (RKKRRQRRR), while the cysteine-rich region contains seven conserved cysteine residues that can form intermolecular disulfide bonds. The second Tat exon contains regions that are important in binding to $\alpha_v\beta_3$ and $\alpha_5\beta_1$ integrins and is thought to contain regulatory elements that influence the relative efficiencies of alternative splicing at the *tat, rev,* and the *env/nef* 3' splice sites (9, 16, 385).

In Tat's role of enhancing mRNA transcription and elongation (180, 188, 212, 240), it functions by binding directly to a bulge region within the TAR element in a one-to-one ratio (85, 309, 386). The TAR element is a 59-nucleotide stem-loop RNA structure formed at the immediate 5' end of all viral transcripts (308, 357). Mutational studies of TAR indicate that the loop, top of the stem, and bulge are necessary for successful transactivation (98, 309). Tat associates with cyclin T1, which binds to both the loop within the TAR element and CDK9 (387, 407), which phosphorylates the C-terminal domain (CTD) of the large subunit of RNA polymerase II

(Pol II) (157, 408). Hyperphosphorylation of the CTD is associated with enhanced processivity during transcription by RNA Pol II (58, 278, 285), preventing the complex from stalling at the 3' end of the TAR element (12, 177, 286). Tat might also function to clear transcription complexes from the promoter and favor the formation of new complexes, thereby indirectly stimulating transcriptional initiation (187, 212).

Lentiviruses other than HIV also use transcriptional activators. These lentiviruses express Tat proteins through mechanisms that either bind viral RNA, similar to the mechanism of HIV-1, or use other processes to regulate transcription. The lentiviral RNA binding Tat proteins all contain an activation domain and a highly basic RNA binding domain, necessary to create a minimal Tat protein (79).

Rev. Rev (for regulator of virion protein expression) is also an essential, early viral protein. This 116-amino-acid, positively charged, two-exon phosphoprotein (152, 256) regulates the switch from early expression of Tat, Rev, and Nef to late, Rev-dependent expression of Gag, Pol, Env, Vif, Vpu, and Vpr and the production of viral genomic RNA for packaging in progeny. This switch is accomplished by allowing the nuclear export of partially spliced and unspliced (genomic) viral mRNA (97, 104, 270, 350). In the absence of Rev, mRNAs that contain introns are generally not exported from the nucleus (136). Rev contains regions specific for nuclear localization, posttranslational activation, protein multimerization, and RNA binding. It associates with a specific mRNA secondary structure, the Rev responsive element (RRE) (10, 61, 154, 160, 161). The RRE consists of multiple overlapping stem-loop structures within the *env* coding region of viral mRNAs (Fig. 2.1) (68, 233, 412). Mutational studies have indicated that the primary binding site of Rev exists within a "bubble" in stem-loop II (234). The interaction between Rev and RRE aids in the stability of mRNAs, the transport of mRNAs out of the nucleus, and the translation of these mRNAs into viral proteins (92, 97, 149, 233, 335).

The binding of Rev to the RRE appears to prevent assembly of functional spliceosomes on viral mRNA (194, 195). Thus, early viral transcripts are fully spliced, leading to expression of Tat, Rev, and the third early protein, Nef. As the Rev level rises, it prevents splicing of a portion of the new viral transcripts, activating the late expression of the structural proteins. A major functional domain in Rev is the N-terminal oligomerization, the nuclear localization and RNA binding domain containing the arginine-rich amino acid motif (RQARRNRRRRWRERQR) (413). The other major functional domain is the C-terminal, leucine-rich effector domain, containing the amino acid motif (LPPLERLTL), which is conserved within the Rev proteins of several other lentiviruses (391). Mutations within the effector domain can create Rev proteins defective in nuclear export (102, 359), whereas intact effector domains induce rapid nuclear export when fused to heterologous proteins (391) and have been shown to function as a nucleocytoplasmic shuttle (174, 175, 258, 300). Attenuating mutations in *rev* have been found to persist in a long-term nonprogressor (LTNP) and thus may be associated with some cases of disease attenuation (167).

Nef. Nef is the third early viral protein, made by up to 80% of the early viral transcripts. It is important for viral replication, pathogenicity, and increased infectivity and is partially responsible for CD4 downregulation in infected cells (50, 78, 123, 124, 203, 261, 414). It is a myristylated phosphoprotein, with the myristyl group, attached to the conserved Gly-2 residue, apparently targeting Nef to the cytoplasmic membrane (409). Nef downregulates cell surface CD4 (3, 14, 123, 124, 145) via induction of endocytosis and subsequent degradation in lysosomes (1, 299, 332). Nef links cell surface CD4 to AP-2 adapter proteins involved in the formation of clathrin-coated pits and then routes internalized CD4 to endosomes via β-COP for lysosomal degradation (13, 137, 236, 290, 318). Domains required for these two activities include the N-terminal myristylation signal, the CD4 binding domain, the AP binding domain, and the lysosomal targeting domain (137, 290).

A second, distinct function of Nef is to downregulate cell surface expression of class I major histocompatibility complex (MHC-I) molecules (333) through linking cell surface MHC-I to AP-1 adapter proteins (138, 215). Downregulation of cell surface MHC-I protects infected cells against attack by cytotoxic T lymphocytes (50). Nef domains required for this phenotype include the N-terminal myristylation signal, a proximal acidic stretch, an SH3-binding motif, and a proximal α-helix (138, 237).

Another property attributed to Nef is its ability to associate with cellular serine kinases (140, 275, 294, 323, 324, 398), including a recently described Nef-associated kinase complex consisting of p56^{lck} and a cellular serine kinase (11). Since the identities and roles of these serine kinases are currently unknown, it is unclear whether they play any role in T-cell modulation or enhancement of virion infectivity. Recently, Nef has been reported to induce the production of CC-chemokines in infected macrophages, and supernatants from Nef-expressing macrophages induced both chemotaxis and activation of resting T cells (358). Several reports suggest that Nef modulates T-cell activation events, but the mechanism and the nature of the modulation (positive or negative) are still controversial.

Importantly, Nef has been reported to enhance viral infectivity, replication, and virulence. The SH3-binding motif has been implicated in this activity (128, 313), leaving it unclear if this activity is distinct from MHC-I downregulation. The demonstration that monkeys challenged with *nef*-deleted strains of SIV failed to progress to AIDS within the expected period of time and had greatly reduced viral loads (6, 81, 193, 310) greatly invigorated the effort to develop a live attenuated vaccine against HIV. The effect of Nef on viral virulence was supported by the fact that an Australian cohort of LTNPs and another individual were identified with defective *nef* genes (69, 193). Unfortunately, the replication of a virus with the ability to persist despite enormous genomic variation (see below) seems inexorably to bring the threat of disease. The first warning was provided by Cranage and colleagues (392), who essentially reiterated the earlier results but also had one animal develop fulminant AIDS. It turned out that the virus in this animal "healed" its deletion and regained its potency by duplication of adjacent sequences. Next, Ruprecht and colleagues found that when infant macaques were inoculated orally with a high dose of SIV (harboring three deletions including in *nef*) they all developed AIDS, while 6 of 15 adults developed some indication of at least impending immunodeficiency or AIDS (7, 310). Finally, recent signs of progression in the LTNPs with Nef-defective HIV-1 infection described above (139, 214) cast great doubt on the notion that Nef-defective viruses are incapable of inducing immunodeficiency disease. Indeed, it was only in the past year that plans for testing live attenuated multiple-gene deleted HIV vaccines in humans were apparently abandoned.

Vpr. Vpr also appears to be involved in multiple events in virus and cell metabolism. It promotes the nuclear localization of the preintegration complex, is involved in cell cycle arrest, and is involved in the induction of cellular differentiation (36, 144, 219, 220, 307). Vpr is a virion-associated protein present at molar ratios equivalent to Gag and thus is an auxiliary gene product an infected cell will encounter in large quantities (47, 48, 411). Vpr possesses two genetically separable functions. In contrast to oncoviruses, lentiviruses can infect infrequently dividing or nondividing cells, such as terminally differentiated macrophages (223, 379). Vpr appears to play a role in this capacity by enhancing translocation of the preintegration complex into the nucleus of nondividing cells, through interactions with importin-α and nucleoporins (114, 155, 291, 377). Vpr-assisted translocation could also be important for hastening the initiation of viral replication in newly infected, short-lived T cells (352).

Another function of Vpr is the induction of cell cycle arrest in the G2 phase of dividing T cells (307). Vpr prevents activation of the p34^{cdc2} kinase by maintaining it in a hyperphosphorylated, inactive state (153, 172). Two hypotheses have been proposed to explain the observation that primate lentiviruses induce a G2 arrest. One is that Vpr prevents activation of p34^{cdc2}, thereby inhibiting cytotoxic T lymphocyte (CTL)-mediated apoptosis of infected cells (91, 249, 342). The other hypothesis is that viral expression may be highest during the G2 phase of the cell cycle (91, 127). Interestingly, the G2 arrest phenotype has also been linked to increased viral transcription in nondividing macrophages (356).

Vpu. Vpu is required for efficient virion maturation and release and is involved in CD4 downregulation (196, 394, 395). It is a late viral protein expressed bicistronically with Env (334). It has two major structural domains: an N-terminal hydrophobic transmembrane region and a C-terminal highly charged region (354). Within the latter are two phosphorylated serines (327, 328). These must be phosphorylated for the C-terminal region of Vpu to target CD4 trapped as CD4-gp160 complexes in the endoplasmic reticulum for degradation, thereby facilitating expression of gp160 (20, 37, 218, 326, 327, 375, 394, 395). Vpu acts as an adapter between CD4 and h-βTrCP, a protein that in turn interacts with Skp1p, a targeting factor for ubiquitin-mediated proteolysis (109, 242, 325). Phosphorylation is not required for the N-terminal region of Vpu to facilitate the release of virions at the plasma membrane (196, 326, 329, 368). Interestingly, Vpu can facilitate the release of a wide variety of retroviruses, such as Moloney murine leukemia virus (Mo-MuLV), SIV, HIV-2, and visna virus (21, 132), which makes it even more curious that only HIV-1 and SIV$_{cpz}$ possess a distinct *vpu* gene (395). Recent evidence suggests that perhaps HIV-2, related to SIV$_{smm}$, does possess the activity of facilitation of virion release, but rather than residing in a distinct gene, the activity may reside in *env* (19, 21).

Vif. Vif influences the infectivity of virus particles and aids in the correct folding of the Gag proteins to form the core complex (159, 312, 380). It is one of the late viral proteins acting during assembly in the host cell to allow formation of progeny competent for some undetermined step, post-entry but preintegration, in the newly infected target cell (18, 347, 380). It seems that Vif influences the stability of the reverse transcriptase complex (106, 344, 346), but it remains unclear whether Vif directly plays a role in reverse transcription or influences Gag processing and core uncoating. Vif from the NL4-3 and HXB2 viral strains were both shown to enhance viral infectivity by two to three orders of magnitude (103, 353). In the absence of Vif, virion cores are morphologically abnormal, although protein composition appears unaffected (18, 106, 159). The requirement for Vif varies with the cell type but is essential for a productive infection in primary T cells (94, 111, 112). Recent work has also found that Vif inhibits an unidentified antiviral activity in cells (231, 345).

Replication. The life cycle of HIV-1 is discussed in terms of processes that take place during the early and late phases of viral replication. The early phase begins with the cellular attachment of the HIV-1 virion and continues until the genomic integration of the HIV-1 provirus. The late phase starts with the transcription of viral mRNA and ends with the release and maturation of new virions (Fig. 2.3).

The HIV-1 virion contains RT, PR, IN, TM, SU, Vpr, Vif, and tRNA[Lys] in addition to a mixture of cellular RNAs and proteins. The attachment of

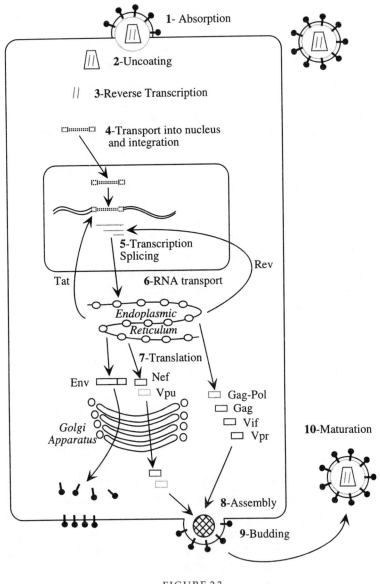

FIGURE 2.3

Viral life cycle

The illustration shows the steps (1–10) involved in the life cycle of HIV-1. Many of the individual steps are described in detail in the text. Viral RNA is represented as black lines, and viral DNA is represented by hatched lines.

the virion to the host cell surface is mediated by interactions between the CD4 and receptors CXCR4 or CCR5 on the cell surface and SU on the surface of the viral particle (2, 60, 88, 99). CD4 is functionally expressed on the surface of T helper lymphocytes and macrophages. Functional CXCR4 coreceptor is expressed on some T cells, while the CCR5 coreceptor is expressed on certain T cells and macrophages. To gain entry into the host cell, viral SU binds to CD4 and one of the coreceptors, producing a conformational change in the SU/TM protein complex (250). This change allows the membranes of the HIV-1 virion and the host cell to fuse and release the viral capsid into the host cell cytoplasm (113, 322). On entry, the viral particles become partially uncoated to produce a nucleoprotein complex. Reverse transcription then takes place using the viral RT with tRNA^{Lys} as a primer, producing a double-stranded linear viral DNA genome (Fig. 2.2). A preintegration complex, containing the viral DNA genome, Vpr, IN, MA, CA, and NC, is then transported to the nucleus, where integration takes place. The viral enzyme IN cleaves the cellular genomic DNA, allowing the viral DNA genome to be inserted (376). The insertion event is completed by host repair enzymes, which ligate the host and viral DNA together (64).

Following the integration of the provirus, transcription of viral mRNA is initiated by the host RNA Pol II (Fig. 2.3). The HIV-1 provirus LTR contains a strong promoter region that includes the TATA box to which RNA Pol II binds as well as other *cis* acting elements including SP1 binding sites and NF-κB enhancer sites, each of which responds to cellular activation signals and can thus activate an otherwise quiescent provirus. The viral mRNA that results is quickly spliced by cellular spliceosomes (141). However, these multiply spliced messages code for the viral proteins Tat and Rev, which control the temporal regulation of HIV-1 protein expression. Tat increases transcription initiation and elongation of transcripts through stabilizing the RNA Pol II complex, enabling more and longer HIV-1 mRNAs to be transcribed (192, 386). These longer HIV-1 messages would be normally targeted by the host cell for splicing and are not able to produce all the HIV-1 proteins needed to create a new virion. Rev solves this splicing problem by interacting with the long messages and directing them out of the nucleus, where they can be translated. Once sufficient levels of Rev are produced to allow transport and translation of singly spliced and unspliced RNA, translation of viral structural components begins, signaling the onset of the late phase of HIV-1 infection.

Following translation, the uncleaved Gag protein complex (Pr55) begins to form the framework for a new virion near the cellular plasma membrane (35). Associated with these previrions are two copies of HIV-1 genomic RNA, which will serve as genomes within new virions. Also associated with the previrions is tRNA^{Lys}, which is used as a primer during reverse transcription (165). During this previrion construction, Env glycoprotein complexes are processed in the endoplasmic reticulum (82, 90). The Env glycoproteins are transported to the Golgi complex, where they are further processed and then finally transported to the cell surface. The new virions bud through areas of the plasma membrane containing these Env surface proteins (SU and TM, cleaved by host cell protease) (148, 262). After budding from the cell, the newly released particles are processed by PR to produce fully infectious virions (Fig. 2.3).

Evolutionary Escape from Antiretroviral Drugs

Some of the first antiviral drugs developed to combat HIV-1 were nucleoside inhibitors that block reverse transcription by chain termination. Although these drugs showed promise by transiently lowering viral loads, they were not effective in stopping the progression to AIDS as the virus evolved resistance to the drugs (210, 363). The next great advancement in antiretroviral therapy came with the development of protease inhibitors, which prevent the maturation of viral particles (186, 245). Current treatment regimens for HIV-1 infections utilize a combination of several drugs (29, 30). These highly active antiretroviral therapy (HAART) regimens generally consist of a protease inhibitor combined with two or more reverse transcriptase inhibitors. HAART has been shown to have the potential to suppress plasma HIV-1 to undetectable levels (142, 143, 150). However, many people on HAART discontinue treatment because of inefficacy or severe toxicity or for other reasons, resulting in treatment failure rates as high as 30% to 44% (67, 95).

Antiretroviral drugs exert selective pressures on HIV, which foster the emergence of drug-resistant variants. Currently there are three classes of antiretroviral drugs, which target the products of two genes in the HIV-1 genome, the protease and reverse transcriptase coding segments. The power of different drugs to suppress viral replication varies. Drugs that markedly reduce HIV-1 replication exert a stronger selective pressure than drugs that have a less profound effect on suppression of viral replication (301). As selective pressure on either of the genes increases, the rate of fixation of mutation in that gene correspondingly increases, resulting in the emergence of drug-resistant strains of virus (52).

One of the chief difficulties in examining the evolution of HIV-1's drug resistance is correlating viral phenotype with viral genotype. How does one discern whether a particular change in the genetic makeup of HIV-1 is responsible for a change in the phenotype of the virus? Typically researchers perform in vitro studies of passaging HIV-1 multiple times in the presence of antiretroviral drugs. Strains that overcome the antiretroviral effect of the drug (i.e., develop phenotypic resistance to the drug) are examined at the nucleotide and amino acid level to determine changes that may have led to the development of the resistant phenotype. This kind of study does not always reliably predict the drug-resistant genotypes found in samples from patients. Typical ex vivo phenotyping assays use patient samples, from which the genes of interest are isolated and inserted into an HIV-1 vector, which is used to examine levels of replication in the presence of various levels of drug. The genotype of the virus may then be correlated with its phenotype. A few studies have been performed that correlate genotypic patterns, phenotypic resistance, and disease progression in HIV-1-infected patients (65, 205). Phenotypic resistance (with its corresponding genotypic pattern) is correlated with increased disease progression (23).

There is a growing body of evidence that ties specific amino acid substitutions in the protease and reverse transcriptase regions to phenotypic resistance to particular antiretroviral drugs (Table 2.1). It is clear that different substitutions confer different levels of resistance (122, 301, 370). Generally, strongly suppressive antiretroviral drugs quickly (in some cases in a week or less) select for single amino acid substitutions that confer high-level resistance (301). Other, more weakly suppressive drugs only slowly (over six months to a year) select for resistance-associated substitutions, and the level of resistance may be low (271). Thus, the more powerful the drug, the stronger the selective pressure to evolve higher-level resistance to the drug.

In most cases, several amino acid substitutions are associated with resistance to a particular drug (183, 211). Although it has been an attractive idea to correlate specific substitutions with phenotypic resistance to specific drugs, it is now known that there is a great deal of cross-resistance associated with most substitutions (77, 185, 282). In addition, certain multidrug resistance substitutions have been observed to confer high-level resistance to entire classes of antiretroviral drugs (166, 336, 397). It is common to separate substitutions into primary and secondary substitutions. Primary substitutions directly affect the ability of the viral protein to evade the effect of the drug, while secondary substitutions compensate for the change in the protein structure caused by the primary substitution. These substitutions tend to have an additive effect—the greater the number of resistance-associated substitutions, the higher the level of resistance (183). Resistance-associated substitutions in the viral genome may hamper the replicative fitness of the virus in comparison with the wild-type counterpart in the absence of the drug (133, 415), and this has been demonstrated for a handful of substitutions to date (404).

Both in vitro and in vivo studies have shown that, once drug pressure is removed, virus bearing wild-type amino acids at resistant sites quickly replace virus with drug resistance–associated substitutions (72). There is evidence that this phenomenon may not be due to further evolution but rather a reemergence of latent virus from its proviral DNA stored in cells in which HIV-1 replication had been suppressed by drug therapy (266). The wild-type virus, being more fit (in the absence of drugs), outgrows the virus with resistance-associated mutations. This observation had led to the hope that patients with resistant virus might be able to discontinue antiretroviral therapy until the wild-type virus reemerged, at which time drug therapy could be again started for greater clinical benefit (72). Unfortunately, resistant strains, like wild-type strains, are archived in a latent state and quickly reemerge when drug pressure is reapplied (266).

The rate of evolution of HIV-1 is directly related to the rate of replication. Combinations of antiretroviral drugs can markedly diminish the level of replication of HIV-1 in patients able to adhere to difficult drug regimens. In best-case scenarios, replication of the virus is suppressed to below the

TABLE 2.1

Drug resistance mutations recognized for NRTI, NNRTI, AND PRI[a]

Nucleoside Reverse Transcriptase Inhibitors (NRTI)

AA (Wild-type mutation[b])	Abacavir	Didanosine	Lamivudine	Stavudine	Zalcitabine	Zidovudine
41 M>L				+		+++
44 E>D/K			***			***
62 A>V	*	*	***	*	*	*
65 K>R	+	++	++	++	++	+
67 D>N	+					++
69 T>D/N	+		++	+	+	++
69 T>Sxx	***	***	***	***	***	***
69 T>Sxx						
70 K>R	+			+	++	++
74 L>V/I	++	+++			+	
75 V>M/A		+				
75 V>T/				++		
75 V>I					+	
77 F>L	*	*	*	*	*	*
115 Y>F	+++	*	*	*		*
116 F>Y	*					
118 V>I			**			
151 Q>M	***	***	***	***	***	***
178 I>M					++	
184 M>V/I	+	+	+++	+	+	
208 H>Y			**			**
210 L>W	+		+	+		++
211 R>K			**			**
214 F>L			**			**
215 T>Y/F	+	+		+	+	+++
219 K>Q/E	+			+		++
333 G>D/E			**			**

Non-Nucleoside Reverse Transcriptase Inhibitors (NNRTI)

AA (Wild-type mutation)	Delavirdine	Efavirenz	Nevirapine
6 E>K	++	++	++
98 A>G	++	++	++
100 L>I	+++	+++	+++
101 K>E/V	+++	++	++
103 K>N	+++	+++	+++
106 V>I/M/A	++	++	++
108 V>I	++	++	++
138 E>K	++	++	++
181 Y>C/I	+++	+	+++
188 Y>L/H/C	+	+++	+++
190 G>A/S	+	+++	+++
227 F>L	++	++	++
236 P>L	++	+	+

Protease Inhibitors (PRI)[b]

AA Wild-type mutation	Amprenavir	Indinavir	Nelfinavir	Ritonavir	Saquinavir
10 L>F/I/R/V	+	+	+	+	+
20 K>M/R		+		+	+
24 L>I	+	+			+
30 D>N	+	+	+++		
32 V>I	+	+		+	
33 L>F/V				+	
36 M>I	+	+	+	+	
46 M>I/L	+	+	+	+	
47 I>V	+				
48 G>V	+	+	+	++	+++
50 I>V	+++	+	+	++	+
54 I>V	+	++	+	++	+
54 I>L	+	+	+	++	+
71 A>V/T	+	+	+	+	+
73 G>S/T	+	+			+
82 V>S/A/F/T	+	+++	++	+++	+
84 I>V	+++	+++	+++	+++	+++
88 N>D/S/T	+	+	+++	+	+
90 L>M	+	+	+++	+	+++

[a]This table is based on data from the Los Alamos Database (http://hiv-web.lanl.gov), the Stanford HIV Database (http://hivd.stanford.edu), and viable presented or published clinical and laboratory studies. For more detailed information concerning resistance, please visit these Web sites.

[b]Amino acids (AA) in the nucleoside and non-nucleoside sections of the table refer to the RT protein; amino acids in the PRI section of the table refer to the PR protein.

+++ Indicates major mutation that is frequently observed with high-level resistance to the drug.

++ Indicates mutation that is frequently observed with low-level resistance to the drug.

+ Indicates mutation that may cause resistance to the drug, usually in combination with other resistance mutations.

*** Q151M is the pivotal mutation in a multidrug complex that includes AAs 62, 75, 77, and 116. This complex will confer high-level resistance to all NRTIs. Mutation of AA69 from T > S followed by the insertion of any two amino acids will confer low-level resistance to the NRTI. Insertions plus ZDV-resistance mutations cause moderate to high-level resistance to the NRTIs.

** H208Y, R211K, F214L, and G333D/E facilitate dual resistance to ZDV and 3TC in association with mutation at AA184 of RT. E44D/K and V118I facilitate resistance to 3TC when accompanied by ZDV resistance mutations (M41L, K70R, T215Y/F).

* A62V, V75I, F77L, and F116Y increase multinucleoside resistance caused by Q151M.

level of detection of current assays. Studies performed on cohorts of these patients show marked slowing in the rate of evolution of HIV-1 and a corresponding lack of development of resistant phenotypes/genotypes (51). Current evidence suggests that low-level replication occurs under HAART, and it is likely that evolution to resistant virus can occur even at very low levels of viral replication (402), albeit at a much slower rate.

Several other proteins and enzymatic activities, including IN, RNase H, and Env, are targets of drug development. Because of the highly error-prone nature of the HIV-1 RT protein, it is likely that resistance-associated substitutions will arise to new antiretroviral drugs. Little is known about the interactions of resistance-associated substitutions in the protease region with mutations causing resistance in the reverse transcriptase encoding region. The regions have largely been studied separately. As more genes of HIV-1 are targeted by drugs, interactions, if any, between resistance-associated substitutions in different genes will become increasingly complex.

Diversity of HIV Genomes

There are currently two known types of HIV: HIV-1 and HIV-2, with HIV-1 found in the majority of the infected individuals worldwide (372). Both are transmitted, though with different rates. Transmission of HIV-2 is more attenuated, from mother to child, through blood interactions and by sexual contact. Both HIV-1 and HIV-2 cause AIDS, but HIV-1 is more virulent (372, 393). HIV-1 and HIV-2 are thought to have originated from separate cross-species infections. HIV-2 is thought to have originated from several independent transmissions from sooty mangabeys (*Cercocebus atys*)[4] to humans (38, 121), and HIV-1 is hypothesized to have originated from chimpanzees (*Pan troglodytes*) (117).

Over the 50 or more years that humans have been infected by primate lentiviruses, considerable sequence diversity has been generated in HIV-1. Examination of this diversity shows that it is not distributed uniformly. To the contrary, it is distributed in clades that may be classified as groups and subtypes. The phylogenetic patterns that we observe in HIV-1 sequences can be used to make inferences about events in the history of the HIV-1 pandemic and possibly to infer current epidemiological incidents.

Viruses involved in the HIV-1 pandemic are grouped into the M (main) group, an O (outlier) group, and an N (non-M/non-O) group. Various genes differ in their capacity to maintain genetic diversity owing to differences in the selective forces operating on them (see below). Phylogenetic analyses of the *env* and *gag* genes of the M group have established 11 distinct subtypes or clades (A through H, J and K) (Fig. 2.4) (118, 200, 202, 229, 371). Current procedures for establishing new subtypes call for obtaining and analyzing three full-length genomes that maintain a distinctive line-

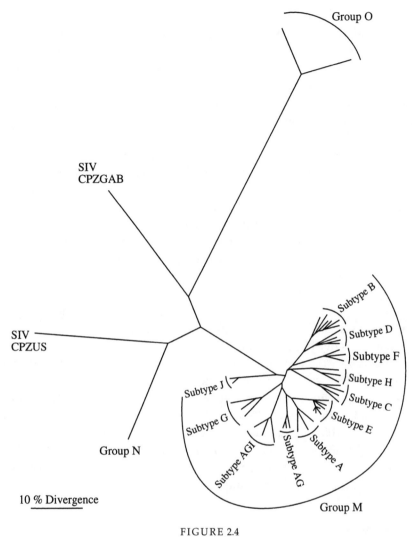

FIGURE 2.4

Phylogenetic classification of HIV-1

Phylogenetic tree of complete HIV-1 genomes showing the evolutionary relationship of the three groups (M, N, and O) and the subtypes in group M (A through J), along with two SIV sequences from chimpanzees.

age within group M and are obtained from individuals who do not have a direct epidemiological linkage (303). Viral variants that do not meet this criteria have been designated "U" until more information is obtained. The amount of genetic diversity seen between groups, between subtypes, between individuals, and even within an individual can be quite large. Regions of the *env* gene can currently differ by up to 35% between subtypes (8, 269), up to 25% between individuals infected with the same subtype (100, 173), and 0 to more than 10% within an individual (75, 382), depending on the length of infection (338). Analysis of complete genomes has shown that different genome regions can vary in the patterns of relationships. For example, the region containing the *gag* gene falls into one subtype, while the remainder falls into another. Observations such as these led to the discovery of intersubtype recombinants that have a genome containing a mosaic of more than one viral subtype (33, 119, 304, 305, 311, 316). Whereas some of these recombinant lineages appear to be restricted to a single individual and have not spread, some appear to have a broader epidemiological impact and have spread widely into many host individuals. These latter lineages have been called circulating recombinant forms (CRFs) (31, 32). Intersubtype recombinants might present a substantial phenotypic change that would not normally be seen in either subtype alone, since they bring together several genetic changes at a single time. Furthermore, the efficacy of subtype-specific vaccines might be lessened by the presence of CRFs, and their spread might even be favored by vaccine usage.

The amount of diversity in HIV-1 varies along the genome. Some regions of the genome, including particularly that containing the *pol* gene, are more conserved, whereas other regions may be highly variable. The *env* gene, with its five hypervariable domains, contains some of the most variable regions in the genome. Env proteins provide the initial contact between the virus and the outside world. Therefore, the Env proteins must be sufficiently conserved to maintain their capacity to engage target cells and facilitate infection, but they must also be sufficiently plastic to accept evolutionary changes that may favor evasion of immune attack. Other regions of the genome experience similarly opposing forces. Even highly conserved gene regions such as RT and PR have the capacity to tolerate changes that confer drug resistance.

Mechanisms for HIV-1 Diversity

HIV-1 achieves great diversity through high mutation rates, rapid viral production, selection, and recombination. The viral enzyme RT is used to transcribe the viral RNA into DNA that is later integrated. As the RT transcribes the DNA strand from the RNA template, it also destroys the RNA template with its RNase H activity, curtailing the possibility of proofreading in the transcription process. The lack of proofreading gives the RT an error rate of approximately 1 in 4,000 nucleotides (238, 239, 295, 302). This high error rate facilitates high viral diversity. The RT also has a high rate of slippage in homopolymeric tracts, which results in insertion and deletion events during reverse transcription. Along with the high error rate of the RT, HIV-1 maintains a very high replication rate, with as many as 10^{10} virions produced daily within an infected individual (46, 158, 288). If one assumes that RT creates on average approximately two point mutations during a single reverse transcription and 10^6 reverse transcription events are taking place each day, then every single point mutation should be produced on a daily basis within an infected individual. Along with these point mutations, HIV-1 is adding insertions/deletions (indels) and recombination events that add to the diversity of the virus population. The viruses within an infected individual come, then, to exist as a quasi species (population) of genetically distinct yet related genotypes. On initial infection, the population within an individual, at least as reflected in the *env* V3 region, has been found to be relatively homogeneous (76, 162, 381, 399, 417, 418), although recent studies have indicated that women harbor a more heterogeneous *env* population early in infection (228, 292). Following viral transmission, viral diversity within the individual increases at a rate of about 0.9% per year in the C2-V5 region of *env* (338) as a result of point mutations. This diversity can also greatly increase through the recombination of divergent viral strains within the population (33, 208, 305). Immune-mediated selection can also increase viral diversity within the host (17, 162). An infected individual's immune system responds to specific epitopes produced by the virus. Variants within the HIV-1 population that are divergent enough to escape immune recognition will replicate until the immune system responds to their novel epitopes, repeating the cycle. Detection of significant immune-mediated selective pressure is, however, difficult (306). Leigh Brown (216) suggests that the effective size of the HIV population in vivo is so small that random genetic drift plays a dominant role in the modulation of diversity. Only very large selective effects will have a stronger influence on diversity than stochastic processes of drift. Other authors suggest that only a relatively small proportion of sites are actually subject to positive selection pressure (272). It is reasonable to posit, as others have done, that the strength and direction of selection are likely to vary over the course of disease (406). It is intuitively appealing to ascribe immune escape, viral persistence, and the evolution of drug resistance at least in part to HIV genetic diversity. Experimental confirmation of this remains the challenge.

Course of Disease

Three prototypic patterns describing the course of disease and relating to the duration of HIV-1 infection have been established. A majority of HIV-1 infected individuals (80–90%) have a survival time of approximately 10 years and are termed "typical progressors" (284). Between 5% and 10% of infected individuals experience a fast course of disease and have a survival time of three to five years (341). These people are classified as "rapid progressors." These people have a weak immune response and produce only low levels of antibodies against HIV-1 proteins and neutralizing antibodies (170). Finally, about 5% of infected people have an extended course of disease and are asymptomatic for 10 or more years with stable CD4+ T-cell levels without the benefit of antiviral therapy. These individuals are termed "long-term nonprogressors" (LTNP) (341). LTNPs often maintain stable, strong CTL responses against HIV-1 proteins (151), while in typical progressors the immune response declines over time (341). Several LTNPs have been identified with viruses containing defective accessory genes (69, 89, 167); however, no common viral factor has been found to account for long-term nonprogression.

The course of disease within an HIV-1 infected individual has three characteristic stages: primary infection, clinical latency, and apparent disease or AIDS. Primary HIV-1 infection is associated with a sudden rise in viremia and often a simultaneous decline of CD4+ T cells (42, 283). These infected individuals sometimes develop flu-like symptoms one to six weeks after the initial infection. Following primary infection and around the time of detectable cellular and humoral immune responses, viral load decreases, and CD4+ cells increase to a level that may remain relatively constant for a time (135, 284, 296). The period of this "stable" phase varies from individual to individual. In some individuals it is nonexistent, with little evidence of immune response and, instead, a rapid progression to AIDS. In others, the stable phase may last indefinitely, with few, if any, signs of immunologic deficit (341). This stage of the infection was once thought by some to be a dormant period for the virus but now has been shown to be a quite active stage, with HIV-1 rapidly producing new virus particles (158, 388). During this stage there are no clinical signs of disease, but there is a progressive decline of CD4+ T cells and continual destruction of the lymphoid tissue (55). The final stage of the infection is the progression to AIDS and clinically apparent disease. This stage is defined by substantial impairment of immune function and the development of opportunistic infections.

A number of hypotheses have been postulated to explain the shift from the stable to the progressive phase of HIV infection. In all instances, these hypotheses postulate a shift in some underlying dynamic or process to account for the change. Some researchers have suggested that changes in viral transcription and replication (54) or immune parameters may be causally related to progression (28, 254). Alternatively, it has been suggested that the emergence of more cytopathic or virulent variants may cause the loss of host cells (39, 55, 265, 267, 281, 365). A model in which viral antigenic diversity increases beyond a threshold, resulting in immune collapse, has also been proposed (264, 273).

Mutations Leading to Different Phenotypes

Many host and viral factors can affect the duration of the asymptomatic interval and potentially contribute to a loss of the T-cell homeostasis found to exist in asymptomatic infection (241). For example, plasma viral load early after the establishment of infection appears to be predictive of the asymptomatic interval (257). It is not known what determines the viral load "set point" early in infection, but viral replication rate and target cell availability are likely to be important (222). The immunogenicity of the virus in a given host and the state of immune function of the host are also important to the control of HIV infection. Host genotype is an important factor that can influence the course of disease. For example, polymorphisms related to HIV coreceptors or their ligands (70, 248, 396) as well as human leukocyte antigen (HLA) gene polymorphisms have been linked to the rate of progression to AIDS (34, 156, 171, 178, 179, 232, 362).

Multiple viral factors may also affect the rate of HIV disease progression. Several studies have found an inverse relationship between rate of viral population diversification and disease progression (74, 75, 115, 226, 230, 343, 400, 401), while others have found a direct relationship (129, 244, 255), and one study found instances of both inverse and direct relationships (253). HIV strains with an SI phenotype on MT-2 cells (now referred to as X4 or R-/X4 for viruses with dual tropism that includes CXCR4) (15) have long been associated with an advanced disease state (5, 39, 101, 364). In most cases, slow-growing, NSI species (now referred to as R5 because of their use of the CCR5 coreceptor) replicate early in infection and persist throughout infection. In contrast, in 2–10% of cases, X4 viruses have been reported to appear early in infection (182, 369). It has long been suggested that X4 viruses play a causal role in the transition from asymptomatic HIV infection to AIDS (268, 281, 365-367). However, the possibility that X4 viruses are required for disease induction has been questioned, primarily because they have been found in only about 50% of people progressing to AIDS (22, 199, 330, 365). Recently, evidence suggests that X4 viruses appear in much more than 50% of progressors but that their abundant representation is only transient and they are often no longer detected by the time of onset of disease (342).

Genomic Recombination

Within an infected individual, HIV exists as a population, in which numerous molecular variants are present at any one time (207). Although it is known that error-prone reverse transcription of the RNA genome of HIV is a major factor in the generation of molecular diversity (295), it has also been suggested that the host environment selects for those variants that can escape immune inactivation (209) or are resistant to antiviral drugs (251). Recent results (163, 184, 263, 304, 311, 315, 419) suggest that a third factor—intrapatient recombination of HIV variants—may operate to increase the genetic diversity of the population in vivo. Indeed, intrapatient viral recombination has the potential to play a major role in the generation of viral genetic diversity, and this diversity has in turn been implicated in neutralization and CTL escape and in the development of antiviral drug resistance (53, 134, 210, 273, 274). Furthermore, recombinant strains make up a surprisingly high 10–20% of all sequences in the HIV Sequence Database (304, 305).

Several conditions are necessary for recombination to be observed within an infected individual (Fig. 2.5). Two viruses must infect a single cell, integrate their genomes into the host's genome, and produce separate RNA genomes that are packaged in the same virion (44). The new virus particle, containing the two different viral genomes, must then infect a new cell in which template switching may occur during reverse transcription of the viral RNA (130, 164, 355, 416). Finally, the new recombinant virus that is produced must be viable for the recombinant variant to spread.

Recombination between different viral subtypes has been observed, producing a genome that is a chimera of multiple subtypes. For this type of recombination to occur, the patient must be dually infected by viruses from two different subtypes in addition to the completion of the other steps required for recombination to take place. Most chimeras described to date have been generated between different sequence subtypes within the M group of HIV-1 (33, 59, 119, 217, 227, 246, 252, 276, 304, 305, 311, 316). Chimeras have also been demonstrated between M and O group strains of HIV-1 (360) and divergent strains of HIV-2 (120, 121). Although intersubtype chimeras have been more frequently documented, intrasubtype

Evolution by genomic chimerization (recombination)

- One person is infected from two sources.
- Two virions from different sources infect the same cell.
- Each virion goes through reverse transcription and integration and produces viral RNA.
- One of each RNA is packaged in a single virion.
- The hybrid virion infects a new cell, reverse transcription occurs, and RT switches between templates, creating a chimeric proviral genome.

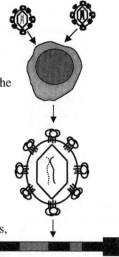

FIGURE 2.5

Evolution of HIV by genomic characterization

Schematic representation of the steps required to generate virus chimeras from previously independent strains of virus. Sequences derived from distinct viral genomes are indicated by black versus gray line shading.

dual infection and presumably recombination are considered to be even more common but more difficult to detect because the higher degree of conservation between the recombining strains tends to obscure these events. However, in regions of the world in which an AIDS epidemic has been established for multiple decades, it is now possible to detect intra-subtype recombinants in vivo (83, 176, 287) and in cell culture (184, 208, 263). The spread of virus chimeras is important in the current spread of HIV-1, accounting for recent outbreaks in Russia and China (225, 339, 410). Chimeras have also been demonstrated within *pol* that lead to enhanced resistance to antiretroviral drugs (184).

Dual infection with HIV has been infrequently documented, but the literature is growing, with examples of several of the possible combinations of infection known. These include early claims of dual infection with HIV-1 and HIV-2 (93, 125, 289, 297), as well as infection with different HIV-1 groups (361), different sequence subtypes from the HIV-1 M group (4, 168, 169), and divergent members of the same subtype (226, 314, 315, 419).

Although dual infections are taking place, the vaccine approach that aims to use live attenuated viruses relies on the assumption that establishment of infection with one strain will induce protection against a second superinfecting strain (63, 80, 247). Resistance to superinfection has also been demonstrated against homologous and heterologous challenges in other primates (383). Otten et al. (280) have recently defined a window of superinfection susceptibility (between four and eight weeks) in macaques infected with HIV-2 strains of comparable infectivity. However, the window of time for the development of superinfection resistance in the macaque model seems to be related to the degree of replication of the initially infecting strain, since resistance takes longer to develop with more attenuated primary infections (49). There are also reported instances of a lack of protection against dual infection during chronic infections, against heterologous HIV-1 infection of chimpanzees (110), and in FIV (277).

Resistance to retrovirus superinfection was initially described to explain a phenomenon that occurs at the level of virus entry within cells, whereby the viral Env protein prevents attachment and entry of additional virions that utilize the same receptor (321, 320), by complex formation and downregulation of available receptor protein from the cell surface. Indeed, a failure to establish superinfection resistance results in a cytopathic retrovirus infection (206, 298, 389, 390). In vitro studies have shown that superinfection resistance can also occur at the level of cellular susceptibility to infection as well as extracellular and intracellular blocking (206, 298) and that this resistance can be different in different people (331). The linkage between these mechanisms and protection of an organism against superinfection is unclear, however, and factors such as maturation of the immune response and the availability of susceptible target cells are likely to play a role in vivo.

HIV Compartmentalization

HIV nucleotide sequences can provide insight into fairly complex virological processes, and recently such analyses have been directed at the study of viral compartmentalization (293, 340). HIV is "compartmentalized" when subpopulations exist in different places within a single host and gene flow between them is restricted. Since the compartmental structure of HIV is likely to affect viral evolution and dynamics, it should affect pathology and treatment strategies alike. In the total absence of compartmentalization, viruses would be expected to flow freely in and out of potential tissue compartments, and an HIV sample obtained from any infected tissue should be a random sample of the entire population at that time. In a noteworthy sense, this assumption underlies every study in which HIV subpopulations are sampled and analyzed to characterize the larger HIV population within a host.

Several studies recognized intrahost compartmentalization when they observed striking dissimilarities among HIV sequences obtained from different tissue compartments. Those observations suggested that intrahost viral gene flow was restricted between blood and semen for HIV-1 subtype B (56, 73, 191), peripheral blood and the female genital tract (293, 337), blood and cerebrospinal fluid (190), brain and blood (201), brain and lymph node (147), brain, spleen, and lymph node (403), and within different regions of brain (340). Distinct variants have also been found in the blood and brain of an HIV-2 infected individual (319).

These studies suggest that compartmentalization plays a role in HIV dynamics. However, in most of the studies cited above, clear cases of compartmentalization are presented along with ambiguous cases, which may or may not lack population structure altogether. Numerous meaningful questions about HIV compartmental structure remain. To name just a few, it will be useful to discover which tissues are affected, how they are affected, and whether compartmentalization patterns correspond to certain pathological profiles, immune profiles, or therapy-response profiles. Last, compartmentalization may influence variant mixtures involved in transmission and thus affect vaccine design and efficacy (73).

ACKNOWLEDGMENTS

We thank Raj Shankarappa and Angelique van't Wout for their helpful comments in preparing this chapter. This work is supported by grants from the University of Washington Center for AIDS Research (CFAR) and by grants awarded from the National Institutes of Health (AI35539, AI47734, and AI32885).

NOTES

1. Retroviruses are pseudodiploid: there is only one copy from which protein expression is derived, but two copies are packaged, such that recombination can occur.

2. The preintegration complex consists of the viral proteins Vpr, IN, MA, CA, and NC and cellular proteins. Vpr is important to the translocation to the nucleus in resting cells.
3. Current potent drug therapies used to treat HIV-1 infections generally include a PR inhibitor combined with RT inhibitors.
4. In regions of Africa, sooty mangabeys and chimpanzees are both kept as pets and hunted for food, which may expose individuals to cross-species viral infections.

REFERENCES

1. Aiken, C., J. Konner, N. R. Landau, M. E. Lenburg, and D. Trono. 1994. Nef induces CD4 endocytosis: requirement for a critical dileucine motif in the membrane-proximal CD4 cytoplasmic domain. Cell 76:853–864.
2. Alkhatib, G., C. Combadiere, C. Broder, Y. Feng, P. E. Kennedy, P. M. Murphy, and E. A. Berger. 1996. CC CKR5: a RANTES, MIP-1a, MIP-1b receptor as a fusion cofactor for macrophage-tropic HIV-1. Science 272:1955–1958.
3. Anderson, S., D. C. Shugars, R. Swanstrom, and J. V. Garcia. 1993. Nef from primary isolates of human immunodeficiency virus type 1 suppresses surface CD4 expression in human and mouse T cells. J. Virol. 67:4923–4931.
4. Artenstein, A. W., T. C. VanCott, J. R. Mascola, J. K. Carr, P. A. Hegerich, J. Gaywee, B.-E. Sanders, M. L. Robb, D. E. Dayhoff, S. Thitivichianlert, S. Nitayaphan, J. G. McNeil, D. L. Birx, R. A. Michael, D. S. Burke, and F. E. McCutchan. 1995. Dual infection with human immunodeficiency virus type 1 of distinct envelope subtypes in humans. J. Infect. Dis. 171:805–810.
5. Asjo, B., L. Morfeldt-Manson, J. Albert, G. Biberfeld, A. Karlsson, K. Lidman, and E. M. Fenyo. 1986. Replicative capacity of human immunodeficiency virus from patients with varying severity of HIV infection. Lancet 2:660–662.
6. Baba, T. W., Y. S. Jeong, D. Pennick, R. Bronson, M. F. Greene, and R. M. Ruprecht. 1995. Pathogenicity of live, attenuated SIV after mucosal infection of neonatal macaques. Science 267:1820–1825.
7. Baba, T. W., V. Liska, A. H. Khimani, N. B. Ray, P. J. Dailey, D. Penninck, R. Bronson, M. F. Greene, H. M. McClure, L. N. Martin, and R. M. Ruprecht. 1999. Live attenuated, multiply deleted simian immunodeficiency virus causes AIDS in infant and adult macaques. Nature Med. 5:194–203.
8. Bachmann, M. H., E. L. Delwart, E. G. Shpaer, P. Lingenfelter, R. Singal, J. I. Mullins, and the WHO Network on HIV-Isolation and Characterization. 1994. Rapid genetic characterization of HIV-1 from four WHO-sponsored vaccine evaluation sites using a heteroduplex mobility assay. AIDS Res. Hum. Retroviruses 10:1343–1351.
9. Barillari, G., R. Gendelman, R. C. Gallo, and B. Ensoli. 1993. The Tat protein of human immunodeficiency virus type 1, a growth factor for AIDS Kaposi sarcoma and cytokine-activated vascular cells, induces adhesion of the same cell types by using integrin receptors recognizing the RGD amino acid sequence. Proc. Natl. Acad. Sci. USA 90:7941–7945.
10. Bartel, D., M. Zapp, M. Green, and J. Szostak. 1991. HIV-1 Rev regulation involves recognition of non-Watson-Crick base pairs in viral RNA. Cell 67:529–536.

11. Baur, A. S., G. Sass, B. Laffert, D. Willbold, C. Cheng-Mayer, and B. M. Peterlin. 1997. The N-terminus of Nef from HIV-1/SIV associates with a protein complex containing Lck and a serine kinase. Immunity 6:283–291.

12. Bengal, E., and Y. Aloni. 1991. Transcriptional elongation by purified RNA polymerase II is blocked at the trans-activation-responsive region of human immunodeficiency virus type 1 in vitro. J. Virol. 65:4910–4918.

13. Benichou, S., M. Bomsel, M. Bodeus, H. Durand, M. Doute, F. Letourneur, J. Camonis, and R. Benarous. 1994. Physical interaction of the HIV-1 Nef protein with beta-COP, a component of non-clathrin-coated vesicles essential for membrane traffic. J. Biol. Chem. 269:30073–30076.

14. Benson, R. E., A. Sanfridson, J. S. Ottinger, C. Doyle, and B. R. Cullen. 1993. Downregulation of cell-surface CD4 expression by simian immunodeficiency virus Nef prevents viral super infection. J. Exp. Med. 177:1561–1566.

15. Berger, E., R. Doms, E. Fenyo, B. Korber, D. Littman, J. Moore, Q. Sattentau, H. Schuitemaker, J. Sodroski, and R. Weiss. 1998. A new classification for HIV-1. Nature 391:240.

16. Bilodeau, P. S., J. K. Domsic, and C. M. Stoltzfus. 1999. Splicing regulatory elements within tat exon 2 of human immunodeficiency virus type 1 (HIV-1) are characteristic of group M but not group O HIV-1 strains. J. Virol. 73: 9764–9772.

17. Bonhoeffer, S., E. C. Holmes, and M. A. Nowak. 1995. Causes of HIV diversity. Nature 376:125.

18. Borman, A. M., C. Quillent, P. Charneau, C. Dauguet, and F. Clavel. 1995. Human immunodeficiency virus type 1 Vif-mutant particles from restrictive cells: role of Vif in correct particle assembly and infectivity. J. Virol. 69:2058–2067.

19. Bour, S., U. Schubert, K. Peden, and K. Strebel. 1996. The envelope glycoprotein of human immunodeficiency virus type 2 enhances viral particle release: a Vpu-like factor? J. Virol. 70:820–829.

20. Bour, S., U. Schubert, and K. Strebel. 1995. The human immunodeficiency virus type 1 Vpu protein specifically binds to the cytoplasmic domain of CD4: implications for the mechanism of degradation. J. Virol. 69:1510–1520.

21. Bour, S., and K. Strebel. 1996. The human immunodeficiency virus (HIV) type 2 envelope protein is a functional complement to HIV type 1 Vpu that enhances particle release of heterologous retroviruses. J. Virol. 70:8285–8300.

22. Broughton, A., J. D. Thrasher, and Z. Gard. 1988. Immunological evaluation of four arc welders exposed to fumes from ignited polyurethane (isocyanate) foam: antibodies and immune profiles. Am. J. Ind. Med. 13:463–472.

23. Brun-Vezinet, F., C. Boucher, C. Loveday, D. Descamps, V. Fauveau, J. Izopet, D. Jeffries, S. Kaye, C. Krzyanowski, A. Nunn, R. Schuurman, J. M. Seigneurin, C. Tamalet, R. Tedder, J. Weber, and G. J. Weverling. 1997. HIV-1 viral load, phenotype, and resistance in a subset of drug-naive participants from the Delta trial. The National Virology Groups. Delta Virology Working Group and Coordinating Committee. Lancet 350:983–990.

24. Bukrinsky, M. I., N. Sharova, M. P. Dempsey, T. L. Stanwick, A. G. Bukrinskaya, S. Haggerty, and M. Stevenson. 1992. Active nuclear import of human immunodeficiency virus type 1 preintegration complexes. Proc. Natl. Acad. Sci. USA 89:6580–6584.

25. Bushman, F. D., and R. Craigie. 1992. Integration of human immunodeficiency virus DNA: adduct interference analysis of required DNA sites. Proc. Natl. Acad. Sci. USA 89:3458–3462.

26. Cann, A. J., M. J. Churcher, M. Boyd, W. O'Brien, J. Q. Zhao, J. A. Zack, and I. S. Y. Chen. 1992. The region of the envelope gene of human immunodeficiency virus type 1 responsible for determination of cell tropism. J. Virol. 66:305–309.

27. Cao, Y., L. Qin, L. Zhang, J. Safrit, and D. D. Ho. 1995. Virologic and immunologic characterization of long-term survivors of HIV-1 infection. N. Engl. J. Med. 332:201–208.

28. Carmichael, A., X. Jin, P. Sissons, and L. Borysiewicz. 1993. Quantitative analysis of the human immunodeficiency virus type 1 (HIV-1)-specific cytotoxic T lymphocyte (CTL) response at different stages of HIV-1 infection: differential CTL responses to HIV-1 and Epstein-Barr virus in late disease. J. Exp. Med. 177:249–256.

29. Carpenter, C. C., M. A. Fischl, S. M. Hammer, M. S. Hirsch, D. M. Jacobsen, D. A. Katzenstein, J. S. Montaner, D. D. Richman, M. S. Saag, R. T. Schooley, M. A. Thompson, S. Vella, P. G. Yeni, and P. A. Volberding. 1996. Antiretroviral therapy for HIV infection in 1996. Recommendations of an international panel. International AIDS Society-USA. JAMA 276:146–154.

30. Carpenter, C. C., M. A. Fischl, S. M. Hammer, M. S. Hirsch, D. M. Jacobsen, D. A. Katzenstein, J. S. Montaner, D. D. Richman, M. S. Saag, R. T. Schooley, M. A. Thompson, S. Vella, P. G. Yeni, and P. A. Volberding. 1997. Antiretroviral therapy for HIV infection in 1997. Updated recommendations of the International AIDS Society-USA panel. JAMA 277:1962–1969.

31. Carr, J. K., B. T. Foley, T. Leitner, M. Salminen, B. Korber, and F. McCutchan. 1999. Reference sequences representing the principal genetic diversity of HIV-1 in the pandemic. http://hiv-web.lanl.gov/ALIGN_CURRENT/SUBTYPE-REF/subtype.html. Los Alamos National Laboratory (Web site), HIV Sequence Database.

32. Carr, J. K., M. O. Salminen, J. Albert, E. Sanders-Buell, D. Gotte, D. L. Birx, and F. E. McCutchan. 1998. Full genome sequences of human immunodeficiency virus type 1 subtypes G and A/G intersubtype recombinants. Virology 247:22–31.

33. Carr, J. K., M. O. Salminen, C. Koch, D. Gotte, A. W. Artenstein, P. A. Hegerich, D. St. Louis, D. S. Burke, and F. E. McCutchan. 1996. Full length sequence and mosaic structure of a HIV-1 isolate from Thailand. J. Virol. 70:5935–5943.

34. Carrington, M., G. W. Nelson, M. P. Martin, T. Kissner, D. Vlahov, J. J. Goedert, R. Kaslow, S. Buchbinder, K. Hoots, and S. J. O'Brien. 1999. HLA and HIV-1: heterozygote advantage and B*35-Cw*04 disadvantage. Science 283:1748–1752.

35. Chazal, N., B. Gay, C. Carriere, J. Tournier, and P. Boulanger. 1995. Human immunodeficiency virus type 1 MA deletion mutants expressed in baculovirus-infected cells: cis and trans effects on the Gag precursor assembly pathway. J. Virol. 69:365–375.

36. Chen, M., R. T. Elder, M. Yu, M. G. O'Gorman, L. Selig, R. Benarous, A. Yamamoto, and Y. Zhao. 1999. Mutational analysis of Vpr-induced G2 arrest, nuclear localization, and cell death in fission yeast. J. Virol. 73:3236–3245.

37. Chen, M.Y., F. Maldarelli, M. K. Karczewski, R. L. Willey, and K. Strebel. 1993. Human immunodeficiency virus type 1 Vpu protein induces degradation of CD4 in vitro: the cytoplasmic domain of CD4 contributes to Vpu sensitivity. J. Virol. 67:3877–3884.

38. Chen, Z., P. Telfier, A. Gettie, P. Reed, L. Zhang, D. D. Ho, and P. A. Marx. 1996. Genetic characterization of new West African simian immunodeficiency virus SIVsm: geographic clustering of household-derived SIV strains with human immunodeficiency virus type 2 subtypes and genetically diverse viruses from a single feral sooty mangabey troop. J. Virol. 70:3617–3627.

39. Cheng-Mayer, C., D. Seto, M. Tateno, and J. A. Levy. 1988. Biological features of HIV-1 that correlate with virulence in the host. Science 240:80–82.

40. Chesebro, B., K. Wehrly, J. Nishio, and S. Perryman. 1992. Macrophage-tropic human immunodeficiency virus isolates from different patients exhibit un-usual V3 envelope sequence homogeneity in comparison with T-cell-tropic isolates: definition of critical amino acids involved in cell tropism. J. Virol. 66:6547–6554.

41. Chiu, I.-M., A. Yaniv, J. E. Dahlberg, A. Gazit, S. F. Skuntz, S. R. Tronick, and S. A. Aaronson. 1985. Nucleotide sequence evidence for relationshiop of AIDS retrovirus to lentiviruses. Nature 317:366.

42. Clark, S. J., M. S. Saag, W. D. Decker, S. Campbell-Hill, J. L. Roberson, P. J. Veldkamp, J. C. Kappes, B. H. Hahn, and G. M. Shaw. 1991. High titers of cytopathic virus in plasma of patients with symptomatic primary HIV-1 infec-tion. N. Engl. J. Med. 324:954–960.

43. Cocchi, F., A. L. DeVico, A. Garzino-Demo, A. Cara, R. C. Gallo, and P. Lusso. 1996. The V3 domain of the HIV-1 gp120 envelope glycoprotein is critical for chemokine-mediated blockade of infection. Nature Med. 2:1244–1247.

44. Coffin, J. M. 1979. Structure, replication, and recombination of retrovirus genomes: some unifying hypotheses. J. Gen. Virol. 42:1–26.

45. Coffin, J. M. 1990. Retroviridae and their replication, p. 1437–1500. In B. N. Fields, D. M. Knipe, R. M. Chanock, M. S. Hirsch, J. L. Melnick, T. P. Monath, and B. Roizman (ed.), Fields virology, 2d ed., vol. 2. Raven Press, New York.

46. Coffin, J. M. 1995. HIV population dynamics in vivo: implications for genetic variation, pathogenesis and therapy. Science 267:483–489.

47. Cohen, E. A., G. Dehni, J. G. Sodroski, and W. A. Haseltine. 1990. Human im-munodeficiency virus vpr product is a virion-associated regulatory protein. J. Virol. 64:3097–3099.

48. Cohen, E. A., E. F. Terwilliger, Y. Jalinoos, J. Proulx, J. G. Sodroski, and W. A. Haseltine. 1990. Identification of HIV-1 vpr product and function. J. Acquired Immune Defic. Syndr. 3:11–18.

49. Cole, K. S., J. L. Rowles, B. A. Jagesrski, M. Murphey-Corb, T. Unangst, J. E. Clements, J. Robinson, M. S. Wyand, R. C. Desrosiers, and R. C. Montelaro. 1997. Evolution of envelope-specific antibody responses in monkeys experi-mentally infected or immunized with simian immunodeficiency virus and its association with the development of protective immunity. J. Virol. 71:5069–5079.

50. Collins, K. L., B. K. Chen, S. A. Kalams, B. D. Walker, and D. Baltimore. 1998. HIV-1 Nef protein protects infected primary cells against killing by cytotoxic T lymphocytes. Nature 391:397–401.

51. Condra, J. H., D. J. Holder, and W. A. Schief. 1996. Bi-directional inhibition of HIV-1 drug resistance selection by combination therapy with indinavir and reverse transcriptase inhibitors. Presented at the XIth International Conference on AIDS, Vancouver, B.C.

52. Condra, J. H., D. J. Holder, W. A. Schleif, O. M. Blahy, R. M. Danovich, L. J. Gabryelski, D. J. Graham, D. Laird, J. C. Quintero, A. Rhodes, H. L. Robbins, E. Roth, M. Shivaprakash, T. Yang, J. A. Chodakewitz, P. J. Deutsch, R. Y. Leavitt, F. E. Massari, J. W. Mellors, K. E. Squires, R. T. Steigbigel, H. Teppler, and E. A. Emini. 1996. Genetic correlates of in vivo viral resistance to indinavir, a human immunodeficiency virus type 1 protease inhibitor. J. Virol. 70:8270–8276.

53. Condra, J. H., W. A. Schleif, O. M. Blahy, L. J. Gabryelski, D. J. Graham, J. C. Quintero, A. Rhodes, H. L. Robbins, E. Roth, M. Shivaprakash, D. Titus, T. Tang, H. Teppler, K. E. Squires, P. J. Deutsch, and E. A. Emini. 1995. In vivo emergence of HIV-1 variants resistant to multiple protease inhibitors. Nature 374:569–571.

54. Connor, R. I., and D. D. Ho. 1994. Human immunodeficiency virus type 1 variants with increased replicative capacity develop during the asymptomatic stage before disease progression. J. Virol. 68:4400–4408.

55. Connor, R. I., H. Mohri, Y. Cao, and D. D. Ho. 1993. Increased viral burden and cytopathicity correlate temporally with CD4+ T-lymphocyte decline and clinical progression in human immunodeficiency virus type 1-infected individuals. J. Virol. 67:1772–1777.

56. Coombs, R. W., C. E. Speck, J. P. Hughes, W. Lee, R. Sampoleo, S. O. Ross, J. Dragavon, G. Peterson, T. M. Hooton, A. C. Collier, L. Corey, L. Koutsky, and J. N. Krieger. 1998. Association between culturable human immunodeficiency virus type 1 (HIV-1) in semen and HIV-1 RNA levels in semen and blood: evidence for compartmentalization of HIV-1 between semen and blood. J. Infect. Dis. 177:320–330.

57. Copeland, T. D., and S. Oroszlan. 1988. Genetic locus, primary structure, and chemical synthesis of human immunodeficiency virus protease. Gene Analysis Techniques 5:109–115.

58. Corden, J. L. 1990. Tails of RNA polymerase II. Trends Biochem. Sci. 15: 383–387.

59. Cornelissen, M., G. Kampinga, F. Zorgdrager, and J. Goudsmit. 1996. Human immunodeficiency virus type 1 subtypes defined by env show high frequency of recombinant gag genes. The UNAIDS Network for HIV Isolation and Characterization. J. Virol. 70:8209–8212.

60. Dalgleish, A. G., P. C. Beverley, P. R. Clapham, D. H. Crawford, M. F. Greaves, and R. A. Weiss. 1984. The CD4 (T4) antigen is an essential component of the receptor for the AIDS retrovirus. Nature 312:763–767.

61. Daly, T. J., K. S. Cook, T. E. Malone, and J. R. Rusche. 1989. Specific binding of HIV-1 recombinant Rev protein to the Rev-responsive element in vitro. Nature 342:714–716.

62. Damgaard, C. K., H. Dyhr-Mikkelsen, and J. Kjems. 1998. Mapping the RNA binding sites for human immunodeficiency virus type-1 gag and NC proteins within the complete HIV-1 and -2 untranslated leader regions. Nucleic Acids Res. 26:3667–3676.

63. Daniel, M. D., F. Kirchhoff, S. C. Czajak, P. K. Sehgal, and R. C. Desrosiers. 1992. Protective effects of a live attenuated SIV vaccine with a deletion in the nef gene. Science 258:1938–1941.

64. Daniel, R., R. A. Katz, and A. M. Skalka. 1999. A role for DNA-PK in retroviral DNA integration. Science 284:644–647.

65. D'Aquila, R. T., V. A. Johnson, S. L. Welles, A. J. Japour, D. R. Kuritzkes, V. DeGruttola, P. S. Reichelderfer, R. Coombs, W. C. S. Crumpacker, J. O. Kahn, AIDS Clinical Trials Group Protocol 116B/117 Team, and Virology Committee Resistance Working Group. 1995. Zidovudine resistance and HIV-1 disease progression during antiretroviral therapy. Ann. Intern. Med. 122: 401–408.

66. Darlix, J. L., C. Gabus, M. T. Nugeyre, F. Clavel, and F. Barre-Sinoussi. 1990. Cis elements and trans-acting factors involved in the RNA dimerization of the human immunodeficiency virus HIV-1. J. Mol. Biol. 216:689–699.

67. d'Arminio Monforte, A., L. Testa, F. Adorni, E. Chiesa, T. Bini, G. C. Moscatelli, C. Abeli, S. Rusconi, S. Sollima, C. Balotta, M. Musicco, M. Galli, and M. Moroni. 1998. Clinical outcome and predictive factors of failure of highly active antiretroviral therapy in antiretroviral-experienced patients in advanced stages of HIV-1 infection. AIDS 12:1631–1637.

68. Dayton, E. T., D. M. Powell, and A. I. Dayton. 1989. Functional analysis of CAR, the target sequence for the Rev protein of HIV-1. Science 246:1625–1629.

69. Deacon, N. J., A. Tsykin, A. Solomon, K. Smith, M. Ludford-Menting, D. J. Hooker, D. A. McPhee, A. L. Greenway, A. Ellett, C. Chatfield, J. S. Lawson, A. Cunningham, D. Dwyer, D. Dowton, and J. Mills. 1995. Genomic structure of an attenuated quasi species of HIV-1 from a blood transfusion donor and recipients. Science 270:988–991.

70. Dean, M., M. Carrington, C. Winkler, G. A. Huttley, M. W. Smith, R. Allikmets, J. J. Goedert, S. P. Buchbinder, E. Vittinghoff, E. Gomperts, S. Donfield, D. Vlahov, R. Kaslow, A. Saah, C. Rinaldo, R. Detels, and S. J. O'Brien. 1996. Genetic restriction of HIV-1 infection and progression to AIDS by a deletion allele of the CKR5 structural gene. Science 273:1856–1862.

71. Debouck, C., J. G. Gorniak, J. E. Strickler, T. D. Meek, B. W. Metcalf, and M. Rosenberg. 1987. Human immunodeficiency virus protease expressed in Escherichia coli exhibits autoprocessing and specific maturation of the gag precursor. Proc. Natl. Acad. Sci. USA 84:8903–8906.

72. Deeks, S. G. 2000. Virologic and immunologic evaluation of structured treatment interruptions (STI) in patients experiencing long-term virologic failure. Presented at the Seventh Conference on Retroviruses and Opportunistic Infections, San Francisco.

73. Delwart, E. L., J. I. Mullins, P. Gupta, G. H. Learn, Jr., M. Holodniy, D. Katzenstein, B. D. Walker, and M. K. Singh. 1998. Human immunodeficiency virus type 1 populations in blood and semen. J. Virol. 72:617–623.

74. Delwart, E. L., H. Pan, H. W. Sheppard, D. Wolpert, A. U. Neumann, B. Korber, and J. I. Mullins. 1997. Slower evolution of human immunodeficiency virus type 1 quasispecies during progression to AIDS. J. Virol. 71:7498–7508.

75. Delwart, E. L., H. W. Sheppard, B. D. Walker, J. Goudsmit, and J. I. Mullins. 1994. Human immunodeficiency virus type 1 evolution in vivo tracked by DNA heteroduplex mobility assays. J. Virol. 68:6672–6683.

76. Delwart, E. L., E. G. Shpaer, F. E. McCutchan, J. Louwagie, M. Grez, H. Rübsamen-Waigmann, and J. I. Mullins. 1993. Genetic relationships determined by a DNA heteroduplex mobility assay: analysis of HIV-1 *env* genes. Science 262:1257–1261.

77. Demeter, L. M., T. Nawaz, G. Morse, R. Dolin, A. Dexter, P. Gerondelis, and R. C. Reichman. 1995. Development of zidovudine resistance mutations in patients receiving prolonged didanosine monotherapy. J. Infect. Dis. 172: 1480–1485.

78. de Ronde, A., B. Klaver, W. Keulen, L. Smit, and J. Goudsmit. 1992. Natural HIV-1 NEF accelerates virus replication in primary human lymphocytes. Virology 188:391–395.

79. Derse, D., M. Carvalho, R. Carroll, and B. M. Peterlin. 1991. A minimal lentivirus Tat. J. Virol. 65:7012–7015.

80. Desrosiers, R. C. 1992. HIV with multiple gene deletions as a live attenuated vaccine for AIDS. AIDS Res. Hum. Retroviruses 8:411–421.

81. Desrosiers, R. C., J. D. Lifson, J. S. Gibbs, S. C. Czajak, A. Y. Howe, L. O. Arthur, and R. P. Johnson. 1998. Identification of highly attenuated mutants of simian immunodeficiency virus. J. Virol. 72:1431–1437.

82. Dewar, R. L., M. B. Vasudevachari, V. Natarajan, and N. P. Salzman. 1989. Biosynthesis and processing of human immunodeficiency virus type 1 envelope glycoproteins: effects of monensin on glycosylation and transport. J. Virol. 63:2452–2456.

83. Diaz, R. S., E. C. Sabino, A. Mayer, J. W. Mosley, and M. P. Busch. 1995. Dual human immunodeficiency virus type 1 infection and recombination in a dually exposed transfusion recipient. The Transfusion Safety Study Group. J. Virol. 69:3272–3281.

84. Di'Marzo-Veronese, F., T. D. Copeland, A. L. DeVico, R. Rahman, S. Oroszlan, R. C. Gallo, and M. G. Sarngadharan. 1986. Characterization of highly immunogenic p66/p51 as the reverse transcriptase of HTLV-III/LAV. Science 231:1289–1291.

85. Dingwall, C., I. Ernberg, M. J. Gait, S. M. Green, S. Heaphy, J. Karn, A. D. Lowe, M. Singh, and M. A. Skinner. 1990. HIV-1 tat protein stimulates transcription by binding to a U-rich bulge in the stem of the TAR RNA structure. EMBO J. 9:4145–4153.

86. Dorfman, T., A. Bukovsky, A. Ohagen, S. Hoglund, and H. G. Gottlinger. 1994. Functional domains of the capsid protein of human immunodeficiency virus type 1. J. Virol. 68:8180–8187.

87. Dorfman, T., J. Luban, S. P. Goff, W. A. Haseltine, and H. G. Gottlinger. 1993. Mapping of functionally important residues of a cysteine-histidine box in the human immunodeficiency virus type 1 nucleocapsid protein. J. Virol. 67:6159–6169.

88. Dragic, T., V. Litwin, G. P. Allaway, S. R. Martin, Y. Huang, K. A. Nagashima, C. Cayanan, P. J. Maddon, R. A. Koup, J. P. Moore, and W. A. Paxton. 1996. HIV-1 entry into CD4+ cells is mediated by the chemokine receptor CC-CKR-5. Nature 381:667–673.

89. Dyer, W. B., A. F. Geczy, S. J. Kent, L. B. McIntyre, S. A. Blasdall, J. C. Learmont, and J. S. Sullivan. 1997. Lymphoproliferative immune function in the Sydney Blood Bank Cohort, infected with natural nef/long terminal repeat

mutants, and in other long-term survivors of transfusion-acquired HIV-1 infection. AIDS 11:1565–1574.

90. Earl, P. L., R. W. Doms, and B. Moss. 1990. Oligomeric structure of the human immunodeficiency virus type 1 envelope glycoprotein. Proc. Natl. Acad. Sci. USA 87:648–652.

91. Emerman, M. 1996. HIV-1, Vpr and the cell cycle. Curr. Biol. 6:1096–1103.

92. Emerman, M., R. Vazeux, and K. Peden. 1989. The rev gene product of the human immunodeficiency virus affects envelope-specific RNA localization. Cell 57:1155–1165.

93. Evans, L. A., J. Moreau, K. Odehouri, D. Seto, G. Thomson-Honnebier, H. Legg, A. Barboza, C. Cheng-Mayer, and J. A. Levy. 1988. Simultaneous isolation of HIV-1 and HIV-2 from an AIDS patient. Lancet 2:1389–1391.

94. Fan, L., and K. Peden. 1992. Cell-free transmission of Vif mutants of HIV-1. Virology 190:19–29.

95. Fatkenheuer, G., A. Theisen, J. Rockstroh, T. Grabow, C. Wicke, K. Becker, U. Wieland, H. Pfister, M. Reiser, P. Hegener, C. Franzen, A. Schwenk, and B. Salzberger. 1997. Virological treatment failure of protease inhibitor therapy in an unselected cohort of HIV-infected patients. AIDS 11:F113–116.

96. Fauci, A. S. 1988. The human immunodeficiency virus: infectivity and mechanisms of pathogenesis. Science 239:617–622.

97. Felber, B. K., M. Hadzopoulou-Cladaras, C. Cladaras, T. Copeland, and G. N. Pavlakis. 1989. rev protein of human immunodeficiency virus type 1 affects the stability and transport of the viral mRNA. Proc. Natl. Acad. Sci. USA 86:1495–1499.

98. Feng, S. H., and E. C. Holland. 1988. HIV-1 tat trans-activation requires the loop sequence within tar. Nature 334:165–167.

99. Feng, Y., C. C. Broder, P. E. Kennedy, and E. A. Berger. 1996. HIV-1 entry cofactor: functional cDNA cloning of a seven-transmembrane, G protein-coupled receptor. Science 272:872–877.

100. Fenyö, E. M. 1994. Antigenic variation of primate lentiviruses in humans and experimentally infected macaques. Immunol. Rev. 140:131–146.

101. Fenyö, E. M., L. Morfeldt-Månson, F. Chiodi, B. Lind, A. Von Gegerfelt, J. Albert, E. Olausson, and B. Åsjö. 1988. Distinct replicative and cytopathic characteristics of human immunodeficiency virus isolates. J. Virol. 62:4414–4419.

102. Fischer, U., J. Huber, W. C. Boelens, I. W. Mattaj, and R. Luhrmann. 1995. The HIV-1 Rev activation domain is a nuclear export signal that accesses an export pathway used by specific cellular RNAs. Cell 82:475–483.

103. Fisher, A. G., B. Ensoli, L. Ivanoff, M. Chamberlain, S. Petteway, L. Ratner, R. C. Gallo, and F. Wong-Staal. 1987. The sor gene of HIV-1 is required for efficient virus transmission in vitro. Science 237:888–893.

104. Fornerod, M., M. Ohno, M. Yoshida, and I. W. Mattaj. 1997. CRM1 is an export receptor for leucine-rich nuclear export signals. Cell 90:1051–1060.

105. Fouchier, R. A., M. Brouwer, S. M. Broersen, and H. Schuitemaker. 1995. Simple determination of human immunodeficiency virus type 1 syncytium-inducing V3 genotype by PCR. J. Clin. Microbiol. 33:906–911.

106. Fouchier, R. A., J. H. Simon, A. B. Jaffe, and M. H. Malim. 1996. Human immunodeficiency virus type 1 Vif does not influence expression or virion incorporation of gag-, pol-, and env-encoded proteins. J. Virol. 70:8263–8269.

107. Fouchier, R. A. M., M. Groenink, N. A. Kootstra, M. Tersmette, H. G. Huisman, F. Miedema, and H. Schuitemaker. 1992. Phenotype-associated sequence variation in the third variable domain (V3) of the human immunodeficiency virus type 1 gp120 molecule. J. Virol. 66:3183–3187.

108. Freed, E. O., J. M. Orenstein, A. J. Buckler-White, and M. A. Martin. 1994. Single amino acid changes in the human immunodeficiency virus type 1 matrix protein block virus particle production. J. Virol. 68:5311–5320.

109. Fujita, K., S. Omura, and J. Silver. 1997. Rapid degradation of CD4 in cells expressing human immunodeficiency virus type 1 Env and Vpu is blocked by proteasome inhibitors. J. Gen. Virol. 78:619–625.

110. Fultz, P. N., A. Srinivasan, C. R. Greene, D. Butler, R. B. Swenson, and H. M. McClure. 1987. Superinfection of a chimpanzee with a second strain of human immunodeficiency virus. J. Virol. 61:4026–4029.

111. Gabuzda, D. H., K. Lawrence, E. Langhoff, E. Terwilliger, T. Dorfman, W. A. Haseltine, and J. Sodroski. 1992. Role of vif in replication of human immunodeficiency virus type 1 in CD4+ T lymphocytes. J. Virol. 66:6489–6495.

112. Gabuzda, D. H., H. Li, K. Lawrence, B. S. Vasir, K. Crawford, and E. Langhoff. 1994. Essential role of vif in establishing productive HIV-1 infection in peripheral blood T lymphocytes and monocyte/macrophages. J. Acquired Immune Defic. Syndr. 7:908–915.

113. Gallaher, W. R. 1987. Detection of a fusion peptide sequence in the transmembrane protein of human immunodeficiency virus. Cell 50:327–328.

114. Gallay, P., V. Stitt, C. Mundy, M. Oettinger, and D. Trono. 1996. Role of the karyopherin pathway in human immunodeficiency virus type 1 nuclear import. J. Virol. 70:1027–1032.

115. Ganeshan, S., R. E. Dickover, B. T. Korber, Y. J. Bryson, and S. M. Wolinsky. 1997. Human immunodeficiency virus type 1 genetic evolution in children with different rates of development of disease. J. Virol. 71:663–677.

116. Ganser, B. K., S. Li, V. Y. Klishko, J. T. Finch, and W. I. Sundquist. 1999. Assembly and analysis of conical models for the HIV-1 core. Science 283: 80–83.

117. Gao, F., E. Bailes, D. L. Robertson, Y. Chen, C. M. Rodenburg, S. F. Michael, L. B. Cummins, L. O. Arthur, M. Peeters, G. M. Shaw, P. M. Sharp, and B. H. Hahn. 1999. Origin of HIV-1 in the chimpanzee Pan troglodytes troglodytes. Nature 397:436–441.

118. Gao, F., D. L. Robertson, C. D. Carruthers, S. G. Morrison, B. Jian, Y. Chen, F. Barre-Sinoussi, M. Girard, A. Srinivasan, A. G. Abimiku, G. M. Shaw, P. M. Sharp, and B. H. Hahn. 1998. A comprehensive panel of near-full-length clones and reference sequences for non-subtype B isolates of human immunodeficiency virus type 1. J. Virol. 72:5680–5698.

119. Gao, F., D. L. Robertson, S. G. Morrison, H. Hui, S. Craig, J. Decker, P. N. Fultz, M. Girard, G. M. Shaw, B. H. Hahn, and P. M. Sharp. 1996. The heterosexual human immunodeficiency virus type 1 epidemic in Thailand is caused by an intersubtype (A/E) recombinant of African origin. J. Virol. 70:7013–7029.

120. Gao, F., L. Yue, D. L. Robertson, S. C. Hill, H. Hui, R. J. Biggar, A. E. Neequaye, T. M. Whelan, D. D. Ho, G. M. Shaw, et al. 1994. Genetic diversity of human immunodeficiency virus type 2: evidence for distinct sequence subtypes with differences in virus biology. J. Virol. 68:7433–7447.

121. Gao, F., L. Yue, A. T. White, P. G. Pappas, J. Barchue, A. P. Hanson, B. M. Greene, P. M. Sharp, G. M. Shaw, and B. H. Hahn. 1992. Human infection by genetically diverse SIVsm-related HIV-2 in West Africa. Nature 358:495–499.

122. Gao, Q., Z. Gu, M. A. Parniak, J. Cameron, N. Cammack, C. Boucher, and M. A. Wainberg. 1993. The same mutation that encodes low-level human immunodeficiency virus type 1 resistance to 2′,3′-dideoxyinosine and 2′,3′-dideoxycytidine confers high-level resistance to the (-) enantiomer of 2′,3′-dideoxy-3′-thiacytidine. Antimicrob. Agents Chemother. 37:1390–1392.

123. Garcia, J. V., J. Alfano, and A. D. Miller. 1993. The negative effect of human immunodeficiency virus type 1 Nef on cell surface CD4 expression is not species specific and requires the cytoplasmic domain of CD4. J. Virol. 67:1511–1516.

124. Garcia, J. V., and A. D. Miller. 1991. Serine phosphorylation-independent downregulation of cell-surface CD4 by nef. Nature 350:508–511.

125. George, J. R., C. Y. Ou, B. Parekh, K. Brattegaard, V. Brown, E. Boateng, and K. M. De Cock. 1992. Prevalence of HIV-1 and HIV-2 mixed infections in Cote d'Ivoire. Lancet 340:337–339.

126. Gibbs, J. S., D. A. Regier, and R. C. Desrosiers. 1994. Construction and in vitro properties of SIV mac mutants with deletions in "nonessential" genes. AIDS Res. Hum. Retroviruses 10:607–616.

127. Goh, W. C., M. E. Rogel, C. M. Kinsey, S. F. Michael, P. N. Fultz, M. A. Nowak, B. H. Hahn, and M. Emerman. 1998. HIV-1 Vpr increases viral expression by manipulation of the cell cycle: a mechanism for selection of Vpr in vivo. Nature Med. 4:65–71.

128. Goldsmith, M. A., M. T. Warmerdam, R. E. Atchison, M. D. Miller, and W. C. Greene. 1995. Dissociation of the CD4 downregulation and viral infectivity enhancement functions of human immunodeficiency virus type 1 Nef. J. Virol. 69:4112–4121.

129. Goodenow, M., T. Huet, W. Saurin, S. Kwok, J. Sninsky, and S. Wain-Hobson. 1989. HIV-1 isolates are rapidly evolving quasispecies: evidence for viral mixtures and preferred nucleotide substitutions. J. Acquired Immune Defic. Syndr. 2:344–352.

130. Goodrich, D. W., and P. H. Duesberg. 1990. Retroviral recombination during reverse transcription. Proc. Natl. Acad. Sci. USA 87:2052–2056.

131. Gorelick, R. J., T. D. Gagliardi, W. J. Bosche, T. A. Wiltrout, L. V. Coren, D. J. Chabot, J. D. Lifson, L. E. Henderson, and L. O. Arthur. 1999. Strict conservation of the retroviral nucleocapsid protein zinc finger is strongly influenced by its role in viral infection processes: characterization of HIV-1 particles containing mutant nucleocapsid zinc-coordinating sequences. Virology 256:92–104.

132. Göttlinger, H. G., T. Dorfman, E. A. Cohen, and W. A. Haseltine. 1993. Vpu protein of human immunodeficiency virus type 1 enhances the release of capsids produced by gag gene constructs of widely divergent retroviruses. Proc. Natl. Acad. Sci. USA 90:7381–7385.

133. Goudsmit, J. 2000. In vivo selection, fitness, and virulence of HIV-1 resistant to multiple nucleoside analogs. Presented at the Seventh Conference on Retroviruses and Opportunistic Infections, San Francisco.

134. Goulder, P. J. R., R. E. Phillips, R. A. Colbert, S. McAdam, G. Ogg, M. A. Nowak, P. Giangrande, G. Luzzi, B. Morgan, A. Edwards, A. J. McMichael,

and S. Rowland-Jones. 1997. Late escape from an immunodominant cytotoxic T-lymphocyte response associated with progression to AIDS. Nature Med. 3:212–217.

135. Graziosi, C., G. Pantaleo, L. Butini, J. F. Demarest, M. S. Saag, G. M. Shaw, and A. S. Fauci. 1993. Kinetics of human immunodeficiency virus type 1 (HIV-1) DNA and RNA synthesis during primary HIV-1 infection. Proc. Natl. Acad. Sci. USA 90:6405–6409.

136. Green, M. R. 1991. Biochemical mechanisms of constitutive and regulated pre-mRNA splicing. Annu. Rev. Cell Biol. 7:559–599.

137. Greenberg, M. E., S. Bronson, M. Lock, M. Neumann, G. N. Pavlakis, and J. Skowronski. 1997. Co-localization of HIV-1 Nef with the AP-2 adaptor protein complex correlates with Nef-induced CD4 down-regulation. EMBO J. 16:6964–6976.

138. Greenberg, M. E., A. J. Iafrate, and J. Skowronski. 1998. The SH3 domain-binding surface and an acidic motif in HIV-1 Nef regulate trafficking of class I MHC complexes. EMBO J. 17:2777–2789.

139. Greenough, T. C., J. L. Sullivan, and R. C. Desrosiers. 1999. Declining CD4 T-cell counts in a person infected with nef-deleted HIV-1. N. Engl. J. Med. 340:236–237.

140. Greenway, A., A. Azad, J. Mills, and D. McPhee. 1996. Human immunodeficiency virus type 1 Nef binds directly to Lck and mitogen-activated protein kinase, inhibiting kinase activity. J. Virol. 70:6701–6708.

141. Gruss, P., C. J. Lai, R. Dhar, and G. Khoury. 1979. Splicing as a requirement for biogenesis of functional 16S mRNA of simian virus 40. Proc. Natl. Acad. Sci. USA 76:4317–4321.

142. Gulick, R. M., J. W. Mellors, D. Havlir, J. J. Eron, C. Gonzalez, D. McMahon, L. Jonas, A. Meibohm, D. Holder, W. A. Schleif, J. H. Condra, E. A. Emini, R. Isaacs, J. A. Chodakewitz, and D. D. Richman. 1998. Simultaneous vs. sequential initiation of therapy with indinavir, zidovudine, and lamivudine for HIV-1 infection: 100-week follow-up. JAMA 280:35–41.

143. Gulick, R. M., J. W. Mellors, D. Havlir, J. J. Eron, C. Gonzalez, D. McMahon, D. D. Richman, F. T. Valentine, L. Jonas, A. Meibohm, E. A. Emini, and J. A. Chodakewitz. 1997. Treatment with indinavir, zidovudine, and lamivudine in adults with human immunodeficiency virus infection and prior antiretroviral therapy. N. Engl. J. Med. 337:734–739.

144. Gummuluru, S., and M. Emerman. 1999. Cell cycle- and Vpr-mediated regulation of human immunodeficiency virus type 1 expression in primary and transformed T-cell lines. J. Virol. 73:5422–5430.

145. Guy, B., M. P. Kieny, Y. Riviere, C. Le Peuch, K. Dott, M. Girard, L. Montagnier, and J. P. Lecocq. 1987. HIV F/3' orf encodes a phosphorylated GTP-binding protein resembling an oncogene product. Nature 330:266–269.

146. Haase, A. T. 1986. Pathogenesis of lentivirus infections. Nature 322:130–136.

147. Haggerty, S., and M. Stevenson. 1991. Predominance of distinct viral genotypes in brain and lymph node compartments of HIV-1-infected individuals. Viral Immunol. 4:123–131.

148. Hallenberger, S., V. Bosch, H. Angliker, E. Shaw, H. D. Klenk, and W. Garten. 1992. Inhibition of furin-mediated cleavage activation of HIV-1 glycoprotein gp160. Nature 360:358–361.

149. Hammarskjold, M. L., J. Heimer, B. Hammarskjold, I. Sangwan, L. Albert, and D. Rekosh. 1989. Regulation of human immunodeficiency virus env expression by the rev gene product. J. Virol. 63:1959–1966.

150. Hammer, S. M., K. E. Squires, M. D. Hughes, J. M. Grimes, L. M. Demeter, J. S. Currier, J. J. Eron, Jr., J. E. Feinberg, H. H. Balfour, Jr., L. R. Deyton, J. A. Chodakewitz, and M. A. Fischl. 1997. A controlled trial of two nucleoside analogues plus indinavir in persons with human immunodeficiency virus infection and CD4 cell counts of 200 per cubic millimeter or less. AIDS Clinical Trials Group 320 Study Team. N. Engl. J. Med. 337:725–733.

151. Harrer, T., E. Harrer, S. A. Kalams, T. Elbeik, S. I. Staprans, M. B. Feinberg, Y. Cao, D. D. Ho, T. Yilma, A. M. Caliendo, R. P. Johnson, S. P. Buchbinder, and B. D. Walker. 1996. Strong cytotoxic T cell and weak neutralizing antibody responses in a subset of persons with stable nonprogressing HIV type 1 infection. AIDS Res. Hum. Retroviruses 12:585–592.

152. Hauber, J., M. Bouvier, M. H. Malim, and B. R. Cullen. 1988. Phosphorylation of the rev gene product of human immunodeficiency virus type 1. J. Virol. 62:4801–4804.

153. He, J., S. Choe, R. Walker, P. Di Marzio, D. O. Morgan, and N. R. Landau. 1995. Human immunodeficiency virus type 1 viral protein R (Vpr) arrests cells in the G2 phase of the cell cycle by inhibiting p34cdc2 activity. J. Virol. 69:6705–6711.

154. Heaphy, S., C. Dingwall, I. Ernberg, M. J. Gait, S. M. Green, J. Karn, A. D. Lowe, M. Singh, and M. A. Skinner. 1990. HIV-1 regulator of virion expression (Rev) protein binds to an RNA stem-loop structure located within the Rev response element region. Cell 60:685–693.

155. Heinzinger, N. K., M. I. Bukinsky, S. A. Haggerty, A. M. Ragland, V. Kewalramani, M. A. Lee, H. E. Gendelman, L. Ratner, M. Stevenson, and M. Emerman. 1994. The Vpr protein of human immunodeficiency virus type 1 influences nuclear localization of viral nucleic acids in nondividing host cells. Proc. Natl. Acad. Sci. USA 91:7311–7315.

156. Hendel, H., S. Caillat-Zucman, H. Lebuanec, M. Carrington, S. O'Brien, J. M. Andrieu, F. Schachter, D. Zagury, J. Rappaport, C. Winkler, G. W. Nelson, and J. F. Zagury. 1999. New class I and II HLA alleles strongly associated with opposite patterns of progression to AIDS. J. Immunol. 162:6942–6946.

157. Herrmann, C. H., and A. P. Rice. 1995. Lentivirus Tat proteins specifically associate with a cellular protein kinase, TAK, that hyperphosphorylates the carboxyl-terminal domain of the large subunit of RNA polymerase II: candidate for a Tat cofactor. J. Virol. 69:1612–1620.

158. Ho, D. D., A. U. Neumann, A. S. Perelson, W. Chen, J. M. Leonard, and M. Markowitz. 1995. Rapid turnover of plasma virions and CD4 lymphocytes in HIV-1 infection. Nature 373:123–126.

159. Höglund, S., A. Öhagen, K. Lawrence, and D. Gabuzda. 1994. Role of vif during packing of the core of HIV-1. Virology 201:349–355.

160. Holland, S. M., N. Ahmad, R. K. Maitra, P. Wingfield, and S. Venkatesan. 1990. Human immunodeficiency virus rev protein recognizes a target sequence in rev-responsive element RNA within the context of RNA secondary structure. J. Virol. 64:5966–5975.

161. Holland, S. M., M. Chavez, S. Gerstberger, and S. Venkatesan. 1992. A specific sequence with a bulged guanosine residue(s) in a stem-bulge-stem structure of Rev-responsive element RNA is required for trans activation by human immunodeficiency virus type 1 Rev. J. Virol. 66:3699–3706.

162. Holmes, E. C., L. Q. Zhang, P. Simmonds, C. A. Ludlam, and A. J. Leigh Brown. 1992. Convergent and divergent sequence evolution in the surface envelope glycoprotein of HIV-1 within a single infected patient. Proc. Natl. Acad. Sci. USA 89:4835–4839.

163. Howell, R. M., J. E. Fitzgibbon, M. Noe, Z. Ren, D. Gocke, T. A. Schwartzer, and D. T. Dubin. 1991. In vivo sequence variation of the human immunodeficiency virus type 1 env gene: evidence for recombination among variants found in a single individual. AIDS Res. Hum. Retroviruses 7:869–876.

164. Hu, W. S., and H. M. Temin. 1990. Retroviral recombination and reverse transcription. Science 250:1227–1233.

165. Huang, Y., J. Mak, Q. Cao, Z. Li, M. A. Wainberg, and L. Kleiman. 1994. Incorporation of excess wild-type and mutant tRNA(3Lys) into human immunodeficiency virus type 1. J. Virol. 68:7676–7683.

166. Iversen, A. K., R. W. Shafer, K. Wehrly, M. A. Winters, J. I. Mullins, B. Chesebro, and T. C. Merigan. 1996. Multidrug-resistant human immunodeficiency virus type 1 strains resulting from combination antiretroviral therapy. J. Virol. 70:1086–1090.

167. Iversen, A. K. N., E. G. Shpaer, A. G. Rodrigo, M. S. Hirsch, B. D. Walker, H. W. Sheppard, T. C. Merigan, and J. I. Mullins. 1995. Persistence of attenuated Rev genes in an HIV-1 infected asymptomatic individual. J. Virol. 69: 5743–5753.

168. Janini, L. M., D. Pieniazek, J. M. Peralta, M. Schechter, A. Tanuri, A. C. Vicente, N. Dela Torre, N. J. Pieniazek, C. C. Luo, M. L. Kalish, G. Schochetman, and M. A. Rayfield. 1996. Identification of single and dual infections with distinct subtypes of human immunodeficiency virus type 1 by using restriction fragment length polymorphism analysis. Virus Genes 13:69–81.

169. Janini, L. M., A. Tanuri, M. Schechter, J. M. Peralta, A. C. Vicente, N. Dela Torre, N. J. Pieniazek, C. C. Luo, A. Ramos, V. Soriano, G. Schochetman, M. A. Rayfield, and D. Pieniazek. 1998. Horizontal and vertical transmission of human immunodeficiency virus type 1 dual infections caused by viruses of subtypes B and C. J. Infect. Dis. 177:227–231.

170. Janvier, B., F. Mallet, V. Cheynet, P. Dalbon, G. Vernet, J. M. Besnier, P. Choutet, A. Goudeau, B. Mandrand, and F. Barin. 1993. Prevalence and persistence of antibody titers to recombinant HIV-1 core and matrix proteins in HIV-1 infection. J. Acquired Immune Defic. Syndr. 6:898–903.

171. Jeffery, K. J., K. Usuku, S. E. Hall, W. Matsumoto, G. P. Taylor, J. Procter, M. Bunce, G. S. Ogg, K. I. Welsh, J. N. Weber, A. L. Lloyd, M. A. Nowak, M. Nagai, D. Kodama, S. Izumo, M. Osame, and C. R. Bangham. 1999. HLA alleles determine human T-lymphotropic virus-I (HTLV-I) proviral load and the risk of HTLV-I-associated myelopathy. Proc. Natl. Acad. Sci. USA 96:3848–3853.

172. Jowett, J. B., V. Planelles, B. Poon, N. P. Shah, M. L. Chen, and I. S. Chen. 1995. The human immunodeficiency virus type 1 vpr gene arrests infected T cells in the G2 + M phase of the cell cycle. J. Virol. 69:6304–6313.

173. Kalish, M. L., A. Baldwin, S. Raktham, C. Wasi, C. C. Luo, G. Schochetman, T. D. Mastro, N. Young, S. Vanichseni, H. Rubsamen-Waigmann, H. von Briesen, J. I. Mullins, E. Delwart, B. Herring, J. Esparza, W. L. Heyward, and S. Osmanov. 1995. The evolving molecular epidemiology of HIV-1 envelope subtypes in injecting drug users in Bangkok, Thailand: implications for HIV vaccine trials. AIDS 9:850–856.

174. Kalland, K. H., A. M. Szilvay, K. A. Brokstad, W. Saetrevik, and G. Haukenes. 1994. The human immunodeficiency virus type 1 Rev protein shuttles between the cytoplasm and nuclear compartments. Mol. Cell. Biol. 14:7436–7444.

175. Kalland, K. H., A. M. Szilvay, E. Langhoff, and G. Haukenes. 1994. Subcellular distribution of human immunodeficiency virus type 1 Rev and colocalization of Rev with RNA splicing factors in a speckled pattern in the nucleoplasm. J. Virol. 68:1475–1485.

176. Kampinga, G. A., A. Simonon, P. Van de Perre, E. Karita, P. Msellati, and J. Goudsmit. 1997. Primary infections with HIV-1 of women and their offspring in Rwanda: findings of heterogeneity at seroconversion, coinfection, and recombinants of HIV-1 subtypes A and C. Virology 227:63–76.

177. Kao, S. Y., A. F. Calman, P. A. Luciw, and B. M. Peterlin. 1987. Anti-termination of transcription within the long terminal repeat of HIV-1 by tat gene product. Nature 330:489–493.

178. Kaslow, R. A., M. Carrington, R. Apple, L. Park, A. Muñoz, A. J. Saah, J. J. Goedert, C. Winkler, S. J. O'Brien, C. Rinaldo, R. Detels, W. Blattner, J. Phair, H. Erlich, and D. L. Mann. 1996. Influence of combinations of human major histocompatibility complex genes on the course of HIV-1 infection. Nature Med. 2:405–411.

179. Kaslow, R. A., and J. M. McNicholl. 1999. Genetic determinants of HIV-1 infection and its manifestations. Proc. Assoc. Am. Physicians 111:299–307.

180. Kato, H., H. Sumimoto, P. Pognonec, C. H. Chen, C. A. Rosen, and R. G. Roeder. 1992. HIV-1 Tat acts as a processivity factor in vitro in conjunction with cellular elongation factors. Genes Dev. 6:655–666.

181. Kato, K., H. Sato, and Y. Takebe. 1999. Role of naturally occurring basic amino acid substitutions in the human immunodeficiency virus type 1 subtype E envelope V3 loop on viral coreceptor usage and cell tropism. J. Virol. 73:5520–5526.

182. Keet, I. P. M., P. Krijnen, M. Koot, J. M. A. Lange, F. Miedema, J. Goudsmit, and R. A. Coutinho. 1993. Predictors of rapid progression to AIDS in HIV-1 seroconverters. AIDS 7:51–57.

183. Kellam, P., C. A. Boucher, and B. A. Larder. 1992. Fifth mutation in human immunodeficiency virus type 1 reverse transcriptase contributes to the development of high-level resistance to zidovudine. Proc. Natl. Acad. Sci. USA 89:1934–1938.

184. Kellam, P., and B. A. Larder. 1995. Retroviral recombination can lead to linkage of reverse transcriptase mutations that confer increased zidovudine resistance. J. Virol. 69:669–674.

185. Kemp, S. D., C. Shi, S. Bloor, P. R. Harrigan, J. W. Mellors, and B. A. Larder. 1998. A novel polymorphism at codon 333 of human immunodeficiency virus

type 1 reverse transcriptase can facilitate dual resistance to zidovudine and L-2′,3′-dideoxy-3′-thiacytidine. J. Virol. 72:5093–5098.

186. Kempf, D. J., K. C. Marsh, J. F. Denissen, E. McDonald, S. Vasavanonda, C. A. Flentge, B. E. Green, L. Fino, C. H. Park, X. P. Kong, et al. 1995. ABT-538 is a potent inhibitor of human immunodeficiency virus protease and has high oral bioavailability in humans. Proc. Natl. Acad. Sci. USA 92:2484–2488.

187. Kessler, M., and M. B. Mathews. 1991. Tat transactivation of the human immunodeficiency virus type 1 promoter is influenced by basal promoter activity and the simian virus 40 origin of DNA replication. Proc. Natl. Acad. Sci. USA 88:10018–10022.

188. Kessler, M., and M. B. Mathews. 1992. Premature termination and processing of human immunodeficiency virus type 1-promoted transcripts. J. Virol. 66:4488–4496.

189. Kestler, H. W. I., D. J. Ringler, K. Mori, D. P. Panicali, P. K. Sehgal, M. D. Daniel, and R. C. Desrosiers. 1991. Importance of the nef gene for maintenance of high virus loads and for the development of AIDS. Cell 65:651–662.

190. Keys, B., J. Karis, B. Fadeel, A. Valentin, G. Norkrans, L. Hagberg, and F. Chiodi. 1993. V3 sequences of paired HIV-1 isolates from blood and cerebrospinal fluid cluster according to host and show variation related to the clinical stage of disease. Virology 196:475–483.

191. Kiessling, A. A., L. M. Fitzgerald, D. Zhang, H. Chhay, D. Brettler, R. C. Eyre, J. Steinberg, K. McGowan, and R. A. Byrn. 1998. Human immunodeficiency virus in semen arises from a genetically distinct virus reservoir. AIDS Res. Hum. Retroviruses 14(Suppl. 1):S33–41.

192. Kim, J. B., Y. Yamaguchi, T. Wada, H. Handa, and P. A. Sharp. 1999. Tat-SF1 protein associates with RAP30 and human SPT5 proteins. Mol. Cell. Biol. 19:5960–5968.

193. Kirchhoff, F., T. C. Greenough, D. B. Brettler, J. L. Sullivan, and R. C. Desrosiers. 1995. Absence of intact nef sequences in a long-term survivor with nonprogressive HIV-1 infection. N. Engl. J. Med. 332:228–232.

194. Kjems, J., A. D. Frankel, and P. A. Sharp. 1991. Specific regulation of mRNA splicing in vitro by a peptide from HIV-1 Rev. Cell 67:169–178.

195. Kjems, J., and P. A. Sharp. 1993. The basic domain of Rev from human immunodeficiency virus type 1 specifically blocks the entry of U4/U6.U5 small nuclear ribonucleoprotein in spliceosome assembly. J. Virol. 67:4769–4776.

196. Klimkait, T., K. Strebel, M. D. Hoggan, M. A. Martin, and J. M. Orenstein. 1990. The human immunodeficiency virus type 1-specific protein vpu is required for efficient virus maturation and release. J. Virol. 64:621–629.

197. Kohl, N. E. E., E. A. Schleif, W. A. Davis, L. J. Heimbach, J. C. Dixon, R. A. F. Scolnick, E. M. Sigal. 1988. Active human immunodeficiency virus protease is required for viral infectivity. Proc. Natl. Acad. Sci. USA 85:4686–4690.

198. Koito, A., G. Harrowe, J. A. Levy, and C. Cheng-Mayer. 1994. Functional role of the V1/V2 region of human immunodeficiency virus type 1 envelope glycoprotein gp120 in infection of primary macrophages and soluble CD4 neutralization. J. Virol. 68:2253–2259.

199. Koot, M., I. Keet, A. Vos, R. deGoede, M. Roos, R. Coutinho, F. Miedema, P. Schellekens, and M. Tersmette. 1993. Prognostic value of HIV-1 syncytium-

inducing phenotype for rate of CD4+ cell depletion and progression to AIDS. Ann. Intern. Med. 118:681–688.

200. Korber, B. T. M., C. Brander, B. D. Walker, R. Koup, J. P. Moore, B. F. Haynes, and G. Myers (ed.). 1999. HIV molecular immunology database. http://hiv-web.lanl.gov/immuno/ctl.

201. Korber, B. T. M., K. J. Kunstman, B. K. Patterson, M. Furtado, M. M. McEvilly, R. Levy, and S. M. Wolinsky. 1994. Genetic differences between blood- and brain-derived viral sequences from HIV-1-infected patients: evidence of conserved elements in the V3 region of the envelope protein of brain-derived sequences. J. Virol. 68:7467–7481.

202. Kostrikis, L. G., E. Bagdades, Y. Cao, L. Zhang, D. Dimitriou, and D. D. Ho. 1995. Genetic analysis of human immunodeficiency virus type 1 strains from patients in Cyprus: identification of a new subtype designated subtype I. J. Virol. 69:6122–6130.

203. Kotov, A., J. Zhou, P. Flicker, and C. Aiken. 1999. Association of Nef with the human immunodeficiency virus type 1 core. J. Virol. 73:8824–8830.

204. Kowalski, M., J. Potz, L. Basiripour, T. Dorfman, W. C. Goh, E. Terwilliger, A. Dayton, C. Rosen, W. Haseltine, and J. Sodroski. 1987. Functional regions of the envelope glycoprotein of human immunodeficiency virus type 1. Science 4820:1351–1355.

205. Kozal, M. J., R. W. Shafer, M. A. Winters, D. A. Katzenstein, E. Aguiniga, J. Halpern, and T. C. Merigan. 1994. HIV-1 syncytium-inducing phenotype, virus burden, codon 215 reverse transcriptase mutation and CD4 cell decline in zidovudine-treated patients. J. Acquired Immune Defic. Syndr. 7:832–838.

206. Kristal, B. S., T. A. Reinhart, E. A. Hoover, and J. I. Mullins. 1993. Interference with superinfection and with cell killing and determination of host range and growth kinetics mediated by feline leukemia virus surface glycoproteins. J. Virol. 67:4142–4153.

207. Kuiken, C. L., K. Nieselt-Struwe, G. F. Weiller, and J. Goudsmit. 1994. Quasispecies behavior of HIV-1: a sample analysis of sequence data. Methods in Molecular Genetics 4:not listed.

208. Kuwata, T., Y. Miyazaki, T. Igarashi, J. Takehisa, and M. Hayami. 1997. The rapid spread of recombinants during a natural in vitro infection with two human immunodeficiency virus type 1 strains. J. Virol. 71:7088–7091.

209. Lamers, S., J. W. Sleasman, J. X. She, K. A. Barrie, S. M. Pomeroy, D. J. Barrett, and M. M. Goodenow. 1993. Independent variation and positive selection in env V1-V2 domains within maternal-infant strains of human immunodeficiency virus type-1 in vivo. J. Virol. 67:3951–3960.

210. Larder, B. A., G. Darby, and D. D. Richman. 1989. HIV with reduced sensitivity to zidovudine (AZT) isolated during prolonged therapy. Science 243:1731–1734.

211. Larder, B. A., and S. D. Kemp. 1989. Multiple mutations in HIV-1 reverse transcriptase confer high-level resistance to zidovudine (AZT). Science 246:1155–1158.

212. Laspia, M. F., A. P. Rice, and M. B. Mathews. 1989. HIV-1 Tat protein increases transcriptional initiation and stabilizes elongation. Cell 59:283–292.

213. Learmont, J., B. Tindall, L. Evans, A. Cunningham, P. Cunningham, J. Wells, R. Penny, J. Kaldor, and D. A. Cooper. 1992. Long-term symptomless HIV-1

infection in recipients of blood products from a single donor. Lancet 340:863–867.

214. Learmont, J. C., A. F. Geczy, J. Mills, L. J. Ashton, C. H. Raynes-Greenow, R. J. Garsia, W. B. Dyer, L. McIntyre, R. B. Oelrichs, D. I. Rhodes, N. J. Deacon, and J. S. Sullivan. 1999. Immunologic and virologic status after 14 to 18 years of infection with an attenuated strain of HIV-1. A report from the Sydney Blood Bank Cohort. N. Engl. J. Med. 340:1715–1722.

215. Le Gall, S., L. Erdtmann, S. Benichou, C. Berlioz-Torrent, L. Liu, R. Benarous, J. M. Heard, and O. Schwartz. 1998. Nef interacts with the mu subunit of clathrin adaptor complexes and reveals a cryptic sorting signal in MHC I molecules. Immunity 8:483–495.

216. Leigh Brown, A. J. 1997. Analysis of HIV-1 env gene sequences reveals evidence for a low effective number in the viral population. Proc. Natl. Acad. Sci. USA 94:1862–1865.

217. Leitner, T., D. Escanilla, S. Marquina, J. Wahlberg, C. Brostrom, H. B. Hansson, M. Uhlen, and J. Albert. 1995. Biological and molecular characterization of subtype D, G, and A/D recombinant HIV-1 transmissions in Sweden. Virology 209:136–146.

218. Lenburg, M. E., and N. R. Landau. 1993. Vpu-induced degradation of CD4: requirement for specific amino acid residues in the cytoplasmic domain of CD4. J. Virol. 67:7238–7245.

219. Levy, D. N., L. S. Fernandes, W. V. Williams, and D. B. Weiner. 1993. Induction of cell differentiation by human immunodeficiency virus 1 vpr. Cell 72:541–550.

220. Levy, D. N., Y. Refaeli, and D. B. Weiner. 1995. Extracellular Vpr protein increases cellular permissiveness to human immunodeficiency virus replication and reactivates virus from latency. J. Virol. 69:1243–1252.

221. Levy, J. A. 1993. Pathogenesis of human immunodeficiency virus infection. Microbiol. Rev. 57:183–289.

222. Levy, J. A., B. Ramachandran, E. Barker, J. Guthrie, T. Elbeik, and J. M. Coffin. 1996. Plasma viral load, CD4+ cell counts, and HIV-1 production by cells. Science 271:670–671.

223. Li, G., M. Simm, M. J. Potash, and D. J. Volsky. 1993. Human immunodeficiency virus type 1 DNA synthesis, integration, and efficient viral replication in growth-arrested T cells. J. Virol. 67:3969–3977.

224. Liang, C., L. Rong, Y. Quan, M. Laughrea, L. Kleiman, and M. A. Wainberg. 1999. Mutations within four distinct gag proteins are required to restore replication of human immunodeficiency virus type 1 after deletion mutagenesis within the dimerization initiation site. J. Virol. 73:7014–7020.

225. Liitsola, K., I. Tashkinova, T. Laukkanen, G. Korovina, T. Smolskaja, O. Momot, N. Mashkilleyson, S. Chaplinskas, H. Brummer-Korvenkontio, J. Vanhatalo, P. Leinikki, and M. O. Salminen. 1998. HIV-1 genetic subtype A/B recombinant strain causing an explosive epidemic in injecting drug users in Kaliningrad. AIDS 12:1907–1919.

226. Liu, S. L., T. Schacker, L. Musey, D. Shriner, M. J. McElrath, L. Corey, and J. I. Mullins. 1997. Divergent patterns of progression to AIDS after infection from the same source: human immunodeficiency virus type 1 evolution and antiviral responses. J. Virol. 71:4284–4295.

227. Lole, K. S., R. C. Bollinger, R. S. Paranjape, D. Gadkari, S. S. Kulkarni, N. G. Novak, R. Ingersoll, H. W. Sheppard, and S. C. Ray. 1999. Full-length human immunodeficiency virus type 1 genomes from subtype C-infected sero-converters in India, with evidence of intersubtype recombination. J. Virol. 73: 152–160.

228. Long, E. M., H. L. Martin, Jr., J. K. Kreiss, S. M. Rainwater, L. Lavreys, D. J. Jackson, J. Rakwar, K. Mandaliya, and J. Overbaugh. 2000. Gender differences in HIV-1 diversity at time of infection. Nature Med. 6:71–75.

229. Louwagie, J., F. E. McCutchan, M. Peeters, T. P. Brennan, E. Sanders-Buell, G. A. Eddy, G. van der Groen, K. Fransen, G.-M. Gershy-Damet, R. Deleys, and D. S. Burke. 1993. Phylogenetic analysis of gag genes from seventy international HIV-1 isolates provides evidence for multiple genotypes. AIDS 7: 769–780.

230. Lukashov, V. V., C. L. Kuiken, and J. Goudsmit. 1995. Intrahost human immunodeficiency virus type 1 evolution is related to length of the immunocompetent period. J. Virol. 69:6911–6916.

231. Madani, N., and D. Kabat. 1998. An endogenous inhibitor of human immunodeficiency virus in human lymphocytes is overcome by the viral Vif protein. J. Virol. 72:10251–10255.

232. Magierowska, M., I. Theodorou, P. Debre, F. Sanson, B. Autran, Y. Riviere, D. Charron, and D. Costagliola. 1999. Combined genotypes of CCR5, CCR2, SDF1, and HLA genes can predict the long-term nonprogressor status in human immunodeficiency virus-1-infected individuals. Blood 93:936–941.

233. Malim, M. H., J. Hauber, S. Y. Le, J. V. Maizel, and B. R. Cullen. 1989. The HIV-1 rev trans-activator acts through a structured target sequence to activate nuclear export of unspliced viral mRNA. Nature 338:254–257.

234. Malim, M. H., L. S. Tiley, D. F. McCarn, J. R. Rusche, J. Hauber, and B. R. Cullen. 1990. HIV-1 structural gene expression requires binding of the Rev trans-activator to its RNA target sequence. Cell 60:675–683.

235. Mammano, F., A. Ohagen, S. Hoglund, and H. G. Gottlinger. 1994. Role of the major homology region of human immunodeficiency virus type 1 in virion morphogenesis. J. Virol. 68:4927–4936.

236. Mangasarian, A., M. Foti, C. Aiken, D. Chin, J. L. Carpentier, and D. Trono. 1997. The HIV-1 Nef protein acts as a connector with sorting pathways in the Golgi and at the plasma membrane. Immunity 6:67–77.

237. Mangasarian, A., V. Piguet, J. K. Wang, Y. L. Chen, and D. Trono. 1999. Nef-induced CD4 and major histocompatibility complex class I (MHC-I) down-regulation are governed by distinct determinants: N-terminal alpha helix and proline repeat of Nef selectively regulate MHC-I trafficking. J. Virol. 73: 1964–1973.

238. Mansky, L. M. 1996. Forward mutation rate of human immunodeficiency virus type 1 in a T lymphoid cell line. AIDS Res. Hum. Retroviruses 12:307–314.

239. Mansky, L. M., and H. M. Temin. 1995. Lower in vivo mutation rate of human immunodeficiency virus type 1 than that predicted from the fidelity of purified reverse transcriptase. J. Virol. 69:5087–5094.

240. Marciniak, R. A., and P. A. Sharp. 1991. HIV-1 Tat protein promotes formation of more-processive elongation complexes. EMBO J. 10:4189–4196.

241. Margolick, J. B., A. Muñoz, A. D. Donnenberg, L. P. Park, N. Galai, J. V. Giorgi, R. G. O'Gorman, and J. Ferbas, for the Multicenter AIDS Cohort Study. 1995. Failure of T-cell homeostasis preceding AIDS in HIV-1 infection. Nature Med. 1:674–680.

242. Margottin, F., S. P. Bour, H. Durand, L. Selig, S. Benichou, V. Richard, D. Thomas, K. Strebel, and R. Benarous. 1998. A novel human WD protein, h-beta TrCp, that interacts with HIV-1 Vpu connects CD4 to the ER degradation pathway through an F-box motif. Mol. Cell 1:565–574.

243. Mariani, R., F. Kirchhoff, T. C. Greenough, J. L. Sullivan, R. C. Desrosiers, and J. Skowronski. 1996. High frequency of defective nef alleles in a long-term survivor with nonprogressive human immunodeficiency virus type 1 infection. J. Virol. 70:7752–7764.

244. Markham, R. B., W. C. Wang, A. E. Weisstein, Z. Wang, A. Munoz, A. Templeton, J. Margolick, D. Vlahov, T. Quinn, H. Farzadegan, and X. F. Yu. 1998. Patterns of HIV-1 evolution in individuals with differing rates of CD4 T cell decline. Proc. Natl. Acad. Sci. USA 95:12568–12573.

245. Markowitz, M., M. Saag, W. G. Powderly, A. M. Hurley, A. Hsu, J. M. Valdes, D. Henry, F. Sattler, A. La Marca, J. M. Leonard, et al. 1995. A preliminary study of ritonavir, an inhibitor of HIV-1 protease, to treat HIV-1 infection. N. Engl. J. Med. 333:1534–1539.

246. Marquina, S., T. Leitner, R. D. Rabinovich, J. Benetucci, O. Libonatti, and J. Albert. 1996. Coexistence of subtypes B, F, and a B/F env recombinant of HIV-1 in Buenos Aires, Argentina. AIDS Res. Hum. Retroviruses 12:1651–1654.

247. Marthas, M. L., S. Sujipto, J. Higgins, B. Lohman, J. Torten, P. A. Luciw, P. A. Marx, and N. C. Pederson. 1990. Immunization with a live, attenuated simian immunodeficiency virus (SIV) prevents early disease but not infection in rhesus macaques challenged with pathogenic SIV. J. Virol. 64:3694–3700.

248. Martin, M. P., M. Dean, M. W. Smith, C. Winkler, B. Gerrard, N. L. Michael, B. Lee, R. W. Doms, J. Margolick, S. Buchbinder, J. J. Goedert, T. R. O'Brien, M. W. Hilgartner, D. Vlahov, S. J. O'Brien, and M. Carrington. 1998. Genetic acceleration of AIDS progression by a promoter variant of CCR5. Science 282:1907–1911.

249. Martin, S. J., A. J. McGahon, W. K. Nishioka, D. LaFace, X. Guo, J. Th'ng, E. M. Bradbury, and D. R. Green. 1995. p34cdc2 and apoptosis. Science 269:106–107.

250. Matthews, T. J., C. Wild, C. H. Chen, D. P. Bolognesi, and M. L. Greenberg. 1994. Structural rearrangements in the transmembrane glycoprotein after receptor binding. Immunol. Rev. 140:93–104.

251. Mayers, D. L., F. E. McCutchan, E. E. Sanders-Buell, L. I. Merritt, S. Dilworth, A. K. Fowler, C. A. Marks, N. M. Ruiz, D. D. Richman, and C. R. Roberts. 1992. Characterization of HIV isolates arising after prolonged zidovudine therapy. J. Acquired Immune Defic. Syndr. 5:749–759.

252. McCutchan, F. E., J. K. Carr, M. Bajani, E. Sanders-Buell, T. O. Harry, T. C. Stoeckli, K. E. Robbins, W. Gashau, A. Nasidi, W. Janssens, and M. L. Kalish. 1999. Subtype G and multiple forms of A/G intersubtype recombinant human immunodeficiency virus type 1 in Nigeria. Virology 254:226–234.

253. McDonald, R. A., D. L. Mayers, R. C.-Y. Chung, K. F. Wagner, S. Ratto-Kim, D. L. Birx, and N. L. Michael. 1997. Evolution of human immunodeficiency

virus type 1 *env* sequence variation in patients with diverse rates of disease progression and T-cell function. J. Virol. 71:1871–1879.

254. McDougal, J. S., M. S. Kennedy, J. K. A. Nicholson, T. J. Spira, H. W. Jaffe, J. E. Kaplan, D. B. Fishbein, P. O'Malley, C. H. Aloisio, C. M. Black, M. Hubbard, and C. B. Reimer. 1987. Antibody response to human immunodeficiency virus in homosexual men. Relation of antibody specificity, titer, and isotype to clinical status, severity of immunodeficiency, and disease progression. J. Clin. Invest. 80:316–324.

255. McNearney, T., Z. Hornickova, R. Markham, A. Birdwell, M. Arens, A. Saah, and L. Ratner. 1992. Relationship of human immunodeficiency virus type 1 sequence heterogeneity to stage of disease. Proc. Natl. Acad. Sci. USA 89: 10247–10251.

256. Meggio, F., D. M. D'Agostino, V. Ciminale, L. Chieco-Bianchi, and L. A. Pinna. 1996. Phosphorylation of HIV-1 Rev protein: implication of protein kinase CK2 and pro-directed kinases. Biochem. Biophys. Res. Commun. 226:547–554.

257. Mellors, J. W., A. Muñoz, J. V. Giorgi, J. B. Margolick, C. J. Tassoni, P. Gupta, L. A. Kingsley, J. A. Todd, A. J. Saah, R. Detels, J. P. Phair, and C. R. Rinaldo, Jr. 1997. Plasma viral load and CD4+ lymphocytes as prognostic markers of HIV-1 infection. Ann. Intern. Med. 126:946–954.

258. Meyer, B. E., and M. H. Malim. 1994. The HIV-1 Rev trans-activator shuttles between the nucleus and the cytoplasm. Genes Dev. 8:1538–1547.

259. Michael, N. L., G. Chang, L. A. d'Arcy, P. K. Ehrenberg, R. Mariani, M. P. Busch, D. L. Birx, and D. H. Schwartz. 1995. Defective accessory genes in a human immunodeficiency virus type 1-infected long-term survivor lacking recoverable virus. J. Virol. 69:4228–4236.

260. Miller, M., J. Schneider, B. K. Sathyanarayana, M. V. Toth, G. R. Marshall, L. Clawson, L. Selk, S. B. Kent, and A. Wlodawer. 1989. Structure of complex of synthetic HIV-1 protease with a substrate-based inhibitor at 2.3 Å resolution. Science 246:1149–1152.

261. Miller, M. D., M. T. Warmerdam, K. A. Page, M. B. Feinberg, and W. C. Greene. 1995. Expression of the human immunodeficiency virus type 1 (HIV-1) nef gene during HIV-1 production increases progeny particle infectivity independently of gp160 or viral entry. J. Virol. 69:579–584.

262. Morikawa, Y., E. Barsov, and I. Jones. 1993. Legitimate and illegitimate cleavage of human immunodeficiency virus glycoproteins by furin. J. Virol. 67: 3601–3604.

263. Moutouh, L., J. Corbeil, and D. D. Richman. 1996. Recombination leads to the rapid emergence of HIV-1 dually resistant mutants under selective drug pressure. Proc. Natl. Acad. Sci. USA 93:6106–6111.

264. Mullins, J. I. 1988. Molecular aspects of the FeLV and SIV AIDS models, p. 43–49. *In* M. Girard and L. Valette (ed.), Retroviruses of human AIDS and related animal diseases, vol. 3. Pasteur Vaccins, Paris.

265. Mullins, J. I. 1994. Virologic determinants of the progression to AIDS: are Lilliputians to blame?, p. 77–81. Neuvieme Colloque Des Cent Gardes, Paris.

266. Mullins, J. I., and L. M. Frenkel. Unpublished data.

267. Mullins, J. I., E. A. Hoover, M. L. Poss, S. L. Quackenbush, P. N. Fultz, P. A. Donahue, T. A. Reinhart, and S. Dewhurst. 1990. Genetic and biochemical

mechanisms of disease induction in animal models for AIDS, p. 57–60. Cinquieme Colloque Des Cent Gardes, Paris.

268. Mullins, J. I., E. A. Hoover, S. L. Quackenbush, and P. R. Donahue. 1991. Disease progression and viral genome variants in experimental feline leukemia virus-induced immunodeficiency syndrome. J. Acquired Immune Defic. Syndr. 4:547–557. (Erratum, 4(9):925.)

269. Myers, G. 1994. Tenth anniversary perspectives on AIDS: HIV: between past and future. AIDS Res. Hum. Retroviruses 10:1317–1325.

270. Neville, M., F. Stutz, L. Lee, L. I. Davis, and M. Rosbash. 1997. The importin-beta family member Crm1p bridges the interaction between Rev and the nuclear pore complex during nuclear export. Curr. Biol. 7:767–775.

271. Nielsen, C., L. Bruun, L. R. Mathiesen, C. Pedersen, and J. Gerstoft. 1996. Development of resistance to zidovudine (ZDV) and didanosine (ddI) in HIV from patients in ZDV, ddI, and alternating ZDV/ddI therapy. AIDS 10:625–633.

272. Nielsen, R., and Z. Yang. 1998. Likelihood models for detecting positively selected amino acid sites and applications to the HIV-1 envelope gene. Genetics 148:929–936.

273. Nowak, M. A., R. M. Anderson, A. R. McLean, T. F. Wolfs, J. Goudsmit, and R. M. May. 1991. Antigenic diversity thresholds and the development of AIDS. Science 254:963–969.

274. Nowak, M. A., R. M. May, R. E. Phillips, S. Rowland-Jones, D. G. Lalloo, S. McAdam, P. Klenerman, B. Koppe, K. Sigmund, C. R. M. Bangham, and A. J. McMichael. 1995. Antigenic oscillations and shifting immunodominance in HIV-1 infections. Nature 375:606–611.

275. Nunn, M. F., and J. W. Marsh. 1996. Human immunodeficiency virus type 1 Nef associates with a member of the p21-activated kinase family. J. Virol. 70:6157–6161.

276. Oelrichs, R. B., C. Workman, T. Laukkanen, F. E. McCutchan, and N. J. Deacon. 1998. A novel subtype A/G/J recombinant full-length HIV type 1 genome from Burkina Faso. AIDS Res. Hum. Retroviruses 14:1495–1500.

277. Okada, S., R. Pu, E. Young, W. V. Stoffs, and J. K. Yamamoto. 1994. Superinfection of cats with feline immunodeficiency virus subtypes A and B. AIDS Res. Hum. Retroviruses 10:1739–1747.

278. Okamoto, H., C. T. Sheline, J. L. Corden, K. A. Jones, and B. M. Peterlin. 1996. Trans-activation by human immunodeficiency virus Tat protein requires the C-terminal domain of RNA polymerase II. Proc. Natl. Acad. Sci. USA 93: 11575–11579.

279. Olshevsky, U., E. Helseth, C. Furman, J. Li, W. Haseltine, and J. Sodroski. 1990. Identification of individual human immunodeficiency virus type 1 gp120 amino acids important for CD4 receptor binding. J. Virol. 64:5701–5707.

280. Otten, R. A., D. L. Ellenberger, D. R. Adams, C. A. Fridlund, E. Jackson, D. Pieniazek, and M. A. Rayfield. 1999. Identification of a window period for susceptibility to dual infection with two distinct human immunodeficiency virus type 2 isolates in a Macaca nemestrina (pig-tailed macaque) model. J. Infect. Dis. 180:673–684.

281. Overbaugh, J., P. R. Donahue, S. L. Quackenbush, E. A. Hoover, and J. I. Mullins. 1988. Molecular cloning of a feline leukemia virus that induces fatal immunodeficiency disease in cats. Science 239:906–910.

282. Palmer, S., R. W. Shafer, and T. C. Merigan. 1999. Highly drug-resistant HIV-1 clinical isolates are cross-resistant to many antiretroviral compounds in current clinical development. AIDS 13:661–667.

283. Pantaleo, G., C. Graziosi, J. F. Demarest, L. Butini, M. Montroni, C. H. Fox, J. M. Orenstein, D. P. Kotler, and A. S. Fauci. 1993. HIV infection is active and progressive in lymphoid tissue during the clinically latent stage of disease. Nature 362:355–358.

284. Pantaleo, G., S. Menzo, M. Vaccarezza, C. Graziosi, O. J. Cohen, J. F. Demarest, D. Montefiori, J. M. Orenstein, C. Fox, L. K. Schrager, J. B. Margolick, S. Buchbinder, J. V. Giorgi, and A. S. Fauci. 1995. Studies in subjects with long-term nonprogressive HIV infection. N. Engl. J. Med. 332:209–216.

285. Parada, C. A., and R. G. Roeder. 1996. Enhanced processivity of RNA polymerase II triggered by Tat-induced phosphorylation of its carboxy-terminal domain. Nature 384:375–378.

286. Parada, C. A., J. B. Yoon, and R. G. Roeder. 1995. A novel LBP-1-mediated restriction of HIV-1 transcription at the level of elongation in vitro. J. Biol. Chem. 270:2274–2283.

287. Pedroza Martins, L., N. Chenciner, and S. Wain-Hobson. 1992. Complex intrapatient sequence variation in the V1 and V2 hypervariable regions of the HIV-1 gp 120 envelope sequence. Virology 191:837–845.

288. Perelson, A. S., A. U. Neumann, M. Markowitz, J. M. Leonard, and D. D. Ho. 1996. HIV-1 dynamics in vivo: virion clearance rate, infected cell life-span, and viral generation time. Science 271:1582–1586.

289. Pieniazek, D., J. M. Peralta, J. A. Ferreira, J. W. Krebs, S. M. Owen, F. S. Sion, C. F. Filho, A. B. Sereno, C. A. de Sa, B. G. Weniger, et al. 1991. Identification of mixed HIV-1/HIV-2 infections in Brazil by polymerase chain reaction. AIDS 5:1293–1299.

290. Piguet, V., F. Gu, M. Foti, N. Demaurex, J. Gruenberg, J. L. Carpentier, and D. Trono. 1999. Nef-induced CD4 degradation: a diacidic-based motif in Nef functions as a lysosomal targeting signal through the binding of beta-COP in endosomes. Cell 97:63–73.

291. Popov, S., M. Rexach, G. Zybarth, N. Reiling, M. A. Lee, L. Ratner, C. M. Lane, M. S. Moore, G. Blobel, and M. Bukrinsky. 1998. Viral protein R regulates nuclear import of the HIV-1 pre-integration complex. EMBO J. 17:909–917.

292. Poss, M., and J. Overbaugh. 1999. Variants from the diverse virus population identified at seroconversion of a clade A human immunodeficiency virus type 1-infected woman have distinct biological properties. J. Virol. 73: 5255–5264.

293. Poss, M., A. G. Rodrigo, J. J. Gosink, G. H. Learn, D. de Vange Panteleeff, H. L. Martin, Jr., J. Bwayo, J. K. Kreiss, and J. Overbaugh. 1998. Evolution of envelope sequences from the genital tract and peripheral blood of women infected with clade A human immunodeficiency virus type 1. J. Virol. 72: 8240–8251.

294. Poulin, L., and J. A. Levy. 1992. The HIV-1 nef gene product is associated with phosphorylation of a 46 kD cellular protein. AIDS 6:787–791.

295. Preston, B. D., B. J. Poiesz, and L. A. Loeb. 1988. Fidelity of HIV-1 reverse transcriptase. Science 242:1168–1171.

296. Ratner, L. 1989. Review: measurement of human immunodeficiency virus load and its relation to disease progression. AIDS Res. Hum. Retroviruses 5:115–119.

297. Rayfield, M., K. De Cock, W. Heyward, L. Goldstein, J. Krebs, S. Kwok, S. Lee, J. McCormick, J. M. Moreau, K. Odehouri, et al. 1988. Mixed human immunodeficiency virus (HIV) infection in an individual: demonstration of both HIV type 1 and type 2 proviral sequences by using polymerase chain reaction. J. Infect. Dis. 158:1170–1176.

298. Reinhart, T. A., A. K. Ghosh, E. A. Hoover, and J. I. Mullins. 1993. Distinct superinfection interference properties yet similar receptor utilization by cytopathic and noncytopathic feline leukemia viruses. J. Virol. 67:5153–5162.

299. Rhee, S. S., and J. W. Marsh. 1994. Human immunodeficiency virus type 1 Nef-induced down-modulation of CD4 is due to rapid internalization and degradation of surface CD4. J. Virol. 68:5156–5163.

300. Richard, N., S. Iacampo, and A. Cochrane. 1994. HIV-1 Rev is capable of shuttling between the nucleus and cytoplasm. Virology 204:123–131.

301. Richman, D. D., D. Havlir, J. Corbeil, D. Looney, C. Ignacio, S. A. Spector, J. Sullivan, S. Cheeseman, K. Barringer, D. Pauletti, et al. 1994. Nevirapine resistance mutations of human immunodeficiency virus type 1 selected during therapy. J. Virol. 68:1660–1666.

302. Roberts, J. D., K. Bebenek, and T. A. Kunkel. 1988. The accuracy of reverse transcriptase from HIV-1. Science 242:1171–1173.

303. Robertson, D. L., J. P. Anderson, J. A. Bradac, J. K. Carr, B. Foley, F. Gao, B. H. Hahn, C. Kuiken, G. H. Learn, T. Leitner, F. McCutchan, S. Osmanov, M. Peeters, D. Pieniazek, M. Salminen, S. Wolinsky, and B. Korber. 1999. HIV-1 subtype and recombinant nomenclature proposal. Presented at the HIV Nomenclature Meeting, Santa Fe, N.M.

304. Robertson, D. L., B. H. Hahn, and P. M. Sharp. 1995. Recombination in AIDS viruses. J. Mol. Evol. 40:249–259.

305. Robertson, D. L., P. M. Sharp, F. E. McCutchan, and B. H. Hahn. 1995. Recombination in HIV-1. Nature 374:124–126.

306. Rodrigo, A. G., and J. I. Mullins. 1996. HIV-1 molecular evolution and the measure of selection. AIDS Res. Hum. Retroviruses 12:1681–1685.

307. Rogel, M. E., L. I. Wu, and M. Emerman. 1995. The human immunodeficiency virus type 1 vpr gene prevents cell proliferation during chronic infection. J. Virol. 69:882–888.

308. Rosen, C. A., J. G. Sodroski, and W. A. Haseltine. 1985. Location of cis-acting regulatory sequences in the human T-cell leukemia virus type I long terminal repeat. Proc. Natl. Acad. Sci. USA 82:6502–6506.

309. Roy, S., N. T. Parkin, C. Rosen, J. Itovitch, and N. Sonenberg. 1990. Structural requirements for trans activation of human immunodeficiency virus type 1 long terminal repeat-directed gene expression by tat: importance of base pairing, loop sequence, and bulges in the tat-responsive sequence. J. Virol. 64:1402–1406.

310. Ruprecht, R. M. 1999. Live attenuated AIDS viruses as vaccines: promise or peril? Immunol. Rev. 170:135–149.

311. Sabino, E. C., E. G. Shpaer, M. G. Morgado, B. T. M. Korber, R. Diaz, V. Bongertz, S. Cavalcante, B. Galvao-Castro, J. I. Mullins, and A. Mayer. 1994.

Identification of human immunodeficiency virus type 1 envelope genes recombinant between subtypes B and F in two epidemiologically linked individuals in Brazil. J. Virol. 68:6340–6346.

312. Sakai, H., R. Shibata, J. Sakuragi, S. Sakuragi, M. Kawamura, and A. Adachi. 1993. Cell-dependent requirement of human immunodeficiency virus type 1 Vif protein for maturation of virus particles. J. Virol. 67:1663–1666.

313. Saksela, K., G. Cheng, and D. Baltimore. 1995. Proline-rich (PxxP) motifs in HIV-1 Nef bind to SH3 domains of a subset of Src kinases and are required for the enhanced growth of Nef+ viruses but not for down-regulation of CD4. EMBO J. 14:484–491.

314. Sala, M., E. Pelletier, and S. Wain-Hobson. 1995. HIV-1 gp120 sequences from a doubly infected drug user. AIDS Res. Hum. Retroviruses 11:653–655.

315. Sala, M., G. Zambruno, J.-P. Vartanian, A. Marconi, U. Bertazzoni, and S. Wain-Hobson. 1994. Spatial discontinuities in human immunodeficiency virus type 1 quasispecies derived from epidermal Langerhans cells of a patient with AIDS and evidence for double infection. J. Virol. 68:5280–5283.

316. Salminen, M. O., J. K. Carr, D. L. Robertson, P. Hegerich, D. Gotte, C. Koch, E. Sanders-Buell, F. Gao, P. M. Sharp, B. H. Hahn, D. S. Burke, and F. E. McCutchan. 1997. Evolution and probable transmission of intersubtype recombinant human immunodeficiency virus type 1 in a Zambian couple. J. Virol. 71:2647–2655.

317. Salvi, R., A. R. Garbuglia, A. Di Caro, S. Pulciani, F. Montella, and A. Benedetto. 1998. Grossly defective nef gene sequences in a human immunodeficiency virus type 1-seropositive long-term nonprogressor. J. Virol. 72:3646–3657.

318. Sanfridson, A., S. Hester, and C. Doyle. 1997. Nef proteins encoded by human and simian immunodeficiency viruses induce the accumulation of endosomes and lysosomes in human T cells. Proc. Natl. Acad. Sci. USA 94:873–878.

319. Sankale, J. L., R. S. De La Tour, R. G. Marlink, R. Scheib, S. Mboup, M. E. Essex, and P. J. Kanki. 1996. Distinct quasi-species in the blood and the brain of an HIV-2-infected individual. Virology 226:418–423.

320. Sarma, P. S., and T. Log. 1971. Viral interference in feline leukemia-sarcoma complex. Virology 44:352–358.

321. Sarma, P. S., and T. Log. 1973. Subgroup classification of feline leukemia and sarcoma viruses by viral interference and neutralization tests. Virology 54:160–169.

322. Sattentau, Q. J., and J. P. Moore. 1991. Conformational changes induced in the human immunodeficiency virus envelope glycoprotein by soluble CD4 binding. J. Exp. Med. 174:407–415.

323. Sawai, E. T., A. Baur, H. Struble, B. M. Peterlin, J. A. Levy, and C. Cheng-Mayer. 1994. Human immunodeficiency virus type 1 Nef associates with a cellular serine kinase in T lymphocytes. Proc. Natl. Acad. Sci. USA 91:1539–1543.

324. Sawai, E. T., A. S. Baur, B. M. Peterlin, J. A. Levy, and C. Cheng-Mayer. 1995. A conserved domain and membrane targeting of Nef from HIV and SIV are required for association with a cellular serine kinase activity. J. Biol. Chem. 270:15307–15314.

325. Schubert, U., L. C. Antón, I. Bacík, J. H. Cox, S. Bour, J. R. Bennink, M. Orlowski, K. Strebel, and J. W. Yewdell. 1998. CD4 glycoprotein degradation induced by human immunodeficiency virus type 1 Vpu protein requires the function of proteasomes and the ubiquitin-conjugating pathway. J. Virol. 72:2280–2288.

326. Schubert, U., S. Bour, A. V. Ferrer-Montiel, M. Montal, F. Maldarell, and K. Strebel. 1996. The two biological activities of human immunodeficiency virus type 1 Vpu protein involve two separable structural domains. J. Virol. 70: 809–819.

327. Schubert, U., P. Henklein, B. Boldyreff, E. Wingender, K. Strebel, and T. Porstmann. 1994. The human immunodeficiency virus type 1 encoded Vpu protein is phosphorylated by casein kinase-2 (CK-2) at positions Ser52 and Ser56 within a predicted alpha-helix-turn-alpha-helix-motif. J. Mol. Biol. 236:16–25.

328. Schubert, U., T. Schneider, P. Henklein, K. Hoffmann, E. Berthold, H. Hauser, G. Pauli, and T. Porstmann. 1992. Human-immunodeficiency-virus-type-1-encoded Vpu protein is phosphorylated by casein kinase II. Eur. J. Biochem. 204:875–883.

329. Schubert, U., and K. Strebel. 1994. Differential activities of the human immunodeficiency virus type 1-encoded Vpu protein are regulated by phosphorylation and occur in different cellular compartments. J. Virol. 68:2260–2271.

330. Schuitemaker, H., M. Koot, N. A. Kootstra, M. W. Dercksen, R. E. de Goede, R. P. van Steenwijk, J. M. Lange, J. K. Schattenkerk, F. Miedema, and M. Tersmette. 1992. Biological phenotype of HIV-1 clones at different stages of infection: progression of disease is associated with a shift from monocytotropic to T-cell-tropic virus population. J. Virol. 66:1354–1360.

331. Schwartz, D. H., R. C. Castillo, S. Arango-Jaramillo, U. K. Sharma, H. F. Song, and G. Sridharan. 1997. Chemokine-independent in vitro resistance to human immunodeficiency virus (HIV-1) correlating with low viremia in long-term and recently infected HIV-1-positive persons. J. Infect. Dis. 176:1168–1174.

332. Schwartz, O., A. Dautry-Varsat, B. Goud, V. Maréchal, A. Subtil, J. M. Heard, and O. Danos. 1995. Human immunodeficiency virus type 1 Nef induces accumulation of CD4 in early endosomes. J. Virol. 69:528–533.

333. Schwartz, O., V. Maréchal, S. Le Gall, F. Lemonnier, and J. M. Heard. 1996. Endocytosis of major histocompatibility complex class I molecules is induced by the HIV-1 Nef protein. Nature Med. 2:338–342.

334. Schwartz, S., B. K. Felber, E. M. Fenyö, and G. N. Pavlakis. 1990. Env and Vpu proteins of human immunodeficiency virus type 1 are produced from multiple bicistronic mRNAs. J. Virol. 64:5448–5456.

335. Schwartz, S., B. K. Felber, and G. N. Pavlakis. 1992. Distinct RNA sequences in the gag region of human immunodeficiency virus type 1 decrease RNA stability and inhibit expression in the absence of Rev protein. J. Virol. 66:150–159.

336. Shafer, R. W., M. J. Kozal, M. A. Winters, A. K. Iversen, D. A. Katzenstein, M. V. Ragni, W. A. R. Meyer, P. Gupta, S. Rasheed, R. Coombs, et al. 1994. Combination therapy with zidovudine and didanosine selects for drug-resistant human immunodeficiency virus type 1 strains with unique patterns of pol gene mutations. J. Infect. Dis. 169:722–729.

337. Shaheen, F., A. V. Sison, L. McIntosh, M. Mukhtar, and R. J. Pomerantz. 1999. Analysis of HIV-1 in the cervicovaginal secretions and blood of pregnant and nonpregnant women. J. Hum. Virol. 2:154–166.

338. Shankarappa, R., J. B. Margolick, S. J. Gange, A. G. Rodrigo, D. Upchurch, H. Farzadegan, P. Gupta, C. R. Rinaldo, G. H. Learn, X. He, X. L. Huang, and J. I. Mullins. 1999. Consistent viral evolutionary changes associated with the progression of human immunodeficiency virus type 1 infection. J. Virol. 73:10489–10502.

339. Shao, Y., F. Zhao, W. Yang, et al. 1999. The identification of recombinant HIV-1 strains in IDUs in Southwest and Northwest China. Chinese J. Exp. Clin. Virol. 13:109–112.

340. Shapshak, P., D. M. Segal, K. A. Crandall, R. K. Fujimura, B. T. Zhang, K. Q. Xin, K. Okuda, C. K. Petito, C. Eisdorfer, and K. Goodkin. 1999. Independent evolution of HIV type 1 in different brain regions. AIDS Res. Hum. Retroviruses 15:811–820.

341. Sheppard, H. W., W. Lang, M. S. Ascher, E. Vittinghoff, and W. Winkelstein. 1993. The characterization of non-progressors: long term HIV-1 infection with stable CD4+ T-cell levels. AIDS 7:1159–1166.

342. Shi, L., W. K. Nishioka, J. Th'ng, E. M. Bradbury, D. W. Litchfield, and A. H. Greenberg. 1994. Premature p34cdc2 activation required for apoptosis. Science 263:1143–1145.

343. Shioda, T., S. Oka, X. Xin, H. Liu, R. Harukuni, A. Kurotani, M. Fukushima, M. K. Hasan, T. Shiino, Y. Takebe, A. Iwamoto, and Y. Nagai. 1997. In vivo sequence variability of human immunodeficiency virus type 1 envelope gp120: association of V2 extension with slow disease progression. J. Virol. 71:4871–4881.

344. Simm, M., M. Shahabuddin, W. Chao, J. S. Allan, and D. J. Volsky. 1995. Aberrant Gag protein composition of a human immunodeficiency virus type 1 vif mutant produced in primary lymphocytes. J. Virol. 69:4582–4586.

345. Simon, J. H., N. C. Gaddis, R. A. Fouchier, and M. H. Malim. 1998. Evidence for a newly discovered cellular anti-HIV-1 phenotype. Nature Med. 4:1397–1400.

346. Simon, J. H., and M. H. Malim. 1996. The human immunodeficiency virus type 1 Vif protein modulates the postpenetration stability of viral nucleoprotein complexes. J. Virol. 70:5297–5305.

347. Sova, P., and D. J. Volsky. 1993. Efficiency of viral DNA synthesis during infection of permissive and nonpermissive cells with vif-negative human immunodeficiency virus type 1. J. Virol. 67:6322–6326.

348. Spearman, P., J. J. Wang, N. Vander Heyden, and L. Ratner. 1994. Identification of human immunodeficiency virus type 1 Gag protein domains essential to membrane binding and particle assembly. J. Virol. 68:3232–3242.

349. Speck, R. F., K. Wehrly, E. J. Platt, R. E. Atchison, I. F. Charo, D. Kabat, B. Chesebro, and M. A. Goldsmith. 1997. Selective employment of chemokine receptors as human immunodeficiency virus type 1 coreceptors determined by individual amino acids within the envelope V3 loop. J. Virol. 71:7136–7139.

350. Stade, K., C. S. Ford, C. Guthrie, and K. Weis. 1997. Exportin 1 (Crm1p) is an essential nuclear export factor. Cell 90:1041–1050.

351. Stammers, D. K., D. O. Somers, C. K. Ross, I. Kirby, P. H. Ray, J. E. Wilson, M. Norman, J. S. Ren, R. M. Esnouf, E. F. Garman, et al. 1994. Crystals of HIV-1 reverse transcriptase diffracting to 2.2 Å resolution. J. Mol. Biol. 242: 586–588.

352. Stark, L. A., and R. T. Hay. 1998. Human immunodeficiency virus type 1 (HIV-1) viral protein R (Vpr) interacts with Lys-tRNA synthetase: implications for priming of HIV-1 reverse transcription. J. Virol. 72:3037–3044.

353. Strebel, K., D. Daugherty, K. Clouse, D. Cohen, T. Folks, and M. A. Martin. 1987. The HIV "A" (sor) gene product is essential for virus infectivity. Nature 328:728–730.

354. Strebel, K., T. Klimkait, F. Maldarelli, and M. A. Martin. 1989. Molecular and biochemical analyses of human immunodeficiency virus type 1 vpu protein. J. Virol. 63:3784–3791.

355. Stuhlmann, H., and P. Berg. 1992. Homologous recombination of copackaged retrovirus RNAs during reverse transcription. J. Virol. 66:2378–2388.

356. Subbramanian, R. A., A. Kessous-Elbaz, R. Lodge, J. Forget, X. J. Yao, D. Bergeron, and E. A. Cohen. 1998. Human immunodeficiency virus type 1 Vpr is a positive regulator of viral transcription and infectivity in primary human macrophages. J. Exp. Med. 187:1103–1111.

357. Sumner-Smith, M., S. Roy, R. Barnett, L. S. Reid, R. Kuperman, U. Delling, and N. Sonenberg. 1991. Critical chemical features in trans-acting-responsive RNA are required for interaction with human immunodeficiency virus type 1 Tat protein. J. Virol. 65:5196–5202.

358. Swingler, S., A. Mann, J. Jacque, B. Brichacek, V. G. Sasseville, K. Williams, A. A. Lackner, E. N. Janoff, R. Wang, D. Fisher, and M. Stevenson. 1999. HIV-1 Nef mediates lymphocyte chemotaxis and activation by infected macrophages. Nature Med. 5:997–1003.

359. Szilvay, A. M., K. A. Brokstad, R. Kopperud, G. Haukenes, and K. H. Kalland. 1995. Nuclear export of the human immunodeficiency virus type 1 nucleocytoplasmic shuttle protein Rev is mediated by its activation domain and is blocked by transdominant negative mutants. J. Virol. 69:3315–3323.

360. Takehisa, J., L. Zekeng, E. Ido, Y. Yamaguchi-Kabata, I. Mboudjeka, Y. Harada, T. Miura, L. Kaptue, and M. Hayami. 1999. Human immunodeficiency virus type 1 intergroup (M/O) recombination in Cameroon. J. Virol. 73:6810–6820.

361. Takehisa, J., L. Zekeng, T. Miura, E. Ido, M. Yamashita, I. Mboudjeka, L. G. Gurtler, M. Hayami, and L. Kaptue. 1997. Triple HIV-1 infection with group O and group M of different clades in a single Cameroonian AIDS patient. J. Acquired Immune Defic. Syndr. Hum. Retrovirol. 14:81–82.

362. Tang, J., C. Costello, I. P. Keet, C. Rivers, S. Leblanc, E. Karita, S. Allen, and R. A. Kaslow. 1999. HLA class I homozygosity accelerates disease progression in human immunodeficiency virus type 1 infection. AIDS Res. Hum. Retroviruses 15:317–324.

363. Tantillo, C., J. Ding, A. Jacobo-Molina, R. G. Nanni, P. L. Boyer, S. H. Hughes, R. Pauwels, K. Andries, P. A. Janssen, and E. Arnold. 1994. Locations of anti-AIDS drug binding sites and resistance mutations in the three-dimensional structure of HIV-1 reverse transcriptase. Implications for mechanisms of drug inhibition and resistance. J. Mol. Biol. 243:369–387.

364. Tersmette, M., R. E. Y. de Goede, B. J. M. Al, I. N. Winkel, R. A. Gruters, H. T. Cuypers, H. G. Huisman, and F. Miedema. 1988. Differential syncytium-inducing capacity of HIV isolates: frequent detection of syncytium-inducing isolates in patients with AIDS and AIDS-related complex. J. Virol. 62:2026–2032.

365. Tersmette, M., R. A. Gruters, F. de Wolf, R. E. de Goede, J. M. Lange, P. T. Schellekens, J. Goudsmit, H. G. Huisman, and F. Miedema. 1989. Evidence for a role of virulent human immunodeficiency virus (HIV) variants in the pathogenesis of acquired immunodeficiency syndrome: studies on sequential HIV isolates. J. Virol. 63:2118–2125.

366. Tersmette, M., J. M. Lange, R. E. de Goede, F. de Wolf, J. K. Eeftink-Schattenkerk, P. T. Schellekens, R. A. Coutinho, H. G. Huisman, J. Goudsmit, and F. Miedema. 1989. Association between biological properties of human immunodeficiency virus variants and risk for AIDS and AIDS mortality. Lancet 1:983–985.

367. Tersmette, M., and H. Schuitemaker. 1993. Virulent HIV strains? AIDS 7:1123–1125.

368. Terwilliger, E. F., E. A. Cohen, Y. C. Lu, J. G. Sodroski, and W. A. Haseltine. 1989. Functional role of human immunodeficiency virus type 1 vpu. Proc. Natl. Acad. Sci. USA 86:5163–5167.

369. Tien, P. C., T. Chiu, A. Latif, S. Ray, M. Batra, C. H. Contag, L. Zejena, M. Mbizvo, E. L. Delwart, J. I. Mullins, and D. A. Katzenstein. 1999. Primary subtype C HIV-1 infection in Harare, Zimbabwe. J. Acquired Immune Defic. Syndr. Hum. Retrovirol. 20:147–153.

370. Tisdale, M., S. D. Kemp, N. R. Parry, and B. A. Larder. 1993. Rapid in vitro selection of human immunodeficiency virus type 1 resistant to 3′-thiacytidine inhibitors due to a mutation in the YMDD region of reverse transcriptase. Proc. Natl. Acad. Sci. USA 90:5653–5656.

371. Triques, K., A. Bourgeois, N. Vidal, E. Mpoudi-Ngole, C. Mulanga-Kabeya, N. Nzilambi, N. Torimiro, E. Saman, E. Delaporte, and M. Peeters. 2000. Near-full-length genome sequencing of divergent African HIV type 1 subtype F viruses leads to the identification of a new HIV type 1 subtype designated K. AIDS Res. Hum. Retroviruses 16:139–151.

372. UNAIDS. 1999. Joint United Nations Programme on HIV/AIDS report on HIV variability. UNAIDS.

373. Unge, T., S. Knight, R. Bhikhabhai, S. Lovgren, Z. Dauter, K. Wilson, and B. Strandberg. 1994. 22 Å resolution structure of the amino-terminal half of HIV-1 reverse transcriptase (fingers and palm subdomains). Structure 2:953–961.

374. Varmus, H. 1988. Retroviruses. Science 240:1427–1435.

375. Vincent, M. J., N. U. Raja, and M. A. Jabbar. 1993. Human immunodeficiency virus type 1 Vpu protein induces degradation of chimeric envelope glycoproteins bearing the cytoplasmic and anchor domains of CD4: role of the cytoplasmic domain in Vpu-induced degradation in the endoplasmic reticulum. J. Virol. 67:5538–5549.

376. Vink, C., and R. H. Plasterk. 1993. The human immunodeficiency virus integrase protein. Trends Genet. 9:433–438.

377. Vodicka, M. A., D. M. Koepp, P. A. Silver, and M. Emerman. 1998. HIV-1 Vpr interacts with the nuclear transport pathway to promote macrophage infection. Genes Dev. 12:175–185.

378. von der Helm, K. 1996. Retroviral proteases: structure, function and inhibition from a non-anticipated viral enzyme to the target of a most promising HIV therapy. Biol. Chem. 377:765–774.

379. von Schwedler, U., R. S. Kornbluth, and D. Trono. 1994. The nuclear localization signal of the matrix protein of human immunodeficiency virus type 1 allows the establishment of infection in macrophages and quiescent T lymphocytes. Proc. Natl. Acad. Sci. USA 91:6992–6996.

380. von Schwedler, U., J. Song, C. Aiken, and D. Trono. 1993. Vif is crucial for human immunodeficiency virus type 1 proviral DNA synthesis in infected cells. J. Virol. 67:4945–4955.

381. Wain-Hobson, S. 1993. The fastest genome evolution ever described: HIV variation in situ. Curr. Biol. 3:878–883.

382. Wain-Hobson, S. 1995. Virological mayhem. Nature 373:102.

383. Wakrim, L., R. Le Grand, B. Vaslin, A. Cheret, F. Matheux, F. Theodoro, P. Roques, I. Nicol-Jourdain, and D. Dormont. 1996. Superinfection of HIV-2-preinfected macaques after rectal exposure to a primary isolate of SIVmac251. Virology 221:260–270.

384. Wang, C. T., H. Y. Lai, and C. C. Yang. 1999. Sequence requirements for incorporation of human immunodeficiency virus gag-beta-galactosidase fusion proteins into virus-like particles. J. Med. Virol. 59:180–188.

385. Watson, K., and R. J. Edwards. 1999. HIV-1-trans-activating (Tat) protein: both a target and a tool in therapeutic approaches. Biochem. Pharmacol. 58:1521–1528.

386. Weeks, K. M., C. Ampe, S. C. Schultz, T. A. Steitz, and D. M. Crothers. 1990. Fragments of the HIV-1 Tat protein specifically bind TAR RNA. Science 249:1281–1285.

387. Wei, P., M. E. Garber, S. M. Fang, W. H. Fischer, and K. A. Jones. 1998. A novel CDK9-associated C-type cyclin interacts directly with HIV-1 Tat and mediates its high-affinity, loop-specific binding to TAR RNA. Cell 92:451–462.

388. Wei, X., S. K. Ghosh, M. E. Taylor, V. A. Johnson, E. A. Emini, P. Deutsch, J. D. Lifson, S. Bonhoeffer, M. A. Nowak, B. H. Hahn, M. S. Saag, and G. M. Shaw. 1995. Viral dynamics of HIV-1 infection. Nature 373:117–122.

389. Weller, S. K., A. E. Joy, and H. M. Temin. 1980. Correlation between cell killing and massive second-round superinfection by members of some subgroups of avian leukosis virus. J. Virol. 33:494–506.

390. Weller, S. K., and H. M. Temin. 1981. Cell killing by avian leukosis viruses. J. Virol. 39:713–721.

391. Wen, W., J. L. Meinkoth, R. Y. Tsien, and S. S. Taylor. 1995. Identification of a signal for rapid export of proteins from the nucleus. Cell 82:463–473.

392. Whatmore, A. M., N. Cook, G. A. Hall, S. Sharpe, E. W. Rud, and M. P. Cranage. 1995. Repair and evolution of nef in vivo modulates simian immunodeficiency virus virulence. J. Virol. 69:5117–5123.

393. Whittle, H. C., K. Ariyoshi, and S. Rowland-Jones. 1998. HIV-2 and T cell recognition. Curr. Opin. Immunol. 10:382–387.

394. Willey, R. L., F. Maldarelli, M. A. Martin, and K. Strebel. 1992. Human immunodeficiency virus type 1 Vpu protein induces rapid degradation of CD4. J. Virol. 66:7193–7200.

395. Willey, R. L., F. Maldarelli, M. A. Martin, and K. Strebel. 1992. Human immunodeficiency virus type 1 Vpu protein regulates the formation of intracellular gp160-CD4 complexes. J. Virol. 66:226–234.

396. Winkler, C., W. Modi, M. W. Smith, G. W. Nelson, X. Wu, M. Carrington, M. Dean, T. Honjo, K. Tashiro, D. Yabe, S. Buchbinder, E. Vittinghoff, J. J. Goedert, T. R. O'Brien, L. P. Jacobson, R. Detels, S. Donfield, A. Willoughby, E. Gomperts, D. Vlahov, J. Phair, ALIVE Study, Hemophilia Growth and Development Study, Multicenter AIDS Cohort Study, San Francisco City Cohort, and S. J. O'Brien. 1998. Genetic restriction of AIDS pathogenesis by an SDF-1 chemokine gene variant. Science 279:389–393.

397. Winters, M. A., K. L. Coolley, Y. A. Girard, D. J. Levee, H. Hamdan, R. W. Shafer, D. A. Katzenstein, and T. C. Merigan. 1998. A 6-basepair insert in the reverse transcriptase gene of human immunodeficiency virus type 1 confers resistance to multiple nucleoside inhibitors. J. Clin. Invest. 102:1769–1775.

398. Wiskerchen, M., and C. Cheng-Mayer. 1996. HIV-1 Nef association with cellular serine kinase correlates with enhanced virion infectivity and efficient proviral DNA synthesis. Virology 224:292–301.

399. Wolfs, T. F., G. Zwart, M. Bakker, and J. Goudsmit. 1992. HIV-1 genomic RNA diversification following sexual and parenteral virus transmission. Virology 189:103–110.

400. Wolfs, T. F. W., J. J. de Jong, H. van den Berg, J. M. G. H. Tijnagel, W. J. A. Krone, and J. Goudsmit. 1990. Evolution of sequences encoding the principal neutralization epitope of human immunodeficiency virus 1 is host dependent, rapid, and continuous. Proc. Natl. Acad. Sci. USA 87:9938–9942.

401. Wolinsky, S. M., B. T. M. Korber, A. U. Neumann, M. Daniels, K. J. Kuntsman, A. J. Whetsell, M. R. Furtado, Y. Cao, D. D. Ho, J. T. Safrit, and R. A. Koup. 1996. Adaptive evolution of HIV-1 during the natural course of infection. Science 272:537–542.

402. Wong, J. K., M. Hezareh, H. F. Günthard, D. V. Havlir, C. C. Ignacio, C. A. Spina, and D. D. Richman. 1997. Recovery of replication-competent HIV despite prolonged suppression of plasma viremia. Science 278:1291–1300.

403. Wong, J. K., C. C. Ignacio, F. Torriani, D. Havler, N. J. S. Fitch, and D. D. Richman. 1997. In vivo compartmentalization of human immunodeficiency virus: evidence from the examination of pol sequences from autopsy tissues. J. Virol. 71:2059–2071.

404. Wrin, T. 2000. Measuring the replicative fitness of recombinant HIV-1 vectors expressing protease and reverse transcriptase derived from patient viruses. Presented at the Seventh Conference on Retroviruses and Opportunistic Infections, San Francisco.

405. Wyatt, R., P. D. Kwong, E. Desjardins, R. W. Sweet, J. Robinson, W. A. Hendrickson, and J. G. Sodroski. 1998. The antigenic structure of the HIV gp120 envelope glycoprotein. Nature 393:705–711.

406. Yamaguchi, Y., and T. Gojobori. 1997. Evolutionary mechanisms and population dynamics of the third variable envelope region of HIV within single hosts. Proc. Natl. Acad. Sci. USA 94:1264–1269.

407. Yang, X., M. O. Gold, D. N. Tang, D. E. Lewis, E. Aguilar-Cordova, A. P. Rice, and C. H. Herrmann. 1997. TAK, an HIV Tat-associated kinase, is a member of the cyclin-dependent family of protein kinases and is induced by activation of peripheral blood lymphocytes and differentiation of promonocytic cell lines. Proc. Natl. Acad. Sci. USA 94:12331–12336.

408. Yang, X., C. H. Herrmann, and A. P. Rice. 1996. The human immunodeficiency virus Tat proteins specifically associate with TAK in vivo and require the carboxyl-terminal domain of RNA polymerase II for function. J. Virol. 70:4576–4584.

409. Yu, G., and R. L. Felsted. 1992. Effect of myristoylation on p27 nef subcellular distribution and suppression of HIV-LTR transcription. Virology 187:46–55.

410. Yu, X. F., J. Chen, Y. Shao, C. Beyrer, and S. Lai. 1998. Two subtypes of HIV-1 among injection-drug users in southern China. Lancet 351:1250.

411. Yuan, X., Z. Matsuda, M. Matsuda, M. Essex, and T. H. Lee. 1990. Human immunodeficiency virus vpr gene encodes a virion-associated protein. AIDS Res. Hum. Retroviruses 6:1265–1271.

412. Zapp, M. L., and M. R. Green. 1989. Sequence-specific RNA binding by the HIV-1 Rev protein. Nature 342:714–716.

413. Zapp, M. L., T. J. Hope, T. G. Parslow, and M. R. Green. 1991. Oligomerization and RNA binding domains of the type 1 human immunodeficiency virus Rev protein: a dual function for an arginine-rich binding motif. Proc. Natl. Acad. Sci. USA 88:7734–7738.

414. Zazopoulos, E., and W. A. Haseltine. 1993. Effect of nef alleles on replication of human immunodeficiency virus type 1. Virology 194:20–27.

415. Zennou, V., F. Mammano, S. Paulous, D. Mathez, and F. Clavel. 1998. Loss of viral fitness associated with multiple Gag and Gag-Pol processing defects in human immunodeficiency virus type 1 variants selected for resistance to protease inhibitors in vivo. J. Virol. 72:3300–3306.

416. Zhang, J., and H. M. Temin. 1993. Rate and mechanism of nonhomologous recombination during a single cycle of retroviral replication. Science 259:234–238.

417. Zhang, L. Q., P. MacKenzie, A. Cleland, E. C. Holmes, A. J. Leigh Brown, and P. Simmonds. 1993. Selection for specific sequences in the external envelope protein of HIV-1 upon primary infection. J. Virol. 67:3345–3356.

418. Zhu, T., H. Mo, N. Wang, D. S. Nam, Y. Cao, R. A. Koup, and D. D. Ho. 1993. Genotypic and phenotypic characterization of HIV-1 in patients with primary infection. Science 261:1179–1181.

419. Zhu, T., N. Wang, A. Carr, S. Wolinsky, and D. D. Ho. 1995. Evidence for co-infection by multiple strains of HIV-1 subtype B in an acute seroconvertor. J. Virol. 69:1324–1327.

Nucleoside Inhibitors of HIV Reverse Transcriptase and the Problem of Drug Resistance

3

MATTHIAS GÖTTE
SHALOM SPIRA
MARK A. WAINBERG

The reverse transcriptase (RT) enzyme of HIV-1 is an important target in antiviral chemotherapeutic strategies. A number of important nucleoside analogs have been developed that antagonize the function of RT by causing the chain termination of elongating strands of viral DNA. In this manner, nucleoside analogs function as competitive inhibitors of naturally occurring nucleosides for incorporation into RT-catalyzed viral DNA strands. Unfortunately, resistance to each of these drugs has occurred in every instance, owing to a series of mutations in the RT gene that result in altered RT proteins that can discriminate against incorporation of the incoming analog. These mutations are located in different regions of the p66 subunit of RT and in some cases may cause cross-resistance among various numbers of the nucleoside analog family of compounds. Because of the high error rate of RT and the fact that viral replication occurs at high titer, all single point mutations that are compatible with viral survival, including resistance-conferring mutations in RT, preexist as part of the viral quasi species before treatment with antiviral drugs is ever initiated.

Among the formidable challenges in the clinical management of HIV disease is the need to prevent and overcome the development of HIV-1 resistance against the drugs that antagonize the function of the viral RT and protease (PR) enzymes. The RT of HIV has an astonishingly high error rate of approximately 10^{-4} (i.e., several orders of magnitude higher than those of cellular polymerases). This virtually guarantees that mutations will occur during each replication cycle of the 9.2 kb retroviral genome. Since mutagenesis is an ongoing process in the viral RT and PR genes, the virus is easily able to adapt to the use of single antiviral agents. Thus, HIV can render itself resistant to drugs that are designed to interfere with its replication. Not all HIV mutations will produce this result; indeed, most mutations may go unnoticed (e.g., when no substitution in amino acid sequence occurs), and some mutations may be lethal, resulting in inability of the viral particle to multiply.

HIV mutagenesis can be effectively recognized under conditions of selective pressure that are imposed by treatment of an infected individual with antiretroviral drugs (ARVs). This antiviral pressure will preferentially allow the replication of mutated viruses that become resistant as a result of mutations in either the RT or PR genes, as a consequence of the high error rate of the viral RT. It can thus be inferred that all single mutations that are compatible with viral survival are already present as part of the viral quasi species even before treatment with ARVs is commenced. Of course, natural selection is also exerted by the body's own immune system, with the appearance of mutant HIV variants whose epitopes are no longer recognized by neutralizing and other antibodies and/or cytotoxic T lymphocytes. Selective pressure creates an environment in which mutated forms of HIV can become the dominant presence in the quasi species. This implies that HIV variants containing single point mutations, associated with drug resistance, are present as only a tiny minority in untreated patients and are unable to replicate as quickly as wild-type viruses.

Inhibition of Reverse Transcription

An important subject of HIV research has been the RT enzyme that is responsible for the transcription of double-stranded proviral DNA from viral genomic RNA. Two categories of drugs have been developed to block RT: dideoxy nucleoside analogs (ddNTPs), which act to short-circuit DNA chain elongation and act as competitive inhibitors of RT, and non-nucleoside RT inhibitors (NNRTIs), which bind to the catalytic site of RT and act as noncompetitive antagonists of enzyme activity. The dideoxy nucleoside analogs and other members of this class are termed nucleoside RT inhibitors (NRTIs).

NRTIs are administered to patients as precursor compounds that are phosphorylated to their active triphosphate form by cellular enzymes. The ddNTPs lack a 3' hydroxyl group (OH) necessary for the nucleophilic attack to the α-phosphate of an incoming nucleotide that results in its addition to a growing chain of DNA. These analogs can compete effectively with normal dNTP substrates for binding to RT and, once incorporated, can terminate transcription (29, 43, 78, 121,137).

The mechanism of NNRTI action is less clear but is known to involve the binding of these highly specific noncompetitive inhibitors to a hydrophobic pocket at or near the catalytic site of RT (19, 56, 135). Kinetic studies confirm that NNRTI inhibition reduces the catalytic rate of polymerization without affecting nucleotide binding or nucleotide-induced conformational change (117). NNRTIs act particularly efficiently at template positions at which the RT enzyme naturally pauses (33). NNRTIs have scarcely any effect on primer/template interactions and do not seem to influence the competition between ddNTPs and the naturally occurring dNTPs for insertion into the growing proviral DNA chain (40, 103).

Both classes of RT inhibitors have been shown to diminish successfully the plasma viral burden of HIV-1 infected hosts (26, 27, 136, 138). However, protracted monotherapy with all drugs will lead to drug resistance and to clinical deterioration (27, 66, 82, 105). In contrast, patients who receive combinations of three or more drugs are less likely to develop drug resistance, since these "cocktails" can suppress viral replication to a far greater extent. Although mutagenesis is far less likely to occur in this circumstance, the emergence of breakthrough viruses has been demonstrated in patients receiving highly active antiviral therapy (HAART) (42, 90). Another major impediment to currently applied anti-HIV chemotherapy is the persistence of reservoirs of latently infected cells (25). Despite an efficient reduction of viral burden, which can reach levels below limits of detection, replication of HIV might be recovered once therapy is stopped or interrupted (134). Eradication of a latent reservoir of 10^5 cells could take as long as 60 years (25).

NRTIs

The common structural feature shared by all clinically available NRTIs is the missing 3' OH group of the sugar moiety of the drug. This type of chemical modification ensures that DNA synthesis is prematurely terminated once the phosphorylated active form of the inhibitor has successfully competed for incorporation with natural nucleoside triphosphates. However, any structural changes in the sugar ring of a given nucleoside can potentially affect its ability to compete with its natural counterpart in multiple ways. These include the efficiency of phosphorylation of the prodrug and the efficiency of incorporation of the active form of the compound by the RT enzyme.

Currently used NRTIs may be divided into five subgroups, based on structural distinctions of their sugar moieties (Fig. 3.1). Group 1 represents the simplest example of a chain terminator, in which the 3' OH group is simply replaced by hydrogen. Didanosine (ddI, or ddATP as active anabolite) and zalcitabine (ddC) are examples of this type of inhibitor. Drugs that belong to group 2 are characterized by a chemical substitution of the 3' OH group. Zidovudine (ZDV), which contains a bulky azido group at this position, was the first approved anti-AIDS drug and is still a very important component of currently used drug regimens. Lamivudine (3TC) is a member of a third class of NRTIs. These compounds contain an oxathiolane ring, in which the sulfur atom is located at the 3' position of the sugar moiety.

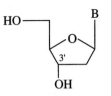

Natural nucleoside structure

Type of NRTI   **Example**

Group 1

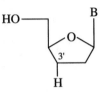   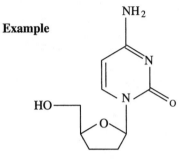

Zalcitabine (ddC)

Group 2

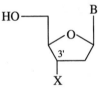   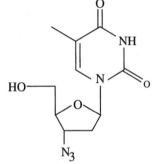

Zidovudine (ZDV)

Group 3

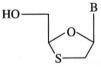   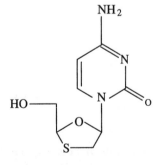

Lamivudine (3TC)

FIGURE 3.1
Structures of various categories of NRTIs

Group 4

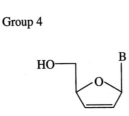

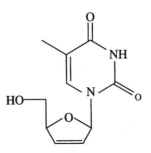

Stavudine (d4T)

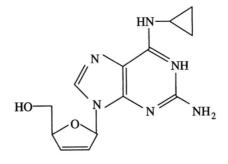

Abacavir (ABC)

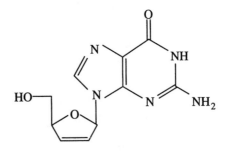

Carbovir (CBV)

FIGURE 3.1 (*continued*)

Compounds that belong to group 4, such as stavudine (d4T) or abacavir (ABC), contain a double bond between positions 2′ and 3. It is noteworthy that abacavir is an NRTI with unique intracellular activity properties that affect the base moiety as well. In brief, the prodrug abacavir is initially phosphorylated to its monophosphate (MP), which undergoes conversion to Carbovir (CBV)-MP. The latter anabolite is further phosphorylated to its triphosphate (CBV-TP), which ultimately serves as a chain terminator.

Group 5

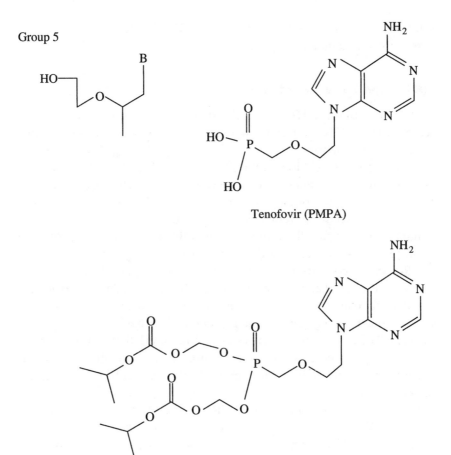

Tenofovir (PMPA)

bis-POC PMPA (oral prodrug of PMPA)

FIGURE 3.1 (*continued*)

Group 5 represents acyclic NRTIs. Although these types of compounds, such as tenofovir (PMPA), lack a sugar moiety, the RT enzyme can still efficiently accept the phosphorylated active form of the drug.

Both tenofovir and the only other member of this family, adefovir, already contain a phosphate and are best referred to as nucleotides rather than nucleosides. NRTIs are important components of currently used multidrug regimens in the treatment of HIV infections. Triple-drug cocktails have been shown to suppress replication of HIV over long periods. These combinations often contain NRTIs together with NNRTIs or PR inhibitors or both. Additive or even synergistic antiviral effects may increase the clinical activity of each of these drugs. However, the therapeutic success of a particular treatment strategy will critically depend on the emergence of mutant viruses that may confer resistance to one or more drugs of the regimen used. In the following, we discuss the various patterns of phenotypic and genotypic resistance to NRTIs in regard to biochemical mechanisms and biological phenotype.

NRTIs and Drug Resistance

With the exception of 3TC [(–)–2′,3′-dideoxy-3′-thiacytidine, lamivudine], resistance to NRTIs commonly appears after about six months of therapy. Phenotypic resistance is detected by comparing the IC_{50} (or drug concentration capable of blocking viral replication by 50%) of pretreatment viral isolates with those obtained after therapy. Thus, higher IC_{50} values obtained after several months of treatment reflect a loss in viral susceptibility to ARVs. Selective polymerase chain reaction (PCR) analysis of the RT genome confirms that the number of mutations associated with drug resistance increases concomitantly with increases in IC_{50} values.

Resistance-conferring mutations have been reported to date in response to the use of any single RT inhibitor from any drug class. However, not all drugs elicit the same mutagenic response; sensitivity and resistance patterns must be considered on an individual drug basis. For example, patients on 3TC monotherapy may develop high-level, that is, 1,000-fold, resistance within weeks, whereas six months or more are often required in order for ZDV sensitivity to drop by 50- to 100-fold. In contrast, HIV may appear to remain reasonably sensitive, even after prolonged monotherapy, to four of the other commonly used NRTIs: ddI, ddC, d4T, and ABC. In the case of ZDV, increases in IC_{50} below threefold are regarded as nonsignificant, a 10- to 50-fold increase represents partial resistance, and increases above 50-fold denote high-level resistance. In vivo resistance to NRTIs can often develop independently of the dose of drug that is administered.

In cell culture, HIV-1 resistance can be easily demonstrated against each of the NRTIs, NNRTIs, and PR inhibitors by gradually increasing the concentration of compound in the tissue culture medium (20, 30, 65, 76, 101). Cell lines are especially useful in this regard, since HIV replication occurs very efficiently in such hosts. Because the same resistance-conferring mutations that arise in cell culture also appear clinically (30, 65, 101), tissue culture selection provides an effective preclinical means of studying HIV mutagenesis.

As mentioned above, RTs in general, and that of HIV-1 in particular, are highly error prone by the standards of other DNA polymerases found in prokaryotes and eukaryotes. A number of biomolecular explanations for this phenomenon have been forwarded, including RT's unique lack of a 3′-5′ exonuclease proofreading activity (104) and its wide catalytic cleft and DNA binding channel (48, 56), which may hamper accurate substrate binding or encourage abnormal strand transfers during reverse transcription or both. Moreover, the relatively low processivity of RT may allow for a higher frequency of mutations at pause sites, that is, points along the template at which the enzyme may temporarily dissociate before rebinding takes place (7). It should be noted that the error rate of HIV in vivo may, in fact, be lower than that predicted from cell-free biochemical assays performed with purified RT (73).

Drug-resistance-conferring mutations are spontaneously generated as a consequence of this high RT error rate and, as well, because HIV turnover in the body is extremely rapid. As such, drug-resistant variants are selected (rather than induced) by pharmacological pressure. Owing to the high turnover and mutation rate of HIV-1, the retroviral quasi species (45, 131) will also include defective particles (11). As stated, singly mutated drug-resistant variants are present in vivo prior to commencement of therapy. Multiply mutated variants appear later and are less commonly found in the retroviral pool of untreated patients. Patients with advanced infection have a higher viral load and possibly a broader range of quasi species than newly infected individuals. Such patients are often immunosuppressed and may also have diminished ability to control viral replication immunologically; this may also lead to a more rapid development of drug resistance.

The kinetics of appearance of drug resistance also vary with the HIV phenotype (e.g., syncytium inducing [SI] versus non–syncytium inducing [NSI]), possibly because of differential viral turnover in cells of lymphocyte versus monocyte origin. Pretreatment isolates usually have a narrow range of IC_{50} values, regardless of disease stage, since it is the selective pressure that is imposed by ARVs that expands the initially small quasi species of resistant particles. For this reason, resistant viruses cannot commonly be detected in vivo when performing drug susceptibility assays of viruses from treatment-naive individuals. In certain cases, drug-resistant quasi species may revert to wild type after long-term growth in the absence of drug, both in vivo and in vitro. Addition of the same drug on a second occasion will commonly lead to the more rapid appearance of resistance and of relevant mutations than was initially seen. This is because the resistance-conferring mutations never disappear but continue to be present at higher levels than seen in nontreated individuals (120).

Initiation of effective treatment at times prior to the development of high viral burden, when quasi species may be less diverse, may help to restrict the development of drug resistance (44).

Molecular Basis of HIV Resistance to NRTIs

It has been shown by site-directed mutagenesis that a variety of RT mutations encode HIV resistance to both NRTIs and NNRTIs (18, 28, 37, 39, 68, 85, 101, 102, 114, 120). Crystallographic and biochemical data have demonstrated that mutations conferring resistance to NNRTIs are found in the peptide residues that make contact with these compounds within their binding pocket (18, 19, 56, 83, 98).

The mature RT exists as a p66/p51 heterodimer that is cleaved from an initially generated p160$^{gag\text{-}pol}$ precursor protein. Mutated RTs, which are purified from *Escherichia coli* expression systems, can be shown to display reduced sensitivity to 2',3'-ddNTPs and to NNRTIs in cell-free enzyme assays (72). Resistance-encoding mutations against the former are found in different regions of the RT enzyme, probably owing to the complexity of nucleoside incorporation, which involves each of several steps, that is, recognition/binding, formation of a phosphodiester bond, release of pyrophosphate, and translocation of the enzyme. Mutations affecting any of the above steps can decrease RT susceptibility to NRTIs, albeit via mechanisms that are poorly understood. A summary of prominent mutations is featured in Table 3.1, and a more exhaustive list of mutations that confer resistance against RT and PR inhibitors can be found elsewhere (108).

Multimutational Basis of Resistance to ZDV

Crystallographic studies suggest that residues in the p66 subunit are mainly responsible for resistance to NRTIs (47, 107, 123). There is a general absence of cross-resistance among NRTIs and NNRTIs; this implies that resistance-conferring mutations act in discrete, unrelated manners. Distinct patterns of resistance emerge in patients treated with ZDV as opposed to those on ddI, ddC, 3TC, d4T, or ABC. ZDV selects for a variety of RT mutations, and the detection of resistance to ZDV normally requires the accumulation of at least two mutations. Loss of susceptibility to the other compounds is usually effected by a single mutation. This distinction can be explained by considering the unique nature of ZDV, in that the 3' OH has been replaced by an azido group, which likely gives this compound unique qualities of inhibition and resistance.

Five major genetic substitutions commonly appear within one year of initiation of ZDV monotherapy; these mutations, which may act additively or synergistically to confer differing levels of resistance, are methionine → leucine at codon 41 (M41L), aspartate → asparagine at codon 67 (D67N), lysine → arginine at codon 70 (K70R), threonine → tyrosine/phenylalanine at codon 215 (T215Y/F), and lysine → glutamine at codon 219 (K219Q). The function of these mutations in drug resistance has been confirmed by site-directed mutagenesis, whereby wild-type residues are replaced with selected mutated nucleosides following identification of the latter by sequencing of the RT gene from viral isolates that manifest resistance to ARVs (53, 68).

Increased levels of resistance to ZDV are associated with an orderly manner of accumulation of these mutations (10, 53, 65). Thus, low levels of resistance, which are associated with initial appearance of K70R, are followed by higher resistance levels and the T215Y/F or D67N mutations, followed in turn by M41L and K219Q. Of these, T215Y and K70R are the most

TABLE 3.1

Important substitutions responsible for HIV resistance to nucleoside drugs

	Amino acid		Position of mutation in RT crystal structure[a]	Drugs against which resistance has been shown using:	
RT position	Wild-type virus	Mutant virus		Viral growth assay[a]	Cell-free RT assay[a]
41	Met (M)	Leu (L)	αA	ZDV	
62	Ala (A)	Val (V)	β3	ZDV, ddI, ddC, d4T, ddG	ZDVTP
65	Lys (K)	Arg (R)	β3-β4 loop	ddC, 3TC, ddI, PMEA, ABC, PMPA	ddCTP, 3TCTP, ddATP, ddITP, PMEApp, ZDVTP
67	Asp (D)	Asn (N)	β3-β4 loop	ZDV	ZDVTP[b]
69	Thr (T)	Asp (D)	β3-β4 loop	ddC	
70	Lys (K)	Arg (R)	β3-β4 loop	ZDV	ZDVTP[b]
74	Leu (L)	Val (V)	β4	ddI, ddC, ABC	ddATP, ddCTP, AZTTP
75	Val (V)	Thr (T)	β4	d4T	
75	Val (V)	Ile (I)	β4	ZDV, ddI, ddC, d4T, ddG	ZDVTP
77	Phe (F)	Leu (L)	β4	ZDV, ddI, ddC, d4T, ddG	ZDVTP
89	Glu (E)	Gly (G)	β5a		ddGTP
116	Phe (F)	Tyr (Y)	αC	ZDV, ddI, ddC, d4T, ddG	ZDVTP
151	Gln (Q)	Met (M)	β8-αE loop	ZDV, ddI, ddC, d4T, ddG	ZDVTP
184	Met (M)	Val /Ile (V/I)	β9-β10 turn	ddI, ddC, 3TC, ABC	3TCTP
215	Thr (T)	Tyr/Phe (Y/F)	β11a	ZDV	ZDVTP[b]
219	Lys (K)	Gln (Q)	β11b	ZDV	ZDVTP[b]

[a]ZDV (zidovudine) (azidothymidine); ZDVTP, ZDV 5'-triphosphate; ddATP, 2',3'-dideoxyadenosine triphosphate; 2',3'-dideoxycytidine (zalcitabine); ddCTP, ddC triphosphate; ddG, 2',3'-dideoxyguanosine; ddGTP, ddG triphosphate; ddI, 2',3'-dideoxyinosine (didanosine); d4T, 2'3'-didehydro-2',3'-dideoxythymidine (stavudine); PMEA (adefovir), PMEApp, 9 (2-phosphonylmethoxyethyl) adenine diphosphate; 3TC, 2',3'-dideoxy-3'-thiacytidine (lamivudine); 3TCTP, 3TC triphosphate; ABC (abacavir); PMPA (tenofovir).

[b]Increased rates of rescue of chain-terminated DNA synthesis in the presence of pyrophosphate or nucleoside triphosphates.

prevalent substitutions found in ZDV-treated patients. Interestingly, cross-resistance is generally found only among 2',3'-ddNDPs that also bear a 3'-azido group, such as 3'-azido-2',3'-dideoxyguanosine (AZG) but not other analogs such as ddC or ddI (64, 129).

K70R was initially thought to be a temporary substitution, serving only as a facilitator for the development of other mutations, but more recent plasma viral load studies indicate that K70R can itself reduce HIV susceptibility to ZDV. The detection of mutations that confer resistance to ZDV can persist for as long as a year following termination of therapy. The appearance of K70R is often superseded by that of the 215 mutation, followed by M41L in clinical samples.

A number of studies have demonstrated that the rate at which resistance emerges is correlated with disease stage (16). In one study, it was shown that it took as long as four years for 60% of asymptomatic individuals to develop resistance (81). In two other studies, patients harboring ZDV-resistant viruses were more than twice as likely to progress to a new AIDS-defining event or death. In the first of these studies, ACTG 116B/117, patients with advanced disease who had received ZDV monotherapy for at least 16 weeks were switched to ddI, whereupon disease progression and likelihood of death were diminished (16, 50). Similar findings were obtained in a Canadian study, which followed relatively asymptomatic patients who were switched from ZDV to ddI and who were subsequently followed over a two-year period (80). Finally, researchers have observed that disease progression is most frequent in patients who harbor drug-resistant forms of HIV-1. One study reported high-level resistance to ZDV in only 7% of patients with high CD4 counts, compared with 28% of patients with CD4 counts below 50 cells/μl (16).

Although high-level ZDV resistance was predictive of increased morbidity and mortality in these monotherapy studies, a switch to ddI was found to be significantly beneficial even in patients without high-level ZDV resistance, such as those lacking either the M41L or T215Y/F mutations or both (16). The Canadian study, as well, demonstrated a general increase in CD4 counts for individuals who switched to ddI compared with a decrease in CD4 counts in patients who continued on ZDV monotherapy (80). Baseline resistance to ZDV was associated with a subsequent diminution in CD4 count. But in those who switched to ddI, only low-level resistance to the new drug was detected, coupled with stabilized or even decreased resistance against ZDV. By contrast, patients continuing on ZDV monotherapy displayed increased levels of resistance and a propensity to develop opportunistic illness or die of HIV-related illness.

The structure of HIV-1 RT bound to a DNA primer/template substrate and an incoming nucleotide suggests that amino acid substitutions associated with ZDV resistance can affect the RT-dNTP/ddNTP interaction (47). Residues D67 and K70 are located in the "β3-β4 loop" of the fingers subdomain that traps the incoming dNTP. The 3′-hydroxyl group of the bound dNTP projects into a site that is designated the "3′ pocket." This structural feature is of particular interest in regard to resistance to NRTIs, since this class of compounds is modulated at the 3′ position of the sugar ring. The pocket of the wild-type enzyme is large enough to accommodate the azido group of ZDV, but the T215 F/Y mutation may change the geometry of the 3′ pocket, presumably inducing alterations of the RT-ZDV-TP interaction. In addition, these specific mutated RTs can affect the interaction with primer/template, since amino acid substitutions at residues 215 and 219 increase processivity of the enzyme (3, 4, 14).

Despite these implications for mechanisms of ZDV resistance, previous kinetic studies using a homopolymeric template/primer have surprisingly shown that both wild-type RTs and RTs containing mutations associated with ZDV resistance have similar enzymatic efficiencies for natural substrate dNTPs as well as similar recognition efficiencies for ZDV 5′-triphosphate (ZDVTP) and other ddNTPs. This is true for RTs that have been purified from both *E. coli* as well as ZDV-resistant viruses. Likewise, in chain elongation/dNTP incorporation assays, using synthetic heteropolymeric template/primer, no differences were observed between wild-type and mutated RTs containing ZDV resistance-associated mutations in regard to chain termination efficiency (60, 62).

A solution to this apparent contradiction between the resistance to ZDV of mutated HIV virus particles and the apparent nonresistance of mutated RTs was recently provided by studies showing that the same enzymes had greatly increased rates of the reverse reaction of DNA polymerization, that is, pyrophosphorolysis. This reaction involves the removal of the incorporated ddNTP from a blocked DNA chain and in turn allows rescue of DNA synthesis. Such rescue of the polymerization reaction was demonstrated in cell-free assays using pyrophosphate (3) and ATP (77), respectively. In these experiments, ZDV-resistant enzymes showed increased rates of primer unblocking when compared with wild-type RT. In agreement with these results are binding studies that showed increased affinities of resistant mutant enzymes to ZDV-terminated primers (3, 5).

Resistance to 3TC

The initial report of a methionine → valine mutation at RT residue 184 (M184V) was in HIV that was selected for resistance in tissue culture to ddI (39). Subsequent findings showed that this substitution could indeed encode low-level resistance to both ddI and ddC and could sometimes be detected in patients receiving therapy with these drugs. Of greatest significance, however, is that the M184V substitution is rapidly selected both in tissue culture and in vivo by 3TC and encodes high-level resistance, that is, 500–1,000 fold, to this drug (8, 31, 32, 111, 125, 128).

The M184V mutation has a number of unique properties in regard to both HIV and RT:

1. It affords high-level resistance to 3TC (IC_{50} levels 1,000-fold above wild type) but low-level resistance against ddI and ddC. This is the only mutation known to encode resistance as high as 1,000-fold to a single nucleoside drug.
2. The mutation rapidly appears both in cell culture and in vivo on administration of 3TC but appears only slowly in the case of ddI or ddC (8, 52, 111, 125).
3. It is located at or nearby the polymerase active site within a conserved YMDD motif that is found in almost all retroviral RTs (130).
4. Recombinant RT containing M184V exhibits a 50-fold diminished sensitivity to 3TC 5'-triphosphate (3TCTP) but has similar K_m and V_{max} values with respect to ddCTP as compared with wild-type RT (23, 94).

A similar mutation, methionine → isoleucine at the same codon (M184I), likewise encodes for high-level resistance to 3TC (8). M184I has been observed in patients receiving 3TC prior to appearance of M184V; however, the latter becomes dominant within weeks because it affords greater fitness to HIV and permits faster growth (23, 94). When compared with wild-type virus, HIV with M184V exhibits diminished RT processivity and decreased viral fitness (5, 23, 69, 94).

As stated, the MI84 residue lies in the center of a highly conserved YMDD motif (residues 183–186), in which the two DD residues are believed to participate in polymerase activity (31, 39, 109). The disparity in levels of resistance to 3TC versus ddI, ddC, and ABC may be explained by molecular differences between the two 2',3'-dideoxy derivatives of deoxycytidine; 3TC has a sulfur in place of the 3'-carbon of ddC. This suggests that the sugar moiety is important in NRTI-RT interactions. In fact, crystallographic studies suggested a steric hindrance between the side chains of RTs containing either 184V or I substitutions and the sugar ring of 3TCTP.

Researchers are currently debating the exact mechanism and impact of M184V-induced resistance. 3TCTP is about 50 times less effective against M184V-mutated than wild-type RT, yet little difference exists between these enzymes in regard to recognition of dNTP substrates (23, 94). A 200-fold resistance to 3TCTP is seen in endogenous RT assays (94, 95). Although the level of resistance seen in cell-free assays is lower than the 1,000-fold increase in IC_{50} values measured in tissue culture, the biochemical data clearly indicate diminished rates of incorporation of 3TC-MP. However, the probability of 3TC-MP being added by the RT-M184V in vivo is not negligible. Biochemical studies have shown that the incorporation efficiency of 3TC-MP is as high as the formation of frequently occurring G:T mismatches by the same mutant enzyme (24).

Despite harboring M184V-mutated HIV, patients treated with 3TC maintained a relatively low plasma RNA copy number over protracted periods (111). The reasons for this observation are largely unknown. However, it should be noted that the mutant enzyme is not capable of removing incorporated 3TC-MP via pyrophosphorolysis or nucleotide-dependent primer unblocking reactions (34). Thus, 3TC-MP, if eventually incorporated, may block DNA synthesis in irreversible fashion and may contribute to a reduction of viral burden. In contrast, as stated above, increased rates of removal of the chain terminator are seen with ZDV-resistant mutant enzymes. These observations suggest that ZDV and 3TC-resistance patterns are not compatible (34), which helps to explain why the M184V mutation can resensitize viruses containing ZDV-resistance-associated mutations to the latter drug, at least on a transient basis (69).

The sustained antiviral effect of ZDV makes the selection of resistance to ZDV by viruses containing the 184V mutation a difficult task (69, 127). Interestingly, M184V may also increase the fidelity of the polymerization reaction by causing a conformational change at the RT catalytic site (24, 46, 88, 99, 127). This could have the effect of helping to limit genetic variation in some cases (91, 124, 127). This concept might prove significant in hosts with early-stage disease, in whom immune responses might be effective at holding viral load at bay. Viral load rebound in formerly suppressed hosts can be correlated with the rapid development of high-level resistance to 3TC (111). The combination of 3TC and ZDV produced greater and more sustainable increases in CD4 counts and superior reductions in viral load than either drug alone (22, 51, 118). The performance of these two drugs also exceeded that of ddC plus ZDV in raising the CD4 count, although both combinations resulted in similar drops in viral load. After 24 weeks in these studies, viral isolates were sensitive to ZDV but not to 3TC. 3TC may be effective in concert with other drugs, as well, if the lower fitness of M184V-mutant HIV is involved in the success of 3TC plus ZDV. However, it should be noted that viruses resistant to both ZDV and 3TC have emerged in patients on prolonged therapy with both these agents. Multiple-drug resistance can also be the result of recombination (38).

Mutations Encoding Resistance to Other NRTIs

Resistance to ddC

Many of the mutations that encode resistance against other nucleosides, such as ddI, ddC, and d4T, are located on the β3-β4 and p4 strand loop of RT of the p66 fingers subdomain; these are commonly mutations of a single residue (47, 83, 107, 123). These substitutions confer moderate levels of resistance and decrease the sensitivity of recombinant RT enzymes to NRTI triphosphates in cell-free RT assays. These alterations do not confer cross-resistance to ZDV but do against other 2′,3′-dideoxynucleoside analogs in tissue culture assays. Such mutations appear infrequently in viral samples taken from hosts on protracted drug therapy.

K65R (lysine → arginine at codon 65) has been found in viruses grown in culture in the presence of ddC and has also been implicated in cross-resistance among ddI, 3TC, and 9(2-phosphonylmethoxyethyl) adenine (PMEA) (37, 41, 139) and PMPA. Viral samples from patients on ddC or ddI for prolonged periods may have the K65R mutation (37, 139), which is located in a conserved IKKK (amino acids 63–66) motif within the β3-β4 connecting loop of the fingers subdomain of RT. In addition, T69D (threonine → aspartic acid at codon 69) has been shown to encode resistance against ddC after prolonged treatment. This mutation can also confer cross-resistance to other nucleosides.

The crystal structure of the ternary RT-DNA-dNTP complex showed that residue K65 interacts with the β-phosphate of an incoming dNTP. The mechanism of resistance of K65R has been widely analyzed, and kinetic experiments show that recombinant mutated RT containing K65R had an increased K_m value for dCTP and dATP, relative to wild-type RT, but not for dTTP or dGTP. This research, involving the four natural nucleoside bases of DNA, was performed using either synthetic homopolymeric template/primers or a heteropolymeric HIV-1 genomic RNA-derived template containing primer-binding sequences as well as repeated (R) and 5' unique (U5) regions. A two- to threefold increase in the V_{max}/K_m ratio (an index of enzymatic efficiency) was found for dCTP and dATP. Furthermore, in comparison with wild-type RT standards, the K_i and K_i/K_m values for K65R RT, calculated to normalize changes in regard to substrate recognition, increased between 10- and 20-fold for ddCTP, 3TCTP, and ddA 5'-triphosphate (the intracellular active form of ddI) (36). Thus, this mutation selectively distorts catalytic recognition of dNTPs/ddNTPs, resulting in resistance. K65R also resulted in an increase in K_i for ZDVTP, indicating potential interaction of the enzyme with dNTPs/ddNTPs (direct or indirect) during polymerization. This may account for the cross-resistance conferred by K65R.

Dideoxynucleoside analog triphosphates competitively inhibit the activity of RT polymerase by competing with their homologous dNTPs in the context of a complementary template (36). Presumably, chain termination is the primary consequence of this interaction. Studies of chain elongation/dNTP incorporation have further demonstrated that K65R-mutated RT was less susceptible to various NTP analogs, including ddCTP, 3TCTP, ddATP, ddI 5'-triphosphate (ddITP), PMEA diphosphate (PMEApp), and ZDVTP in reactions employing an HIV-1 genome–derived template plus either a deoxyoligonucleotide or tRNA[Lys3] as a cognate primer to initiate RT activity (35, 41).

When compared with its wild-type counterpart, K65R-mutated RT displayed unusual chain termination frequencies at different complementary RNA template bases (35). This might be caused by the template's secondary structure or by pausing or both. Another peculiarity of the mutated RT was that pausing frequencies were lessened at certain sites with increased ddNTP concentration despite its similar processivity to wild-type RT. This, too, might be explained by the fact that K65R encodes drug resistance. Areas of decreased frequency of chain termination and diminished pausing may also be important in K65R-mediated resistance to NRTIs; this mutation may indirectly alter template-RT interactions.

Resistance to ddI

The clinical significance of ddI resistance is still unknown, as such diminished sensitivity is usually moderate (5- to 10-fold increase in IC_{50}) and is not always correlated with the L74V mutation, which encodes resistance to this drug (1, 2).

The L74V mutation was described in patients who were switched from ZDV to ddI; this mutation resulted in a 6- to 24-fold decrease in ddI sensitivity after 6–12 months of therapy. It also resensitized ZDV-resistant virus to the latter drug (120). However, mutations at codons 65, 74, and 181 (encoding resistance to NNRTIs) and 184 can all confer resistance to single agents while partially restoring ZDV susceptibility.

The antiviral affect of ddI was found to be significantly increased in the presence of the anticancer agent hydroxyurea (HU). Possible mechanisms that help to explain the antiviral effects of HU alone and in combination with NRTIs have recently been summarized (70). Briefly, HU inhibits the cellular enzyme ribonucleotide reductase, which ultimately results in reduced dNTP pools in the cytoplasm. Since NRTIs compete with natural dNTPs for incorporation, it is currently thought that the augmented antiviral effect of HU is attributable to increased NRTI/dNTP ratios that will facilitate incorporation of the chain terminator. Combining ddI, PMPA, or PMEA with HU is particularly efficient because of the pronounced reduction of cellular dATP pools (89). However, the presence of HU does not prevent the emergence of resistance-conferring mutations in the RT enzyme.

Although resistance to ddI is moderate and slow to develop, its emergence is often a function of disease stage. ZDV-experienced patients with high viral loads and CD4 counts in the 100–150/µl range who were switched to ddI exhibited the L74V mutation as early as eight weeks after a change in therapy (96, 97). This is illustrative of the rapid generation of mutations in patients with high viral burden, due to more extensive HIV replication, and contrasts with the infrequent resistance to ddI found in early-stage patients. A study of 50 patients with a median CD4 count of 320/µl who switched from ZDV monotherapy to ddI revealed only one case of high-level resistance (80).

L74V also encodes cross-resistance to ddC (120). Patients who had formerly received ZDV and later developed resistance to ddI became resensitized to ZDV in some cases. Their viral RTs were sequenced and found to contain both L74V and T215Y, a hallmark of ZDV resistance. The joint presence of both mutations within a recombinant HIV-1 clone reversed ZDV resistance, although not that of ddI or ddC (120), suggesting that RT subdomain interactions are complex. It is unclear how L74V reverses the ZDV-resistance effect of T215Y, since residues 74 and 215 are distant from each other in the RT crystal structure; the former is in the β4 fingers subdomain and the latter in the β11a palm subdomain (123).

The altered recognition of natural substrate deoxynucleotides and dideoxynucleotide inhibitors by L74V-mutant RT helps to explain the mechanism of resistance against these agents. Mutated RTs also behave differently than wild type in interaction with templates of various lengths. Wild-type RT is especially sensitive to ddNTP analogs when long templates are employed and is especially resistant when the template overhang is three nucleotides or shorter. L74V-mutant RT was resistant to template extensions of any length (13), suggesting that distorted RT template interactions may afford partial resistance to NRTIs. In fact, the RT-DNA-dNTP structure shows interactions between residue 74 and the template nucleoside that is base-paired with the incoming dNTP. Moreover, both the L74V and the M184V substitution showed diminished processivity, which may, at least in part, explain the reduced replication fitness of these HIV variants (5, 113).

Surprisingly, recombinant HIV containing K65R and L74V did not show any ZDV resistance in tissue culture assays, despite the increased K_i values for ZDVTP in cell-free assays using RTs containing these same mutations (36, 74). Thus, other factors may also be involved such as the viral nucleocapsid protein that plays a key role in initiation of reverse transcription and in template switching in cell-free RT reactions (6, 70).

Resistance to d4T

V75T (valine → threonine at codon 75) has been shown to confer about sevenfold resistance to d4T by molecular mutagenesis (61). V75T did not afford cross-resistance to ZDV (even though the latter is chemically related to the thymidine-derived d4T) but did to other 2′,3′-dideoxynucleoside analogs.

However, the V75T mutation is rarely observed in patients receiving d4T, even in cases in which some degree of phenotypic resistance to this drug is present. Typical viral isolates from patients on d4T show low-level resistance (e.g., three- to fivefold), and one study located V75T in only one of five viral isolates taken from patients who had developed d4T resistance (71). The same study found only a low degree of reduced sensitivity to d4T after long-term monotherapy. Only 2 out of 32 patients treated with d4T between 6 and 30 months harbored V75T. In these cases, d4T susceptibility was reduced by only twofold. In fact, a patient who did not have V75T registered the greatest degree of resistance to d4T in this study, that is, 12-fold after 1.5 years of monotherapy (71).

Isolates from 5 out of 11 patients on d4T monotherapy in the same trial showed decreased susceptibility to ZDV, indicating possible cross-resistance between the two drugs. Even so, HIV containing ZDV-resistance-encoding mutations (codons 67, 70, 215, and 219) remained susceptible to both ddI and d4T. d4T-resistant viruses may sometimes exhibit a nonreciprocated cross-resistance to other agents.

Other Mutations

E89G (glutamate → glycine at codon 89) can reduce viral sensitivity to ddGTP as well as to other ddNTPs and to the pyrophosphate analog phosphonoformic acid (foscarnet, PFA). This mutation was initially identified in vitro during screening of bacterially expressed RT in regard to various ddNTPs (93). However, E89G only effects resistance to PFA in tissue culture (55). Although this mutation has also been seen in cell cultures containing 3TC-resistant virus, it did not itself confer resistance to 3TC, nor does it affect the normal resistance patterns of M184V containing viruses or RTs. Exceptionally, E89G may encode some cross-resistance to NNRTIs (54). E89G is found on the β5a strand in the palm subdomain, two or three amino acids downstream of the polymerase active site, where the template strand makes contact with the enzyme "template grip" (123). Besides altering the recognition of RT for dNTP/ddNTPs, E89G also increased enzymatic activation of dNTPs and processivity. Substrate utilization was also affected by the presence of this mutation on the p66 subunit, while reaction velocity was increased by its presence on both the p66 and p51 subunits (55). E89G can also alter the dependence of RT on template length relative to wild-type RT, as was found with L74V. Finally, E89G caused RT to lose divalent cation preference (93). Recently, a novel drug-resistant point mutation, P157S, which is also located in the "template grip," has been described. This mutation confers low-level resistance to 3TC and shows increased sensitivity to ZDV and PMPA (116).

Multidrug Resistance to NRTIs

Resistance to a variety of 2',3'-dideoxynucleoside analogs, including ZDV, ddI, ddC, d4T, 3TC, and ddG (but not to NNRTIs or PFA) is encoded by five other RT mutations: A62V (alanine → valine), V75I (valine → isoleucine), F77L (phenylalanine → leucine), F116Y (alanine → tyrosine), and Q151M (glutamine → methionine) (114). These mutations were observed in viral isolates from patients taking ZDV plus either ddI or ddC for more than one year. These isolates did not display other substitutions associated with resistance against ZDV, ddI, or ddC in monotherapy.

Limitations of RT function and structure or induced genotypic features of the virus, or both, may account for the failure of certain mutations to appear sometimes (112). The above-mentioned five mutations developed sequentially, beginning with Q151M (notwithstanding the double nucleotide substitution required to produce it), followed by F116Y and F77L in hosts receiving ZDV/ddC or ZDV/ddI combinations (18, 114). Q151M alone resulted in low-level resistance against the analogs listed above, while combinations of mutations cumulatively increased resistance to these agents.

Residues Q151 and F116 are found within the highly conserved α and β motifs of RT, respectively. Both codons are located in close proximity to the dNTP-binding site. V75, F79, and Q151 are near the first template base according to crystallographic studies, which lends credence to the idea that these three amino acids form part of the "template grip" (114, 123). Mutations at these three codons may simulate the same pattern of drug resistance as seen with mutations at residues E89, L74, and K65, since both of these trios are neighbors in the crystal structure of the enzyme. When compared with wild-type RT, enzymes containing these substitutions displayed increased K_i values for ZDVTP, while both types of RT displayed similar enzymatic efficiency (44). Finally, it has recently been shown that a family of insertion mutations between codons 67 and 70 cause resistance to a variety of NRTIs, including ZDV, 3TC, ddI, ddC, and d4T. Usually, these insertion mutations confer multidrug resistance in a ZDV-resistant background (63, 122, 133). Biochemical data suggest that the additional residues are also responsible for low-level resistance to ddI (12).

Multidrug Resistance and Combination Therapy

The use of combinations of anti-HIV drugs (e.g., NRTIs plus NNRTIs), both in vitro and in vivo, will commonly result in a synergistic inhibition of viral replication. The different modes of action of these two classes of drugs may, at least in part, explain the synergy that emerges from the use of various dNTPs and NNRTIs in combination (100). In contrast, mostly additive effects are seen in regard to inhibition of RT polymerase activity when ddNTPs and NNRTIs are studied in cell-free assays (40, 132). This suggests that ARVs may block HIV replication by somewhat different mechanisms in infected cells versus cell-free reactions.

This issue of synergy in culture versus additive effects in biochemical assays may relate to the blocking of integrase and the RT-associated RNase H activity by ddNTP metabolites (75). Disease stage and cell activation state may also be important factors. NRTIs may be phosphorylated more rapidly in some cell types than in others and in actively infected cells more so than in latently infected T cells or monocytes. Consistent with the fact that various NRTIs are metabolized differently and do not, in general, affect phosphorylation pathways of other drugs, simultaneous therapy with different NRTIs is commonly effective. The exception to this rule is the joint use of d4T and ZDV, in which case the simultaneous use of both drugs can reduce phosphorylation efficiency, since similar enzymatic pathways are involved.

Even with the success of combination therapy, all multidrug trials have yielded some degree of resistance, including multiple-drug resistance, both in vivo and in culture (22, 32, 42, 67, 114). Alternating regimens with single agents have commonly led to multiple resistance and should be discouraged (32). Multidrug resistance may also result from the fusion of cells that are infected by different drug-resistant strains, generating particles that contain hybrid genomic strands of RNA (38). In this case, reverse transcription may allow for strand transfer to recombine the retroviral genome. Recombination protocols in culture have yielded multiple resistance to ZDV, 3TC, other dNTPs, and PR inhibitors.

Peculiar RT phenotypes can be generated by the differential presence of resistance-conferring substitutions. Combinations of both L74V- and ZDV-resistance-conferring mutations increased susceptibility to ZDV but not ddI. HIV containing M184V as well as T215Y and M41L had decreased resistance to ZDV alone (but not to ddI or 3TC) (67, 125). The combination of M41L and T215Y and/or L74V together with V106A (encoding NNRTI resistance) did not affect levels of resistance to ZDV, ddI, or nevirapine, whereas the addition of M184V reduced ZDV resistance (69). HIV containing M41L, L74V, T215Y, and Y181C (encoding resistance to most NNRTIs) had almost no resistance to ZDV while still remaining insensitive to nevirapine and ddI.

At the same time, the presence of multiple mutations does not change all enzyme characteristics. Recombinant RTs containing both M184V and K65R performed comparably to K65R RT in reactions that tested chain termination (37, 61). In addition, recombinant HIV containing both M184V and either K65R or V75T displayed similar levels of drug resistance as singly mutated viruses (35).

Combinations of ZDV and either ddI or NNRTIs postponed the development of resistance to ddI and nevirapine without altering the emergence of ZDV resistance in either alternating or simultaneous treatment protocols (57, 119). This might be due to the dependence of ZDV phosphorylation on cell activation, a factor that may not be germane in the case of ddI, since plasma HIV-1 is likely produced in large part by activated CD4+ T lymphocytes. ZDV sensitivity was increased when either L74V- or NNRTI-resistance-encoding mutations were combined with ZDV-resistant mutations, suggesting that infected activated CD4+ cells with the aforementioned RT mutations may be inhibited by ZDV.

Moreover, it has recently been shown that multidrug resistance is not necessarily associated with mutations in the RT gene or other parts of the viral genome (87, 110, 115). An increased efflux of NRTIs is found associated with excess levels of multidrug-resistance-associated proteins (MRPs). MRP4 was identified as a ZDV-dependent drug transporter that is linked to the efflux of nucleoside MP analogs from human cells (115).

Clinical Significance of HIV Drug Resistance

NRTI therapy lowers patient viral load, boosts CD4 levels, and curbs the risk of opportunistic infection. Many studies have associated increased plasma viral burden with drug resistance (9, 58, 81, 114). After treatment, certain patients harbored mostly drug-resistant HIV, but viral titer did not always rise. Elevated viremic levels can often be correlated with the development of drug-resistant strains (79). In regard to multidrug resistance, plasma viral RNA levels were not always correlated with IC_{50} values. An appearance of the Q151M or K70R mutation was often followed by increased viral burden over pretreatment levels (114). In contrast, no further increase in viral RNA copy number occurred owing to the generation of viruses containing multiple-resistance-associated mutations, conferring synergistic or additive effects (53, 114). Such outcomes might be underpinned by differences in disease stage, phenotypic and genotypic features of individual viruses, and the state of immune responsiveness in various hosts. The T215Y mutation may confer a harmful prognosis (49). The presence of the SI phenotype may also cut $CD4^+$ levels during ZDV treatment to a greater extent than seen with NSI variants (59).

CD4 cell count declines, incidence of opportunistic disease, and rates of death have shown that ZDV-resistant children apparently suffered a more rapid disease progression than children who remained ZDV sensitive (84, 86, 126). Children with low CD4s were also more likely to have ZDV-resistant strains, a likely reflection of elevated viral burden and disease progression. Children receiving combination therapy showed less evidence of disease progression than those on ZDV monotherapy.

In adults as well as children, increases in viral load and reductions in $CD4^+$ count did not always correlate with resistance to 3TC and the presence of M184V. When 3TC was combined with other agents in culture, cross-resistance to 3TC and other analogs and/or NNRTIs was not observed. This may be due to slower growth of M184V mutant virus as mentioned above (5, 69).

Other Considerations

Another important consideration is the concept of "genetic barrier." The lengthy time delay (6–24 months) between the initiation of ZDV treatment and development of resistance may, in part, be a function of the number of mutations that must be present and selected in order for resistance to be detected. This is also true in regard to PR inhibitors such as indinavir. On the other hand, resistance can develop swiftly to drugs such as 3TC owing to single point mutations such as M184V.

One must further consider that some primary infections may themselves be caused by drug-resistant forms of HIV, as mutant virus can be transmitted intravenously or sexually to new hosts. Incomplete patient compliance with drug regimens may result in suboptimal levels of ARVs in the blood and suboptimal antiviral pressure, leading to drug resistance. These considerations are of obvious public health importance.

In the absence of drug pressure, wild-type viruses are those that are most fit for replication. Drugs select for the proliferation of mutant resistant viruses. Effective inhibition of viral replication by a combination of antiretroviral agents should reduce the incidence of resistance, since non-replicating HIV cannot mutate.

REFERENCES

1. Abrams, D. I., A. I. Goldman, C. Launer, et al. 1994. A comparative trial of didanosine or zalcitabine after treatment with zidovudine in patients with human immunodeficiency virus infection. N. Engl. J. Med. 330:657–662.
2. Antonelli, G., F. Dianzani, D. Bellarosa, et al. 1994. Drug combination of AZT and ddI synergism of action and prevention of appearance of AZT-resistance. Antiviral Chem. Chemother. 5:51–55.
3. Arion, D., N. Kaushik, S. McCosmic, et al. 1998. Phenotypic mechanism of HIV-1 resistance to 3'-azido-3' deoxythymidine (AZT): increased polymerization processivity and enhanced sensitivity to pyrophosphate of the mutant viral reverse transcriptase. Biochemistry 37:15908–15917.
4. Arts, E. J., and M. A. Wainberg. 1996. Mechanisms of nucleoside analog antiviral activity and resistance during human immunodeficiency virus reverse transcription. Antimicrob. Agents Chemother. 40:527–540.
5. Back, N. K., M. Nijhuis, W. Keulen, et al. 1996. Reduced replication of 3TC-resistant HIV-1 variants in primary cells due to a processivity defect of the reverse transcriptase enzyme. EMBO J. 15:4040–4049.
6. Barat, C., V. Lullien, O. Schatz, et al. 1989. HIV-1 reverse transcriptase specifically interacts with the anticodon domain of its cognate primer tRNA. EMBO J. 8:3279–3285.
7. Bebenek, K., J. Abbotts, S. H. Wilson, et al. 1993. Error-prone polymerization by HIV-1 reverse transcriptase: contribution of template-primer misalignment, miscoding, and termination probability to mutational spots. J. Biol. Chem. 268:10324–10334.
8. Boucher, C. A. B., N. Cammack, P. Schipper, et al. 1993. High-level resistance to (−)enantiomeric 2'-deoxy-3'-thiacytidine in vitro is due to one amino acid substitution in the catalytic site of human immunodeficiency virus type 1 reverse transcriptase. Antimicrob. Agents Chemother. 37:B2231–2234.

9. Boucher, C. A. B., J. M. A. Lange, F. F. Miedema, et al. 1992. HIV-1 biological phenotype and the development of zidovudine resistance in relation to disease progression in asymptomatic individuals during treatment. AIDS 6:1259–1264.

10. Boucher, C. A. B., E. O'Sullivan, J. W. Mulder, et al. 1992. Ordered appearance of zidovudine (AZT) resistance mutations during treatment. J. Infect. Dis. 165:105–110.

11. Boulerice, F., S. Bour, R. Geleziunas, et al. 1990. High frequency of isolation of defective human immunodeficency virus type 1 and heterogeneity of viral gene expression in clones of infected U-937 cells. J. Virol. 64:1745–1755.

12. Boyer, P. L., J. Lisziewicz, F. Lori, et al. 1999. Analysis of amino insertion mutations in the fingers subdomain of HIV-1 reverse transcriptase. J. Mol. Biol. 286:995–1008.

13. Boyer, P. L., C. Tantill, A. Jacobo-Molina, et al. 1994. The sensitivity of wild-type human immunodeficiency virus type 1 reverse transcriptase to dideoxynucleotides depends on template length; the sensitivity of drug-resistant mutations does not. Proc. Natl. Acad. Sci. USA 91:4882–4886.

14. Caliendo, A., A. Savara, D. An, et al. 1995. ZDV resistance mutations increase replication in drug-free PBMC stimulated after infection. Fourth International Workshop on HIV Drug Resistance, Sardinia, Italy, abstr. 4:4.

15. Canard, B., S. R. Sarfati, and C. C. Richardson. 1998. Enhanced binding of azidothymidine-resistant human immunodeficency virus 1 reverse transcriptase to the 3'-azido-3'-deoxythymidine 5'-mono-phosphate-terminated primer. J. Biol. Chem. 273:14596–14604.

16. D'Aquila, R. T., V. A. Johnson, S. L. Welles, et al. 1995. Zidovudine resistance and HIV-1 disease progression during antiretroviral therapy. Ann. Intern. Med. 122:401–408.

17. De Boer, R. J., C. A. B. Boucher, and A. S. Perelson. 1998. Target cell availability and the successful suppression of HIV by hydroxyurea and didanosine. AIDS 12:1567–1570.

18. De Clercq, E. 1994. HIV resistance to reverse transcriptase inhibitors. Biochem. Pharmacol. 47:155–169.

19. Ding, J., K. Das, H. Moereels, et al. 1995. Structure of HIV-1 RT/TIBO R 86183 complex reveals similarity in the binding of diverse non-nucleoside inhibitors. Nat. Struct. Biol. 2:407–415.

20. El-Farrash, M. A., M. J. Kuroda, T. Kitazaki, et al. 1994. Generation and characterization of a human immunodeficiency virus type 1 (HIV-1) mutant resistant to an HIV-1 protease inhibitor. J. Virol. 68:233–239.

21. Eron, J. J., S. L. Benoit, J. Jemsek, et al. 1995. Treatment with lamivudine, zidovudine, or both in HIV-positive patients with 200 to 500 CD4+ cells per cubic millimeter. N. Engl. J. Med. 333:1662–1669.

22. Eron, J. J., Y. K. Chow, A. M. Caliendo, et al. 1993. pol mutations conferring zidovudine and didanosine resistance with different effects in vitro yield multiply resistant human immunodeficiency virus type 1 isolates in vivo. Antimicrob. Agents Chemother. 37:1480–1487.

23. Faraj, A., L. A. Agrofoglio, J. K. Wakefield, et al. 1994. Inhibition of human immunodeficiency virus type 1 reverse transcriptase by the 5'-triphosphate

β enantiomers of cytidine analogs. Antimicrob. Agents Chemother. 38:2300–2305.

24. Feng, J. Y., and K. S. Anderson. 1999. Mechanistic studies examining the efficiency and fidelity of DNA synthesis by the 3TC-resistant mutant (184V) of HIV-1 reverse transcriptase. Biochemistry 38:9440–9448.

25. Finzi, D., J. Blankson, J. D. Siliciano, et al. 1997. Latent infection of CD4$^+$ T cells provides a mechanism for lifelong persistence of HIV-1, even in patients on effective combination therapy. Nature Med. 5:512–7.

26. Fischl, M. A., D. D. Richman, D. M. Causey, et al. 1989. Prolonged zidovudine therapy in patients with AIDS and advanced AIDS-related complex. JAMA 262:2405–2410.

27. Fischl, M. A., D. D. Richman, M. H. Grieco, et al. 1987. The efficacy of azidothymidine (AZT) in the treatment of patients with AIDS and AIDS-related complex: a double-blind placebo-controlled trial. N. Engl. J. Med. 317:185–191.

28. Fitzgibbon, J. E., R. M. Howell, C. A. Haberzettl, et al. 1992. Human immunodeficiency virus type 1 pol gene mutations which cause decreased susceptibility to 2′,3′-dideoxycytidine. Antimicrob. Agents Chemother. 36:153–157.

29. Furman, P. A., J. A. Fyfe, M. H. St. Clair, et al. 1986. Phosphorylation of 3′-azido-3′ deoxythymidine and selective interactions of the 5′-triphosphate with human immunodeficiency virus reverse transcriptase. Proc. Natl. Acad. Sci. USA 83:8333–8337.

30. Gao, Q., Z. Gu, M. A. Parniak, et al. 1992. In vitro selection of variants of human immunodeficiency virus type 1 resistant to 3′-azido-3′-deoxythymidine and 2′,3′-dideoxyinosine. J. Virol. 66:12–19.

31. Gao, Q., Z. Gu, M. A. Parniak, et al. 1993. The same mutation that encodes low-level human immunodeficiency virus type 1 resistance to 2′,3′-dideoxyinosine and 2′,3′ dideoxycytidine confers high-level resistance to the (−)enantiomer of 2′,3′-dideoxy-3′-thiacytidine. Antimicrob. Agents Chemother. 37:1390–1392.

32. Gao, Q., Z. Gu, H. Salomon, et al. 1994. Generation of multiple drug resistance by sequential in vitro passage of the human immunodeficiency virus type 1. Arch. Virol. 136:111–122.

33. Götte, M., D. Arion, L. Cellai, et al. 1999. Effects of nucleoside and non-nucleoside analogue RT inhibitors on the initiation of HIV-1 plus-strand DNA synthesis. Antiviral Therapy 4:18, abstr. 23.

34. Götte, M., D. Arion, M. A. Parniak, et al. 1999. Mechanisms of HIV-1 resistance to zidovudine and lamivudine. Antiviral Therapy 4:18, abstr. 22.

35. Gu, Z., E. J. Arts, M. A. Parniak, et al. 1995. Mutated K65R recombinant HIV-1 reverse transcriptase shows diminished chain termination in the presence of 2′,3′-dideoxycytidine-5′-triphosphate and other drugs. Proc. Natl. Acad. Sci. USA 92:2760–2764.

36. Gu, Z., R. S. Fletcher, E. J. Arts, et al. 1994. The K65R mutant reverse transcriptase of HIV-1 cross resistance to 2′,3′-dideoxycytidine, 2′,3′-dideoxy-3′-thiacytidine, and 2′,3′-dideoxyinosine shows reduced sensitivity to specific dideoxynucleoside triphosphate inhibitors in vitro. J. Biol. Chem. 269:28118–28122.

37. Gu, Z., Q. Gao, H. Fang, et al. 1994. Identification of a mutation at condon 65 in the IKKK motif of reverse transcriptase that encodes human immunodeficiency virus resistance to 2',3'-dideoxycytidine, 2',3'-dideoxy-3'-thiacytidine. Antimicrob. Agents Chemother. 38:275–281.

38. Gu, Z., Q. Gao, E. A. Faust, et al. 1995. Possible involvement of cell fusion and viral recombination in generation of human immunodeficiency virus variants that display dual drug resistance. J. Gen. Virol. 76:2601–2605.

39. Gu, Z., Q. Gao, X. Li, et al. 1992. Novel mutation in the human immunodeficiency virus type 1 reverse transcriptase gene that encodes crossresistance to 2',3'-dideoxyinosine and 2',3'-dideoxycytidine. J. Virol. 66:7128–7135.

40. Gu, Z., Y. Quan, Z. Li, et al. 1995. Effects of non-nucleosides inhibitors of human immunodeficiency virus type 1 in cell-free recombinant reverse transcriptase assay. J. Biol. Chem. 270:31046–31051.

41. Gu, Z., H. Salomon, J. M. Cherrington, et al. 1995. The K65R mutation of human immunodeficiency virus type 1 reverse transcriptase encodes resistance to 9-(2-phosphonyl-methoxyethyl)adenine. Antimicrob. Agents Chemother. 38:1888–1891.

42. Gunthard, H. F., J. K. Wong, C. C. Ignacio, et al. 1998. Human immunodeficiency virus replication and genotypic resistance in blood and lymph nodes after a year of potent antiretroviral therapy. J. Virol. 72:2422–2428.

43. Hart, G. J., D. C. Orr, C. R. Penn, et al. 1992. Effects of (–) 2'-deoxy-3'-thiacytidine (3TC) 5'-triphosphate on human immunodeficiency virus reverse transcriptase and mammalian DNA polymerases alpha, beta and gamma. Antimicrob. Agents Chemother. 37:918–920.

44. Ho, D. D. 1995. Time to hit HIV, early and hard. N. Engl. J. Med. 333:450–451.

45. Ho, D. D., A. U. Neumann, A. S. Perelson, et al. 1995. Rapid turnover of plasma virions and CD4 lymphocytes in HIV-1 infection. Science 273:123–126.

46. Hsu, M., P. Inouye, L. Rezende, et al. 1997. Higher fidelity of RNA-dependent DNA mispair extension by M184V drug-resistant reverse transcriptase of human immunodeficiency virus type 1. Nucleic Acids Res. 25:4532–4536.

47. Huang, H., R. Chopra, G. L. Verdine, et al. 1998. Structure of a covalently trapped catalytic complex of HIV-1 reverse transcriptase: implications for drug resistance. Science 282:1669–1675.

48. Jacobo-Molina, A., J. Ding, R. G. Nanni, et al. 1993. Crystal structure of human immunodeficiency virus type 1 reverse transcriptase complexed with double-stranded DNA at 3.0 Å resolution shows bent DNA. Proc. Natl. Acad. Sci. USA 90:6320–6324.

49. Japour, A. J., S. Welles, R. T. D'Aquila, et al. 1995. Prevalence and clinical significance of zidovudine resistance mutations in human immunodeficiency virus isolated from patients after long-term zidovudine treatment. J. Infect. Dis. 171:1172–1179.

50. Kahn, J. O., S. W. Lagakos, D. D. Richman, et al. 1992. A controlled trial comparing continued zidovudine with didanosine in human immunodeficiency virus infection: the NIAID AIDS Clinical Trials Group. N. Engl. J. Med. 327:581–587.

51. Katlama, C., D. Ingrand, C. Loveday, et al. 1996. Safety and efficacy of lamivudine-zidovudine combination therapy in antiretroviral-naive patients: a ran-

domized controlled comparison with zidovudine monotherapy. JAMA 276:118–125.

52. Kavlick, M. F., T. Shirasaka, E. Kojima, et al. 1995. Genotypic and phenotypic characterization of HIV-1 isolated from patients receiving (–)2′,3′-dideoxy-3′-thiacytidine. Antiviral Res. 28:133–146.

53. Kellam, P., C. A. B. Boucher, and B. A. Larder. 1992. Fifth mutation in human immunodeficiency virus type 1 reverse transcriptase contributes to the development of high-level resistance to zidovudine. Proc. Natl. Acad. Sci. USA 89:1934–1938.

54. Kew, Y., H. Salomon, L. R. Olsen, et al. 1996. The nucleoside analog-resistant E89G mutant of human immunodeficiency virus type 1 reverse transcriptase displays a broader cross-resistance that extends to nonnucleoside inhibitors. Antimicrob. Agents Chemother. 40:1711–1714.

55. Kew, Y., Q. Song, and V. R. Prasad. 1994. Subunit-selective mutagenesis of Glu-89 residue in human immunodeficiency virus reverse transcriptase. J. Biol. Chem. 269:15331–15336.

56. Kohlstaedt, L. A., J. Wang, J. M. Friedman, et al. 1992. Crystal structure at 3.5 Å resolution of HIV-1 reverse transcriptase complexed with an inhibitor. Science 256:1783–1790.

57. Kojima, E., T. Shirasaka, B. D. Anderson, et al. 1995. Human immunodeficiency virus type 1 (HIV-1) viremia changes and development of drug-related mutations in patients with symptomatic HIV-1 infection receiving alternating or simultaneous zidovudine and didanosine therapy. J. Infect. Dis. 171:1152–1158.

58. Kozal, M. J., R. W. Shafer, M. A. Winters, et al. 1993. A mutation in human immunodeficiency virus reverse transcriptase and decline in CD4 lymphocyte numbers in long-term zidovudine recipients. J. Infect. Dis. 167:526–532.

59. Kozal, M. J., R. W. Shafer, M. A. Winters, et al. 1994. HIV-1 syncytium-inducing phenotype, virus burden, codon 215 reverse transcriptase mutation, and CD4 cell decline in zidovudine-treated patients. J. Acquired Immune Defic. Syndr. 7:832–838.

60. Krebs, R., U. Immendörfer, T. Thrall, et al. 1997. Single-step kinetics of HIV-1 reverse transcriptase mutants responsible for virus resistance to nucleoside inhibitors zidovudine and 3-TC. Biochemistry 36:10292–10300.

61. Lacey, S., and B. A. Larder. 1994. Novel mutation (V75T) in human immunodeficiency virus type 1 reverse transcriptase confers resistance to 2′,3′-didehydro-2′, 3′-dideoxythimidine in cell culture. Antimicrob. Agents Chemother. 38:1428–1432.

62. Lacey, S. F., J. E. Reardon, E. S. Furfine, et al. 1992. Biochemical studies on the reverse transcriptase and RNase H activities from human immunodeficiency virus strains resistant to 3′-azido-3′-deoxythymidine. J. Biol. Chem. 267:15789–15794.

63. Larder, B. A., S. Bloor, S. D. Kemp, et al. 1999. A family of insertion mutations between codons 67 and 70 of human immunodeficiency virus type 1 reverse transcriptase confer multinucleoside analog resistance. Antimicrob. Agents Chemother. 43:1961–1967.

64. Larder, B. A., B. Chesebro, and D. D. Richman. 1990. Susceptibility of zidovudine-susceptible and resistance human immunodeficiency virus isolates to

antiviral agents determined by using a quantitative plaque reduction assay. Antimicrob. Agents Chemother. 34:436–441.

65. Larder, B. A., K. E. Coates, and S. D. Kemp. 1991. Zidovudine-resistant human immunodeficiency virus selected by passage in cell culture. J. Virol. 65:5232–5236.

66. Larder, B. A., G. Darby, and D. D. Richman. 1989. HIV with reduced sensitivity to zidovudine (AZT) isolated during prolonged therapy. Science 243: 1731–1734.

67. Larder, B. A., P. Kellam, and S. D. Kemp. 1993. Convergent combination therapy can select viable multidrug-resistance HIV-1 in vitro. Nature 365: 451–453.

68. Larder, B. A., and S. D. Kemp. 1989. Multiple mutations in HIV-1 reverse transcriptase confer high level resistance to zidovudine (AZT). Science 246: 1155–1158.

69. Larder, B. A., S. D. Kemp, and P. R. Harrigan. 1995. Potential mechanism for sustained antiretroviral efficacy of AZT-3TC combination therapy. Science 269:696–699.

70. Li, X., Y. Quan, E. J. Arts, et al. 1996. HIV-1 nucleocapsid protein (NCp7) directs specific initiation of minus strand DNA synthesis primed by human tRNA^{Lys3} in vitro: studies of viral RNA molecules mutated in regions that flank the primer binding site. J. Virol. 70:4996–5004.

71. Lin, P.-F., H. Samanta, R. E. Rose, et al. 1994. Genotypic and phenotypic analysis of human immunodeficiency virus type 1 isolates from patients on prolonged stavudine therapy. J. Infect. Dis. 170:1157–1164.

72. Loya, S., M. Bakhanashvili, R. Tal, et al. 1994. Enzymatic properties of two mutants of reverse transcriptase of human immunodeficiency virus type 1 (tyrosine 181- and tyrosine 188-Leucine), resistant to non-nucleoside inhibitors. AIDS Res. Hum. Retroviruses 10:939–946.

73. Mansky, L. M., and H. M. Temin. 1995. Lower in vitro mutation rate of human immunodeficiency virus type 1 that predicted from the fidelity of purified reverse transcriptase. J. Virol. 69:5087–5094.

74. Martin, J. L., J. E. Wilson, R. L. Haynes, et al. 1993. Mechanism of resistance of human immunodeficiency virus type 1 to 2′, 3′-dideoxyinosine. Proc. Natl. Acad. Sci. USA 90:6135–6139.

75. Mazumder, A., D. Cooney, R. Agbaria, et al. 1994. Inhibition of human immunodeficiency virus type 1 integrase by 3′-azido-3′-deoxy-thymidine. Proc. Natl. Acad. Sci. USA 91:5771–5775.

76. Mellors, J. W., G. E. Dutschman, G. J. Im, et al. 1992. In vitro selection and molecular characterization of human immunodeficiency virus-1 resistance to non-nucleoside inhibitor of reverse transcriptase. Mol. Pharmacol. 41: 446–451.

77. Meyer, P. R., S. E. Matsuura, A. M. Mian, et al. 1999. A mechanism of AZT resistance: an increase in nucleotide-dependent primer unblocking by mutant HIV-1 reverse transcriptase. Mol. Cell 43:35–43.

78. Mitsuya, H., and S. Broder. 1986. Inhibition of the in vitro infectivity and cytopathic effect of human T-lymphotropic virus type III/lymphadenopathy-associated virus (HTLV-III/LAV) by 2′,3′-dideoxynucleosides. Proc. Natl. Acad. Sci. USA 83:1911–1915.

79. Mohri, H., M. K. Singh, W. T. Ching, et al. 1993. Quantitation of zidovudine-resistant human immunodeficiency virus type 1 in the blood of treated and untreated patients. Proc. Natl. Acad. Sci. USA 90:250–290.

80. Montaner, J. S. G., M. T. Schechter, A. Rachlis, et al. 1995. Didanosine compared with continued zidovudine therapy for HIV-infected patients with 200 to 500 CD4 cells/mm^3: a double-blind, randomized, controlled trial. Ann. Intern. Med. 123:561–571.

81 Montaner, J. S. G., J. Singer, M. T. Schechter, et al. 1993. Clinical correlates of in vitro HIV-1 resistance to zidovudine. Results of the multicentre Canadian AZT trial (MCAT). AIDS 7:189–196.

82. Moore, R. D., J. Hildago, B. W. Sugland, et al. 1991. Zidovudine and the natural history of the acquired immunodeficiency syndrome. N. Engl. J. Med. 324:1412–1416.

83. Nanni, R. G., J. Ding, A. Jacobo-Molina, et al. 1993. Review of HIV-1 reverse transcriptase three-dimensional structure: implication for drug design. Perspect. Drug Design 1:129–150.

84. Nielsen, K., L. S. Wei, M. S. Sim, et al. 1995. Correlation of clinical progression in human immunodeficiency virus-infected children with in vitro zidovudine resistance measured by a direct quantitative peripheral blood lymphocyte assay. J. Infect. Dis. 172:359–364.

85. Nunberg, J. H., W. A. Schleif, E. J. Boots, et al. 1991. Viral resistance to human immunodeficiency virus type 1-specific pyridinone reverse transcriptase inhibitors. J. Virol. 65:4887–4892.

86. Ogino, M. T., W. M. Dankner, S. A. Spector, et al. 1993. Development of zidovudine resistance in children infected with human immunodeficiency virus. J. Pediatr. 123:1–8.

87. Ouar, Z., R. Lacave, M. Bens, et al. 1999. Mechanisms of altered sequestration and efflux of chemotherapeutic drugs by multidrug-resistant cells. Cell Biol. Toxicol. 15:91–100.

88. Oude Essnik, B. B., N. K. Back, and B. Berkhout. 1997. Increased polymerase fidelity of the 3TC-resistant variants of HIV-1 reverse transcriptase. Nucleic Acids Res. 25:3212–3217.

89. Palmer, S., R. W. Shafer, and T. C. Merigan. 1999. Hydroxyurea enhances the activities of didanosine, 9-[2-(phosphonylmethoxy) ethyl] adenine, and 9-[2-(phosphonylmethoxy) propyl] adenine against drug-susceptible and drug-resistant human immunodeficiency virus isolates. Antimicrob. Agents Chemother. 43:2046–2050.

90. Palmer, S., R. W. Shafer, and T. C. Merigan. 1999. Highly drug-resistant HIV-1 clinical isolates are cross-resistant to many antiretroviral compounds in current clinical development. AIDS 13:661–667.

91. Pandey, V. N., N. Kaushik, N. Rege, et al. 1996. Role of methionine 184 of human immunodeficiency virus type-1 transcriptase in the polymerase function and fidelity of DNA synthesis. Biochemistry 35:2168–2179.

92. Pokholok, D. K., S. O. Gudima, D. S. Yesipov, et al. 1993. Interactions of the HIV-1 reverse transcriptase AZT-resistant mutant with substrates and AZTTP. FEBS Lett. 325:237–241.

93. Prasad, V. R., I. Lowy, T. D. L. Santos, et al. 1991. Isolation and characterization of a dideoxyguanosine triphosphate-resistant mutant of human immuno-

deficiency virus reverse transcriptase. Proc. Natl. Acad. Sci. USA 88:11363–11367.

94. Quan, Y., Z. Gu, X. Li, et al. 1996. Mutated HIV-1 M184V reverse transcriptase displays resistance to the triphosphate of (–)2′,3′-dideoxy-3′-thiacytidine (3TC) in both endogenous and cell-free enzyme assays. J. Virol. 70:5642–5645.

95. Quan, Y., Z. Gu, X. Li, C. Liang, et al. 1998. Endogenous reverse transcriptase assays reveal synergy between combinations of the M184V and other drug resistance-conferring mutations in interactions with nucleoside analog triphosphates. J. Mol. Biol. 47:227–237.

96. Reichman, R., N. Tejani, J. Strussenberg, et al. 1992. Antiviral susceptibilities of HIV isolates obtained from long-term recipients of dideoxyinosine (ddI). Presented at the XIII International Conference on AIDS, Amsterdam, July 19–24.

97. Reichman, R. C., N. Tejani, J. L. Lambert, et al. 1993. Didanosine (ddI) and zidovudine (ZDV) susceptibilities of human immunodeficiency virus (HIV) isolates from long-term recipients of ddI. Antiviral Res. 20:267–277.

98. Ren, J., R. Esnouf, E. Garman, et al. 1995. High resolution structures of HIV-1 RT from four RT-inhibitor complexes. Nat. Struct. Biol. 2:293–302.

99. Ricchetti, M., and H. Buc. 1990. Reverse transcriptase and genomic variability: the accuracy of DNA replication is enzyme specific and sequence dependent. EMBO J. 9:1583–1593.

100. Richman, D., A. S. Rosenthal, M. Skoog, et al. 1991. BI-587 is active against zidovudine-resistant human immunodeficiency virus type 1 and synergistic with zidovudine. Antimicrob. Agents Chemother. 35:305–308.

101. Richman, D., C. K. Shih, I. Lowy, et al. 1991. Human immunodeficiency virus type 1 mutants resistant to non-nucleoside inhibitors of reverse transcriptase arise in cell culture. Proc. Natl. Acad. Sci. USA 88:11241–11245.

102. Richman, D. D., D. Havlir, J. Corbeil, et al. 1994. Neviparine resistance mutations of human immunodeficiency virus type 1 selected during therapy. J. Virol. 68:1660–1666.

103. Rittinger, K., G. Divita, and R. S. Goody. 1995. Human immunodeficiency virus reverse transcriptase substrate-induced conformational changes and the mechanism of inhibition by non-nucleoside inhibitors. Proc. Natl. Acad. Sci. USA 92:8046–8049.

104. Roberts, J. D., K. Bebenek, and T. A. Kunkel. 1988. The accuracy of reverse transcriptase from HIV-1. Science 242:1171–1173.

105. Rooke, R., M. Tremblay, H. Soudeyns, et al. 1989. Isolation of drug-resistant variants of HIV-1 from patients on long-term zidovudine (AZT) therapy. AIDS 3:411–415.

106. Sarafianos, S. G., K. Das, A. D. Clark, et al. 1999. Lamivudine (3TC) resistance in HIV-1 reverse transcriptase involves steric hindrance with beta-branched amino acids. Proc. Nat. Acad. Sci. USA 96:10027–10032.

107. Sarafianos, S. G., K. Das, J. Ding, et al. 1999. Touching the heart of HIV-1 drug resistance: the fingers close down on the dNTP at the polymerase active site. Chemistry and Biology 6:R137–146.

108. Schinazi, R. F., B. A. Larder, and J. W. Mellors. 1996. Mutations in retroviral genes associated with drug resistance. International Antiviral News 4:95–107.

109. Schinazi, R. F., R. M. Lloyd, Jr., M. H. Nguyen, et al. 1993. Characterization of human immunodeficiency viruses resistant to oxathiolane-cytosine nucleosides. Antimicrob. Agents Chemother. 37:875–881.

110. Schuetz, J. D., M. C. Connelly, D. X. Sun, et al. 1999. MRP4: a previously unidentified factor in resistance to nucleoside-based antiviral drugs. Nature Med. 5:1048–1051.

111. Schuurman, R., M. Nijhuis, R. V. Leeuwen, et al. 1995. Rapid changes in human immunodeficiency virus type 1 RNA load and appearance of drug-resistant virus populations in persons treated with lamivudine (3TC). J. Infect. Dis. 171:1411–1419.

112. Shafer, R. W., M. J. Kozal, M. A. Winters, et al. 1994. Combination therapy with zidovudine and didanosine selects for drug-resistant human immunodeficiency virus type 1 strains with unique patterns of pol gene mutations. J. Infect. Dis. 169:722–729.

113. Sharma, P. L., and C. S. Crumpacker. 1999. Decreased processivity of human immunodeficiency virus type 1 reverse transcriptase (RT) containing didanosine-selected mutation leu74Val: a comparative analysis of RT variants Leu74Val and lamivudine-selected Met184Val. J. Virol. 73 :8448–8456.

114. Shirasaka, T., M. F. Kavlick, T. Ueno, et al. 1995. Emergence of human immunodeficiency virus type 1 variants with resistance to multiple dideoxynucleosides in patients receiving therapy with dideoxynucleosides. Proc. Natl. Acad. Sci. USA 92:2398–2402.

115. Signoretti, C., G. Romagnoli, O. Turriziani, et al. 1997. Induction of the multidrug-transporter P-glycoprotein by 3′-azido-3′-deoxythymidine (AZT) treatment in tumor cell lines. J. Exp. Clin. Cancer Res. 16:29–32.

116. Smith, R. A., G. J. Klarmann, K. M. Stray, et al. 1999. A new point mutation (P157S) in the reverse transcriptase of human immunodeficiency virus type 1 confers low-level resistance to (−)-beta-2′,3′-dideoxy-3′-thiacytidine. Antimicrob. Agents Chemother. 43:2077–2080.

117. Spence, R. A., W. M. Kati, K. S. Anderson, et al. 1995. Mechanism of inhibition of HIV-1 reverse transcriptase by non-nucleoside inhibitors. Science 267:988–992.

118. Staszewski, S., C. Loveday, J. J. Picazo, et al. 1996. Safety and efficacy of lamivudine-zidovudine combination therapy in zidovudine-experienced patients: a randomized controlled comparison with zidovudine monotherapy. JAMA 276:111–117.

119. Staszewski, S., F. E. Massari, A. Kober, et al. 1995. Combination therapy with zidovudine prevents selection of human immunodeficiency virus type 1 variants expressing high-level resistance to L-6097,661, a non-nucleoside reverse transcriptase inhibitor. J. Infect. Dis. 171:1159–1165.

120. St. Clair, M. H., J. L. Martin, G. Tudor-Williams, et al. 1991. Resistance to ddI and sensitivity to AZT induced by a mutation in HIV-1 reverse transcriptase. Science 253:1557–1559.

121. St. Clair, M. H., C. A. Richards, T. Spector, et al. 1987. 3′-azido-3′-deoxythymidine triphosphate as an inhibitor and substrate of purified human immunodeficiency virus reverse transcriptase. Antimicrob. Agents Chemother. 3:1972–1977.

122. Sugiura, W., M. Matsuda, Z. Matsuda, et al. 1999. Identification of insertion mutations in HIV-1 reverse transcriptase causing multiple drug resistance to nucleoside analogue reverse transcriptase inhibitors. J. Human Virol. 2: 146–153.

123. Tantillo, C., J. Ding, A. Jacobo-Molina, et al. 1994. Location of anti-AIDS drug binding sites and resistance mutations in the three-dimensional structure of HIV-1 reverse transcriptase. J. Mol. Biol. 243:369–387.

124. Temin, H. M. 1993. Retrovirus variation and reverse transcription: abnormal strand transfer results in retrovirus genetic variation. Proc. Natl. Acad. Sci. USA 90:6900–6903.

125. Tisdale, M., S. D. Kemp, N. R. Parry, et al. 1993. Rapid in vitro selection of human immunodeficiency virus type 1 resistance to 3'-thiacytidine inhibitors due to a mutation in the YMDD region of reverse transcriptase. Proc. Natl. Acad. Sci. USA 90:5653–5656.

126. Tudor-Williams, G., M. H. St. Clair, R. E. McKinney, et al. 1992. HIV-1 sensitivity to zidovudine and clinical outcome in children. Lancet 339:15–19.

127. Wainberg, M. A., W. C. Drosopoulos, H. Salomon, et al. 1996. Enhanced fidelity of 3TC-selected mutant HIV-1 reverse transcriptase. Science 271: 1282–1285.

128. Wainberg, M. A., H. Salomon, Z. Gu, et al. 1995. Development of HIV-1 resistance to (–)2'-deoxy-3'-thiacytidine in patients with AIDS or advanced AIDS-related complex. AIDS 9:351–357.

129. Wainberg, M. A., M. Tremblay, R. Rooke, et al. 1990. Characterization of reverse transcriptase activity and susceptibility to other nucleosides of AZT-resistant variants of HIV-1, p. 616:346–352. In V. St. Georgiev and J. J. McGowan (ed.), AIDS: Anti-HIV agents, therapies, and vaccines. Ann. N.Y. Acad. Sci., New York.

130. Wakefield, J. K., S. A. Jablonski, and C. D. Morrow. 1992. In vitro enzymatic activity of human immunodeficiency virus type 1 reverse transcriptase mutants in the highly conserved YMDD amino acid motif correlates with the infectious potential of the proviral genome. J. Virol. 66:6806–6812.

131. Wei, X., S. K. Ghosh, M. E. Taylor, et al. 1995. Viral dynamics in human immunodeficiency virus type 1 infection. Science 273:117–122.

132. White, E. L., W. B. Parker, S. J. Ross, et al. 1993. Lack of synergy in the inhibition of HIV-1 reverse transcriptase by combinations of the 5' triphosphates of various anti-HIV nucleoside analogs. Antiviral Res. 22:295–308.

133. Winters, M. A., K. L. Coolley, Y. A. Girard, et al. 1998. A 6-basepair insert in the reverse transcriptase gene of human immunodeficiency virus type 1 confers resistance to multiple nucleoside. J. Clin. Invest. 102:1769–1775.

134. Wong, J. K., M. Hezareh, H. F. Gunthard, et al. 1997. Recovery of replication-competent HIV despite prolonged suppression of plasma viremia. Science 278:1291–1295.

135. Wu, J. C., T. C. Warren, J. Adams, et al. 1991. A novel dipyridodiazepinone inhibitor of HIV-1 reverse transcriptase acts through a nonsubstrate binding site. Biochemistry 30:2022–2026.

136. Yarchoan, R., R. W. Klecker, K. J. Weinhold, et al. 1986. Administration of 3'-azido-3'-deoxythymidine, an inhibitor of HTLV-III.LAV replication, to patients with AIDS or AIDS-related complex. Lancet 1:575–580.

137. Yarchoan, R., H. Mitsuya, C. E. Myers, et al. 1989. Clinical pharmacology of 3'-azido-2',3'-dideoxythymidine (zidovudine) and related dideoxynucleosides. N. Engl. J. Med. 321:726–738.

138. Yarchoan, R., C. F. Perno, R. V. Thomas, et al. 1988. Phase I studies of 2',3'-dideoxythymidine in severe human immunodeficiency virus infection as a single agent and alternating with zidovudine (AZT). Lancet 1:76–81.

139. Zhang, D., A. M. Caliendo, E. J. Eron, et al. 1994. Resistance to 2',3'-dideoxycytidine conferred by a mutation in condon 65 of the human immunodeficiency virus type 1 reverse transcriptase. Antimicro. Agents Chemother. 38:282–287.

Non-Nucleoside Reverse Transcriptase Inhibitors of HIV-1

4

JAN BALZARINI

Approximately one decade ago, the first leads of highly specific anti–human immunodeficiency virus type 1 (HIV-1) inhibitors were identified (8, 99, 107). Later, numerous other—at the first glance unrelated—structural classes of HIV-1-specific compounds were reported (for an overview, see reference 43). No other lentiviruses (e.g., HIV-2, simian immunodeficiency virus [SIV], feline immunodeficiency virus [FIV], visna virus [VV]), oncoviruses (i.e., murine sarcoma virus [MSV], Moloney murine leukemia virus [Mo-MuLV]), DNA viruses, or RNA viruses were sensitive to the inhibitory effects of these compounds. Since HIV-1 reverse transcriptase (RT) has been identified as the target for their antiviral activity, and since their chemical structure is unrelated to the nucleoside structure, the different families of HIV-1-specific drugs were designated "non-nucleoside RT inhibitors," or NNRTIs. More than 30 different structural classes of NNRTIs have been described (43).

The NNRTIs differ from the nucleoside RT inhibitors (designated NRTIs, namely, the clinically approved zidovudine [AZT], zalcitabine [ddC], didanosine [ddI], stavudine [d4T], lamivudine [3TC], abacavir [ABC]) in a number of aspects (Table 4.1):

1. Whereas the NRTIs have a typical dideoxynucleoside structure, the NNRTIs consist of a variety of compound families that are not related to nucleosides (namely, the clinically approved nevirapine, delavirdine, and efavirenz). Two exceptions exist—TSAO derivatives and HEPT derivatives. However, although these NNRTIs have a (modified) nucleoside structure, they do not functionally behave as NRTIs (see below) and thus should be classified as NNRTIs.

2. NRTIs need to be intracellularly activated to their 5′-triphosphate metabolites upon three distinct phosphorylation steps catalyzed by

TABLE 4.1
General properties and differences between NRTIs and NNRTIs

NRTIs	*NNRTIs*
Nucleoside structure	Non-nucleoside structure
Intracellularly converted to active metabolite	Do not need metabolic activation
Broad-spectrum antiretroviral agents	Highly HIV-1-specific
Interact with substrate binding site on RT (at catalytic Asp triad)	Interact with non–substrate binding site on RT (at lipophylic pocket)
Competitive inhibitors against dNTPs	Noncompetitive inhibitors against dNTPs and template/primer
Incorporate into viral DNA chain leading to DNA chain termination	Do not incorporate into growing DNA chain but slow down catalytic activity of RT
Often select for mutant virus strains at moderate speed	Rapidly select for mutant virus strains
Resistant virus strains keep full sensitivity to NNRTIs	Resistant virus strains keep full sensitivity to NRTIs
Moderate selectivity index and usually more severe side effects in humans than NNRTIs	High in vivo therapeutic index and usually moderate side effects in humans

cellular enzymes. NNRTIs are active as such, and they do not need intracellular metabolic activation to be inhibitory to HIV-1.

3. Both NRTIs and NNRTIs are targeted at the virus-encoded RNA-dependent DNA polymerase (RDDP). NRTIs do not markedly discriminate between RTs from different origins (e.g., HIV-1, HIV-2, SIV, FIV, VV, MSV, Mo-MuLV). They even recognize the DNA polymerase of human hepatitis B virus (HBV) that also has RDDP activity. In contrast, the NNRTIs are highly specific for HIV-1 RT and do not recognize RTs from other origins. This property explains the highly selective anti-HIV-1 activity of the NNRTIs.

4. Whereas the NRTIs (as their 5'-triphosphates) compete with the natural substrates (i.e., 2'-deoxynucleotide 5'-triphosphates, or dNTPs) of the RT reaction in a competitive manner, the NNRTIs act as noncompetitive inhibitors of HIV-1 RT by interacting at a non–substrate binding site distinct from the substrate binding site.

5. The principal mechanism of antiviral activity of NRTIs is the incorporation of the NRTIs into the growing viral DNA chain and subsequent DNA chain termination, preventing the further elongation of the viral DNA chain. In contrast, the NNRTIs act by considerably slowing down the viral DNA synthesis as a result of conformational

changes within parts of the HIV-1 RT, which affect the positioning of the catalytic site toward the template/primer.

6. NRTI and NNRTI exposure to HIV-1 selects for virus variants that are less susceptible to the inhibitory effects of these compounds. The locations of the amino acid mutations that arise in the HIV RT upon NRTI and NNRTI exposure and that lead to partial or high-level drug resistance are distinct between both groups of RT inhibitors. Whereas the NNRTI-specific mutations are clustered within the NNRTI-characteristic binding pocket, the NRTI-specific mutations appear at several other sites of the RT. Interestingly and importantly, virus strains that are NRTI-resistant keep full sensitivity to the NNRTIs and, vice versa, virus strains that contain characteristic NNRTI-specific amino acid mutations in their RT keep their sensitivity to NRTIs.

7. Toxic side effects of NRTIs and NNRTIs are usually nonoverlapping. This property may represent one of the arguments to combine NRTIs and NNRTIs in one drug cocktail.

The first NNRTI that was approved by the Food and Drug Administration (FDA) in June 1996 was nevirapine (95) (Viramune, Boehringer Ingelheim). This drug was followed by delavirdine mesylate (51, 114) (Rescriptor, Pharmacia and Upjohn), which was approved in April 1997, and efavirenz (136) (Sustiva, DuPont), approved in September 1998. Another five NNRTIs—the HEPT derivative MKC-442 (emivirine) (9) (Triangle Pharmaceuticals), calanolide A (75) (Sarawak MediChem Pharmaceuticals), quinoxaline GW420867X (5, 15) (GlaxoWellcome), MIV-150 (PETT-5) (1, 127) (Medivir), and AG1549 (previously designated S1153) (60) (Agouron Pharmaceuticals)—were in 2000 the subject of phase I, II, or III clinical trials. Quinoxaline has now been suspended. The current combinations of anti-HIV drugs may contain an NNRTI, one or two NRTIs, and one or two protease inhibitors (PIs). Given the actual concern about the long-term toxicity of PIs, the NNRTIs recently gained more importance to become included in a variety of drug regimen schedules used in the highly active antiretroviral therapy (HAART).

Overview of the Structural Classes of NNRTIs

To qualify as an NNRTI, the drug should inhibit the RT of HIV-1 strains but not HIV-2 or any other lentivirus RT. Consequently, the NNRTIs should be solely active against HIV-1 replication in cell culture at concentrations that are well below their toxicity threshold. Owing to their unique specificity, the NNRTIs are usually endowed with a pronounced selectivity index (SI), which is the ratio of the 50% cytotoxic concentration (50% CC_{50}) over the 50% antivirally effective concentration (EC_{50}). To date, more than 30 different structural classes of NNRTIs have been reported (Table 4.2) (for

TABLE 4.2
Overview of NNRTI families

NNRTI families	General class abbreviation	Prototype drug	Commercial name	Reference
Hydroxyethoxymethylphenylthiothymine 1-(ethoxymethyl)-5-isopropyl-6-benzyl-uracil	HEPT	MKC-442 (I-EBU)	Emivirine	8, 99 9
Tetrahydroimidazobenzodiazepin-one and -thiones (+)-(5S)-4,5,6,7-tetrahydro-9-chloro-5-methyl-6-(3-methyl-2-butenyl)imidazo[4,5,1jk]-[benzo-diazepin-2(1H)-thione]	TIBO	9-Cl-TIBO (R82,913)	—	107 107
(+)-(5S)-4,5,6,7-tetrahydro-8-chloro-5-methyl-6-(3-methyl-2-butenyl)imidazo[4,5,1JK]-[benzo-diazepin-2(1H)-thione]		8-Cl-TIBO (R86,183)	Tivirapine	106
Dipyridodiazepinones 11-cyclopropyl-5,11-dihydro-4-methyl-6H-dipyridol[3,2-b:2′,3′-e]diazepin-6-one		BI-RG-587	Nevirapine	95
Pyridinones 3-[[(4,7-dichloro-1,3-benzoxazol-2-yl)methyl] amino]-5-ethyl-6-methylpyridin-2(1H)-one		L-697,661		61
Bis(heteroaryl)piperazines 1-[3-[(ethylamino)-2-pyridinyl]-4-[[5-methoxy-amino]-1H-indol-2-yl-carbonyl]-piperazine	BHAP	U-87201E	Atevirdine mesylate	114 114
1-[3-[(1-methylethyl)amino]-2-pyridinyl]-4-[[5-[(methylsulphony)amino]-1H-indol-2yl] carbonyl]-piperazine		U-90152S	Delavirdine mesylate	51

(continued)

TABLE 4.2 (continued)

NNRTI families	General class abbreviation	Prototype drug	Commercial name	Reference
Tertbutyldimethylsilylspiroaminooxathioledioxidethymines [2′,5′-bis-O-(tert-butyldimethylsilyl)-3′-spiro-5′-(4″-amino-1″2″-oxathiole-2″2″-dioxide)]-β-D-pento-furanosyl-N-methyl-thymine	TSAO	TSAO-m^{3}T		22, 23, 34, 108
α-Anilinophenylacetamides [(2-acetyl,5-methyl)anilino]-[2,6-dichlorophenyl]-acetamide	α-APA	R89,439	Loviride	106 106
Phenylethylthiazolylthioureas N-(2-pyridyl)ethyl-N′-(5-bromo-2-pyridyl)thiourea	PETT	LY 300046.HCl	Trovirdine	1 25, 138
New PETT derivatives urea PETT derivative	PETT	MSC-204 (PETT-4 metabolite)		127
urea PETT derivative		MIV-150 (MSH-372 (PETT-5))		127
Thiocarboxanilides N-[4-chloro-3-(3-methyl-2-butenyloxy)phenyl]-2-methyl-3-furancarbothioamide	TCA	UC-781		20
Quinoxalines 6-chloro-3,3-dimethyl-4-(isopropenyloxy-carbonyl)-3,4-dihydro-quinoxalin-2(1H)thione		S-2720		79 79
(S)-4-isopropoxycarbonyl-6-methoxy-3-(methylthio-methyl)-3,4-dihydroquinoxaline-2(1H)-thione		HBY 097		79, 80

Name	Abbrev.	Code		References
(S)-4-isopropoxycarbonyl-6-fluoro-3-ethyl-3,4-dihydro-quinoxalino-2(1H)-oe		GW420867X		5
Thiazolobenzimidazoles	TBZ			
1-(2′,6′-difluorophenyl)-1H,3H-thiazolo[3,4-a]benzimidazole		NSC-625487		31, 39
Thiazoloisoindolinones				
(R)?(+)-9b-(3,S-dimethylphenyl)-2,3-dihydrothiazolo [2,3-a]isoindol-5(9bH)-on		BM+51.0836		90, 96
Indolecarboxamides				
5-chloro-3-(phenylsulfonyl)indole-2-carboxamide		L-737,126		130
Benzothiadiazines				
Benzothiadiazine-1-oxide derivative		NSC 287474		30
Quinazolinones				124
4-(2-pyridinylethynyl)-6-chloro-4-cyclopropyl-3,4-dihydroquinazoline-2(1H)-one		L-738,372		37
Benzoxazinones				
(−)-6-chloro-4-cyclopropylethynyl-4-trifluoromethyl-1,4-dihydro-2H-3,1-benzoxazin-2-one		DMP 266 (L-743,726)	Efavirenz	136
Calanolide A				75, 137
Imidazodipyridodiazepines				
Imidazo[2′,3′:6,5]dipyrido[3,2-b:2′,3′-e]-1,4-diazepine		UK-129485		123
Imidazopyridazines				
7-[2-(1H-imidazol-1-yl)-5-methylimidazo[1,5-b] pyridazin-7-yl]-1-phenyl-1-heptanone				87
Thiadiazolyldialkylcarbamates	TDA			
4-(2,6-dichlorophenyl)-1,2,5-thiadiazol-3-yl-N,N(methyl,isopropyl)carbamate		RD-4-2024		67, 68
Arylpyridodiazepine- and thiodiazepines				
6,7-dihydro-7-methyl-12-ethyl-pyrido[2,3-b]pyrido [2,3-4,5]thieno[2,3-f][1,4]diazepin-6(12H)-thione		MEN 10979		26

(continued)

TABLE 4.2 (continued)

NNRTI families	General class abbreviation	Prototype drug	Commercial name	Reference
Dihydroalkoxybenzyloxopyrimidines	DABO			7, 91
HEPT-pyridinone hybrids				49
Benzyloxymethylpyridinones				73
Alkoxy(arylthio)uracils				78
Indolyldipyridodiazepinones				76
Pyrrolobenzoxazepinones				35
Highly substituted pyrroles				4
Benzylthiopyrimidines				
4-amino-2-(benzylthio)-6-chloropyrimidine		U-31355		3
Pyridazinobenzoxazepinones				24
Imidazobenzodiazepine and imidazoquinazolines				85
(Pyrrolo)benzothiadiazepines				40, 43, 48
Indolobenzothiazepines				116
Furopyridinylthiopyrimidinamines				
(−)-6-chloro-2-[(1-furo[2,3-c]pyridin-5-yl-ethyl)thio]-4-pyrimidinamine		PNU-142721		133
Pyrido[1,2a]indoles				
Pyrido[1,2a]indole derivative		BCH-4989		122
Highly substituted imidazoles				
5-(3,5-dichlorophenyl)thio-4-isopropyl-1-(4-pyridyl) methyl-1H-imidazol-2-ylmethyl carbamate		S-1153/AG-1549		60
Trioxothienothiadiazines	TTD			6, 134

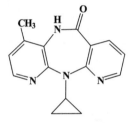

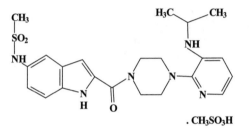

Nevirapine (BI-RG-587)
Viramune®

BHAP (U-90152)
Delavirdine
Rescriptor®

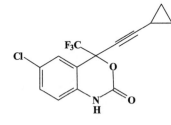

Benzoxazinone
DMP 266
Efavirenz
Sustiva™

FIGURE 4.1

NNRTIs approved by the FDA for HIV-1 treatment

an overview, see reference 43). The structures of the NNRTIs that are clin-
ically approved (nevirapine, delavirdine, and efavirenz) are depicted in
Fig. 4.1. The structures of the NNRTIs that are the subject of clinical phase
I (PETT-5), phase II (quinoxaline GW420867X, calanolide A, AG1549), and
phase III (emivirine) trials but not officially approved yet are depicted in
Fig. 4.2. In the past, a number of other NNRTIs (9-chloro-TIBO, 8-chloro-
TIBO [tivirapine], pyridinone L697,661, BHAP U-87201E [atevirdine],
α-APA [loviride], LY-300046.HCl [trovirdine], quinoxaline HBY 097, and
GW420867X) have been the subject of clinical trials, but continuation of
these studies has been suspended for several reasons.

For the structures of the different classes of NNRTIs listed in Table 4.2,
see reference 43. The most potent and selective NNRTIs (efavirenz, tivi-
rapine, emivirine, loviride, quinoxaline GW420867X, PETT-5, AG1549, and
the thiocarboxanilide UC-781) inhibit HIV-1 replication at the lower
nanomolar range of drug concentrations. Their selectivity indices (ratio
CC_{50}/EC_{50}) amount up to 10,000–100,000 or even higher. These drugs are
also highly inhibitory to HIV-1 RT, and there is usually a good correlation

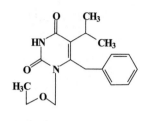

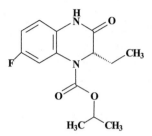

HEPT derivative
I-EBU (MKC-442)
Emivirine

Quinoxaline GW420867X

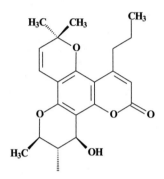

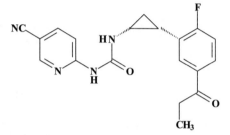

Calanolide A

MSH-372
(PETT-5)

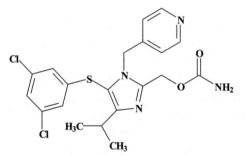

Dichlorophenylthio(pyridyl)imidazole derivative
AG 1549

FIGURE 4.2

NNRTIs currently the subject of phase I, II, and III clinical trials

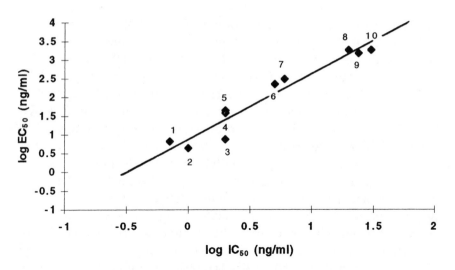

FIGURE 4.3

Correlation between the inhibitory activity of NNRTIs against
HIV-1(III$_B$) in cell culture (EC$_{50}$) and their inhibitory activity
against HIV-1 RT

Symbols: 1, efavirenz; 2, quinoxaline HBY 097; 3, the thiocarboxanilide UC-781; 4,
emivirine; 5, 8-chloro-TIBO; 6, loviride; 7, delavirdine; 8, 9-chloro-TIBO; 9, TSAO-m^{3}T;
10, nevirapine.

between antiviral potency of the NNRTIs in cell culture and their inhibitory activity against purified HIV-1 RT (Fig. 4.3).

Mechanism of Action of NNRTIs

The NNRTIs are targeted at HIV-1 RT. This enzyme is encoded by the virus
and fulfills three different functions that are closely related to one another
(104). The RT is endowed with an RDDP activity that catalyzes the polymerization of 2′-deoxynucleotides using the viral genomic single-stranded
RNA as the template. The original RNA strand of the resulting RNA/DNA
hybrid is then hydrolyzed by the RNase H function of the RT enzyme to
generate a single-stranded DNA chain that is then converted to a double-
stranded DNA by the DNA-dependent DNA polymerase (DDDP) activity
of the RT enzyme. The resulting proviral DNA is subsequently transported
to the nucleus of the infected cell for incorporation into the cellular genome
by a virus-encoded integrase.

In contrast to the NRTIs, all the NNRTIs show a unique specificity for
the HIV-1 RT, noncompetitive kinetics with respect to the dNTP substrates,
and noncompetitive or uncompetitive inhibitory kinetics with respect to
the template/primer (14, 21, 42, 59, 61, 79, 129, 135, 138). These character-

istics strongly suggest a specific interaction of these inhibitors with an HIV-1 RT site that is clearly distinct from the substrate binding site of the enzyme and that must be absent in the HIV-2 RT or any other retroviral RT or cellular DNA polymerase. In addition, the binding of the enzyme to the polynucleotide template is not influenced by the inhibitor. Thus, NNRTIs must interact with a unique non–substrate binding site of the HIV-1 RT. NNRTIs usually show a pronounced preference for poly(C)·oligo(dG) as the homopolymeric template/primer, although inhibition of the RT reaction in the presence of other homopolymeric template/primers, such as poly(A)·oligo(dT), poly(U)·oligo(dA), or poly(I)·oligo(dC), or heteropolymeric template/primers such as primed 16S/23S rRNA or activated (gapped duplex) DNA has been demonstrated (101). Most NNRTIs also show a preferential inhibition of the RDDP function of HIV-1 RT. The inhibition of the DDDP function is often inferior compared with inhibition of the RDDP function of HIV-1 RT. The observed differences can range from two- to threefold to more than 50-fold depending on the nature of the NNRTI and on the particular reaction conditions (59, 101, 129).

As already mentioned, the NNRTIs are inactive against the RT of HIV-2 and the RTs of MSV, Mo-MuLV, SIV, FIV, and feline leukemia virus. In addition to the RTs from retroviruses other than HIV-1, human DNA polymerases α, β, and γ are also refractory to inhibition by NNRTIs. Another clear distinction between these types of HIV-1 RT inhibitors and the NRTIs is the fact that the NNRTIs do not act as DNA chain terminators and do not have to be incorporated into the growing DNA chain to act as an inhibitor of the RT reaction. Frank et al. (59) noted an increase in the proportion of shorter DNA fragments and a decrease in the proportion of longer DNA chains when HIV-1 RT reaction mixtures to which TIBO had been added were examined in sequencing gels. From these data and other experimental evidence, it was concluded that TIBO and related NNRTIs considerably slow down the rate of DNA chain elongation, and this represents the principal mechanism of antiviral action of NNRTIs (59, 118).

It has often been observed that the antiviral potency of the NNRTIs in cell culture is higher than their affinity (IC_{50} or K_i) for HIV-1 RT. Such sometimes marked differences in the inhibitory action of the NNRTIs against HIV-1 replication and HIV-1 RT activity have been observed by several investigators and are most likely due to the artificial experimental conditions used to measure RT inhibition in cell-free assays. However, there is usually a fairly good correlation between the IC_{50} values of the NNRTIs for HIV-1 replication in cell culture and their K_i/K_m values or IC_{50} values in the presence of primed rRNA or poly(C)·oligo(dG) (Fig. 4.3).

Fletcher et al. (57, 58) have shown that several NNRTIs might selectively inhibit different mechanistic forms of the RT. This interesting conclusion was based on the observation that the oxathiin carboxanilide derivative UC-84 (Fig. 4.4) was able to afford complete photoprotection of the

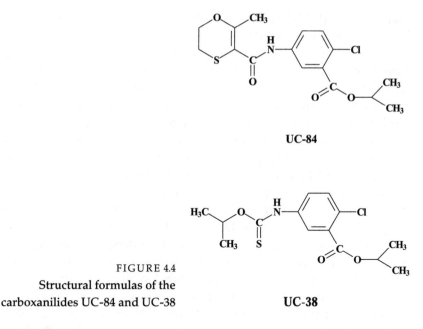

UC-84

UC-38

binary RT-primer/template complex in the presence of the irreversible HIV-1 RT photoinactivating azido-substituted nevirapine analog, whereas the thiocarboxanilide UC-38 (Fig. 4.4) was unable to do so. In addition, UC-84 was quite effective in protecting free RT enzyme from irreversible photoinactivation by the azido-substituted nevirapine, whereas UC-38 was not. In contrast, UC-38 but not UC-84 showed very efficient photoprotection profiles against the ternary complex of RT in the presence of poly(C)·oligo(dG) and dGTP. Based on these observations, it was not unexpected that the combination of UC-84 and UC-38 resulted in synergistic inhibition of both HIV-1 RT activity and HIV-1 replication in cell culture. This supports the view that NNRTIs can sometimes preferentially inhibit different conformational forms of the RT.

The NNRTI-Characteristic Lipophilic Pocket in HIV-1 RT

Structure of HIV-1 RT in Relation to the NNRTI-Specific Pocket

The HIV-1 RT is a heterodimeric enzyme of 1,000 amino acid residues and consists of a p66 subunit containing 560 amino acid residues and a p51 subunit containing 440 amino acid residues. The p51 subunit is identical to the first part of the p66 and formed after cleavage of the p66 subunit to p51 (+ p15) by the virus-encoded protease. The last 120 residues of the p66 subunit (p15) encode the RNase H domain of HIV-1 RT. The first report on the complete structure of HIV-1 RT was based on the complex between the enzyme and nevirapine (84). Since then, numerous RT structures complexed with a variety of NNRTIs (119) but also unliganded RT (64, 110, 125) and recently also HIV-1 RT complexed with a modified oligonucleotide and a dNTP have been reported (66).

The HIV-1 RT has an asymmetric nine-domain structure. The three-dimensional structure of the p66 subunit has been compared with a right hand containing a finger, palm, thumb, and connection domain (84). The rather open structure of p66 contrasts with the compact p51 structure in which the arrangements of the different domains are quite different. The p51 interacts with the p66 subunit through the connection domains but also through several other parts of the RT peptide chain. Whereas the core domains of the HIV-1 are represented by the p66 connection domain and p51 fingers and p51 connection domain and hardly differ in conformation in the different available crystal structures (54, 110), the p66 fingers domain and p66 thumb domain are rather flexible. In the majority of crystal structures, the p66 fingers and palm domains are quite spread, mimicking an open hand with a large cleft. The nucleic acid is bound in this cleft passing behind the fingers and in front of the thumb domains (69). However, in the RT enzyme complexed with a dNTP, the fingers have shown to be folded down into the palm domain (66). In the latter structure, a catalytic pocket is created, and the template/primer now passes in front of both the fingers and thumb domains. The catalytic site in the HIV-1 RT is represented by three highly conserved Asp110, Asp185, and Asp186 residues located in the p66 palm domain. The corresponding Asp residues in the p51 subunit are buried in the p51 structure and have no catalytic function.

All NNRTIs bind at a single site within the p66 palm domain (105, 108, 110). This binding site is represented by a lipophilic pocket at the base of a three-stranded β-sheet (β4, β7, and β8). At the top of this sheet, the three catalytic Asp residues are approximately 10–15 Å distant from the bound NNRTIs. The pocket is further formed from the β4, β7, β8 sheet (amino acid residues 105–110 and 179–191); the β9, β10, β11 sheet (amino acid residues 224–241); the structure preceding β4 (amino acid residues 98–104); and amino acid residues 318, 138, 139, and 141. The mouth of the pocket contains the Pro225 and Pro236 residues that are able to "close the door" behind the inhibitor after the NNRTI has entered (55). Interestingly, the NNRTI-characteristic pocket does not physically exist in unliganded RT but is created upon NNRTI binding (53, 110). Indeed, the pocket undergoes a conformational shift upon NNRTI binding by moving the Tyr 181 and Tyr 188 residues into the direction of the catalytic amino acid residues (98). Concomitantly, the whole β sheet comprising β4, β7, and β8 and the three catalytic Asp residues shift by about 2 Å (Fig. 4.5). This important and consistent shift upon NNRTI binding in the lipophilic pocket is assumed to result in a dramatic slowing down of the catalytic activity of the enzyme and most likely represents the molecular basis of the inhibitory action of the NNRTIs (53) (Fig. 4.5). This structural explanation of NNRTI inhibition is consistent with the kinetic mechanistic studies of Spence et al. (118).

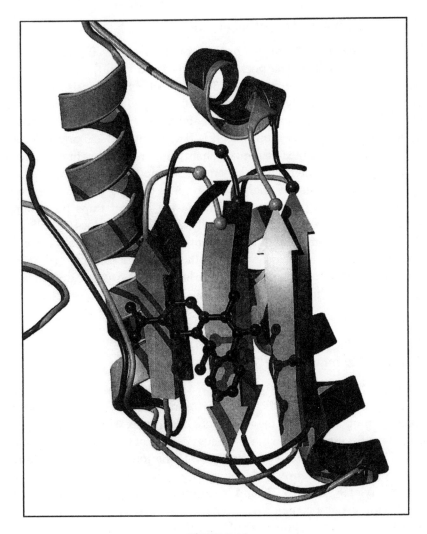

FIGURE 4.5

Mode of inhibition of RT by an NNRTI (stick-and-ball model in black)

The pale gray structure shows a part of the unliganded enzyme. When the inhibitor binds (dark gray enzyme structure), there is a movement of this part of the structure by 2 Å. This movement is most pronounced for the three catalytic aspartate residues: 110, 185, and 186 (Cα positions marked by spheres).

The total volume of the NNRTI pocket is roughly between 620 and 720 Å^3, whereas most NNRTIs have a volume of 220 to 320 Å^3. Delavirdine (volume about 380 Å^3) and TSAO (volume > 500 Å^3) are exceptions. From delavirdine, it is known that part of it protrudes from the mouth of the pocket (55), and for TSAO, there is compelling evidence that the thymine part of the molecule (in particular the N-3 side) is exposed to the solvent.

Structure of the NNRTI-Specific Pocket

The roof of the pocket is formed by the aromatic residues Tyr 181, Tyr 188, and Trp 229 (Fig. 4.6). The pocket walls are lined with the hydrophobic residues Leu 100, Val 106, and Leu 234. The pocket floor consists of main-chain atoms of several lysines in the Lys 101 → Lys 103 domain preceding β4. Toward the pocket mouth, two aromatic residues (Phe 227 and Tyr 318) are in place. The pocket mouth itself is flanked by Pro 225 and Pro 236, which are located on flexible peptide chains and are instrumental in allowing the NNRTIs to enter the pocket and in closing the pocket mouth again behind the NNRTI. Interestingly, delavirdine is too long to fit entirely into the NNRTI pocket; it protrudes from the pocket and traps the proline residues in the open conformation. Finally, amino acid residues Glu 138 and Thr 139 derived from the p51 (and not from the p66 subunit) are positioned to the left of the pocket, just beyond residues Leu 100 and Tyr 181 (Fig. 4.6). Their counterparts on the p66 subunit are located in the fingers domain and do not play a structural role in the formation of the NNRTI pocket.

Structure of the NNRTIs in Relation to Their Binding into the NNRTI Pocket

Although the variety of NNRTIs show quite remarkable differences in structure and molecular weights, they are much more similar in conformational properties when their structure in complex with the HIV-1 RT is compared. Several investigators have suggested that the shape of the bound NNRTIs resembles that of a butterfly (47). The top wing of the butterfly often contains a π-electron system to interact with the aromatic residues of Tyr 181, Tyr 188, and Trp 229 and is closest to the catalytic Asp triad. The other wing usually contains an aromatic ring and may form a hydrogen bridge to the main peptide chain of Lys 101. The tail of the butterfly is close to Tyr 181 and results in a marked movement of the functional group (hydroxyphenyl) of this amino acid. Although most NNRTIs adapt such a butterfly shape (i.e., nevirapine, loviride, HEPT), several NNRTIs do not. The top wing is markedly diminished or virtually absent with quinoxalines and (thio)carboxanilides, whereas TSAOs and delavirdine look quite different from the butterfly shape. For TSAO, no crystal structure has even been available so far, and it is currently unclear how TSAOs may fit into the NNRTI pocket. It has recently been suggested that TSAOs may affect the stability of the dimerization between p66 and p51 (62). This observation is not surprising, as there is compelling evidence that TSAOs interfere with Glu 138 of the p51 subunit and thus may interact at the interphase between both p66 and p51 subunits of the HIV-1 RT (22, 28, 72).

    Comparison of the structural features of the numerous NNRTIs revealed that the more rigid the inhibitors (namely, nevirapine), the less they

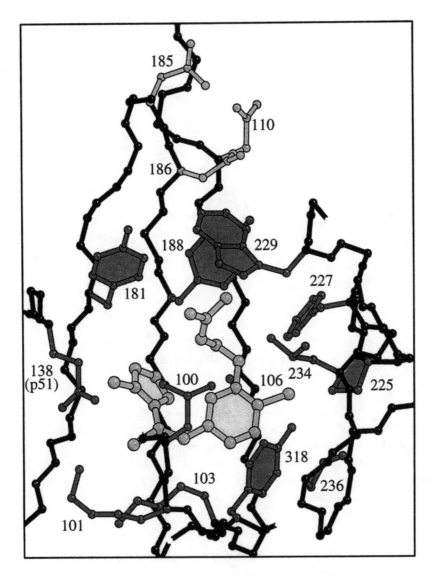

FIGURE 4.6

Amino acids lining the NNRTI-specific pocket in HIV-1 RT

The main chain atoms are shown in black. The aspartic acid triad (110, 185, 186) is shown in light gray. The NNRTI (UC-781) is also shown in light gray. The functional groups of the amino acids lining the pocket are shown in dark gray.

are able to adapt to changes that may occur in the pocket upon mutation of one or several amino acids lining the pocket. More flexible NNRTIs such as PETTs and thiocarboxanilides (i.e., UC-781) can better adapt their structure in concert with a changed conformation of the pocket. Fig. 4.7 displays the structural features of UC-781 and the interaction of this drug with amino acids of the HIV-1 NNRTI pocket. UC-781 contains two rings where

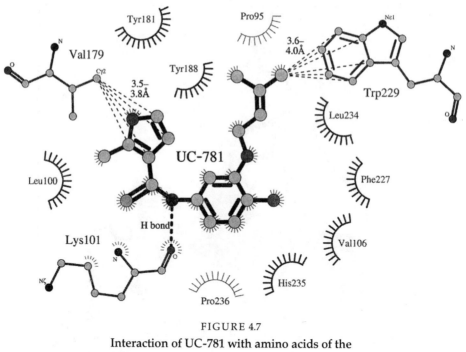

FIGURE 4.7

Interaction of UC-781 with amino acids of the
NNRTI-characteristic pocket of HIV-1 RT

the furanyl ring acts like the butterfly's tail and where the top wing is replaced by a relatively small pentenyloxyether moiety (109). It has been assumed that the flexibility of UC-781 and the relatively small number of interactions with the amino acids of the pocket may facilitate alterations in
the inhibitors' binding mode upon conformational changes in the NNRTI
pocket.

Nature of the Interactions between NNRTIs and Amino Acids of the NNRTI-Characteristic Lipophilic Pocket

A variety of interactions between the NNRTIs and the amino acids lining
the NNRTI-specific pocket may occur (Table 4.3). There are subtle differences between the different NNRTIs in their eventual interactions with
amino acids of the NNRTI-characteristic pocket, which determines not
only their inhibitory potential against the wild-type HIV-1 RT but also, at
least partially, their inhibitory activity against mutant HIV-1 RTs. Among
the most important interactions of the NNRTIs in the pocket of RT are the
aromatic stacking interactions between aromatic rings of the NNRTI drugs
and protein residues Tyr 181, Tyr 188, Trp 229, and Tyr 318 of the lipophilic
pocket. Electrostatic forces, particularly significant for Lys 101 and Lys 103

TABLE 4.3

Overview of resistance mutations found to appear in HIV-1 RT under selective drug pressure by nevirapine, delavirdine, and efavirenz[a]

Amino acid number	Amino acid mutation	Codon mutation	NNRTI that may select for the mutation[b]	Reference
98	Ala → Gly	GCA → GGA	Nev	33, 112
100	Leu → Ile	TTA → ATA	Nev, Del, Efa	16, 33, 113, 126, 136
101	Lys → Glu	AAA → GAA	Efa	136
103	Lys → Asn	AAA → AAC	Nev, Del, Efa	16, 112, 136
103	Lys → Thr	AAA → ACA	Del	13
106	Val → Ala	GTA → GCA	Nev, Del	16, 112, 113, 126
108	Val → Ile	GTA → ATA	Nev, Efa	33, 131, 132
135	Ile → Met/Thr/Leu	ATA → ?	Efa	10, 136
179	Val → Asp	GTT → GAT	Efa	33, 131, 132
179	Val → Glu	GTT → GAG	Efa	33, 131, 132
181	Tyr → Cys	TAT → TGT	Nev, Del, Efa	112, 126, 131, 132, 136
181	Tyr → Ile	TAT → ATT	Nev, Del	18
188	Tyr → Cys	TAT → TGT	Nev	112
188	Tyr → His	TAT → CAT	Del	56
188	Tyr → Leu	TAT → TTA	Efa	136
190	Gly → Glu	GGA → GAA	Del, Efa	103
190	Gly → Ala	GGA → GCA	Nev, Efa	112
190	Gly → Ser	GGA → ?	Efa	10, 11
225	Pro → His	CCT → CAT	Efa	10, 11
233	Glu → Val	GAA → GTA	Del	52
236	Pro → Leu	CCT → CTT	Del	52
238	Lys → Thr	AAA → ACA	Del	52

[a]For an overview, see references 12 and 94.

[b]Nev, nevirapine; Del, delavirdine; Efa, efavirenz.

and for Glu 138, may also add to the binding affinity of the NNRTIs for the RT. In addition, van der Waals interactions with Leu 100, Val 106, Val 179, Tyr 181, Gly 190, Trp 229, Leu 234, and Tyr 318 and, last but not least, hydrogen bonding between the NNRTIs and the main chain (carbonyl/imino) peptide bonds (i.e., main chain -CONH- between Lys 101 and Lys 102 or between Lys 103 and Lys 104) contribute to the interaction and binding affinities of the NNRTIs in the lipophilic pocket.

Resistance Development of HIV-1 against NNRTIs

Selection of Drug-Resistance Mutations

Failure of long-term efficacy of NRTIs, NNRTIs, and PIs is often associated with the appearance of dose-limiting side effects or, more important, with the emergence of drug-resistant virus strains. Indeed, under drug pressure, the RT inhibitors (both NRTIs and NNRTIs) may select for virus strains that show reduced susceptibility to the particular drugs. These mutations easily appear in HIV-1-infected cell cultures and in NNRTI drug-treated HIV-1-infected individuals. Interestingly, the mutations that appear under NRTI drug treatment of HIV-1 are different from those that emerge under NNRTI drug treatment (12, 94). Moreover, the mutant virus strains resistant to NRTIs keep full sensitivity to the inhibitory action of NNRTIs, and vice versa, HIV-1 strains containing NNRTI-characteristic amno acid mutations in their RT keep full sensitivity to NRTIs. In contrast with NRTI-specific and multi-NRTI drug resistance mutations that are scattered over several parts of the RT enzyme, the NNRTI-specific mutations are clustered in a lipophilic NNRTI-specific pocket (Fig. 4.8) (12). For the NNRTIs, a cluster of mutations consists of Ala 98 Gly, Leu 100 Ile, Lys 101 Glu/Gln/Ile, Lys 103 Asn/Thr/Gln/Arg, Val 106 Ala/Ile/Leu, and Val 108 Ile in the β-sheet comprising β5b and β6 and of Val 179 Asp/Glu, Tyr 181 Cys/Ile, Tyr 188 Cys/His/Leu, Val 189 Ile, and Gly 190 Glu/Thr/Glu/Ala/Ser in the β sheet comprising β9 and β10. In addition, Ile 135 Met/Thr/Leu, Glu 138 Lys, Thr 139 Ile, and Gly 141 Glu mutations have been reported and are located at the interphase between p51 and p66. Furthermore, Pro 225 His, Phe 227 Leu, Glu 233 Val, Pro 2136 Leu, and Lys 238 Thr are also found to play a role in NNRTI resistance development (Tables 4.3, 4.4). All these mutations conferring resistance at varying degrees to NNRTIs are very well clustered and are part of the lipophilic pocket in HIV-1 RT (Fig. 4.8). A characteristic property of these amino acid mutations is that a single amino acid change may result in a marked degree of resistance to first-generation NNRTIs (namely, nevirapine, TIBO, loviride, delavirdine) (17). This degree of NNRTI resistance caused by single amino acid mutations in the NNRTI-characteristic pocket is usually much more pronounced than that observed for single NRTI-specific amino acid mutations. In addition, significant cross-resistance to a variety of other NNRTIs against a single amino acid mutation is more common within the class of the NNRTIs than of the NRTIs. However, the cross-resistance is highly determined by the nature of the amino acid mutation and the type of NNRTI (17). Even different amino acid changes at one single amino acid location can have markedly different effects on the sensitivity of the RT for an NNRTI. For example, whereas Gly 190 Ala hardly confers resistance to quinoxaline HBY 097, Gly 190 Glu results in a more than 100-fold degree of resistance to this drug (82). Moreover, Tyr 181 Ile and Tyr 188 Leu usu-

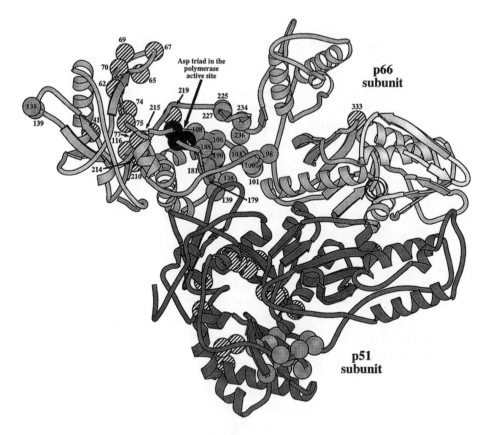

FIGURE 4.8

Clustering of NNRTI-specific mutations in
the NNRTI-specific lipophilic pocket

The light gray peptide chain represents the p66 subunit, and the dark gray peptide chain represents the p51 subunit. The aspartic acid triad is represented by black circles. The NRTI-characteristic mutations are represented by dashed circles. The NNRTI-characteristic mutations are represented by gray circles. The amino acids at positions 138 and 139 in the p66 subunit do not play a role in the formation of the lipophilic pocket. Instead, the amino acids at positions 138 and 139 in the p51 subunit play a role in the formation of the NNRTI-specific pocket.

ally cause a much higher level of resistance against most, if not all, NNRTIs than the Tyr 181 Cys and Tyr 188 Cys mutations. It is important to realize that the currently most active (second-generation) NNRTIs, such as efavirenz, quinoxaline GW420867X, MIV-150 (PETT-5), AG1549, and UC-781, can usually deal very well with single mutations in the RT and need several (two or more) NNRTI-specific mutations in the RT to achieve a high level of resistance against these NNRTIs (i.e., combinations of Lys 103 Asn with other NNRTI-specific mutations or double mutations located in one codon [i.e., Tyr 181 Ile or Tyr 188 Leu]) (12).

TABLE 4.4

Reasons for changes of NNRTI drug affinity to HIV-1 RT

Steric hindrance

Gly 190 Glu (for most NNRTIs)
Gly 190 Ala (for nevirapine)

Loss of contact

Tyr 181 Cys (for 9-chloro-TIBO and other NNRTIs)
Tyr 188 Leu (for quinoxaline HBY 097)

Gain of contact

Tyr 181 Cys (for calanolide B)

Change or introduction of charge

Glu 138 Lys (for TSAOs)
Gly 190 Glu (for most, if not all, NNRTIs)

Slower binding rate

Lys 103 Asn (for most, if not all, NNRTIs)

It should also be mentioned that the individual effects of NNRTI-specific mutations on drug resistance are not always additive when combined with each other. For example, whereas the Val 108 Ile and Pro 225 His mutations did not confer measurable resistance of HIV-1 RT to efavirenz as single mutations, addition of the Lys 103 Asn amino acid change to these mutations increased the efavirenz resistance 17- to more than 100-fold. Even more, the Leu 100 Ile mutation, while conferring 21-fold resistance to efavirenz, resulted in a more than 4,000-fold resistance to efavirenz when combined with Lys 103 Asn, which itself gives only about 20-fold resistance to efavirenz.

Sensitization of Drugs against HIV-1 RT

Amino acid mutations in the NNRTI-specific pocket do not always result in resistance development of the RT against NNRTIs. A number of NNRTI-specific mutations in the HIV-1 RT have been identified to sensitize HIV-1 to a number of well-defined NRTIs and NNRTIs. The best known example is the Tyr 181 Cys mutation, which is able to reverse the phenotypic resistance of virus strains that contain typical NRTI (AZT) resistance mutations by 30- to 35-fold (86). The Leu 100 Ile mutation is also able to reverse phenotypic AZT resistance when added to an AZT-resistance background (Lys 70 Arg: about 4-fold [103]; Met 41 Leu + Thr 215 Tyr: 1,000-fold [32]; Asp 67 Asn + Lys 70 Arg + Thr 215 Tyr + Lys 219 Gln: 4,000-fold [32]). Interestingly, the Tyr 181 Cys mutation has also proven to sensitize the activity of the NNRTI (-)-7,8-dihydro-calanolide B by about 10-fold (65). Likewise, the Pro 225 His and the Pro 236 Leu mutations, both located at the mouth of the NNRTI-specific pocket, are able to increase the inhibitory effect of delavirdine (Pro 225 His) or a variety of other NNRTIs (Pro 236 Leu), including nevirapine, pyridinone, and 9-chloro-TIBO. In addition, in some cases, mutations that are selected under PFA (foscarnet) pressure (i.e., Gln 161 Leu and Gln 161 Leu + His 208 Tyr) have been shown to sensitize the RT for the inhibitory effects of NNRTIs such as nevirapine and 9-chloro-TIBO by 11- to 20-fold (93, 121).

Appearance of Compensatory Mutations in an NNRTI-Resistance Background

In a number of cases, the NNRTI-resistance mutation compromises the catalytic efficacy of the enzyme. Such a mutant (drug-resistant) enzyme is clearly catalytically less active and the associated virus less fit than other mutant enzymes and cannot compete against wild-type or other mutant viruses, except the replication fitness is increased again. The Gly 190 Glu RT mutated virus, which has shown to emerge under specific experimental conditions in the presence of quinoxaline HBY 097 or GW420867X, is an example of such a virus that has been demonstrated to contain an RT that displays only approximately 5% of the catalytic activity of wild-type RT (82). Interestingly, upon prolonged exposure of this mutant virus in the presence of the quinoxaline, additional mutations appeared that did not further enhance the level of drug resistance but markedly increased the catalytic efficacy of the enzyme and concomitant fitness of the virus again. In the case of the Gly 190 Glu RT mutant virus, the appearance of additional mutations at amino acid positions 74 and 75 has been observed (29, 81). It has been shown that these mutations indeed increased the catalytic efficiency of the enzyme, rather than further increasing drug resistance. Thus, not all mutations in the HIV-1 RT that appear under NNRTI pressure are aimed to afford decreased sensitivity against the NNRTI drugs. The phenomenon of the appearance of compensatory mutations to increase fitness of mutant HIV-1 strains has also been recognized to occur in both NRTI- and PI-resistant viruses and thus seems to represent a common mechanism of the virus to restore the replication competence of mutated virus strains under drug pressure.

In Vivo Administration and Activity of NNRTIs

Pharmacological Properties

The three NNRTIs that are currently approved in the clinic are endowed with a high oral bioavailability (Table 4.5). They can be administered once or twice daily (nevirapine, efavirenz) or twice or three times daily (delavirdine) to obtain steady-state trough drug levels of approximately 16 μM (4.7 μg/ml) for nevirapine, 15.9 μM (7.3 μg/ml) for delavirdine, and 4.2 μM

TABLE 4.5

Summary of the pharmacological properties of clinically approved NNRTIs[a]

	Nevirapine	Delavirdine	Efavirenz
Total daily dose (mg)	400 mg	1,200 mg	600 mg
Frequency of administration	Once or twice daily	Twice or three times daily	Once or twice daily
Steady-state trough drug levels	4.7 µg/ml	7.3 µg/ml	1.9 µg/ml
Plasma half-life	25–30 hr	7–21 hr	40–55 hr
Bioavailability	> 90%	> 50%	> 60%
Protein binding	60%	98%	> 99%
Metabolic properties	P450 inducer	P450 inhibitor	P450 inducer

[a]Data taken from reference 72.

(1.9 µg/ml) for efavirenz. These levels are 300-fold (nevirapine), 2,000-fold (delavirdine), and 7,000-fold (efavirenz) higher than the EC_{50} (50% antivirally effective concentrations) of these NNRTIs in cell culture. An interesting property, allowing only one or two administrations per day for nevirapine and efavirenz, is their long pharmacological half-life (25–30 hours and 40–55 hours, respectively). NNRTIs are extensively metabolized in the liver through cytochrome P450. Nevirapine leads to an acute induction of cytochrome P450 enzymes, resulting in a 1.5- to 2-fold increased clearance of this drug during the first two to four weeks of dosing. In contrast with nevirapine and efavirenz, delavirdine is an inhibitor of cytochrome P450 and has opposite effects on drug metabolism and clearance than nevirapine and efavirenz. In particular, delavirdine markedly increases plasma levels of PIs. The effect on PI metabolism by the NNRTIs highly depends on the nature of the PI (72).

Therapeutic Efficacy

Monotherapy with nevirapine and delavirdine showed a transient antiviral efficacy (38, 41). After 12 weeks of treatment, the viral load returned to baseline. This loss of antiviral efficacy was due to the emergence of mutant virus strains that proved resistant to the particular drugs (38, 44, 63). The rapid emergence of resistant virus strains under NNRTI treatment argued for incorporation of an NNRTI in a drug treatment schedule that already contains at least one or preferably two or three other drugs. Therefore, the NNRTIs have been combined in several clinical studies with one or two NRTIs, in addition to one or two PIs.

In general, addition of nevirapine to heavily NRTI (AZT, ddI)-pretreated patients resulted in a slightly higher efficacy of the treatment. However, when nevirapine was part of a drug cocktail (containing AZT and ddI) given to antiretroviral naive patients (Italy, the Netherlands, Canada, Australia Study Group [INCAS] trial), the triple drug arm proved clearly superior to the double combinations (i.e., AZT + nevirapine or AZT + ddI) (40, 88, 100). At week 52, 51% of patients had HIV RNA levels below 20 copies/ml for the triple drug combination arm, versus 12% and 0% in the AZT + ddI and AZT + nevirapine arms.

Likewise, patients treated with AZT + ddI + delavirdine demonstrated more sustained HIV RNA drops than patients treated with AZT + ddI or AZT + delavirdine (41). In addition, AZT + 3TC + delavirdine triple therapy proved more effective than AZT + 3TC or AZT + delavirdine treatment in drug-naive patients (115).

When efavirenz was combined with AZT + 3TC, a potent antiviral effect was noted that proved at least as effective as a conventional triple drug therapy containing two NRTIs and one PI (101). Inclusion of an NNRTI in treatment schedules consisting of one NRTI (e.g., 3TC, d4T) and one PI (e.g., nelfinavir, indinavir) resulted in a substantial virologic (and immunologic) effect (74). Moreover, quadruple combination therapy, including efavirenz, the PI nelfinavir, and two NRTIs, suppressed plasma viral load below 50 copies/ml in 75% of the cases and was more efficient than the triple drug arm combining nelfinavir with the two NRTIs (2). NNRTIs (i.e., delavirdine) have also shown to display activity in patients failing triple drug therapy with PIs (27). It is not clear whether the beneficial effect of delavirdine is due to the positive pharmacokinetic interactions between delavirdine and the PIs or to its intrinsic antiviral efficacy or both (89).

Small pilot studies have shown that NNRTIs may be useful as second-line therapy (71). However, it is recommended that these drugs not be added to current failing antiviral regimens but combined with drugs to which the patient is still naive or for which no cross-resistance is expected to the drugs that were used in the previous treatment schedule. Such cross-resistance will decrease the efficacy of the salvage (second-line) therapy and will allow the virus to gain NNRTI-specific resistance mutations rapidly.

It should be mentioned that NNRTIs may be well suited to prevent vertical transmission between mother and child or to prevent productive virus infection upon accidental HIV-1 exposure (e.g., needle sticks) because of their safety profile. Clinical trials to explore these issues are ongoing (50).

In Vivo Tolerance of NNRTIs

Because of their high antiviral selectivity, the NNRTIs usually display less severe toxic side effects than NRTIs. The major toxicity associated with nevirapine is maculopapular rash (17% of the patients), which has a characteristic onset within the first six weeks of therapy (83). When the rash is extensive or involves mucous membranes, nevirapine administration should be discontinued (71). Several cases of Stevens-Johnson syndrome have been reported and estimated to have an incidence of approximately 0.3% (128). Hepatitis has been rarely associated with nevirapine. Other side effects noticed in nevirapine-treated patients include diarrhea, fever (sometimes associated with the rash), fatigue, depression, and headache (125).

The most common toxicity associated with delavirdine is a diffuse, pruritic maculopapular rash (18% of patients) and occurs usually within the first four weeks of treatment (70). Severe rash (6% in nevirapine treatment) is less frequent in delavirdine-treated patients (3.8%). Steven-Johnson syndrome occurs very rarely. Other side effects, such as headache, gastrointestinal complaints, and hepatic transaminase elevation, have been reported (125).

The major adverse reactions reported for efavirenz are central nervous system complaints such as dizziness. These complaints are usually mild or moderate and often resolve after a few weeks. Rash is reported less frequently than for nevirapine or delavirdine and is usually mild (71, 92).

Emergence of Drug Resistance in NNRTI-Treated Patients

In the initial clinical studies, it was shown that the Tyr 181 Cys mutation most frequently appeared under nevirapine monotherapy (111). Interestingly, when combined with AZT, nevirapine infrequently selects for Tyr 181 Cys. For the pyridinone L-697661, similar observations were reported (120). Instead, a variety of other mutations at the amino acid locations 98, 100, 103, 106, 108, 181, 188, and 190 emerged. In particular, the emergence of Lys 103 Asn, Tyr 188 Cys, and Gly 190 Ala was favored (71). These observations are in line with the in vitro findings that Tyr 181 Cys reverses phenotypic AZT resistance owing to the presence of the 215 mutation (12, 86). For delavirdine monotherapy, the Lys 103 Asn mutation was the predominant amino acid mutation, followed by Tyr 181 Cys and Pro 236 Leu (as single mutations or combined with Lys 103 Asn) (46). In addition, the Lys 103 Asn mutant virus is most frequently observed in efavirenz-treated patients, conferring approximately 20-fold resistance to the drug (10). Whereas viruses containing Tyr 188 Cys or Gly 190 Ala mutations have only 4-fold decreased sensitivity to efavirenz, Tyr 188 Leu or Gly 190 Ser mutated viruses were found to be 100- to 200-fold resistant to efavirenz. The codons for 188 Leu and 190 Ser require two mutations when compared with wild-type Tyr 188 and Gly 190, whereas formation of the 188 Cys and 190 Ala RT virus mutants requires only one mutation in their codon (136). Thus, efavirenz (as well as other second-generation NNRTIs) requires more than one mutation in the HIV-1 RT gene before losing its pronounced inhibitory potential against HIV-1 (11, 72, 136).

A survey of more than 5,000 patient samples of NNRTI (nevirapine, delavirdine, and efavirenz)-treated individuals has recently been analyzed and genotypically and phenotypically characterized (77). Of the virus isolates, 56% proved cross-resistant to all three NNRTIs, 34% were cross-resistant to two NNRTIs, and only 18% proved resistant to one NNRTI. All efavirenz-resistant virus strains proved cross-resistant to nevirapine, whereas many nevirapine-resistant virus strains kept sensitivity to efavirenz or delavirdine. The most common mutations seen in the drug-treated individuals were the Lys 103 Asn mutation (29%), the Tyr 181 Cys mutation (14%), and the Gly 190 Ala mutation (17%). The most common double mutations were Lys 103 Asn + Tyr 181 Cys, and the most common triple mutations were Lys 103 Asn + Tyr 181 Cys + Gly 190 Ala. Sole nevirapine resistance was often due to the appearance of the 98 Gly and 108 Ile mutations.

Because patients failing on any of the NNRTIs are likely to possess one or multiple NNRTI-characteristic resistance mutations in the RT gene, it would be unwise to treat such patients with another, even second-generation, NNRTI, since such a treatment schedule is probably equivalent to sequential monotherapy and will likely lead to rapid emergence of NNRTI-resistant virus strains. However, if data on genotypic/phenotypic testing of the virus isolates of such patients are available, a better estimate can be made with regard to the feasibility of replacing the first NNRTI by another (second-generation) NNRTI in the treatment schedule. In contrast, for NNRTI-naive patients who failed NRTI or PI treatment or both, the use of an NNRTI with new NRTIs/PIs can be recommended. In addition, switching PIs for NNRTIs as part of the triple drug combination in patients with undetectable viral load can be an interesting strategy to offer the best conditions to the NNRTIs for a potent and sustained antiviral efficacy owing to the lack of measurable viral replication at the time of drug initiation, minimizing the risk of viral resistance and avoiding the emergence of long-term toxicity (i.e., hyperglycemia, hyperlipidemia, lipodystrophy, and visceral fat accumulation) associated with PIs (36, 97).

Conclusion

It has become increasingly clear that NNRTIs represent several structurally different families of HIV-1-specific RT inhibitors that are endowed with a number of unique properties; because of these properties, NNRTIs are of particular interest for inclusion in the current triple or quadruple drug cocktails used in HAART. The rapid drug-resistance development is clearly the Achilles' heel of these types of compounds. However, the NNRTIs have been proven beneficial in a number of clinical studies, especially when they are part of a triple drug combination regimen that contains two additional NRTIs or one NRTI and one PI. Since subtle changes in the structures of NNRTIs can markedly affect their resistance profile and antiviral efficacy, continuous efforts should be devoted to develop additional NNRTIs to be added to the current armamentarium of anti-HIV drugs to optimize the antiretroviral therapy further.

ACKNOWLEDGMENTS

The author thanks Christiane Callebaut, Inge Aerts, and Chantal Biernaux for dedicated editorial help. The research of the author is partially supported by grants from the European Commission.

REFERENCES

1. Ahgren, C., K. Backro, F. W. Bell, A. S. Cantrell, M. Clemens, J. M. Colacino, J. B. Deeter, J. A. Engelhardt, M. Hogberg, S. R. Jaskunas, N. G. Johansson, C. L. Jordan, J. S. Kasher, M. D. Kinnick, P. Lind, C. Lopez, J. M. Morin, Jr., M. A. Muesing, R. Noreen, B. Öberg, C. J. Paget, J. A. Palkowitz, C. A. Parrish, P. Pranc, M. K. Rippy, C. Rydergard, C. Sahlberg, S. Swanson, R. J. Ternasky, T. Unge, R. T. Vasileff, L. Vrang, S. J. West, H. Zhang, and X. X. Zhou. 1995. The PETT series, a new class of potent nonnucleoside inhibitors of human immunodeficiency virus type 1 reverse transcriptase. Antimicrob. Agents Chemother. 39:1329–1335.
2. Albrecht, M., D. Katzenstein, R. Bosch, S. H. Liou, and S. M. Hammer. 1998. ACTG 364: virologic efficacy of nelfinavir and/or efavirenz in combination with new nucleoside analogs in nucleoside experienced subjects. Abstracts of the 12th World AIDS Conference, Geneva, June 28–July 3, 1998, no. 12203.
3. Althaus, I. W., K.-C. Chou, R. J. Lemay, K. M. Franks, M. R. Deibel, F. J. Kezdy, L. Resnick, M. E. Busso, A. G. So, K. M. Downey, D. L. Romero, R. C. Thomas, P. A. Aristoff, W. G. Tarpley, and F. Reusser. 1996. The benzylthiopyrimidine U-31,355, a potent inhibitor of HIV-1 reverse transcriptase. Biochem. Pharmacol. 51:743–750.
4. Antonucci, T., J. S. Warmus, J. C. Hodges, and D. G. Nickell. 1995. Characterization of the antiviral activity of highly substituted pyrroles: a novel class of non-nucleoside HIV-1 reverse transcriptase inhibitor. Antiviral Chem. Chemother. 6:98–108.
5. Arasteh, K., M. Mueller, R. Wood, L. Cass, K. H. P. Moore, N. Dallow, A. Jones, V. Burt, J. P. Kleim, and W. Prince. 1999. Preliminary tolerability, pharmacokinetics (PK), and initial effect on plasma HIV-1 RNA following administration of GW420867X once-daily (50 mg, 100 mg and 200 mg) for 28 days to patients infected with HIV-1. Interscience Conference for Antimicrobial Agents and Chemotherapy (ICAAC), abstr. 504.
6. Arranz, E., J. A. Díaz, S. T. Ingate, M. Witvrouw, C. Pannecouque, J. Balzarini, E. De Clercq, and S. Vega. 1998. Novel 1,1,3-trioxo-2H,4H-thieno[3,4-e]-[1,2,4]thiadiazine (TTD) derivatives as non-nucleoside reverse transcriptase inhibitors that inhibit the human immunodeficiency virus type 1 (HIV-1) replication. J. Med. Chem. 41:4103–4117.

7. Artico, M., S. Massa, A. Mai, M. E. Marongiu, G. Piras, E. Tramontano, and P. La Colla. 1993. 3,4-Dihydro-2-alkoxy-6-benzyl-4-oxopyrimidines (DABOs): a new class of specific inhibitors of human immunodeficiency virus type 1. Antiviral Chem. Chemother. 4:361–368.

8. Baba, M., H. Tanaka, E. De Clercq, R. Pauwels, J. Balzarini, D. Schols, H. Nakashima, C.-F. Perno, R. T. Walker, and T. Miyasaka. 1989. Highly specific inhibition of human immunodeficiency virus type 1 by a novel 6-substituted acyclouridine derivative. Biochem. Biophys. Res. Commun. 165:1375–1381.

9. Baba, M. M., S. Shigeta, S. Yuasa, H. Takashima, K. Sekiya, M. Ubasawa, H. Tanaka, T. Miyasaka, R. T. Walker, and E. De Clercq. 1994. Preclinical evaluation of MKC-442, a highly potent and specific inhibitor of human immunodeficiency virus type 1 *in vitro.* Antimicrob. Agents Chemother. 38:688–692.

10. Bacheler, L., O. Weislow, S. Snyder, and P. G. Hanna. 1998. Virological resistance to efavirenz. Abstracts of the 12th World AIDS Conference, Geneva, June 28–July 3, 1998, no. 41213.

11. Bacheler, L. T., E. Anton, S. Jeffrey, H. George, G. Hollis, A. Abremski, and Sustiva Resistance Study Team. 1998. RT gene mutations associated with resistance to efavirenz. Abstracts of the Second International Workshop on HIV Drug Resistance and Treatment Strategies, June 24–27, 1998, Lake Maggiore, Italy, no. 19.

12. Balzarini, J. 1999. Strategies to suppress resistance to drugs targeted at human immunodeficiency virus reverse transcriptase by combination therapy. Commentary Biochem. Pharmacol. 58:1–27.

13. Balzarini, J., W. G. Brouwer, E. E. Felauer, E. De Clercq, and A. Karlsson. 1995. Activity of various thiocarboxanilide derivatives against wild-type and several mutant human immunodeficiency virus type 1 strains. Antiviral Res. 27:219–236.

14. Balzarini, J., and E. De Clercq. 1996. Analysis of inhibition of retroviral reverse transcriptase. Methods Enzymol. 275:472–502.

15. Balzarini, J., E. De Clercq, A. Carbonez, V. Burt, and J.-P. Kleim. 2000. Long-term exposure of combinations of the novel quinoxaline GW420867X with lamivudine, abacavir and a variety of non-nucleoside reverse transcriptase inhibitors to HIV-1-infected cell cultures. AIDS Res. Hum. Retroviruses 16:517–528.

16. Balzarini, J., A. Karlsson, M.-J. Pérez-Pérez, M.-J. Camarasa, W. G. Tarpley, and E. De Clercq. 1993. Treatment of human immunodeficiency virus type 1 (HIV-1)-infected cells by combinations of HIV-1-specific inhibitors results in a different resistance pattern than does treatment with single-drug therapy. J. Virol. 67:5353–5359.

17. Balzarini, J., A. Karlsson, M.-J. Pérez-Pérez, L. Vrang, J. Walbers, H. Zhang, B. Oberg, A.-M. Vandamme, and E. De Clercq. 1993. HIV-1 specific reverse transcriptase inhibitors show differential activity against HIV-1 mutant strains containing different amino acid substitutions in the reverse transcriptase. Virology 192:246–253.

18. Balzarini, J., A. Karlsson, V. V. Sardana, E. A. Emini, M.-J. Camarasa, and E. De Clercq. 1994. Human immunodeficiency virus 1 (HIV-1)-specific reverse transcriptase (RT) inhibitors may suppress the replication of specific drug-

resistant (E138K)RT HIV-1 mutants or select for highly resistant (Y181C → C181I)RT HIV-1 mutants. Proc. Natl. Acad. Sci. USA 91:6599–6603.

19. Balzarini, J., A. Karlsson, A.-M.Vandamme, M.-J. Pérez-Pérez, H. Zhang, L. Vrang, B. Öberg, K. Bäckbro, T. Unge, A. San-Félix, S.Velazquez, M.-J. Camarasa, and E. De Clercq. 1993. Human immunodeficiency virus type 1 (HIV-1) strains selected for resistance against the HIV-1-specific [2′,5′-bis-O-(tert-butyldimethylsilyl)-3′-spiro-5″-(4″-amino-1″,2″-oxathiole-2″,2″-dioxide)]-β-D-pentofuranosyl (TSAO) nucleoside analogues retain sensitivity to HIV-1-specific nonnucleoside inhibitors Proc. Natl. Acad. Sci. USA 90: 6952–6956.

20. Balzarini, J., H. Pelemans, S. Aquaro, C.-F. Perno, M.Witvrouw, D. Schols, E. De Clercq, and A. Karlsson. 1996. Highly favorable antiviral activity and resistance profile of the novel thiocarboxanilide pentenyloxy ether derivatives UC-781 and UC-82 as inhibitors of human immunodeficiency virus type 1 (HIV-1) replication. Mol. Pharmacol. 50:394–401.

21. Balzarini, J., M.-J. Pérez-Pérez, A. San-Félix, M.-J. Camarasa, I. C. Bathurst, P. J. Barr, and E. De Clercq 1992. Kinetics of inhibition of human immunodeficiency virus type 1 (HIV-1) reverse transcriptase by the novel HIV-1-specific nucleoside analogue [2′,5′-bis-O-(tert-butyldimethylsilyl)-β-D-ribofuranosyl]-3′-spiro-5″-(4″-amino-1″,2″-oxathiole-2″,2″-di-oxide)thymine (TSAO-T). J. Biol. Chem. 267:11831–11838.

22. Balzarini, J., M.-J. Pérez-Pérez, A. San-Félix, D. Schols, C.-F. Perno, A.-M. Vandamme, M.-J. Camarasa, and E. De Clercq. 1992. 2′,5′-Bis-O-(tert-butyldimethylsilyl)-3′-spiro-5″-(4″-amino-1″,2″-oxathiole-2″,2″-dioxide)pyrimidine (TSAO) nucleoside analogues: highly selective inhibitors of human immunodeficiency virus type 1 that are targeted at the viral reverse transcriptase. Proc. Natl. Acad. Sci. USA 89:4392–4396.

23. Balzarini, J., M.-J. Pérez-Pérez, S. Vélazquez, A. San-Félix, M.-J. Camarasa, E. De Clercq, and A. Karlsson. 1995. Suppression of the breakthrough of human immunodeficiency virus type 1 (HIV-1) in cell culture by thiocarboxanilide derivatives when used individually or in combination with other HIV-1-specific inhibitors (i.e. TSAO derivatives). Proc. Natl. Acad. Sci. USA 92:5470–5474.

24. Barth, B., M. Dierich, G. Heinisch, V. Jenny, B. Matuszczak, K. Mereiter, R. Planer, I. Schöpf, H. Stoiber, T. Traugott, and P. V. Aufschnaiter. 1996. Pyridazino[3,4-b][1,5]benzoxazepin-5(6H)-ones: synthesis and biological evaluation. Antiviral Chem. Chemother. 7:300–312.

25. Bell, F. W., A. S. Cantrell, M. Högberg, S. R. Jaskunas, N. G. Johansson, C. L. Jordan, M. D. Kinnick, L. Lind, J. M. Morin, Jr., R. Noréen, B. Öberg, J. A. Palkowitz, C. A. Parrish, P. Pranc, C. Sahlberg, R. J. Ternansky, R. T.Vasileff, L. Vrang, S. J. West, H. Zhang, and X.-X. Zhou. 1995. Phenethylthiazolethiourea (PETT) compounds, a new class of HIV-1 reverse transcriptase inhibitors. 1. Synthesis and basic structure-activity relationship studies of PETT analogs. J. Med. Chem. 38:4929–4936.

26. Bellarosa, D., G. Antonelli, F. Bambacioni, D. Giannotti, G.Viti, R. Nannicini, A. Giachetti, F. Dianzani, M. Witvrouw, R. Pauwels, J. Desmyter, and E. De Clercq. 1996. New arylpyrido-diazepine and -thiodiazepine derivatives are

potent and highly selective HIV-1 inhibitors targeted at the reverse transcriptase. Antiviral Res. 30:109–124.

27. Bellman, P. 1998. Clinical experience with adding delavirdine to combination therapy in patients in whom multiple antiretroviral treatment including protease inhibitors has failed. AIDS 12:1333–1340.

28. Boyer, P. L., J. Ding, E. Arnold, and S. H. Hughes. 1994. Subunit specificity of mutations that confer resistance to non-nucleoside inhibitors in human immunodeficiency virus type 1 reverse transcriptase. Antimicrob. Agents Chemother. 38:1909–1914.

29. Boyer, P. L., H.-Q. Gao, and S. H. Hughes. 1998. A mutation at position 190 of human immunodeficiency virus type 1 reverse transcriptase interacts with mutations at positions 74 and 75 via the template primer. Antimicrob. Agents Chemother. 42:447–452.

30. Buckheit, R. W., Jr., V. Fliakas-Boltz, W. D. Decker, J. L. Roberson, C. A. Pyle, E. L. White, B. J. Bowdon, J. B. McMahon, M. R. Boyd, J. P. Bader, D. G. Nickell, H. Barth, and T. K. Antonucci. 1994. Biological and biochemical anti-HIV activity of the benzothiadiazine class of nonnucleoside reverse transcriptase inhibitors. Antiviral Res. 25:43–56.

31. Buckheit, R. W., Jr., M. G. Hollingshead, J. Germany-Decker, E. L. White, J. B. McMahon, L. B. Allen, L. J. Ross, W. D. Decker, L. Westbrook, W. M. Shannon, O. Weislow, J. P. Bader, and M. R. Boyd. 1993. Thiazolobenzimidazole: biological and biochemical anti-retroviral activity of a new nonnucleoside reverse transcriptase inhibitor. Antiviral Res. 21:247–265.

32. Byrnes, V. W., E. A. Emini, W. A. Schleif, J. H. Condra, C. L. Schneider, W. J. Long, J. A. Wolfgang, D. J. Graham, L. Gotlib, A. J. Schlabach, B. S. Wolanski, O. M. Blahy, J. C. Quintero, A. Rhodes, E. Roth, D. L. Titus, and V. V. Sardana. 1994. Susceptibilities of human immunodeficiency virus type 1 enzyme and viral variants expressing multiple resistance-engendering amino acid substitutions to reserve transcriptase inhibitors. Antimicrob. Agents Chemother. 38:1404–1407.

33. Byrnes, V. W., V. V. Sardana, W. A. Schleif, J. H. Condra, J. A. Waterbury, J. A. Wolfgang, W. J. Long, C. L. Schneider, A. J. Schlabach, B. S. Wolanski, D. J. Graham, L. Gotlib, A. Rhodes, D. L. Titus, E. Roth, O. M. Blahy, J. C. Quintero, S. Staszewski, and E. A. Emini. 1993. Comprehensive mutant enzyme and viral variant assessment of human immunodeficiency virus type 1 reverse transcriptase resistance to nonnucleoside inhibitors. Antimicrob. Agents Chemother. 37:1576–1579.

34. Camarasa, M.-J., M.-J. Pérez-Pérez, A. San-Félix, J. Balzarini, and E. De Clercq. 1992. 3'-Spironucleosides (TSAO derivatives), a new class of specific human immunodeficiency virus type 1 inhibitors. Synthesis and antiviral activity of 3'-spiro-5"-[4"-amino-1",2"-oxathiole-2",2"-dioxide]pyrimidine nucleosides. J. Med. Chem. 35:2721–2727.

35. Campiani, G., V. Nacci, I. Fiorini, M. P. De Filippis, A. Garofalo, G. Greco, E. Novellino, S. Altamura, and L. Di Renzo. 1996. Pyrrolobenzothiazepinones and pyrrolobenzoxazepinones: novel and specific non-nucleoside HIV-1 reverse transcriptase inhibitors with antiviral activity. J. Med. Chem. 39: 2672–2680.

36. Carr, A., K. Samaras, S. Burton, J. Freund, D. J. Chisholm, and D. A. Cooper. 1998. A syndrome of peripheral lipodystrophy, hyperlipidemia and insulin resistance due to HIV protease inhibitors. Abstracts of the Fifth Conference on Retroviruses and Opportunistic Infections, Chicago, no. 410.

37. Carroll, S. S., M. Stahlhut, J. Geib, and D. B. Olsen. 1994. Inhibition of HIV-1 reverse transcriptase by a quinazolinone and comparison with inhibition by pyridinones. J. Biol. Chem. 269:32351–32357.

38. Cheeseman, S., D. Havlir, M. M. McLaughlin, T. C. Greenough, J. L. Sullivan, D. Hall, S. E. Hattox, S. A. Spector, D. S. Stein, M. Myers, and D. D. Richman.. 1995. Phase I/II evaluation of nevirapine alone and in combination with zidovudine for infection with human immunodeficiency virus. J. Acquired Immune Defic. Syndr. Hum. Retrovirol. 8:141–151.

39. Chimirri, A., S. Grasso, C. Molica, A.-M. Monforte, P. Monforte, M. Zappalà, G. Bruno, F. Nicolò, M. Witvrouw, H. Jonckheere, J. Balzarini, and E. De Clercq. 1997. Structural features and anti-human immunodeficiency virus (HIV) activity of the isomers of 1-(2′,6′-difluorophenyl)-1H,3H-thiazolo[3,4-a]benzimidazole, a potent non-nucleoside HIV-1 reverse transcriptase inhibitor. Antiviral Chem. Chemother. 8:363–370.

40. D'Aquila, R. T., M. D. Hughes, V. A. Johnson, M. A. Fischl, J. P. Sommadossi, S. H. Liou, J. Timpone, M. Myers, N. Basgoz, M. Niu, and M. S. Hirsch. 1996. Nevirapine, zidovudine and didanosine compared with zidovudine and didanosine in patients with HIV-1 infection. A randomized, double-blind, placebo-controlled trial. Ann. Intern. Med. 124:1019–1030.

41. Davey, R. T., Jr., D. G. Chaitt, G. F. Reed, W. W. Freimuth, B. R. Herpin, J. A. Metcalf, P. S. Eastman, J. Falloon, J. A. Kovacs, M. A. Polis, R. E. Walker, H. Masur, J. Boyle, S. Coleman, S. R. Cox, L. Wathen, C. L. Daenzer, and H. C. Lane. 1996. Randomized, controlled phase I/II trial of combination therapy with delavirdine (U-90152S) and conventional nucleosides in human immunodeficiency virus type 1-infected patients. Antimicrob. Agents Chemother. 40:1657–1664.

42. Debyser, Z., R. Pauwels, K. Andries, and E. De Clercq. 1992. Specific HIV-1 reverse transcriptase inhibitors. J. Enzyme Inhibition 6:47–53.

43. De Clercq, E. 1999. Perspectives of non-nucleoside reverse transcriptase inhibitors (NNRTIs) in the therapy of HIV-1 infection. Il Farmaco 54:26–45.

44. De Jong, M., S. Vella, A. Carr, et al. 1997. High-dose nevirapine in previously untreated human immunodeficiency virus type-1-infected persons does not result in sustained suppression of viral replication. J. Infect. Dis. 175: 966–970.

45. De Lucca, G. V., and M. J. Otto. 1992. Synthesis and anti-HIV activity of pyrrolo-[1,2-d]-(1,4)-benzodiazepin-6-ones. Bioorganic Med. Chem. Lett. 2: 1639–1644.

46. Demeter, L., R. Shafer, M. Para, et al. 1996. Delavirdine (DLV) susceptibility of HIV-1 isolates obtained from patients receiving DLV monotherapy. Abstracts of the Third Conference on Retroviruses and Opportunistic Infections, Washington, no. 323.

47. Ding, J., K. Das, H. Moereels, L. Koymans, K. Andries, P. A. J. Janssen, S. H. Hughes, and E. Arnold. 1995. Structure of HIV-1 RT/TIBO R 86183 complex

reveals similarity in the binding of diverse non-nucleoside inhibitors. Nat. Struct. Biol. 2:407–415.

48. Di Santo, R., R. Costi, M. Artico, S. Massa, M. E. Marongiu, A. G. Loi, A. De Montis, and P. La Colla. 1998. 1,2,5-Benzothiadiazepine and pyrrolo[2,1-d][1,2,5]benzo-thiadiazepine derivatives with specific anti-human immunodeficiency virus type 1 activity. Antiviral Chem. Chemother. 9:127–137.

49. Dollé, V., C. H. Nguyen, A. M. Aubertin, A. Kirn, M. L. Andreola, G. Jamieson, L. Tarrago-Litvak, and E. Bisagni. 1995. A new series of pyridinone derivatives as potent non-nucleoside human immunodeficiency virus type 1 specific reverse transcriptase inhibitors. J. Med. Chem. 38:4679–4686.

50. Dorenbum-Kracer, A., J. Sullivan, R. Gelbert, L. Mofeson, M. Culnane, C. Cunningham, G. Brown, K. Beckerman, and K. Dransfield. 1998. Antiretroviral use in pregnancy in PACTG316; a phase III randomized, blinded study of single-dose intrapartum/neonatal nevirapine to reduce mother to infant HIV transmission. Abstracts of the 12th World AIDS Conference, Geneva, June 28–July 3, 1998, no. 23281.

51. Dueweke, T. J., S. M. Poppe, D. L. Romero, S. M. Swaney, A. G. So, K. M. Downey, I. W. Althaus, F. Reusser, M. Busso, L. Resnick, D. L. Mayers, J. Lane, P. A. Aristoff, R. C. Thomas, and W. G. Tarpley. 1993. U-90152, a potent inhibitor of human immunodeficiency virus type 1 replication. Antimicrob. Agents Chemother. 37:1127–1131.

52. Dueweke, T. J., T. Pushkarskaya, S. M. Poppe, S. M. Swaney, Q. Zhao, S. Y. Chen, M. Stevenson, and W. G. Tarpley. 1993. A mutation in revese transcriptase of bis(heteroaryl)piperazine-resistant human immunodeficiency virus type 1 that confers increased sensitivity to other nonnucleoside inhibitors. Proc. Natl. Acad. Sci. USA 90:4713–4717.

53. Esnouf, R., J. Ren, C. Ross, Y. Jones, D. Stammers, and D. Stuart. 1995. Mechanism of inhibition of HIV-1 reverse transcriptase by non-nucleoside inhibitors. Nat. Struct. Biol. 2:303–308.

54. Esnouf, R. M., J. Ren, E. F. Garman, D. O'N. Somers , C. K. Ross, E. Y. Jones, D. K. Stammers, and D. I. Stuart. 1998. Continuous and discontinuous changes in the unit cell of HIV-1 reverse transcriptase crystals on dehydration. Acta Crystallographica D54:938–953.

55. Esnouf, R. M., J. Ren, A. L. Hopkins, A. K. Ross, E. Y. Jones, D. K. Stammers, and D. I. Stuart. 1997. Unique features in the structure of the complex between HIV-1 reverse transcriptase and the bis(heteroaryl)piperazine (BHAP) U-90152 explain resistance mutations for this nonnucleoside inhibitor. Proc. Natl. Acad. Sci. USA 94:3984–3989.

56. Fan, N., K. B. Rank, D. B. Evans, R. C. Thomas, W. G. Tarpley, and S. K. Sharma. 1995. Simultaneous mutations at Tyr-181 and Tyr-188 in HIV-1 reverse transcriptase prevents inhibition of RNA-dependent DNA polymerase activity by the bisheteroarylpiperazine (BHAP) U-90152s. FEBS Lett. 370:59–62.

57. Fletcher, R. S., D. Arion, G. Borkow, M. A. Wainberg, G. I. Dmitrienko, and M. A. Parniak. 1995. Synergistic inhibition of HIV-1 reverse transcriptase DNA polymerase activity and virus replication in vitro by combinations of carboxanilide nonnucleoside compounds. Biochemistry 34:10106–10112.

58. Fletcher, R. S., K. Syed, S. Mithani, G. I. Dmitrienko, and M. A. Parniak. 1995. Carboxanilide derivative non-nucleoside inhibitors of HIV-1 reverse transcriptase interact with different mechanistic forms of the enzyme. Biochemistry 34:4346–4353.

59. Frank, K. B., G. J. Noll, E. V. Connell, and I. S. Sim. 1991. Kinetic interaction of human immunodeficiency virus type 1 reverse transcriptase with the antiviral tetrahydroimidazo[4,5,1-jk][1,4]-benzodiazepine-2-(1H)-thione compound, R82150. J. Biol. Chem. 266:14232–14236.

60. Fujiwara, T., A. Sato, M. El-Farrash, S. Miki, K. Abe, Y. Isaka, M. Kodama, Y. Wu, L. B. Chen, H. Harada, H. Sugimoto, M. Hatanaka, and Y. Hinuma. 1998. S-1153 inhibits replication of known drug-resistant strains of human immunodeficiency virus type 1. Antimicrob. Agents Chemother. 42:1340–1345.

61. Goldman, M. E., J. H. Nunberg, J. A. O'Brien, J. C. Quintero, W. A. Schleif, K. F. Freund, S. L. Gaul, W. S. Saari, J. S. Wai., J. M. Hoffman, P. S. Anderson, D. J. Hupe, E. A. Emini, and A. M. Stern. 1991. Pyridinone derivatives: specific human immunodeficiency virus type 1 reverse transcriptase inhibitors with antiviral activity. Proc. Natl. Acad. Sci. USA 88:6863–6867.

62. Harris, D., R. Lee, H. S. Misra, P. K. Pandey, and V. N. Pandey. 1998. The p51 subunit of human immunodeficiency virus type 1 reverse transcriptase is essential in loading the p66 subunit on the template primer. Biochemistry 37:5903–5908.

63. Havlir, D., S. H. Cheeseman, M. McLaughin, R. Murphy, A. Erice, S. A. Spector, T. C. Greenough, J. L. Sullivan, D. Hall, and M. Myers. 1995. High-dose nevirapine: safety, pharmacokinetics, and antiviral effect in patients with human immunodeficiency virus infection. J. Infect. Dis. 171:537–545.

64. Hellmig, B., D. J. Woolf, C. Debouck, and S. C. Harrison. 1995. The structure of unliganded reverse transcriptase from the human immunodeficiency virus type 1. Proc. Natl. Acad. Sci. USA 92:1222–1226.

65. Hsiou, Y., K. Das, J. Ding, A. D. Clarck, Jr., P. L. Boyer, P. A. J. Janssen, J.-P. Kleim, M. Rosner, S. H. Hughes, and E. Arnold. 1998. Crystal structures of wild-type and mutant HIV-1 reverse transcriptase and non-nucleoside inhibitors: implications for drug resistance mechanisms. Abstracts of the Second International Workshop on HIV Drug Resistance and Treatment Strategies, June 24–27, 1998, Lake Maggiore, Italy, no. 21.

66. Huang, H. F., R. Chopra, G. L. Verdine, and S. C. Harrison. 1998. Structure of a covalently trapped catalytic complex of HIV-1 reverse transcriptase. Implications of drug resistance. Science 282:1669–1675.

67. Ijichi, K., M. Fujiwara, Y. Hanasaki, H. Watanabe, K. Katsuura, H. Takayama, S. Shirakawa, S.-I. Sakai, S. Shigeta, K. Konno, T. Yokota, and M. Baba. 1995. Potent and specific inhibition of human immunodeficiency virus type 1 replication by 4-(2,6-dichlorophenyl)-1,2,5-thiadiazol-3-Y1 N,N-dialkylcarbamate derivatives. Antimicrob. Agents Chemother. 39:2337–2340.

68. Ijichi, K., M. Fujiwara, H. Nagano, Y. Matsumoto, Y. Hanasaki, T. Ide, K. Katsuura, H. Takayama, S. Shirakawa, N. Aimi, S. Shigeta, K. Konno, M. Matsushima, T. Yokota, and M. Baba. 1996. Anti-HIV-1 activity of thiadiazole derivatives: a structure-activity relationship, reverse transcriptase inhibition, and lipophilicity. Antiviral Res. 31:87–94.

69. Jacobo-Molina, A., J. Ding, R. G. Nanni, A. D. Clarck, X. Lu, C. Tantillo, R. L. Williams, G. Kame, A. L. Ferris, P. Clarck, A. Hitzi, S. H. Hughes, and E. Arnold. 1993. Crystal structure of human immunodeficiency virus type 1 reverse transcriptase complexed with double-stranded DNA at 3.0 Å shows bent DNA. Proc. Natl. Acad. Sci. USA 90:6320–6324.

70. Joly, V., on behalf of the M/3331:013B Study Group. 1998. Tolerance and efficacy of delavirdine mesylate (DLV) and zidovudine (ZDV) therapy in the treatment of HIV infected patients (study M/3331/013B). Abstracts of the Fourth International Congress on Drug Therapy in HIV Infection, Glasgow, United Kingdom, no. P32.

71. Joly, V., and P. Yeni. 1999. Non nucleoside reverse transcriptase inhibitors. AIDS Reviews 1:37–44.

72. Jonckheere, H., J.-M. Taymans, J. Balzarini, S. Velazquez, M.-J. Camarasa, J. Desmyter, E. De Clercq, and J. Anné. 1994. Resistance of HIV-1 reverse transcriptase against [2′,5′-bis-O-(*tert*-butyldimethylsilyl)-3′-spiro-5″-(4″-amino-1″,2″-oxathiole-2″,2″-dioxide)] (TSAO) derivatives is determined by the mutation Glu^{138} → Lys on the p51 subunit. J. Biol. Chem. 269:25255–25258.

73. Jourdan, F., J. Renault, C. Fossey, R. Bureau, D. Ladurée, M. Robba, A. M. Aubertin, and A. Kirn. 1997. Design, synthesis and antiviral activity of new pyridinone derivatives. Antiviral Chem. Chemother. 8:161–172.

74. Kagan, S., J. Jemsek, D. G. Martin, G. Pierone, D. J. Manion, S. R. Lee, N. Ruiz, and the DMP 266-24 Clinical Study Team. 1998. Initial effectiveness and tolerability of nelfinavir (NFV) in combination with efavirenz (EFV, Sustiva, DMP 266) in antiretroviral therapy naïve or nucleoside analogue experience HIV-1 infected patients: characterization in a phase II, open-label, multicenter study at > 36 weeks. 38th Interscience Conference on Antimicrobial Agents and Chemotherapy, San Diego, abstr. I-102.

75. Kashman, Y., K. R. Gustafson, R. W. Fuller, J. H. Cardellina II, J. B. McMahon, M. J. Currens, R. W. Buckheit, Jr., S. H. Hughes, G. M. Cragg, and M. R. Boyd. 1992. The calanolides, a novel HIV-inhibitory class of coumarin derivatives from the tropical rainforest tree, *Calophyllum lanigerum*. J. Med. Chem. 35:2735–2743.

76. Kelly, T. A., D. W. McNeil, J. M. Rose, E. David, C.-K. Shih, and P. M. Grob. 1997. Novel non-nucleoside inhibitors of human immunodeficiency virus type 1 reverse transcriptase. 6. 2-Indol-3-yl- and 2-azaindol-3-yl-dipyrido-diazepinones. J. Med. Chem. 40:2430–2433.

77. Kemp, S., S. Bloor, A. Van Cauwenberghe, I. De Koning, C. Van den Eynde, B. Larder, and K. Hertogs. 1999. Analysis of 5000 HIV-1 clinical samples reveals complex non-nucleoside RT inhibitor resistance patterns. Third International Workshop on HIV Drug Resistance and Treatment Strategies, San Diego, June 23–26. Antiviral Therapy 4(suppl. 1):20, abstr. 26.

78. Kim, D.-K., J. Gam, Y.-W. Kim, J. Lim, H.-T. Kim, and K. H. Kim. 1997. Synthesis and anti-HIV-1 activity of a series of 1-alkoxy-5-alkyl-6-(arylthio)uracils. J. Med. Chem. 40:2363–2373.

79. Kleim, J.-P., R. Bender, U.-M. Billhardt, C. Meichsner, G. Riess, M. Rösner, I. Winkler, and A. Paessens. 1993. Activity of a novel quinoxaline derivative

against human immunodeficiency virus type 1 reverse transcriptase and viral replication. Antimicrob. Agents Chemother. 37:1659–1664.

80. Kleim, J.-P., R. Bender, R. Kirsch, C. Meichsner, A. Paessens, M. Rösner, H. Rübsamen-Waigmann, R. Kaiser, M. Wichers, K. E. Schneweis, I. Winkler, and G. Riess. 1995. Preclinical evaluation of HBY 097, a new nonnucleoside reverse transcriptase inhibitor of human immunodeficiency virus type 1 replication. Antimicrob. Agents Chemother. 39:253–257.

81. Kleim, J.-P., M. Rosner, I. Winkler, A. Paessens, R. Kirsch, Y. Hsiou, E. Arnold, and G. Riess. 1996. Selective pressure of a quinoxaline nonnucleoside inhibitor of human immunodeficiency virus type 1 (HIV-1) reverse transcriptase (RT) on HIV-1 replication results in the emergence of nucleoside RT-inhibitor-specific (RT Leu-74-Val or Ile and Val-75-Leu or Ile) HIV-1 mutants. Proc. Natl. Acad. Sci. USA 93:34–38.

82. Kleim, J.-P., I. Winkler, M. Rosner, R. Kirsch, H. Rubsamen-Waigmann, A. Paessens, and G. Reiss. 1997. In vitro selection for different mutational patterns in the HIV-1 reverse transcriptase using high and low selective pressure on the nonnucleoside reverse transcriptase inhibitor HBY 097. Virology 231:112–118.

83. Kohlbrenner, V., K. Dransfield, D. Cotton, P. Robinson, and M. Myers. 1996. Cutaneous eruptions associated with nevirapine therapy in HIV-A infected individuals. Abstracts of the XI International Conference on AIDS, Vancouver, B.C., no. Mo.B.1202.

84. Kohlstaedt, L. A., J. Wang, J. M. Friedman, P. A. Rice, and T. A. Steitz. 1992. Crystal structure at 3.5Å resolution of HIV-1 reverse transcriptase complexed with an inhibitor. Science 256:1783–1790.

85. Krikorian, D., S. Parushev, V. Tarpanov, P. Mechkarova, B. Mikhova, M. Botta, F. Corelli, G. Maga, and S. Spadari. 1997. Synthesis and biological evaluation of imidazo[1,2-d][1,4]benzodiazepines and related compounds as potential anti-HIV-1 agents. Med. Chem. Res. 7:546–556.

86. Larder, B. A. 1992. 3-Azido-3′-deoxythymidine resistance suppressed by a mutation conferring human immunodeficiency virus type 1 resistance to nonnucleoside reverse transcriptase inhibitors. Antimicrob. Agents Chemother. 36:2664–2669.

87. Livermore, D. G. H., R. C. Bethell, N. Cammack, A. P. Hancock, M. M. Hann, D. V. S. Green, R. B. Lamont, S. A. Noble, D. C. Orr, J. J. Payne, M. V. J. Ramsay, A. H. Shingler, C. Smith, R. Storer, C. Williamson, and T. Willson. 1993. Synthesis and anti-HIV-1 activity of a series of imidazo[1,5-b]pyridazines. J. Med. Chem. 36:3784–3794.

88. Luzuriaga, K., Y. Bryson, P. Krogstad, J. Robinson, B. Stechenberg, M. Lamson, S. Cort, and J. L. Sullivan. 1997. Combination treatment with zidovudine, didanosine, and nevirapine in infants with human immunodeficiency virus type 1 infection. N. Engl. J. Med. 336:1343–1349.

89. Lyle, G. 1998. Effect of nelfinavir/indinavir/delavirdine in HIV+ patients with extensive antiviral experience. Abstracts of the 12th World AIDS Conference, Geneva, June 28–July 3, 1998, no. 12329.

90. Maass, G., U. Immendoerfer, B. Koenig, U. Leser, B. Mueller, R. Goody, and E. Pfaff. 1993. Viral resistance to the thiazolo-iso-indolinones, a new class of

nonnucleoside inhibitors of human immunodeficiency virus type 1 reverse transcriptase. Antimicrob. Agents Chemother. 37:2612–2617.

91. Massa, S., A. Mai, M. Artico, G. Sbardella, E. Tramontano, A. G. Loi, P. Scano, and P. La Colla. 1995. Synthesis and antiviral activity of new 3,4-dihydro-2-alkoxy-6-benzyl-4-oxopyrimidines (DABOs), specific inhibitors of human immunodeficiency virus type 1. Antiviral Chem. Chemother. 6:1–8.

92. Mayers, D., J. Jemesk, E. Eyster, K. Tashima, and M. Thompson. 1998. A double-blind, placebo-controlled study to assess the safety, tolerability and antiretroviral activity of efavirenz in combination with open-label zidovudine and lamivudine in HIV-1 infected patients (DMP-266-004). Abstracts of the 12th World AIDS Conference, Geneva, June 28–July 3, 1998, no. 22340.

93. Mellors, J., H. Bazmi, R. F. Schinazi, B. M. Roy, Y. Hsiou, E. Arnold, J. Weir, and D. Mayers. 1995. Novel mutations in the reverse transcriptase of human immunodeficiency virus type 1 reduce susceptibility to foscarnet in laboratory and clinical isolates. Antimicrob. Agents Chemother. 39:1087–1092.

94. Mellors, J. W., B. A. Larder, and R. F. Schinazi. 1998. Mutations in HIV-1 reverse transcriptase and protease associated with drug resistance. Int. Antiviral News, MediTech Media Ltd.

95. Merluzzi, V. J., K. D. Hargrave, M. Labadia, K. Grozinger, M. Skoog, J. C. Wu, C.-K. Shin, K. Eckner, S. Hattox, J. Adams, A. S. Rosenthal, R. Faanes, R. J. Eckner, R. A. Koup, and J. L. Sullivan. 1990. Inhibition of HIV-1 replication by a nonnucleoside reverse transcriptase inhibitor. Science 250:1411–1413.

96. Mertens, A., H. Zilch, B. Konig, W. Schafer, T. Poll, W. Kampe, H. Seidel, U. Leser, and H. Leinert. 1993. Selective non-nucleoside HIV-1 reverse transcriptase inhibitors. New 2,3-dihydrothiazolo[2,3-a]isoindol-5(9H)-ones and related compounds with anti-HIV-1 activity. J. Med. Chem. 36: 2526–2535.

97. Miller, K. D., E. Jones, J. A. Yanovski, R. Shankar, I. Feuerstein, and J. Falloon. 1998. Visceral abdominal-fat accumulation associated with use of indinavir. Lancet 351:871–875.

98. Miyasaka, C., R. T. Walker, H. Tanaka, D. K. Stammers, and D. I. Stuart. 1996. Complexes of HIV-1 reverse transcriptase with inhibitors of the HEPT series reveal conformational changes relevant to the design of potent non-nucleoside inhibitors. J. Med. Chem. 39:1589–1600.

99. Miyasaka, T., H. Tanaka, M. Baba, H. Hayakawa, R. T. Walker, J. Balzarini, and E. De Clercq. 1989. A novel lead for specific anti-HIV-1 agents: 1-[(2-hydroxyethoxy)methyl]-6-(phenylthio)thymine. J. Med. Chem. 32:2507–2509.

100. Montaner, J., P. Reiss, D. Cooper, S. Vella, M. Harris, B. Conway, M. A. Wainberg, D. Smith, P. Robinson, D. Hall, M. Myers, and J. M. Lange. 1998. A randomized, double-blind trial comparing combinations of nevirapine, didanosine and zidovudine for HIV-infected patients. The INCAS trial. JAMA 279:930–937.

101. Morales-Ramirez, J., K. Tashima, D. Hardy, P. Johnson, M. Nelson, S. Staszewski, D. Farina, N. Ruiz, and the DMP 2666-6 Clinical Study Team. 1998. A phase II, multicenter, randomized, open-label study to compare the antiretroviral activity and tolerability of efavirenz (EFV) + indinavir (IDV), versus EFV + zidovudine (ZDV) + lamivudine (3TC), versus IDV + ZDV +

3TC at 36 weeks (DMP 266-006). 38th Interscience Conference on Antimicrobial Agents and Chemotherapy, San Diego, abstr. I-103.

102. Nanni, R. G., J. Ding, A. Jacobo-Molina, S. H. Hughes, and E. Arnold. 1993. Review of HIV-1 reverse transcriptase three-dimensional structure: implications for drug design. Perspect. Drug Discovery Research 1:129–150.

103. Olmsted, R. A., D. E. Slade, L. A. Kopta, S. M. Poppe, T. J. Poel, S. W. Newport, K. B. Rank, C. Biles, R. A. Morge, T. J. Dueweke, Y. Yagi, D. L. Romero, R. C. Thomas, S. K. Sharma, and W. G. Tarpley. 1996. (Alkylamino)piperidine bis(heteroaryl)piperizine analogs are potent, broad-spectrum nonnucleoside reverse transcriptase inhibitors of drug-resistant isolates of human immunodeficiency virus type 1 (HIV-1) and select for drug-resistant variants of HIV-1IIIB with reduced replication phenotypes. J. Virol. 70:3698–3705.

104. Patel, P. H., A. Jacobo-Molina, J. Ding, C. Tantillo, A. D. Clarck, R. Raag, Jr., R. G. Nanni, S. H. Hughes, and E. Arnold. 1995. Insights into DNA polymerization mechanisms from structure and function analysis of HIV-1 reverse transcriptase. Biochemistry 34:5351–5363.

105. Pauwels, R., K. Andries, Z. Debyser, M.-J. Kukla, D. Schols, H. J. Breslin, R. Woestenborghs, J. Desmyter, M. A. C. Janssen, E. De Clercq, and P. A. J. Janssen. 1994. New tetrahydroimidazo[4,5-1-*jk*][1,4]-benzodiazepin-2(1*H*)-one and -thione derivatives are potent inhibitors of human immunodeficiency virus type 1 replication and are synergistic with 2′,3′-dideoxynucleoside analogs. Antimicrob. Agents Chemother. 38:2863–2870.

106. Pauwels, R., K. Andries, Z. Debyser, P. Van Daele, D. Schols, P. Stoffels, K. De Vreese, R. Woestenborghs, A.-M. Vandamme, C. G. M. Janssen, J. Anné, G. Cauwenbergh, J. Desmyter, J. Heykants, M. A. C. Janssen, E. De Clercq, and P. A. J. Janssen. 1993. Potent and highly selective human immunodeficiency virus type 1 (HIV-1) inhibition by a series of α-anilinophenylacetamide derivatives targeted at HIV-1 reverse transcriptase. Proc. Natl. Acad. Sci. USA 90:1711–1715.

107. Pauwels, R., K. Andries, J. Desmyter, D. Schols, M. J. Kukla, H. J. Breslin, A. Raeymaeckers, J. Van Gelder, R. Woestenborghs, J. Heykants, K. Schellekens, M. A. C. Janssen, E. De Clercq, and P. A. J. Janssen. 1990. Potent and selective inhibition of HIV-1 replication *in vitro* by a novel series of TIBO derivatives. Nature 343:470–474.

108. Pérez-Pérez, M.-J., A. San-Félix, M. J. Camarasa, J. Balzarini, and E. De Clercq. 1992. Synthesis of [1-[2′,5′-bis-*O*-(t-butyldimethylsilyl)-(β-D-xylo- and β-D-ribofuranosyl)thymine]-3′-spiro-5″-[4″-amino-1″,2″-oxathiole-2″,2″-dioxide]] (TSAO). A novel type of specific anti-HIV agents. Tetrahedron Letters 33:3029–3032.

109. Ren, J., R. M. Esnouf, A. L. Hopkins, J. Warren, J. Balzarini, D. I. Stuart, and D. K. Stammers. 1998. Crystal structures of HIV-1 reverse transcriptase in complex with carboxanilide derivatives. Biochemistry 37:14394–14403.

110. Ren, J. S., R. Esnouf, E. Garman, D. Somers, C. Ross, I. Kirby, J. Keeling, G. Darby, Y. Jones, D. Stuart, and D. Stammers. 1995. High resolution structure of HIV-1 RT: insights from four RT-inhibitor complexes. Nat. Struct. Biol. 2:293–302.

111. Richman, D., C.-K. Shih, I. Lowy, J. Rose, P. Prodanovich, S. Goff, and J. Griffin. 1991. Human immunodeficiency virus type 1 mutants resistant to non-

nucleoside inhibitors of reverse transcriptase arise in tissue culture. Proc. Natl. Acad. Sci. USA 88:11241–11245.

112. Richman, D. D. 1993. Resistance of clinical isolates of human immuno-deficiency virus to antiretroviral agents. Antimicrob. Agents Chemother. 37: 1207–1213.

113. Richman, D. D., D. Havlir, J. Corbeil, D. Looney, C. Ignacio, S. A. Spector, J. Sullivan, S. Cheeseman, K. Barringer, D. Pauletti, C.-K. Myers, and J. Griffin. 1994. Nevirapine resistance mutations of human immunodeficiency virus type 1 selected during therapy. J. Virol. 68:1660–1666.

114. Romero, D. L., M. Busso, C.-K. Tan, F. Reusser, J. R. Palmer, S. M. Poppe, P. A. Aristoff, K. M. Downey, A. G. So, L. Resnick, and W. G. Tarpley. 1991. Non-nucleoside reverse transcriptase inhibitors that potently and specifically block human immunodeficiency virus type 1 replication. Proc. Natl. Acad. Sci. USA 88:8806–8810.

115. Sargent, S., S. Green, M. Para, W. Freimuth, L. Wahren, L. Getchel, and C. Greenwald. 1998. Sustained plasma viral burden reductions and CD4 increases in HIV-1-infected patients with rescriptor plus retrovir plus epivir. Fifth Conference on Retroviruses and Opportunistic Infections, Chicago, abstr. 699.

116. Silvestri, R., M. Artico, B. Bruno, S. Massa, E. Novellino, G. Greco, M. E. Marongiu, A. Pani, A. De Montis, and P. La Colla. 1998. Synthesis and biological evaluation of 5H-indolo [3,2-b][1,5]benzothiazepine derivatives, designed as conformationally constrained analogues of the human immuno-deficiency virus type 1 reverse transcriptase inhibitor L-737,126. Antiviral Chem. Chemother. 9:139–148.

117. Smerdon, S. J., J. Jäger, J. Wang, L. A. Kohlstaedt, A. J. Chirino, J. M. Friedman, P. A. Rice, and T. A. Steitz. 1994. Structure of the binding site for non-nucleoside inhibitors of the reverse transcriptase of human immunodefi-ciency virus type 1. Proc. Natl. Acad. Sci. USA. 91:911–915.

118. Spence, R. A., W. M. Kati, K. S. Anderson, and K. A. Johnson. 1995. Mecha-nism of inhibition of HIV-1 reverse transcriptase by non-nucleoside in-hibitors. Science 267:988–993.

119. Stammers, D. K., D. O. Somers, C. K. Ross, I. Kirby, P. H. Ray, J. E. Wilson, M. Norman, J. S. Ren, R. M. Esnouf, E. F. Garman, E. Y. Jones, and D. I. Stuart. 1994. Crystals of HIV-1 reverse transcriptase diffracting to 2.2 Å resolution. J. Mol. Biol. 242:586–588.

120. Staszewski, S., F. E. Massari, A. Kober, R. Gohler, S. Durr, K. W. Anderson, C. L. Schneider, J. A. Waterbury, K. K. Bakshi, V. I. Taylor, C. S. Hildebrand, C. Kreisl, B. Hoffstedt, W. A. Schleif, H. von Briesen, H. Rübsamen-Waigmann, G. B. Calandra, J. L. Ryan, W. Stille, E. A. Emini, and V. W. Byrnes. 1995. Com-bination therapy with zidovudine prevents selection of human immunodefi-ciency virus type 1 variants expressing high level resistance to L-697,661, a non-nucleoside reverse transcriptase inhibitor. J. Infect. Dis. 171:159–165.

121. Tachedjian, G., J. Mellors, H. Bazmi, C. Birch, and J. Mills. 1996. Zidovudine resistance is suppressed by mutations conferring resistance of human im-munodeficiency virus type 1 to foscarnet. J. Virol. 70:7171–7181.

122. Taylor, D. L., P. S. Ahmed, A. S. Tyms, J. Bedard, J. Duchaine, G. Falardeau, J. F. Lavallee, M. Hamel, R. F. Rando, and T. Bowlin. 1998. A pyrido [1,2a] in-

dole derivative identified as a novel non-nucleoside reverse transcriptase inhibitor of HIV-1. Abstracts of the 11th International Conference on Antiviral Research, San Diego, April 5–10, 1998. Antiviral Res. 37:A53, abstr. 44.

123. Terrett, N. K., D. Bojanic, J. R. Merson, and P. T. Stephenson. 1992. Imidazo[2′,3′:6,5]dipyrido[3,2-b:2′,3′-e]-1,4-diazepines: non-nucleoside HIV-1 reverse transcriptase inhibitors with greater enzyme affinity than nevirapine. Bioorganic Med. Chem. Lett. 2:1745–1750.

124. Tucker, T. J., T. A. Lyle, C. M. Wiscount, S. F. Britcher, S. D. Young, W. M. Sanders, W. C. Lumma, M. E. Goldman, J. A. O'Brien, R. G. Ball, C. F. Homnick, W. A. Schleif, E. A. Emini, J. R. Huff, and P. S. Anderson. 1994. Synthesis of a series of 4-(arylethynyl)-6-chloro-4-cyclopropyl-3,4-dihydroquinazolin-2(1H)-ones as novel non-nucleoside HIV-1 reverse transcriptase inhibitors. J. Med. Chem. 37:2437–2444.

125. Vandamme, A.-M., K. Van Vaerenbergh, and E. De Clercq. 1998. Anti-human immunodeficiency virus drug combination strategies. Antiviral Chem. Chemother. 9:187–203.

126. Vasudevachari, M. B., C. Battista, H. C. Lane, M. C. Psallidopoulos, B. Zhao, J. Cook, J. R. Palmer, D. L. Romero, W. G. Tarpley, and N. P. Salzman. 1992. Prevention of the spread of HIV-1 infection with nonnucleoside reverse transcriptase inhibitors. Virology 190:269–277.

127. Vrang, L., C. Ahgren, K. Ekelöf, P. Engelhardt, M. Högberg, R. Noréen, B. Öberg, C. Rydergard, and C. Sahlberg. 1998. Anti-HIV activity of PETT-4 in vitro. Abstracts of the 11th International Conference on Antiviral Research, San Diego, April 5–10, 1998. Antiviral Res. 37:A55, abstr. 51.

128. Warren, K. J., D. E. Boxwell, N. Y. Kim, and B. A. Drolet. 1998. Nevirapine-associated Stevens-Johnson syndrome. Lancet 351:567.

129. White, E. L., R. W. Buckheit, Jr., L. J. Ross, J. M. Germany, K. Andries, R. Pauwels, P. A. J. Janssen, W. M. Shannon, and M. A. Chirigos. 1991. A TIBO derivative, R82913, is a potent inhibitor of HIV-1 reverse transcriptase with heteropolymer templates. Antiviral Res. 26:257–266.

130. Williams, T. M., T. M. Ciccarone, S. C. MacTough, C. S. Rooney, S. K. Balani, J. H. Condra, E. A. Emini, M. E. Goldman, W. J. Greenlee, L. R. Kauffman, J. A. O'Brien, V. V. Sardana, W. A. Schleif, A. D. Theoharides, and P. S. Anderson. 1993. 5-Chloro-3-(phenylsulfonyl)indole-2-carboxamide: a novel, non-nucleoside inhibitor of HIV-1 reverse transcriptase. J. Med. Chem. 36: 1291–1294.

131. Winslow, D. L., S. Garber, C. Reid, H. Scarnati, B. Korant, E. Emini, and E. D. Anton. 1995. Development of high-level resistance to DMP 266 requires multiple mutations in the reverse transcriptase gene. Abstracts of the Fourth International Workshop on HIV Drug Resistance, July 6–9, 1995, Sardinia, Italy, no. 13.

132. Winslow, D. L., C. Reid, S. Garber, H. Scarnati, M. Rayner, and E. Anton. 1996. Selection conditions affect the evolution of specific mutations in the reverse transcriptase gene associated with resistance to DMP 266. Abstracts of the Fifth International Workshop on HIV Drug Resistance, July 7–12, 1996, Whistler, Canada, no. 10.

133. Wishka, D. G., D. R. Graber, L. A. Kopta, R. A. Olmsted, J. M. Friis, J. D. Hosley, W. J. Adams, E. P. Seest, T. M. Castle, L. A. Dolak, B. J. Keiser, Y. Yagi,

A. Jeganathan, S. T. Schlachter, M. J. Murphy, G. J. Cleek, R. A. Nugent, S. M. Poppe, S. M. Swaney, F. Han, W. Watt, W. L. White, T.-J. Poel, R. C. Thomas, R. L. Voorman, K. J. Stefanski, R. G. Stehle, W. G. Tarpley, and J. Morris. 1998. (–)-6-Chloro-2-[(1-furo[2,3-c]pyridin-5-yl-ethyl)thio]-4-pyrimidinamine, PNU-142721, a new broad spectrum HIV-1 non-nucleoside reverse transcriptase inhibitor. J. Med. Chem. 41:1357–1360.

134. Witvrouw, M., M. E. Arranz, C. Pannecouque, R. Declercq, H. Jonckheere, J.-C. Schmit, A. M. Vandamme, J. A. Diaz, S. T. Ingate, J. Desmyter, R. Esnouf, L. Van Meervelt, S. Vega, J. Balzarini, and E. De Clercq. 1998. 1,1,3-Trioxo-2H,4H-thieno[3,4-e][1,2,4]thiadiazine (TTD) derivatives: a new class of non-nucleoside human immunodeficiency virus type 1 (HIV-1) reverse transcriptase inhibitors (NNRTIs) with anti-HIV-1 activity. Antimicrob. Agents Chemother. 42:618–623.

135. Wu, J. C., T. C. Warren, J. Adams, J. Proudfoot, J. Skiles, P. Raghavan, C. Perry, I. Potocki, P. R. Farina, and P. M. Grob. 1991. A novel dipyridodiazepinone inhibitor of HIV-1 reverse transcriptase acts through a nonsubstrate binding site. Biochemistry 30:2022–2026.

136. Young, S. D., S. F. Britcher, L. O. Tran, L. S. Payne, W. C. Lumma, T. A. Lyle, J. R. Huff, P. S. Anderson, D. B. Olsen, S. S. Carroll, D. J. Pettibone, J. A. O'Brien, R. G. Ball, S. K. Balani, J. H. Lin, I.-W. Chen, W. A. Schleif, V. V. Sardana, W. J. Long, V. W. Byrnes, and E. A. Emini. 1995. L-743,726 (DMP-266): a novel, highly potent nonnucleoside inhibitor of the human immunodeficiency virus type 1 reverse transcriptase. Antimicrob. Agents Chemother. 39:2602–2605.

137. Zembower, D. E., S. Liao, M. T. Flavin, Z.-Q. Xu, T. L. Stup, R. W. Buckheit, Jr., A. Khilevich, A. A. Mar, and A. K. Sheinkman. 1997. Structural analogues of the calanolide anti-HIV agents. Modification of the *trans*-10,11-dimethyl-dihydropyran-12-ol ring (ring C). J. Med. Chem. 40:1005–1017.

138. Zhang, H., L. Vrang, K. Backbro, P. Lind, C. Sahlberg, T. Unge, and B. Öberg. 1995. Inhibition of human immunodeficiency virus type 1 wild-type and mutant reverse transcriptases by the phenyl ethyl thiazolyl thiourea derivatives trovirdine and MSC-127. Antiviral Res. 28:31–342.

5

JON H. CONDRA
JOSEPH P. VACCA

HIV-1 Protease
Inhibitors

The past fifteen years have seen an explosion in the number of therapies developed to treat human immunodeficiency virus type 1 (HIV-1) infection. Early drugs such as zidovudine (AZT, ZVD), zalcitabine (ddC), and didanosine (ddI) were developed as competitive, chain-terminating inhibitors of the viral reverse transcriptase (RT) enzyme, which catalyzes an early step in the viral life cycle, the synthesis of viral DNA from a viral RNA template. These early compounds were weak inhibitors and elicited modest and transient clinical effects as single agents. It was not until the nucleoside analog RT inhibitor (NRTI) lamivudine (3TC) was developed and combined with AZT that sustained suppression of viral replication was demonstrated, if only moderately, by today's standards.

Following the discovery of retroviral proteases (146) and the validation of the HIV-1 protease (HIVP) as a therapeutic target in the late 1980s (80), a substantial research effort was mounted to discover orally bioavailable inhibitors of this enzyme. The early nineties saw several of these agents enter clinical trials, and the results were dramatic when these compounds were combined with other agents such as AZT/3TC or stavudine (d4T)/3TC. In November 1995, the first HIV-1 protease inhibitor (PI), Invirase® (saquinavir [SQV]), received U.S. regulatory approval and was followed by Norvir® (ritonavir [RTV], February 1996), Crixivan® (indinavir sulfate [IDV], March 1996), Viracept® (nelfinavir mesylate [NFV], March 1997), Agenerase® (amprenavir [APV], April 1999), and Kaletra™ (lopinavir [LPV]/RTV, September, 2000) (Fig. 5.1). This chapter focuses on the discovery, development, and clinical use of the six currently used agents, as well as on some promising HIV-1 PIs currently in clinical development.

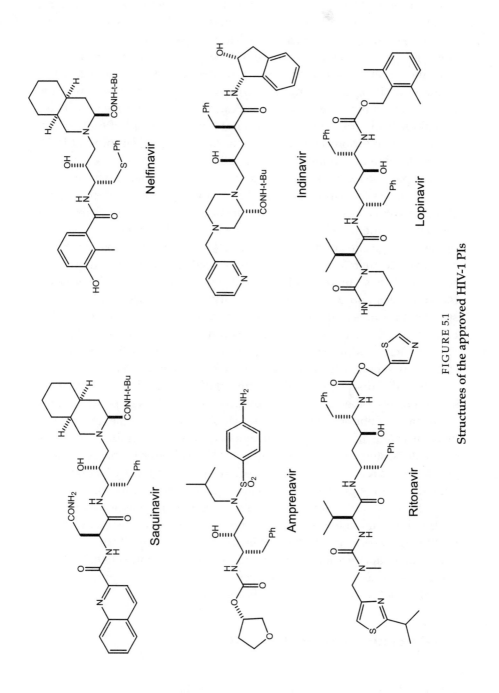

FIGURE 5.1

Structures of the approved HIV-1 PIs

The HIVP as a Therapeutic Target

The HIVP is a 99 amino acid protein that exists as a homodimer to give a symmetrical enzyme. The enzyme belongs to the class known as "aspartic acid proteases," which contain two adjacent aspartic acids in the catalytic site (Fig. 5.2). The enzyme cleaves the *gag-pol* polyprotein precursor to generate the proteins needed for capsid assembly. These cleavages occur late in the viral life cycle, during (or perhaps after) viral budding from the plasma membranes of infected cells. Protease-mediated cleavages are essential for final viral maturation, as viral mutants devoid of protease activity generate virions containing the normal complement of viral RNA and protein but are noninfectious (80, 118).

The peptide substrates for this proteolysis consist of at least eight distinct cleavage sites within the *gag-pol* polyprotein precursor. Each of these cleavage sites consists of eight amino acids, each occupying a "subsite" in the viral enzyme. The four amino acid residues to the amino-terminal side of the cleavage site are designated P1'–P4' residues, and those on the C-terminal side are referred to as the P1–P4 residues. Because each protease cleavage site has a unique amino acid sequence, the affinity of the protease for these sites and its cleavage specificity must be imparted by shared structural features of these sites. These cleavages are mediated by the coordinated addition of a water molecule to an amide bind cleavage site (Fig. 5.2). The initial addition of water goes through a tetrahedral transition-state intermediate, which then resolves to the final cleaved products.

The initial discovery and development of HIV-1 PIs built on earlier research on two other well-known aspartic acid proteases, pepstatin and renin. Early inhibitors of these enzymes took advantage of the catalytic enzyme mechanism by incorporating a nonhydrolyzable, tetrahedral transition-state isostere into a peptide mimetic (44). Although numerous potent pepstatin and renin inhibitors had been developed by many laboratories, none reached the product stage owing to their poor pharmacokinetics in Phase I clinical trials. However, several of these renin inhibitors served as leads in HIVP inhibitor research programs, and because of their availability, the discovery of potent HIV-1 PIs occurred fairly rapidly after the initial identification of the viral protease as a therapeutic target (80). Yet finding compounds that possessed useful pharmacokinetic properties in animal models proved to be a significant challenge.

The Currently Approved HIV-1 PIs

SQV

The first PI to receive regulatory approval for the treatment of HIV-1 infection was SQV (Ro 31-8959) (Table 5.1). Researchers at Hoffmann–La Roche designed SQV (31, 126) based on the sequence of Leu165–Ile169, one

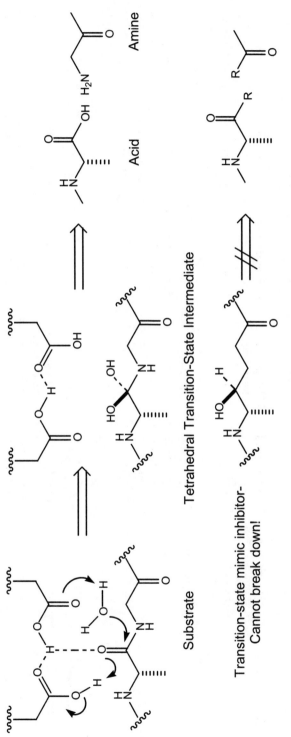

FIGURE 5.2

Mechanism of peptide hydrolysis by aspartic acid proteases

TABLE 5.1

Characteristics of HIV-1 PIs

	Saquinavir (SQV)	Ritonavir (RTV)	Indinavir (IDV)	Nelfinavir (NFV)	Amprenavir (APV)	Lopinavir/Ritonavir (LPV/RTV)
Generic name						
Trade name	Invirase®, Fortovase™	Norvir®	Crixivan®	Viracept®	Agenerase®	Kaletra™
Molecular weight	670.86 (as free base)	720.95 (as free base)	757.94 (as sulfate ethanolate salt)	663.9 (as mesylate salt)	505.64 (as free base)	628.8 (LPV as free base)
Salt	Mesylate salt (Invirase®); free base (Fortovase™)	Free base	Sulfate salt	Mesylate salt	Free base	Free base
Form	200 mg capsules	100 mg soft gelatin capsules; 600 mg/7.5 ml oral solution	200 mg and 400 mg capsules	250 mg tablets; oral powder, 5 mg/g	50 mg and 150 mg soft gelatin capsules containing vitamin E (109 IU/150 mg capsule)	Soft gelatin capsules containing 133.3 mg LPV + 33.3 mg RTV; oral solution containing 80 mg LPV + 20 mg RTV/ml
Route of administration	Oral	Oral	Oral	Oral	Oral	Oral
Approved dosages	600 mg (3 capsules) tid with full meal (Invirase®); 1,200 mg (6 capsules) tid with full meal (Fortovase™)	600 mg (6 capsules or 7.5 ml oral solution) bid (with meal if possible); dose escalation required[a]	800 mg (two 400 mg capsules) q8h (1 hr before or 2 hr after a meal; may take with light meal). Adequate	750 mg (3 tablets) tid with meal or light snack; 1,250 mg (5 tablets) bid with meal or light snack	Adults: 1,200 mg (eight 150 mg capsules) bid with or without meals; should not be taken with high-fat meal. Pediatric patients,	Adults: 3 capsules (400 mg LPV/100 mg RTV total), twice daily with food. Pediatric patients, age 6 months to 12 years: oral solution 12/3 mg/kg

			hydration (at least 1.5 liters per day) recommended	age 4–12 years or <50 kg weight: 20 mg/kg bid or 15 mg/kg tid	for 7 to <15 kg; 10/2.5 mg/kg for 15–40 kg
Oral bioavailability	4% (Invirase®); 12% (Fortovase™)	Not determined	60%	20–80%	Not determined. Solution is 14% less bioavailable than capsule formulation.	Not determined
Serum half-life	1–2 hr	3–5 hr	1.5–2 hr	3.5–5 hr	7.1–10.6 hr	5–6 hr
Fold attenuation of in vitro antiviral activity by 50% human serum (103)	26	20	2	37	7	5–11
Storage	Room temperature (Invirase®); Fortovase™ must be refrigerated (but stable at room temperature up to 3 months)	Soft gelatin capsules must be refrigerated (but stable 30 days below 77°F). Oral solution should not be refrigerated. Protect from light.	Room temperature, protected from moisture	Room temperature	Room temperature	Soft gelatin capsules and oral solution must be refrigerated. If stored at room temperature, should be used within 2 months.
Major adverse events	Diarrhea, nausea, abdominal discomfort, dyspepsia, elevated liver transaminases	Gastrointestinal intolerance: nausea, vomiting, diarrhea; paresthesia:	Nephrolithiasis, abdominal pain, indirect hyperbilirubinemia, hemolytic	Diarrhea, nausea	Nausea, vomiting, diarrhea, rash, paresthesia, depressive/mood disorders, taste	Diarrhea, hyperglyceridemia, hypercholesterolemia, elevated GGT, SGOT/AST, SGPT/ALT

(continued)

TABLE 5.1 (continued)

Generic name	Saquinavir (SQV)	Ritonavir (RTV)	Indinavir (IDV)	Nelfinavir (NFV)	Amprenavir (APV)	Lopinavir/Ritonavir (LPV/RTV)
		circumoral and in extremities; asthenia; hepatitis; taste perversion; triglyceride elevations >200%; liver transaminase elevations; elevated CPK and uric acid	anemia, nausea, headache, asthenia, blurred vision, dizziness, rash, metallic taste		disorders, hyperglycemia, hypertriglyceridemia	
Drug interactions	Inhibits cytochrome P450. SQV levels increased by clarithromycin, IDV, NFV, RTV, delavirdine, ketoconazole. SQV levels decreased by nevirapine, rifabutin, rifampin; possibly by carbamazepine, phenytoin, phenobarbital, dexamethasone. SQV decreases	Potent cytochrome P450 inhibitor. Increases blood levels of clarithromycin, desipramine, IDV, ketoconazole, normeperidine (metabolite of meperidine), rifabutin, SQV, sildenafil. Levels of numerous other drugs may be increased by RTV.[b] Reduces	Inhibits cytochrome P450. IND levels increased by ketoconazole, RTV, delavirdine. IND levels reduced by rifampin, rifabutin, efavirenz, and possibly by phenobarbital, phenytoin, carbamazepine, dexamethasone. IDV increases blood levels of	Inhibits cytochrome P450. NFV levels increased by ketoconazole, RTV, IDV, SQV, and efavirenz. NFV levels reduced by rifampin and rifabutin. NFV increases plasma levels of lamivudine IND, SQV, and rifabutin and decreases levels of zidovudine, ethinyl estradiol, and	Inhibits cytochrome P450. APV levels increased by itraconazole, erythromycin, RTV, warfarin, delavirdine; decreased by rifampin, rifabutin, efavirenz, phenobarbital, phenytoin, carbamazepine. APV increases plasma levels of rifabutin, ketoconazole,	Inhibits cytochrome P450. LPV levels decreased by RTV, efavirenz, nevirapine, carbamazepine, phenobarbital, phenytoin, dexamethasone; increased by ritonavir, delavirdine. Kaletra increases levels of APV, IDV, SQV, ketoconazole, rifabutin, 25-O-desacetyl rifabutin, amiodarone, bepridil, systemic

blood levels of NFV, clarithromycin; increases level of terfenadine (should not be coadministered).

plasma levels of meperidine, methadone, oral contraceptives, theophylline, and possibly also warfarin, phenytoin, ivalproex, lamotrigine, and atovaquone. RTV levels are reduced by rifampin. Dosage of didanosine should be separated from RTV dosing by 2.5 hr to avoid formulation incompatibility.

rifabutin, ethinyl estradiol, and norethindrone.

norethindrone. Caution should be used when co-administering NFV with sildenafil or HMG CoA reductase inhibitors such as atorvastatin and cerivastatin, and others are contraindicated (see below).

zidovudine, atorvastatin, cerivastatin, lovastatin, pravastatin, simvastatin, sildenafil, dapsone, erythromycin, itraconazole, alprazolam, clorazepate, diazepam, flurazepam, diltiazem, nicardipine, nifedipine, nimodipine, clozapine, carbamazepine, loratadine, pimozide, warfarin. Coadministered drug monitoring needed for amiodarone, systemic lidocaine, quinidine, warfarin, tricyclic antidepressants.

lidocaine, quinidine, ketoconazole, itraconazole, clarithromycin, dihydropyridine calcium channel blockers, sildenafil, atorvastatin, cerivastatin, cyclosporine, tacrilimus, rapamycin. Kaletra decreases levels of atovaquone, methadone, ethinyl estradiol.

(continued)

TABLE 5.1 (continued)

Generic name	Saquinavir (SQV)	Ritonavir (RTV)	Indinavir (IDV)	Nelfinavir (NFV)	Amprenavir (APV)	Lopinavir/Ritonavir (LPV/RTV)
Should not be coadministered with:	Terfenadine, astemizole, ergot derivatives, cisapride, midazolam, triazolam	Amiodarone, bepridil, flecainide, propafenone, quinidine, astemizole, terfenadine, dihydro-ergotamine, ergotamine, midazolam, triazolam, cisapride, pimozide	Terfenadine, astemizole, cisapride, triazolam, midazolam, ergot derivatives	Astemizole, cisapride, triazolam, midazolam, ergot derivatives, amiodarone or quinidine, lovastatin or simvastatin	Astemizole, rifampin, midazolam, triazolam, bepridil, dihydroergotamine, ergotamine, cisapride, supplemental vitamin E. Oral solution contraindicated in certain patient populations because of high propylene glycol content.	Rifampin, St. John's wort, lovastatin, simvastatin. Contraindicated with flecainide, propafenone, astemizole, terfenadine, dihydroergotamine, ergonovine, ergotamine, methylergonovine, cisapride, pimozide, midazolam, triazolam.

[a]Dose escalation recommended for Norvir: 300 mg twice daily, increasing by 100 mg twice daily at 2- to 3-day intervals.

[b]Examples of other drugs whose levels may be increased by Norvir: tramadol, propoxyphene, disopyramide, lidocaine, mexiletine, carbamazepine, clonazepam, ethosuximide, bupropion, nefazodone, selective serotonin reuptake inhibitors (SSRIs), tricyclic antidepressants, dronabinol, quinine, metoprolol, timolol, diltiazem, nifedipine, verapamil, atorvastatin, cerivastatin, lovastatin, simvastatin, cyclosporine, tacrolimus, perphenazine, risperidone, thioridazine, clorazepate, diazepam, estazolam, flurazepam, zolpidem, dexamethasone, prednisone, methamphetamine.

of the eight major peptide cleavage sites hydrolyzed by HIVP (33). Several transition-state analog isosteres were inserted into this sequence to settle finally on the amino-alcohol moiety. Subsequent optimization of each of the transition-state flanking groups culminated in the discovery of SQV. It proved to be quite potent in cell culture, with a 95% inhibitory concentration for viral replication (IC_{95}) of about 25 nM. SQV had minimal oral bioavailability in rats (4%) but was still taken into the clinic because of the dire need for new, potent antiviral compounds. However, in patients, the original hard capsule formulation (SQV_{hc}, Invirase®) also suffered from limited bioavailability (ca. 4%; highest with a high-fat meal) (5), high human serum protein binding (103), and rapid first-pass metabolism (5).

As a result, in early clinical studies, the in vivo efficacy of SQV was modest, resulting in small and transient reductions in viral load. At the dosage ultimately approved for clinical use, 600 mg three times daily, maximal vRNA reductions seen in SQV monotherapy were 80% ($-0.7 \log_{10}$) by 8 weeks, returning toward baseline by 16 weeks (79). Similarly, CD4 increases were moderate (ca. 50 cells/mm^3), but these also returned to baseline values after 16 weeks of therapy.

As proved to be the case with subsequently developed HIV-1 PIs, the in vivo antiviral activity of SQV was augmented by combination therapy. When combined with the NRTIs AZT or ddC, treatment with SQV mediated greater viral reductions and CD4 elevations than were observed with any of these drugs alone (20). Similarly, in a clinical endpoint study, combination therapy with SQV + ddC proved superior to either SQV or ddC alone in reducing progression to AIDS-defining illnesses or death (83), although this effect was not compared with standard of care.

In response to the weak in vivo antiviral activity elicited by SQV, efforts were made to increase its efficacy by using higher doses than approved for standard therapy. In a pilot study employing up to 7.2 g/day of SQV monotherapy in six divided doses, viral load reductions and CD4 cell elevations were shown to be superior to those achieved by the approved 1.8 g/day dosage (134). Although this dosing regimen was not practical, it proved that increased drug exposure could improve the in vivo antiviral activity of SQV.

More recently, a new soft gelatin capsule formulation of SQV (SQV_{sgc}, Fortovase™) was approved. This new formulation has about three times the oral bioavailability of the original hard capsule formulation (SQV_{hc}) (5). In a clinical comparison, SQV_{sgc} demonstrated antiviral efficacy superior to that of SQV_{hc}. In an intent-to-treat analysis of therapy-naive patients receiving SQV_{sgc} versus SQV_{hc} + 2 NRTIs, the percentages of patients after 16 weeks with vRNA reductions greater than 400 copies/ml were 67% and 37% for SQV_{sgc} and SQV_{hc}, respectively (100). In a short-term study comparing treatment-naive patients receiving SQV_{sgc} + AZT + 3TC with patients receiving IDV (see below) + AZT + 3TC, no significant difference in vRNA reductions between the regimens was observed after 24 weeks (19). Although the initial antiviral efficacy of SQV_{sgc} is clearly superior to that of SQV_{hc}, its long-term durability remains to be demonstrated.

The most common adverse events associated with SQV therapy are gastrointestinal disturbances (including diarrhea, nausea, and abdominal discomfort) and elevated liver transaminases (5).

RTV

The second PI to receive U.S. regulatory approval for the treatment of HIV-1 disease was RTV (ABT-538, Norvir®) (Table 5.1). RTV was discovered by researchers at Abbott Laboratories (73) and was the third compound they had taken into the clinic. Their first inhibitors were symmetrical dihydroxy-containing analogs that were designed to take advantage of the symmetry found in HIVP (42). The first compound, A-77003 (74), was meant to be given intravenously but proved to have a short human half-life and showed no efficacy in a short-term clinical trial. Their second compound, A-80987 (75), was related to the first but was not symmetrical. It did have good oral bioavailability in animals and humans but still had too short a half-life to be clinically useful.

The human pharmacokinetics of RTV, however, were shown to be greatly improved over previous compounds. Although RTV is less potent than SQV in cell culture (IC_{95} = 200–400 nM) and is highly bound to human serum proteins (35, 60, 103), it achieves sustained high blood levels in humans after oral administration, resulting in potent suppression of HIV-1 replication in vivo. This greater in vivo antiviral activity is largely a result of its inhibition of cytochrome P450 (CYP) 3A4 and 2D5, which mediate the primary routes of RTV metabolism (60, 62, 82). In addition, it has been shown to inhibit the P-glycoprotein multidrug transporter system (8, 39, 52, 78, 86), which mediates its cellular efflux. By inhibiting both its own metabolism and its efflux, therapeutic levels of RTV are maintained throughout the dosing interval when administered at the recommended oral dosage of 600 mg twice daily.

In early clinical studies, RTV proved to have potent in vivo antiviral activity. In monotherapy, it mediated maximal vRNA reductions of 1.4 to 2 log_{10} units in PI-naive patients (3, 32, 93), maintaining reductions of 0.7 to 1.0 log_{10} after 24 weeks of therapy (3, 32). In these studies, CD4 elevations from 90 to more than 200 cells/mm^3 were observed after 24 weeks (3, 32, 93). When used in combination with AZT and ddC, RTV's antiviral effects were improved further, reducing plasma vRNA loads to below 500 copies/ml in about 50% of patients after one year (96). However, in another combination study, Protocol 245, RTV + AZT combination therapy elicited smaller vRNA reductions than observed with RTV alone (3), possibly because of poor tolerability of RTV when combined with AZT.

Nonetheless, combination therapy with RTV and NRTIs was shown to confer significant clinical benefit. Study 247 was a double-blind comparison of RTV + (1 to 2) NRTIs versus (RTV placebo) + (1 to 2) NRTIs in patients with advanced HIV disease (CD4 ≤ 100 cells/mm^3). During the 12-month double-blind period of study, 22% of the RTV group progressed to AIDS-defining illnesses or death, compared with 38% of the control group. Similarly, the cumulative mortality of the RTV group was 18% versus 26% for the placebo group (3, 12). After the double-blind period, an overall survival benefit was observed in RTV-treated patients through 15 months of therapy (12). Therefore, compared with the then standard of care, RTV combination therapy demonstrated significant clinical benefits in the treatment of HIV-1 infection.

Despite its documented antiviral efficacy, RTV is seldom used in single PI regimens because of its poor tolerability at therapeutic doses. However, because of its great potency as a CYP3A4 inhibitor and its MDR-1 inhibitory activity, it is widely used as a pharmacokinetic "enhancer" to boost the levels of other PIs, especially for salvage therapy of PI failures (see below). In this setting, it is often used at subtherapeutic doses (in the interest of tolerability) that are nevertheless sufficient to increase dramatically the exposure to the other PIs with which it is combined.

The principal RTV-associated adverse events include gastrointestinal intolerance (including nausea, vomiting, and diarrhea), asthenia, and circumoral paresthesia (3).

IDV

Licensed shortly after the approval of RTV, IDV (L-735,524, MK-639, Crixivan®) (Table 5.1) became the third HIV-1 PI available to treat HIV-1 infection. IDV was discovered by researchers at Merck Research Laboratories (37, 148) and is structurally related to SQV in that it contains a basic amine group in its backbone to impart good aqueous solubility at the acidic pH found in the stomach. The rest of the compound is structurally related to an earlier series of hydroxyethylene inhibitors that were potent but had poor oral bioavailability in animals.

IDV proved to be highly potent (IC$_{95}$ = 50–100 nM in cell culture) and selective for the HIVP, with excellent bioavailability in humans (60%). Unlike SQV, RTV, and NFV (see below), its human serum protein binding is low (ca. 60%) (4, 103), which substantially improves drug exposure and therefore its in vivo antiviral activity. However, its relatively short plasma half-life when administered alone (T$_{1/2}$ = 1.8 hr) necessitates an eight-hour dosing interval to maintain optimal suppression of viral replication in vivo (4).

The earliest clinical studies of IDV as monotherapy demonstrated its in vivo potency and also established many of the concepts that currently guide treatment practices for HIV disease. Protocol 006 compared the virological responses to monotherapy with either 200 mg or 400 mg of IDV administered four times daily (0.8 or 1.6 g/day, respectively). These patients experienced moderate initial reductions in viral load, but most returned toward baseline within 24 weeks (4, 97). This vRNA rebound was accompanied by the appearance of amino acid substitutions in the viral protease that are associated with resistance to IDV (24, 28, 98). Patients receiving the higher dose experienced greater vRNA reductions than those at the lower dose, but neither was sufficient to maintain suppression over a 24-week period. While this study was in progress, newly acquired safety data permitted a higher dose of IDV to be used, and all patients were switched to 600 mg four times daily (2.4 g/day). Despite this higher dose, the patients experiencing vRNA rebound showed no improved virological response. Therefore, once viral rebound due to resistance had begun, it could not be overcome by this increased dosage of IDV.

In contrast, patients who *initiated* therapy with this same daily dosage of IDV, 2.4 g/day, administered either as 600 mg every six hours (Protocol 019) or 800 mg every eight hours (Protocol 021), exhibited more potent and more sustained virological responses. In these patients, initial vRNA reductions of 2 $\log_{10}$ were sustained over the 24 weeks of observation. Therefore, great initial exposure to IDV elicited potent and sustained suppression of viral replication that was far greater than observed with the same dosages given after the emergence of resistance had begun. These and other studies (51, 76) proved that the durability of therapy is a function of therapeutic potency and that maximally potent *initial* therapy increases that regimen's durability by suppressing the viral replication that is needed for new mutations to arise (21, 25, 41). Moreover, because multiple new mutations are required for IDV resistance (24, 28), a significant amount of residual viral replication would be needed for IDV breakthrough. Thus, both the extent of viral inhibition and the long-term durability of therapy are consequences of a regimen's initial potency and its "genetic barrier" to resistance (21, 24, 25, 28).

Later studies of IDV combination therapy provided additional validation of these concepts. Protocol 035 (48–50) was a comparison of IDV monotherapy versus AZT + 3TC versus IDV + AZT + 3TC in NRTI-experienced patients. During an initial 24-week double-blind period, in an intention-to-treat analysis, triple combination therapy with IDV achieved far greater virological suppression than achieved by IDV monotherapy or AZT + 3TC therapy, with 88% of IDV + AZT + 3TC-treated patients maintaining viral RNA loads below 500 copies/ml (66% < 50 copies/ml). In contrast, 43% (30% < 50 copies/ml) of patients receiving IDV monotherapy maintained that level of suppression, but none of the patients receiving

AZT + 3TC did so. After the double-blind period, all were converted to open-label IDV + AZT + 3TC therapy for long-term follow-up.

Subsequent virological responses to this IDV + AZT + 3TC regimen varied according to the therapy to which the patients had been originally randomized. After 100 weeks, the virological suppression achieved in the patients originally randomized to IDV + AZT + 3TC (78% of patients < 500 copies/ml) was significantly greater than observed in patients who switched to that regimen after initial IDV monotherapy (45% < 500 copies/ml) or AZT + 3TC combination therapy (30% < 500 copies/ml) (48). Therefore, by allowing low-level viral replication and the accumulation of resistance-associated mutations, these initially suboptimal regimens had blunted the antiviral effects of subsequently administered IDV + AZT + 3TC therapy.

Following three years of IDV + AZT + 3TC treatment, in an intention-to-treat analysis, 68% of the patients originally randomized to this regimen maintained viral suppression below 400 copies/ml (65% < 50 copies/ml) (50). The data from this study demonstrated for the first time that long-term suppression of HIV-1 replication was possible, and they validated the concept that optimal suppression requires highly potent initial treatment that imposes a high genetic barrier to drug resistance.

Two independent multicenter, randomized, double-blind studies have demonstrated that these same concepts also translate into clinical benefits. Protocol 028 compared IDV +AZT versus IDV versus AZT in therapy-naive patients with CD4 counts 50–250 cells/mm^3. After a median follow-up of 56 weeks, 18.7% of patients receiving AZT monotherapy experienced progression to AIDS-defining illness or death, compared with 8.1% of patients on IDV monotherapy and 6.3% receiving IDV +AZT combination therapy (4, 87). In this study, both the vRNA reductions and the CD4 elevations achieved in both IDV-containing arms were significantly greater than observed in patients receiving AZT.

A concurrent clinical endpoint study, ACTG 320, compared patients with CD4 greater than 200 cells/mm^3 who received IDV +AZT (or d4T) + 3TC triple combination therapy with patients receiving AZT (or d4T) + 3TC therapy. As was seen in Protocol 028, the proportion of patients progressing to AIDS or death was significantly reduced among the IDV + AZT(d4T) + 3TC-treated patients (6%) relative to that observed in AZT(d4T) + 3TC-treated patients (11%). Mortality rates for the two groups were 1.4% and 3.4%, respectively (55). Therefore, treatment with IDV was shown to confer significant clinical benefits to patients with respect to progression to AIDS and death when compared with the current standard of care.

From these and other results it became clear that if therapy is properly implemented, achieving its stated objective, to suppress viral replication as much as possible and for as long as possible, can translate into long-term virological and clinical benefits.

Adverse events most commonly associated with IDV therapy include nephrolithiasis (flank pain with or without hematuria), asymptomatic hyperbilirubinemia, and nausea (4).

NFV

The fourth PI to be approved for the treatment of HIV-1 infection was NFV (AG1343, Viracept®) (Table 5.1). NFV was designed based on eliminating some of the deficiencies of SQV. SQV is a large molecule that contains several amide bonds in its backbone. Researchers at Agouron Pharmaceuticals and Eli Lilly Laboratories collaborated on a joint research venture and discovered that a small 2-hydroxy-3-methylbenzeneamide was an excellent replacement for the large asparagine-quinoline carbonyl group found in the P2-P3 position of SQV (67). To improve potency as well , they inserted a sulfur group into the P1 benzyl side chain that helped to fill a critical hydrophobic pocket.

As with the other HIV-1 PIs, NFV exhibits potent antiviral activity in cell culture (IC_{95} = 50–100 nM) and is a selective, competitive inhibitor of the viral protease (66, 116). NFV is highly (> 98%) bound to human serum proteins (7), which substantially attenuates its antiviral activity (103). However, it has a relatively long plasma half-life following oral administration to humans (3.5–5 hr), which yields similar pharmacokinetics when administered at 750 mg three times daily or 1,250 mg twice daily (4).

A Phase I/II clinical study of NFV in monotherapy (91) showed that when administered at the approved dose of 750 mg three times daily, NFV mediated vRNA reductions of about 1.5 $\log_{10}$ over a 28-day period. However, virtually all patients experienced a rebound of vRNA to pretreatment levels within six to eight months.

Protocol 506 compared two doses of NFV (500 mg or 750 mg tid) plus d4T, versus d4T monotherapy. Patients receiving either dose of NFV + d4T showed greater antiviral activity than those receiving d4T alone, with 11% of patients receiving NFV (750 mg tid)/d4T (and 8% of patients treated with NFV [500 mg tid] + d4T) exhibiting vRNA reductions below 400 copies/ml at 24 weeks. By contrast, 1% of patients receiving d4T monotherapy achieved similar vRNA reductions.

In Protocol 511, triple combination therapy of antiretroviral therapy–naive patients with NFV (750 mg tid) + AZT + 3TC mediated greater vRNA reductions than observed with AZT + 3TC alone. Over a 48-week period, about 55% of patients receiving NFV (750 mg tid) + AZT + 3TC sustained vRNA reductions below 400 copies/ml, compared with 3% of the patients who received AZT + 3TC therapy (7). During this same time period, CD4 elevations in the two treated populations were 190 cells /mm^3 and 120 cells/mm^3, respectively. Therefore, as had been seen with the previous PIs, the efficacy of NFV was greatest when combined with two or more RT inhibitors.

Because of its relatively long plasma half-life, NFV has received approval for twice-daily administration. Study 542 compared two dosage regimens of NFV (750 mg tid and 1,250 mg bid) in combination with d4T + 3TC in therapy-naive patients. Both the tid and bid groups showed similar vRNA reductions, with 61% and 58% of patients, respectively, achieving vRNA loads below 400 copies/ml at 48 weeks (7). CD4 cell responses were similar in the two groups of patients with mean increases of 150 and 200 cells/mm^3 at weeks 24 and 48, respectively.

Because NFV was approved after the demonstration of a strong association between vRNA load and clinical outcome (99, 107), NFV became the first HIV PI to receive full approval based solely on surrogate marker data. Accordingly, no data are available to assess NFV's potential to reduce progression to AIDS-defining illnesses or mortality.

The most common adverse experiences associated with NFV therapy are diarrhea and nausea (7).

APV

Following its recent U.S. approval, APV (VX-478, 141W94, Agenerase®) (Table 5.1) became the fifth HIV-1 PI available to treat HIV-1 infection. Discovered by researchers at Vertex Laboratories, APV (77) is the lowest molecular weight compound of the six clinically approved HIV PIs. It also contains a hydroxy transition-state group in it but has a tetrahydrofuranyl carbamate for a P2 group and a benzosulfonamide group in the P1' position. The sulfonamide group has a para-amino group to help impart aqueous solubility and facilitate absorption from the GI tract in animals and humans. Like the other PIs, it is active against HIV-1 replication in cell culture, with an IC$_{50}$ between 12 and 80 nM in the absence of human serum. In the presence of 50% human serum, its in vitro potency is reduced approximately sevenfold (103).

When APV entered initial clinical studies, its in vitro potency and pharmacokinetic properties had suggested that it might be effective as a monotherapeutic agent. Accordingly, these early studies compared its efficacy alone or in combination with AZT and 3TC. Unfortunately, its efficacy in monotherapy was disappointing, mediating maximal vRNA reductions of about 1.5 log$_{10}$ by two to four weeks of therapy but returning to less than 1 log$_{10}$ below baseline by eight weeks. In contrast, similar initial responses were seen in patients receiving APV + AZT + 3TC, and vRNA reductions of greater than 2 log$_{10}$ below baseline were sustained through 12 weeks of therapy (105). Similarly, while only about 20% of patients receiving APV monotherapy achieved vRNA levels less than 500 copies/ml by 12 weeks, about 60% of patients receiving APV + AZT + 3TC did so.

Although APV potently suppresses HIV-1 replication when administered in combination therapy, its in vivo efficacy may be limited by intolerability. In study PROAB2002, the antiviral efficacies of different dosages of APV with AZT + 3TC were compared among patients naive to PIs and 3TC. By on-treatment analysis, patients receiving the highest dosages of APV exhibited the greatest antiviral effects, with 86%, 80%, and 65% of treated patients receiving 1,200, 1,050, and 900 mg bid, respectively, achieving vRNA loads less than 400 copies/ml at 60 weeks (57). However, in intent-to-treat analysis (dropouts considered failures), only 20% of patients randomized to the highest dose remained below 400 copies/ml after 60 weeks, whereas 25% and 43% of patients receiving 900 mg and 1,050 mg, respectively, did so. This discordant result was attributed to a high discontinuation rate due to adverse events among patients receiving the highest dosage of APV.

The major adverse reactions associated with APV therapy include gastrointestinal events (nausea, vomiting, diarrhea), rash (severe or life threatening, including Stevens-Johnson syndrome, in 1% of recipients), and paresthesias (2).

LPV/RTV

In September 2000, LPV/RTV (ABT-378/r, Kaletra™) (Table 5.1) received accelerated FDA marketing approval, making it the sixth PI approved for the treatment of HIV disease. LPV was initially designed by researchers at Abbott Laboratories in an effort to find compounds active against some of the more prevalent RTV-resistant clinical isolates (137). Modeling studies showed that the binding of RTV to the HIV protease enzyme was dependent on a hydrophobic interaction that was sterically unfeasible in a mutant bearing a valine-to-phenylalanine substitution at residue 82 (V82F). The goal of the group was to find potent RTV analogs that were not dependent on this interaction. Several iterations of the compound series resulted in the discovery of LPV. This compound was reported to be active against wild-type ($K_i = 1.3$ pM) and mutant (V82A, $K_i = 4.9$ pM; V82F, $K_i = 3.7$ pM; V82T, $K_i = 3.6$ pM) enzymes. In contrast, RTV had been 8- to 80-fold less potent against these enzymes.

In cell culture, LPV exhibits potent anti-HIV-1 activity, with IC_{50} values ranging from 10 to 27 nM against wild-type HIV-1 (6). It is 98–99% bound to human plasma proteins at steady state (6) and shows 5- to 11-fold attenuation of antiviral activity by 50% human serum in vitro (6, 103).

One serious drawback of LPV was its rapid metabolism by CYP3A4, which resulted in low blood levels of drug. Accordingly, LPV was developed to be co-dosed with RTV to take advantage of that drug's potent CYP3A4 inhibitory activity. When 400 mg of LPV was coadministered with 100 mg of RTV, high plasma levels of LPV were observed. The steady-state trough concentration was 5.5 ± 4.0 µg/ml, well above the mean wild-type IC_{50} in the presence of added 50% normal human serum. A 48% increase in mean AUC and a 23% increase in mean C_{max} were observed when LPV/RTV was administered with a moderate fat meal. It is therefore recommended that this combination be given with food.

In its approved form, LPV is coformulated with RTV at a ratio of 400 mg LPV/100 mg RTV. Because of its recent approval, little clinical information is available apart from the studies supporting licensure.

LPV/RTV has demonstrated potent antiretroviral activity in clinical studies. Protocol 863 is an ongoing comparison of LPV/RTV + d4T + 3TC versus NFV (750 mg tid) + d4T + 3TC in antiretroviral-naive patients (mean baseline vRNA: 4.9 $\log_{10}$; mean CD4: 259 cells/mm³). Through week 24, 79% of patients in the LPV/RTV-containing arm achieved vRNA reductions less than 400 copies/ml (65% < 50 copies/ml) , whereas 70% of the NFV-treated patients achieved that level of suppression (60% < 50 copies/ml). CD4 elevations were nearly identical between the two arms, with increases of 154 and 150 cells/mm³ in the patients receiving LPV/RTV and NFV, respectively (6).

In a second study of therapy-naive patients, protocol 720 compared three different dosing regimens of LPV/RTV: (200/100 mg bid and 400/100 bid [Group 1]; 400/100 mg bid and 400/200 mg bid [Group 2]) + d4T + 3TC. Between weeks 48 and 72, all patients were converted to open-label LPV/RTV at 400/100 mg bid. Through 72 weeks of therapy, 75% of patients maintained vRNA loads less than 400 copies/ml, and 58% achieved levels less than 50 copies/ml. Among the 36 patients originally randomized to receive the 400/100 mg bid dose, the mean increase in CD4 count from baseline over 72 weeks was 174 cells/mm³ (6).

LVP/RTV, when combined with efavirenz and NRTIs, has also shown potential to be effective in salvage therapy of non-nucleoside RT inhibitor (NNRTI)–naive patients with prior PI virological failure (see below) (6).

The major adverse events associated with LPV/RTV therapy are diarrhea and elevated cholesterol and triglyceride levels (6).

Metabolic Changes Associated with HIV-1 PIs

Since the introduction of HIV-1 PIs and the widespread use of highly active antiretroviral therapy, several types of metabolic disturbances have been reported in patients receiving long-term therapy (for review, see reference 132). These include abnormalities in fat deposition (including central obesity, increased breast size, and "buffalo hump"), lipoatrophy (particularly wasting of the face, arms, and legs), increased cholesterol and triglyceride levels, and insulin resistance.

Although they were initially described in patients receiving HIV-1 PIs, the fat redistribution syndromes have also been reported in many patients on non-PI-containing regimens. Because of the wide range of clinical definitions, reporting methods, and therapies received by these patients, however, the potential association between PI use and fat redistribution is unclear. It is possible that these syndromes result from multiple contributing factors, including other classes of antiretroviral agents, duration of antiretroviral therapy, changes in viral load, or differences in gender, body weight, or age, and additional research will be needed to define the etiologies of these syndromes unambiguously.

In contrast, available evidence strongly suggests that increases in serum lipids may be associated with PI therapy. Early in HIV infection, high-density lipoprotein (HDL) and low-density lipoprotein (LDL) levels generally decrease, followed by a rise in triglycerides and very-low-density lipoprotein (VLDL) levels with progression to AIDS (46, 47). Several studies have demonstrated substantial rises in triglycerides and cholesterol that may be associated with PI use. In one study, an approximate doubling of triglycerides and a 31% increase in cholesterol were observed in patients on PI therapy, relative to levels in non-PI-treated patients (15). Similarly, other studies showed PI treatment to elevate significantly fasting triglyceride and cholesterol (LDL but not HDL) levels relative to patients not receiving PIs (132).

Similarly, insulin resistance appears to be manifest in some patients receiving HIV-1 PIs. Although hyperinsulinemia has been demonstrated in HIV-infected patients independently of PI treatment (53), impaired glucose tolerance and high insulin-to-glucose ratios developed in some patients who initiated therapy with PIs, relative to values obtained in the same patients prior to PI use (11).

Resistance to HIV-1 PIs

The emergence of resistance to HIV-1 PIs is associated with the appearance of amino acid substitution mutations in the viral protease gene. During in vitro drug selection or during therapy, these substitutions accumulate over time, leading to gradual losses of drug susceptibility.

Because all available HIV-1 PIs are peptidomimetic, competitive inhibitors, they all bind to the same cleft in the enzyme (encompassing the active site and adjacent regions) that is normally occupied by the natural peptide substrates of the protease. As might be expected, many amino acid substitutions involved in PI resistance affect the binding equilibrium between drug and enzyme. However, numerous other substitutions involved in resistance have been shown to map elsewhere in the molecule, and in many cases far removed from the binding site. To date, among the 99 amino acid residues of the protease, 25 or more have been implicated in resistance to the PIs. The involvement of such a large number of amino acid residues in PI resistance testifies to the remarkable plasticity of the viral enzyme and its coding sequences.

General Mechanisms of Resistance

Despite the variability and complexity of mutational patterns observed, the basis of resistance to the HIV-1 PIs is actually quite simple in concept. The many amino acid changes implicated in resistance to PIs can be divided into three functional groups.

First, amino acid substitutions in or near the drug binding site may antagonize the binding of the drug to the protease. This reduced drug affinity is measurable as a K_i increase using purified enzyme. However, because the PIs are substrate mimics, substitutions that antagonize drug binding often antagonize the binding of the enzyme's natural peptide substrates as well. Therefore, while these "resistant" enzymes may have reduced drug binding affinity (a selective advantage for the virus when a PI is present), these same substitutions may inhibit normal enzymatic function (a distinct disadvantage for the virus at a time when its protease activity is already limited by drug). As a result, the overall selective advantages of these changes will be determined by a balance between evolutionary "benefit" and "cost." Because different PIs have different chemical structures and make different physical contacts with the enzyme, the selective advantages conferred by such "active-site" substitutions usually differ from drug to drug—the greater the drug binding antagonism conferred by a given substitution, the more likely that substitution is to be selected by that drug. Consistent with this observation, many amino acid substitutions mapping near the active site can be shown to impair viral replicative capacity (sometimes termed "fitness") in vitro in the absence of drug.

Second, amino acid substitutions that do not affect the drug-enzyme interaction may confer viral replicative advantages in the presence of PIs. Because enzyme inhibition by drug limits the protease activity available to support viral replication, amino acid substitutions in the protease that improve its overall enzymatic activity (irrespective of drug binding) will buffer the enzyme—and therefore the virus—against the inhibitory effects of drug. That is, increased enzymatic activity is an advantage when that activity is limiting. The selection of these substitutions by PIs may occur in the absence of other substitutions (22, 24, 28). This is direct evidence, therefore, that these substitutions may confer advantages in their own right. However, they are often selected following the appearance of "active-site" substitutions known to impair catalytic function. In this latter case, they may play a "compensatory" role by partially offsetting the deleterious effects of substitutions already selected by drug.

The third type of resistance substitution involves mutations outside the protease coding region. Because the protease normally cleaves the *gag-pol* polyprotein into smaller functional units, the peptide substrates themselves may become targets for the selective pressures of PI therapy. Thus, the overall effects of protease inhibition may be offset by changes within the protease, as in the two previous examples, or, alternatively, by modifying its substrates to facilitate their cleavage (38, 156). To date, these "cleavage site" substitutions have only been observed following the appearance of amino acid substitutions in the protease. Further, the specific cleavage site substitutions observed may differ among drugs that select different amino acid substitution patterns in the protease. This is consistent with the interpretation that drug-specific changes within the enzyme alter the enzyme's cleavage specificity, differentially affecting the abilities of the peptide substrates to be cleaved. In response, sequence changes in those substrates may facilitate their cleavage by these altered enzymes.

Although these three functional classes of mutations may be selected by PI therapy, the end result is the same: all give rise to enhanced *gag-pol* substrate cleavage when that activity has been limited by drug.

The Genetic Basis of PI Resistance

The earliest in vitro studies of resistance to the HIV-1 PIs came from cell culture selection of variants resistant to Abbott's c2-symmetrical inhibitor, A-77003 (59) and Roche's SQV (64). In these selection experiments, several active-site and non-active-site amino acid substitutions were identified, but these studies yielded only a limited glimpse of the complexity that would be observed in a clinical setting.

Resistance to IDV. Once the HIV-1 PIs entered clinical trials, the emergence of resistance to these drugs began to be observed. The first reports of clinical resistance to an HIV-1 PI came from studies of resistance to IDV monotherapy using dosages now known to be suboptimal (28, 98). Reduced susceptibility to IDV was shown to be associated with the appearance of multiple amino acid substitutions in the protease, and the accumulation of these substitutions was associated with increasing levels of resistance (24, 28). Resistance was associated with widely varying combinations of substitutions that occurred in no consistent order. Attempts to reconstruct IDV resistance in vitro with recombinant viruses proved challenging because no substitution engendered any measurable loss of drug susceptibility by itself or when paired with another.

An example of the cumulative nature of IDV resistance is shown in Table 5.2. From the mutational pattern observed in one patient whose viruses developed IDV resistance, site-directed viral mutants carrying all possible combinations of substitutions M46I (i.e., methionine at residue 46 replaced by isoleucine), L63P, and V82T were constructed and tested in vitro. None of the single or pairwise combinations of these substitutions engendered any measurable loss of IDV susceptibility. However, when all three substitutions (M46I/L63P/V82T) were combined, susceptibility to IDV was reduced fourfold relative to wild type. Therefore, resistance to IDV was due to the combined effects of multiple substitutions whose ef-

TABLE 5.2

Interactive effects of IDV-resistance-associated amino acid substitutions[a]

(Non-active site) M46	(Non-active site) L63	(Active site) V82	IDV IC$_{95}$ (nM)
(wt)	(wt)	(wt)	100 (1×)
I	**P**	**T**	**400 (4×)**
(wt)	**P**	**T**	100 (1×)
I	(wt)	**T**	100 (1×)
I	**P**	(wt)	50 (0.5×)
I	(wt)	(wt)	50 (0.5×)
(wt)	**P**	(wt)	50 (0.5×)
(wt)	(wt)	**T**	100 (1×)

[a]Site-directed mutants of HIV NL4-3 were constructed to reconstruct protease mutational patterns observed in virus from a single patient (28). IC$_{95}$ = the concentration of IDV (in nM) required to inhibit 95% of HIV-1 spread in cell culture. Amino acid substitutions and phenotypic resistance are indicated in **bold**. Amino acid substitutions from the wild-type ("wt") sequence (the North American/European Clade "B" consensus [106]) are given in single-letter amino acid code.

fects were not apparent alone or in pairs. Further examination revealed that viruses with other combinations of these same substitutions had widely divergent phenotypes, indicating that their effects are critically dependent on the ways in which they are combined.

Among these three substitutions contributing to reduced IDV susceptibility, only one (V82T) maps near the drug binding pocket of the enzyme. The others, M46I and L63P, do not influence drug binding to the enzyme but appear to contribute to resistance by increasing the catalytic efficiency of the enzyme (136). Thus, the viral phenotype was demonstrably affected by both active-site and non-active-site substitutions, and no straightforward relationship between the presence of specific substitutions and IDV resistance could be defined.

Because of this complexity, only a few residues have been directly implicated in IDV resistance based on site-directed mutagenesis studies, and it has been necessary to infer others from statistical associations with changes in viral phenotypes. Based on these studies, at least 11 amino acid residues (positions L10, K20, L24, M46, I54, L63, I64, A71, V82, I84, and L90) have been shown to be associated with phenotypic IDV resistance (24, 28) (see Fig. 5.3).

A further complication was the finding that many substitutions associated with resistance to IDV and other PIs are found naturally, in PI-naive patients (81, 85). These involve residues L10, K20, L63, I64, A71, and very

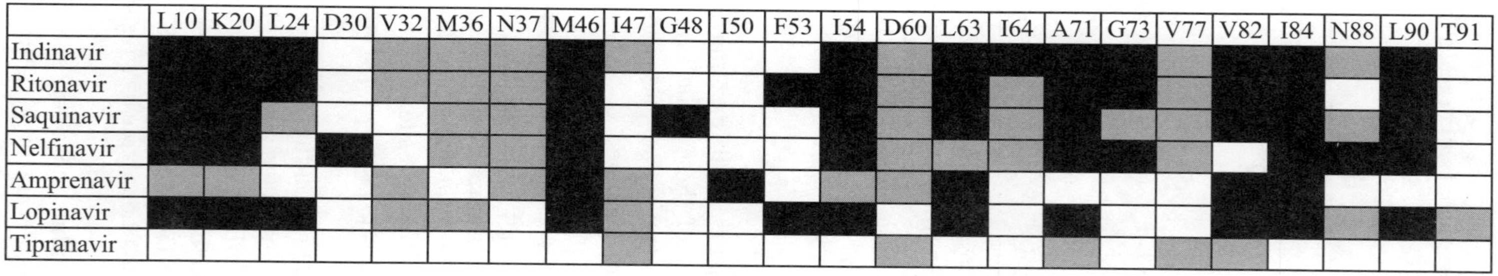

Top table (shaded cells, no values)

	L10	K20	L24	D30	V32	M36	N37	M46	I47	G48	I50	F53	I54	D60	L63	I64	A71	G73	V77	V82	I84	N88	L90	T91
Indinavir																								
Ritonavir																								
Saquinavir																								
Nelfinavir																								
Amprenavir																								
Lopinavir																								
Tipranavir																								

Bottom table (reference numbers)

	L10	K20	L24	D30	V32	M36	N37	M46	I47	G48	I50	F53	I54	D60	L63	I64	A71	G73	V77	V82	I84	N88	L90	T91
Indinavir	(24,28,72)	(72,102,135)	(24,28)		(24,28)	(24,28)	(24,28)	(24,28,72)	(24,28)				(24,28,72)	(24,25)	(24,28,72)	(24,28)	(24,28,72)	(24,72)	(24)	(24,28,72)	(24,28,72)	(24)	(24,28,72)	
Ritonavir	(72,102,135)	(72,102)	(72,102,138)		(135)	(102)	(102,135)	(72,89,102,135,139)				(72,102)	(72,89,102,135,139)	(102)	(72,102,135,139)	(102)	(72,89,102,135)	(72)	(102)	(72,102,135,138)	(72,102,135,138)		(72,102,135)	
Saquinavir	(63,72,89,139)	(72,124)	(30)			(63)	(124)	(28,63)		(63,138,150)			(72,134,139)	(30)	(28,63,72,138,150)	(30)	(63,72,138,150)	(72,138)	(138)	(28,63,138)	(28,63,72,138,150)	(124)	(28,63,138,150)	
Nelfinavir	(23,72)	(23,72,114)		(112,113,117)	(117)	(23,112,113)	(23,114)	(23,72,112,113,117)					(72,114)	(23,114)	(112,117)	(114)	(23,72,112,113,117)	(23,72,114)	(112)	(23,117)	(72,112,117)	(72,112,113)	(23,72,112,113,117)	
Amprenavir	(25,36,111)	(36)			(25,90)		(25)	(25,28,90,111)	(111)		(36,111,145)		(33,145)	(33,111)	(28,36)					(28,33)	(28,33,111)			
Lopinavir	(72,92)	(72)	(72)		(92)	(101)	(72,92)	(72,92)	(92)			(72)	(72)		(72)		(72)			(72)	(72,92)	(101)	(72)	
Tipranavir									(70)					(152)			(152)		(152)	(70)	(72,92)			(92)

FIGURE 5.3

Genetic correlates of reduced susceptibility to HIV-1 PIs

Amino acid residues most strongly implicated in reduced susceptibility to HIV-1 PIs are shown for each drug. In the upper panel, residues are categorized based on the strength of the data implicating them in resistance. No attempt is made to assess the relative "importance" of individual residues for resistance to the various drugs because these effects are highly variable and depend strongly on the protease genetic background. In one background, the amino acid residue at a particular position may demonstrably affect viral phenotype, and in another context, its effect may be immeasurable (and possibly irrelevant). Unshaded boxes represent residues at which no substitutions have been demonstrated to be selected by a given drug, in vitro or in vivo. Light-shaded boxes are residues at which PI-selected substitutions have been shown to occur but for which no clear association with changes in phenotypic susceptibility has been made. In many cases, the appropriate controlled experiments have not yet been done, so this categorization should not imply evidence for a lack of effect. Dark-shaded squares represent residues at which substitutions have been associated with changes in viral phenotype in controlled experiments, either alone or in combination with other substitutions. The lower panel gives literature references for the assignments in the upper panel. In some instances, a reference is cited for an unshaded square. In these cases, in vitro experiments have shown an effect of that substitution (alone or in combination) on viral phenotypic drug susceptibility, although no selection of that change by that drug has been demonstrated to date. It should be noted that more residues have been implicated in resistance to the more thoroughly characterized drugs than have been implicated for those that are less well characterized. Accordingly, especially for the newer drugs, additional residues are likely to be implicated over time.

likely others. Therefore, the presence of such genetic polymorphisms in patients does not necessarily signify PI resistance, and one of the challenges in interpretation of mutational patterns is to discern meaningful contributions to resistance in the face of this genetic background "noise."

The observation that multiple amino acid substitutions are necessary for measurable phenotypic resistance to IDV has important clinical consequences. Owing to the high mutation rate of HIV-1, many, if not most, single amino acid substitution mutations are likely to exist in patients, even before therapy (18). If only one such substitution is sufficient for phenotypic resistance to a therapeutic agent, resistance selection may occur readily. In contrast, the requirement for multiple substitutions greatly reduces the probability that the requisite combinations of substitutions would pre-exist in a patient before therapy. Moreover, should one of these substitutions occur, it would be unlikely to manifest significant resistance to IDV by itself, which would limit its competitive advantages in further evolution toward resistance. Thus, the need for multiple mutations for resistance imposes a formidable "genetic barrier" toward the emergence of resistance (21), and this is believed to be one of the principal reasons for the demonstrated durability of IDV therapy.

Resistance to RTV. Although the determinants of IDV resistance are very similar to those of other PIs, differences between the individual agents can be seen. As RTV resistance evolves, the first substitution that is observed is usually a substitution of residue V82 to A, F, T, or S (102). This can be explained by the observation that single substitutions of residue 82 engender low-level but measurable resistance to RTV, indicating that such single mutants would be at a significant competitive advantage, relative to wild type, in the presence of RTV. Following the selection of that substitution, however, the order of selection of additional substitutions is much less predictable. Although limited information is available to identify the specific mutational combinations contributing to RTV resistance, it is known that alterations of residues 54 and 84 can also affect viral phenotypic resistance to RTV. As in the case with IDV, multiple other substitutions have been shown to be selected in patients by RTV. In aggregate, the amino acid substitutions implicated in resistance to RTV are virtually indistinguishable from those selected by IDV (Fig. 5.3) (24, 102).

Resistance to SQV. In vitro and in patients, resistance to SQV is most often associated with the selection of an L90M substitution, which is sufficient to confer from 4- to 10-fold resistance to SQV in vitro (63) without greatly impairing viral replicative capacity (94, 95). Less frequently, other substitutions implicated in SQV binding are selected, including G48V, V82A, and I84V. In addition to substitutions known to affect drug binding, other substitutions overlapping those selected by other PIs are also selected by SQV, including substitutions of residues L10, K20, M46, L63, I54, A71, G73, V77, and N88 (see Fig. 5.3). It was formerly believed that the original SQV$_{hc}$ formulation was less prone than other PIs to the selection of resistance, but this lower observed incidence of resistance can be explained by its low bioavailability, resulting in minimal selective pressure (149). In patients previously treated with SQV$_{hc}$, subsequent therapy with IDV has been shown to select preferentially L90M or G48V substitutions that were not originally detected during the original SQV therapy (40, 125). This is evidence that the SQV exposure had been adequate to enrich the viral population with these mutants but was still insufficient to bring these mutants to a detectable level until greater selective pressure was applied by IDV. Therefore, it will be of interest to determine if resistance to SQV$_{sgc}$ develops more rapidly under the higher selective pressure exerted by this more bioavailable formulation of the drug.

Resistance to NFV. Low to moderate resistance (five- to nine-fold) to NFV is associated with any of three single amino acid substitutions in the protease, D30N, I84V, or L90M (112, 116). Among these, D30N substitutions are the most commonly observed in association with NFV failure. Although D30N confers moderate resistance to NFV, it does not seem to affect susceptibility to IDV, RTV, SQV, or APV in vitro. However, other amino acid substitutions that are selected by NFV are involved in resistance to other PIs, including residues I13, M36, M46, L63, A71, I84, N88, L90, and others (23, 116). In some patients, NFV failure has been associated with the selection of an L90M substitution, usually in the absence of D30N. L90M substitutions are often associated with varying combinations of additional substitutions of residues L10, I13, L19, K20, M46, D60, A71, G73, and T74 (23). Estimates of the frequency of L90M among NFV failures with genetic evidence of resistance vary, ranging from 15% to 40% (23, 115, 142). The lower frequency of L90M relative to D30N selection by NFV is consistent with that substitution's lesser contribution (ca. fivefold) to NFV resistance relative to the seven- to ninefold loss of NFV susceptibility engendered by D30N (116).

Resistance to APV. APV resistance involves many amino acid substitutions previously associated with resistance to the other PIs, although the most frequently observed substitution, I50V, appears uniquely selected by that inhibitor. By itself, I50V engenders only three-fold APV resistance and significantly greater resistance (about 20-fold) when it is combined with M46I and I47V (90). Other substitutions implicated in APV resistance include residues L10, K20, V32, I54, D60, L63, V77, V82, and I84 (see Fig. 5.3). Interestingly, an N88S substitution, known to be selected in some patients treated with IDV, SQV, or NFV, has been reported to hypersensitize HIV-1 to APV 2.5- to 12.5-fold (157), although the clinical significance of this observation is currently unknown.

Resistance to LPV. Because of the frequent association of V82 substitutions with resistance to IDV, RTV, or SQV, LPV was designed to minimize its interactions with this amino acid residue in the protease (137). It was hoped that this would allow LPV to retain activity among proteases exhibiting resistance to other PIs. During selection in cell culture, these predictions originally appeared to be borne out: resistance to LPV was associated with changes at residues 10, 32, 46, 47, 84, and 91, and no substitutions of residue 82 were observed (16). However, with clinical experience, the resistance pattern associated with LPV therapy revealed substitutions of multiple residues that had not been observed in vitro, including V82A/F/T. In all, substitutions of 11 residues were identified as statistical correlates of clinical resistance to LPV: L10, K20, L24, M46, F53, I54, L63, A71, V82, I84, and L90 (72). Strikingly, among these 11 residues, 10 are shared with the 11 known correlates of IDV resistance (24). In addition, as had been determined for IDV, decreases in phenotypic susceptibility were associated with multiple amino acid substitutions, suggesting that resistance to LPV results from the cumulative effects of multiple substitutions occurring both within and outside the active-site region (16, 72).

Cross-Resistance among PIs

As can be seen from the comparison in Fig. 5.3, most of the substitutions implicated in resistance to the HIV-1 PIs are shared among many (and sometimes all) members of the class. Considerable overlap is evident, not only among the many "non-active-site" residues but also among residues involved in drug-enzyme interaction, especially residues 32, 82, 84, and 90, despite the structural differences among compounds.

Consistent with this observation, as resistance evolves and these substitutions accumulate, resistance to any one PI frequently leads to cross-resistance to other members of the class, either in vitro or in the clinic, (24, 28, 36, 58, 84, 112, 133, 135, 139, 140, 144, 149, 153). Clearly, the incidence of cross-resistance is lowest at the earliest stages of resistance evolution, when only small numbers of substitutions are present. However, as the number of shared substitutions increases, the degree of cross-resistance observed among the PIs increases as well.

As a result of the emergence of cross-resistance, virological failure of PI-containing regimens may blunt the effectiveness of subsequently used PIs. This has been a widely accepted consequence of high-level resistance to either IDV or RTV, but the generality of this conclusion has been called into question for initial virological failures of SQV, NFV, or APV, all of which select some amino acid substitutions not generally associated with other PIs.

Several studies have addressed virological responses of PI-containing therapies in SQV-experienced patients and have demonstrated blunted virological responses to subsequent treatment with IDV, NFV, or combination RTV/SQV therapies (69, 84, 108, 109).

Similarly, patients experiencing failure of initial NFV therapy have demonstrated suboptimal virological responses to salvage therapies with either RTV/SQV plus two NRTIs (142, 158) or IDV/efavirenz (EFV)/adefovir dipivoxil (23, 131). In these studies, the virological responses to these salvage regimens did not appear to be compromised by the presence of the NFV-specific D30N substitution (23, 131, 158); rather, blunted responses were associated with the presence of the NFV-selected L90M substitution (23, 131), which is associated with resistance to multiple PIs (Fig. 5.3). Therefore, the virological responses to PI salvage of NFV failures are likely to depend on the specific mutations selected during the initial treatment with NFV.

To date, the clinical consequences of APV or LPV failures have not been explored. However, given the overlapping resistance patterns between these drugs and other PIs (Fig. 5.3), the selection of these substitutions during APV or LPV therapies would be expected to blunt the efficacy of subsequently administered PIs as well.

Taken together, these data strongly suggest that if any available HIV-1 PI fails as a result of resistance selection, the probability of successful salvage therapy by another PI will be reduced significantly. However, for any of these drugs, the success of such salvage will depend on both the number and the types of resistance-associated substitutions that were selected by the PI that was used initially.

PI Potency, Exposure, and Resistance

The in vivo antiviral efficacies of HIV-1 PIs are determined by the relationship between drug potency, drug exposure, and viral drug susceptibility (27). Drug potency against wild-type virus is generally measured as an IC_{50} or IC_{95}, the drug concentration necessary to inhibit 50% or 95% of viral spread, respectively, in culture. Because of this dose response, the greatest in vivo efficacy will be achieved when the concentration of active drug at the sites of viral replication exceeds that needed to prevent viral replication. Therefore, as long as drug exposure is maintained well above inhibitory levels, viral suppression is expected to be effective.

Whereas the measurement of in vitro potency by IC_{50} or IC_{95} is straightforward, measuring drug exposure in vivo is not. Because clinically important HIV-1 replication occurs in multiple body compartments, many of which are not accessible for sampling, it has been necessary to approximate drug exposure in vivo by measuring plasma drug levels. Typically, blood level measurements reflect total concentrations of drug in the plasma. However, for all the available PIs, a significant amount of drug is tightly bound to proteins, typically albumin or alpha-1-acid glycoprotein or both (10, 103, 155), rendering it unavailable to bind the viral protease and significantly attenuating its antiviral activities. Thus, the addition of 50% human serum to infected cell cultures has been shown to attenuate the antiviral activities of all the available PIs. This attenuation of activity varies over a wide range for the PIs, from a 2-fold reduction in effective potency for IDV up to a 37-fold reduction for NFV (103) (Table 5.2). For practical reasons, it is difficult to measure these effects at higher serum concentrations than 50%; however, the attenuation of activity in vivo, in the presence of 100% human plasma, is expected to be greater. Although the best available data yield only approximations of this effect, it is clearly necessary to correct for the inhibitory effects of human serum protein binding in order to estimate PI efficacy in vivo.

Overall drug exposure is generally assessed by sampling blood levels during the dosing interval. The most reliable blood level measurements come from formal, steady-state pharmacokinetic studies, and exposures are expressed as "peak" (C_{max}), "trough" (C_{min}), and "area under the curve" (AUC) during the dosing interval. Because the point of lowest drug exposure is generally believed to be the point at which the risk of viral replication and the selection of resistance are the greatest, estimates of antiviral efficacy have focused on the ratio of C_{min} to human serum protein binding–corrected IC_{95} (27). By maximizing drug exposure relative to inhibitory concentration, the greatest antiviral efficacy is predicted to be achieved.

Figure 5.4 compares the C_{min}/IC_{95} ratios for the available HIV-1 PIs, derived from formal, steady-state pharmacokinetic measurements when given at approved doses as single agents. Based on these data, most of the available HIV-1 PIs maintain blood levels above that drug's protein binding–corrected IC_{95} against wild-type HIV-1 (27). From these pharmacological considerations, significant suppression of wild-type virus should be achievable by most of these individual PIs in a clinical setting.

PI Intensification and Salvage Therapy

Although the available PIs may effectively suppress wild-type HIV-1, the drug exposures that can be maintained may be insufficient to suppress viruses with reduced PI susceptibility. Even for the most potent of these drugs, with low-level (fourfold) resistance, the new viral IC_{95} would exceed the achievable C_{min} and reduce its potential to suppress viral replication effectively (Fig. 5.4). However, owing to a favorable pharmacological interaction among HIV-1 PIs, it is possible to "intensify" PI exposure by using these drugs in combination.

Because RTV is a potent CYP3A4 inhibitor (60, 62, 82) and also inhibits P-glycoprotein-mediated PI cellular efflux (8, 39, 52, 78, 86), coadministration of RTV with another PI (typically IDV, SQV, or APV) leads to greatly

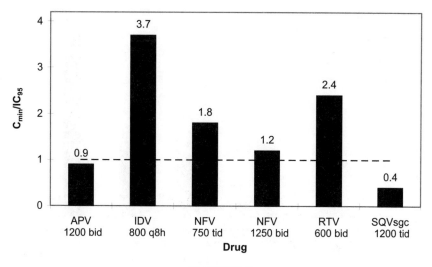

FIGURE 5.4

C_{min}/corrected IC_{95} ratios for individual HIV-1 PIs

Human serum binding–corrected C_{min}/IC_{95} ratios for the available HIV-1 PIs when administered at approved dosages as single agents (27). IC_{95} values were determined for wild-type virus in the ViroLogic PhenoSense assay (119), corrected for the effects of human serum protein binding as previously described (103) and compared with published steady-state C_{min} values determined for each of the indicated regimens: APV 1,200 mg bid (2); IDV 800 mg q8h (4); NFV 750 mg tid (65); NFV 1,250 mg bid (65); RTV 600 mg bid (3); SQV$_{sgc}$ 1,200 mg tid (29). A C_{min}/ IC_{95} ratio of 1.0 is indicated by the horizontal line.

increased blood levels of the second drug. By contrast, RTV levels are increased only slightly by co-dosing with other PIs.

Through this pharmacokinetic interaction with RTV, significant increases in PI exposure can be achieved. Although RTV co-dosing increases C_{max} values, its major effect is to increase the C_{min}, flattening the pharmacokinetic curve and prolonging the allowable dosing interval. This type of PI "intensification" was first explored with SQV, and it has been applied more recently to increase IDV or APV exposure.

A comparison of these RTV-intensified regimens, based on protein binding–corrected C_{min}/IC_{95} ratios, is shown in Fig. 5.5A. When RTV is used in the most commonly employed dosing regimens, the steady-state C_{min} values for SQV$_{sgc}$, APV, or IDV are increased to 1.7, 6.7, or 28–79 times their protein binding–corrected IC_{95} values, respectively, by the coadministration of RTV (27). While this study utilized viral IC_{95} values, some investigators prefer to compare IC_{50} values. To facilitate this comparison, the data from the same experiment are shown in Fig. 5.5B as C_{min}/corrected IC_{50} ratios. Because IC_{95} values are generally about fivefold higher than IC_{50} values, the C_{min}/IC_{50} ratios for SQV$_{sgc}$, APV, and IDV are correspondingly higher, at 13, 47, and 139–393, respectively (26). However, de-

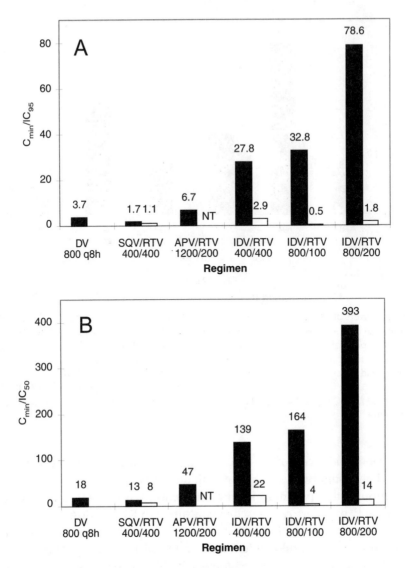

FIGURE 5.5

PI intensification by RTV coadministration

Human serum binding–corrected C_{min}/IC_{95} (Panel A) ratios (27) and C_{min}/IC_{50} (Panel B) ratios (26) for available HIV-1 PIs in the most commonly used RTV-intensified regimens. IC_{95} and IC_{50} values were determined for wild-type virus in the same experiment in the ViroLogic PhenoSense assay (119), corrected for the effects of human serum protein binding as previously described (103) and compared with published steady-state C_{min} values determined for each of the indicated regimens: IDV (approved dose, 800 mg q8h) (4); SQV 400 mg bid + RTV 400 mg bid (13); APV 1,200 mg bid + RTV 200 mg bid (122); IDV 400 mg bid + RTV 400 mg bid (130); IDV 800 mg bid + RTV 100 mg bid (130); IDV 800 mg bid + RTV 200 mg bid (130).

spite these numeric differences, the relative shifts in the C_{min}/IC ratios for the different PI combinations are virtually identical, irrespective of the method of calculation.

The earliest attempts at clinical PI intensification were directed at increasing SQV exposures. SQV-RTV combination therapy has been shown to suppress viral replication effectively in PI-naive patients. In one study, the combination of RTV and SQV_{hc} (with background RT inhibitor therapy) suppressed viral load to less than 200 copies/ml in 82–96% of patients by week 48 in an on-treatment analysis (varying by dosage), or in 65–74% of these patients in an intent-to-treat analysis (13). In a comparison of several different dosing regimens, the best tolerability and antiviral efficacy were achieved at the lowest doses of RTV and SQV examined, 400 mg of each drug twice daily. In the Danish Protease Inhibitor Study, comparing SQV + RTV versus IDV versus RTV in 318 PI-naive patients, treatment with SQV-RTV + two NRTIs yielded equivalent virological suppression over 72 weeks to that observed in patients receiving IDV + two NRTIs but was superior to responses in patients receiving RTV + two NRTIs (68).

The efficacy of SQV-RTV combination therapy has also been investigated in salvage therapy of prior PI failures. In most such studies, SQV-RTV-containing salvage regimens have mediated only modest and transient suppression of viral loads (34, 43, 54, 69, 88), although other investigators found favorable virological responses through 60 weeks in about 50% of treated patients (141). However, in a salvage setting, the most potent suppression was usually observed if SQV-RTV was initiated early after initial treatment failure and at low viral loads (54, 110, 142), and virological failure of SQV-RTV-based regimens has been strongly associated with preexisting genotypic and/or low-level phenotypic SQV resistance (34, 56, 69, 120, 121, 142, 159). Thus, from the available clinical or virological data (27), there is no evidence to suggest that SQV-RTV-based regimens can achieve adequate in vivo drug exposures to overcome measurable levels of resistance to either drug.

More recently, RTV coadministration has been used to increase IDV exposures in the clinic. In addition to the pharmacokinetic increases in IDV levels, combination therapy with RTV eliminates the inhibition of IDV absorption by food (60, 61, 130). Therefore, when given twice daily (with or without meals) with RTV, IDV exposures greatly exceed those achievable by standard eight-hour dosing of IDV as a single agent.

In a clinical setting, IDV-RTV therapy has been shown to be highly efficacious in both PI-naive and experienced patients. In one study, treatment-naive patients and those with more than six months of SQV + RTV + d4T + 3TC therapy were examined for virological responses to IDV 400 mg + RTV 400 mg + d4T + 3TC therapy. Among 12 well-controlled patients with SQV-RTV experience, all maintained their vRNA loads at less than 400 copies after 36 weeks, accompanied by substantial CD4 increases. Similarly, all of 9 treatment-naive patients who had reached week 12 had vRNA reductions to below 400 copies/ml (154). A second study examined virological responses of 90 treatment-naive patients given IDV 400 mg + RTV 400 mg twice daily with two NRTIs. After 24 weeks of therapy, vRNA reductions to less than 500 copies/ml were achieved in 86.7% of patients in an intent-to-treat analysis and in 97.5% by on-treatment analysis (128).

Despite these excellent virological responses to IDV-RTV therapies, significantly greater overall antiviral activity should be achieved at higher IDV dosages, particularly at 800 mg IDV + 200 mg RTV twice daily (Fig. 5.5) (27, 130). Significantly, the increased PI exposure achievable with RTV combination therapy may allow suppression of viruses that exhibit reduced PI susceptibility. Particularly because the IDV C_{min} for twice-daily IDV 800 mg–RTV 200 mg is nearly 80 times the corrected wild-type IC_{95}, this exceeds the IC_{95} values for at least 18 of a panel of 20 genotypically and phenotypically PI-resistant and cross-resistant viruses, most of which had been selected by IDV therapy (27). Therefore, by achieving greatly increased drug exposure, it may be possible to salvage many instances of PI failure, even by using the same drug that had selected the initial resistance.

Several studies currently under way are designed to test this prediction. In two recent reports, IDV 800 mg + RTV 200 mg + RT inhibitors suppressed viral loads to less than 400 copies/ml in the majority of patients with prior virological failure of PI-containing regimens (14, 45), despite the presence of genotypic resistance and high-level phenotypic resistance ($\leq$ 35-fold) to both IDV and RTV (14). In this latter study, adherence to therapy was the best predictor of therapeutic success, and preexisting PI resistance was not associated with failure. Therefore, these data are consistent with the virological studies and suggest that the increased IDV exposure achieved by coadministration of RTV may overcome virological failures of prior PI therapies, including failure of IDV itself.

Similarly, the combination of APV 1,200 mg–RTV 200 mg twice daily may have salvage potential in many cases of PI failure. Against the same panel of viruses, the 12-hour C_{min} for APV was found to exceed the protein binding–corrected IC_{95} for 17 of the 20 (largely IDV-selected) viruses tested (27). However, because this APV C_{min} was only 6.7 times the wild-type IC_{95}, this reflects the observation that most of the IDV-resistant viruses did not exhibit high-level resistance to APV. To date, no clinical data are available to assess the ability of this new PI-PI combination to salvage virological failures of HIV-1 PIs.

With the recent approval of LPV/RTV, another "boosted" PI combination with significant salvage potential has become available. When administered at the approved dosage of LPV 400 mg–RTV 100 mg twice daily, protein binding–corrected C_{min}/IC_{50} ratios for LPV range from 30 to 75 against wild-type viruses (17, 71) , although no estimates of C_{min}/IC_{95} ratio are available. This suggests that LPV/RTV therapy may also be efficacious against some viruses exhibiting resistance to available HIV PIs. In support of this prediction, in Study 957, treatment of multiple PI–experienced, NNRTI-naive patients with LPV/RTV + EFV + NRTIs yielded vRNA reductions to less than 400 copies/ml in the majority of patients. In all, 93% of patients with less than 10-fold reduced susceptibility to LPV and 65% of patients with greater than 10-fold baseline LPV resistance showed this level of viral suppression after 24 weeks of therapy. However, because these patients harbored EFV-susceptible viruses, the relative contributions of LPV and EFV to the overall antiviral effect are difficult to discern, and a clear assessment of the ability of LPV/RTV to suppress highly PI-resistant viruses warrants further investigation. Nonetheless, the high drug exposures achievable by LPV-RTV combination therapy suggest that it should be effective in salvage therapy in many cases of virological failure due to PI resistance.

Investigational HIV-1 PIs

Two additional compounds are in the advanced stages of clinical testing, and their chemical structures are shown in Fig. 5.6.

Tipranavir

Tipranavir (TPV, PNU-140690) was discovered by researchers at Pharmacia-Upjohn Laboratories (123, 143, 147). TPV is unique among the HIV PIs studied to date by virtue of its nonpeptidyl structure. Normally, the peptidomimetic inhibitors occupy active-site hydrophobic "pockets" and interact with the protease beta-turn "flap" region through a shared water molecule. In contrast, TPV interacts directly with the "flap" through its pyrone carbonyl group. The binding of TPV is less dependent than other PIs on interactions with amino acid side chains of the protease, thus reducing its vulnerability to inhibition of binding due to amino acid changes selected by other PIs (9, 129). Despite this novel mode of interaction, amino acid substitutions associated with resistance to other PIs have been shown to diminish TPV susceptibility (Fig. 5.3), but the genetic basis for TPV resistance appears to be complex (70).

When TPV is given to patients as a single agent, very high doses are needed to achieve sufficient exposure to suppress viral replication effectively. Accordingly, clinical studies in progress employ coadministration with RTV to inhibit its metabolism and increase its blood concentration. In early studies, combination therapy of antiretroviral-naive patients with TPV/RTV led to vRNA reductions of 1.4–1.6 $\log_{10}$ after two weeks of therapy (151).

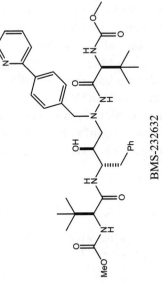

BMS-232632

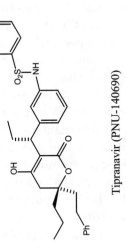

Tipranavir (PNU-140690)

FIGURE 5.6

Structures of investigational HIV-1 PIs

BMS-232632

BMS-232632 is an azapeptide whose design is based on the symmetrical structure of the HIV protease (127). The compound is potent against HIV protease ($K_i = 2.66$ nM) and is highly active in cell culture ($IC_{50} = 2.62$–5.28 nM). Addition of 40% normal human serum to the cell culture assay reduced its antiviral activity by 2.7-fold. The compound was well absorbed in human subjects and is now undergoing clinical evaluation for once-per-day administration.

Challenges for the Future

The introduction of the HIV-1 PIs into the antiretroviral armamentarium in the mid-1990s was followed by the first declines in AIDS-related illnesses and mortality seen in the history of the disease (1, 104). Simultaneously, it became clear that extremely potent PI combination therapies are indeed capable of providing long-term suppression of viral replication and forestalling drug resistance, resulting in long-term clinical benefits. Accordingly, the HIV-1 PIs rapidly became the cornerstones of effective antiretroviral therapy.

As potent as these new antiretroviral agents are, however, the chronic nature of HIV infection is likely to require long-term, if not lifelong, therapy to maintain continued viral suppression and the control of HIV disease. At any time, incomplete suppression and low-level viral replication may permit viral evolution and ultimately compromise the effects of therapy through the emergence of drug resistance. Therefore, it is imperative to continue drug discovery efforts to identify new antiretrovirals with overwhelming potency and high genetic barriers to resistance to provide long-term viral suppression combined with sufficient tolerability and convenience to encourage their long-term use. For this reason, intensive efforts are under way to develop new generations of highly potent HIV PIs, antiretroviral drugs directed at other viral targets, and effective HIV vaccines. With the continued discovery of new therapeutic options and as we learn to optimize the use of the available therapies, we will improve our ability to maintain control of replication and provide lasting clinical benefits to people with HIV disease.

REFERENCES

1. Anonymous. 1997. HIV/AIDS surveillance report. Centers for Disease Control and Prevention.
2. Anonymous. 1999. Agenerase®, US Prescribing Information.
3. Anonymous. 1999. Norvir®, US Prescribing Information.
4. Anonymous. 2000. Crixivan®, US Prescribing Information.

5. Anonymous. 2000. Fortovase™, US Prescribing Information.

6. Anonymous. 2000. Kaletra™, US Prescribing Information.

7. Anonymous. 2000. Viracept®, US Prescribing Information.

8. Aungst, B. J. 1999. P-glycoprotein, secretory transport, and other barriers to the oral delivery of anti-HIV drugs. Adv. Drug Delivery Rev. 39:105–116.

9. Back, N. K. T., A. van Wijk, D. Remmerswaal, M. van Monfort, M. Nijhuis, R. Schuurman, and C. A. B. Boucher. 2000. In-vitro tipranavir susceptibility of HIV-1 isolates with reduced susceptibility to other protease inhibitors. AIDS 14:101–102.

10. Barry, M., S. Gibbons, D. Back, and F. Mulcahy. 1997. Protease inhibitors in patients with HIV disease—clinically important pharmacokinetic considerations. Clin. Pharmacokinetics 32:194–209.

11. Behrens, G., A. Dejam, H. Schmidt, H. J. Balks, G. Brabant, T. Korner, M. Stoll, and R. E. Schmidt. 1999. Impaired glucose tolerance, beta cell function and lipid metabolism in HIV patients under treatment with protease inhibitors. AIDS 13:F63–70.

12. Cameron, D. W., M. Heath-Chiozzi, S. Danner, C. Cohen, S. Kravcik, C. Maurath, E. Sun, D. Henry, R. Rode, A. Potthoff, and J. Leonard. 1998. Randomised placebo-controlled trial of ritonavir in advanced HIV-1 disease. Lancet 351:543–549.

13. Cameron, D. W., A. J. Japour, Y. Xu, A. Hsu, J. Mellors, C. Farthing, C. Cohen, D. Poretz, M. Markowitz, S. Follansbee, J. B. Angel, D. McMahon, D. Ho, V. Devanarayan, R. Rode, M. Salgo, D. J. Kempf, R. Granneman, J. M. Leonard, and E. Sun. 1999. Ritonavir and saquinavir combination therapy for the treatment of HIV infection. AIDS 13:213–224.

14. Campo, R., G. Suarez, N. Miller, J. Moreno, M. Kolber, D. J. Holder, M. Shivaprakash, D. M. DeAngelis, J. L. Wright, K. Holmes, W. A. Schleif, E. A. Emini, and J. H. Condra. 2000. Efficacy of indinavir (IDV)/ritonavir (RTV)-based regimens (IRBR) among patients with prior protease inhibitor failure. Antiviral Therapy 5(Suppl. 2):6, abstr. 7.

15. Carr, A., K. Samaras, S. Burton, M. Law, J. Freund, D. J. Chisholm, and D. A. Cooper. 1998. A syndrome of peripheral lipodystrophy, hyperlipidaemia and insulin resistance in patients receiving HIV protease inhibitors. AIDS 12:F51–58.

16. Carrillo, A., K. D. Stewart, H. L. Sham, D. W. Norbeck, W. E. Kohlbrenner, J. M. Leonard, D. J. Kempf, and A. Molla. 1998. In vitro selection and characterization of human immunodeficiency virus type 1 variants with increased resistance to ABT-378, a novel protease inhibitor. J. Virol. 72:7532–7541.

17. Clumeck, N., P. M. Girard, A. Telenti, J. Rockstroh, S. Becker, A. Lazzarin, S. Brun, E. Sun, and X. U. Yi. 2000. ABT-378/ritonavir (ABT-378/r) and efavirenz: 16 week safety/efficacy evaluation in multiple PI experienced patients. XIII International AIDS Conference, Durban, South Africa, abstr. TuPeB3196.

18. Coffin, J. M. 1995. HIV population dynamics in vivo: implications for genetic variation, pathogenesis, and therapy. Science 267:483–489.

19. Cohen Stuart, J. W., R. Schuurman, D. M. Burger, P. P. Koopmans, H. G. Sprenger, J. R. Juttmann, C. Richter, P. L. Meenhorst, R. M. Hoetelmans, F. P.

Kroon, B. Bravenboer, D. Hamann, C. A. Boucher, and J. C. Borleffs. 1999. Randomized trial comparing saquinavir soft gelatin capsules versus indinavir as part of triple therapy (CHEESE study). AIDS 13:F53–58.

20. Collier, A. C., R. W. Coombs, D. A. Schoenfeld, R. L. Bassett, J. Timpone, A. Baruch, M. Jones, K. Facey, C. Whitacre, V. J. Mcauliffe, H. M. Friedman, T. C. Merigan, R. C. Reichman, C. Hooper, and L. Corey. 1996. Treatment of human-immunodeficiency-virus infection with saquinavir, zidovudine, and zalcitabine. N. Engl. J. Med. 334:1011–1017.

21. Condra, J. H., and E. A. Emini. 1997. Preventing HIV-1 drug resistance. Science and Medicine 4(1):14–23.

22. Condra, J. H., D. J. Holder, D. J. Graham, M. Shivaprakash, D. T. Laird, W. A. Schleif, J. A. Chodakewitz, and E. A. Emini. 1997. Genotypic or phenotypic susceptibility testing may not predict clinical responses to indinavir. Abstracts of the International Workshop on HIV Drug Resistance, Treatment Strategies and Eradication, no. 47:31–32.

23. Condra, J. H., D. J. Holder, W. A. Schleif, K. Bakshi, R. M. Danovich, D. J. Graham, M. Shivaprakash, K. Holmes, A. J. Saah, R. Y. Leavitt, J. A. Chodakewitz, and E. A. Emini. 1999. Genetic correlates of virological response to an indinavir-containing salvage regimen in patients with nelfinavir failure. Antiviral Therapy 4(Suppl. 1):44.

24. Condra, J. H., D. J. Holder, W. A. Schleif, O. M. Blahy, R. M. Danovich, L. J. Gabryelski, D. J. Graham, D. Laird, J. C. Quintero, A. Rhodes, H. L. Robbins, E. Roth, M. Shivaprakash, T. Yang, J. A. Chodakewitz, P. J. Deutsch, R. Y. Leavitt, F. E. Massari, J. W. Mellors, K. E. Squires, R. T. Steigbigel, H. Teppler, and E. A. Emini. 1996. Genetic correlates of in-vivo viral resistance to indinavir a human immunodeficiency virus type-1 protease inhibitor. J. Virol. 70:8270–8276.

25. Condra, J. H., D. J. Holder, W. A. Schleif, J. A. Chodakewitz, F. E. Massari, O. M. Blahy, R. M. Danovich, L. J. Gabryselski, D. J. Graham, D. Laird, J. C. Quintero, A. Rhodes, H. L. Robbins, E. Roth, M. Shivaprakash, T. Yang, and E. A. Emini. 1996. Bi-directional inhibition of HIV-1 drug resistance selection by combination therapy with indinavir and reverse transcriptase inhibitors. Abstracts of XI International Conference on AIDS, July 7–12, 1996, Vancouver, B.C., Program Supplement p. 19, no. Th.B.932.

26. Condra, J. H., C. J. Petropoulos, R. Ziermann, W. A. Schleif, M. Shivaprakash, and E. A. Emini. Unpublished data.

27. Condra, J. H., C. J. Petropoulos, R. Ziermann, W. A. Schleif, M. Shivaprakash, and E. A. Emini. 2000. Drug resistance and predicted virologic responses to human immunodeficiency virus type 1 protease inhibitor therapy. J. Infect. Dis. 182:758–765.

28. Condra, J. H., W. A. Schleif, O. M. Blahy, L. J. Gabryelski, D. J. Graham, J. C. Quintero, A. Rhodes, H. L. Robbins, E. Roth, M. Shivaprakash, D. Titus, T. Yang, H. Teppler, K. E. Squires, P. J. Deutsch, and E. A. Emini. 1995. In vivo emergence of HIV-1 variants resistant to multiple protease inhibitors. Nature (London) 374:569–571.

29. Cox, S., B. Conway, W. Freimuth, E. Berber, L. Paxton, B. Carel, L. Nieto, C. Rivera, M. Wolff, J. Benetucci, P. Cahn, and K. Williams. 2000. Pilot study of

bid and tid combinations of saquinavir-sgc (S), delavirdine (D), zidovudine (ZDV) & lamivudine (3TC) as initial therapy: pharmacokinetic (PK) interaction between S-SGC and D. Abstracts of the 7th Conference on Retroviruses and Opportunistic Infections, January 30–February 2, 2000, San Francisco, no. 82.

30. Craig, C., E. Race, J. Sheldon, L. Whittaker, S. Gilbert, A. Moffatt, J. Rose, S. Dissanayeke, G. W. Chirn, I. B. Duncan, and N. Cammack. 1998. HIV protease genotype and viral sensitivity to HIV protease inhibitors following saquinavir therapy. AIDS 12:1611–1618.

31. Craig, J. C., I. B. Duncan, D. Hockley, C. Grief, N. A. Roberts, and J. S. Mills. 1991. Antiviral properties of Ro 31-8959, an inhibitor of human immunodeficiency virus (HIV) proteinase. Antiviral Res. 16:295–305.

32. Danner, S. A., A. Carr, J. M. Leonard, L. M. Lehman, F. Gudiol, J. Gonzales, A. Raventos, R. Rubio, E. Bouza, V. Pintado, A. G. Aguado, J. G. de Lomas, R. Delgado, J. C. C. Borleffs, A. Hsu, J. M. Valdes, C. A. B. Boucher, and D. A. Cooper for the European-Australian Collaborative Ritonavir Study Group. 1995. A short-term study of the safety, pharmacokinetics, and efficacy of ritonavir, an inhibitor of HIV-1 protease. European-Australian Collaborative Ritonavir Study Group. N. Engl. J. Med. 333:1528–1533.

33. Debouck, C. 1992. The HIV-1 protease as a therapeutic target for AIDS. AIDS Res. Hum. Retroviruses 8:153–164.

34. Deeks, S. G., R. M. Grant, G. W. Beatty, C. Horton, J. Detmer, and S. Eastman. 1998. Activity of a ritonavir plus saquinavir-containing regimen in patients with virologic evidence of indinavir or ritonavir failure. AIDS 12:F97–102.

35. Denissen, J. F., B. A. Grabowski, M. K. Johnson, A. M. Buko, D. J. Kempf, S. B. Thomas, and B. W. Surber. 1997. Metabolism and disposition of the HIV-1 protease inhibitor ritonavir (ABT-538) in rats, dogs, and humans. Drug Metabolism and Disposition 25:489–501.

36. De Pasquale, M. P., R. Murphy, D. Kuritzkes, J. Martinez-Picado, J.-P. Sommadossi, R. Gulick, L. Smeaton, V. DeGruttola, A. Caliendo, L. Sutton, A. V. Savara, R. D'Aquila, for the ACTG 347 Team. 1998. Resistance during early virological rebound on amprenavir plus zidovudine plus lamividine triple therapy or amprenavir monotherapy in ACTG protocol 347. Abstracts of the Second International Workshop on HIV Drug Resistance and Treatment Strategies, June 24–27, 1998, Lake Maggiore, Italy, no. 71.

37. Dorsey, B. D., R. B. Levin, S. L. Mcdaniel, J. P. Vacca, J. P. Guare, P. L. Darke, J. A. Zugay, E. A. Emini, W. A. Schleif, J. C. Quintero, J. H. Lin, I. W. Chen, M. K. Holloway, P. Fitzgerald, M. G. Axel, D. Ostovic, P. S. Anderson, and J. R. Huff. 1994. L-735,524—the design of a potent and orally bioavailable HIV protease inhibitor. J. Med. Chem. 37:3443–3451.

38. Doyon, L., G. Croteau, D. Thibeault, F. Poulin, L. Pilote, and D. Lamarre. 1996. Second locus involved in human immunodeficiency virus type 1 resistance to protease inhibitors. J. Virol. 70:3763–3769.

39. Drewe, J., H. Gutmann, G. Fricker, M. Török, C. Beglinger, and J. Huwyler. 1999. HIV protease inhibitor ritonavir: a more potent inhibitor of P-glycoprotein than the cyclosporine analog SDZ PSC 833. Biochem. Pharmacol. 57:1147–1152.

40. Dulioust, A., S. Paulous, L. Guillemot, A. M. Delavalle, F. Boue, and F. Clavel. 1999. Constrained evolution of human immunodeficiency virus type 1 protease during sequential therapy with two distinct protease inhibitors. J. Virol. 73:850–854.

41. Emini, E. A., D. J. Holder, W. A. Schleif, R. M. Danovich, D. J. Graham, D. T. Laird, M. Shivaprakash, J. A. Chodakewitz, and J. H. Condra. 1997. Evidence for the prevention of new HIV-1 infection cycles in patients treated with indinavir plus zidovudine and lamivudine. Abstracts of the International Workshop on HIV Drug Resistance, Treatment Strategies and Eradication, St. Petersburg, Fla., no. 128.

42. Erickson, J., D. J. Neidhart, J. Vandrie, D. J. Kempf, X. C. Wang, D. W. Norbeck, J. J. Plattner, J. W. Rittenhouse, M. Turon, N. Wideburg, W. E. Kohlbrenner, R. Simmer, R. Helfrich, D. A. Paul, and M. Knigge. 1990. Design, activity, and 2.8 Å crystal-structure of a c2 symmetrical inhibitor complexed to HIV-1 protease. Science 249:527–533.

43. Fätkenheuer, G., R. M. W. Hoetelmans, N. Hunn, A. Schwenk, C. Franzen, M. Reiser, A. Jutte, J. Rockstroh, V. Diehl, and B. Salzberger. 1999. Salvage therapy with regimens containing ritonavir and saquinavir in extensively pretreated HIV-infected patients. AIDS 13:1485–1489.

44. Greenlee, W. J. 1990. Renin inhibitors. Med. Res. Rev. 10:173–236.

45. Grossman, H., A. Luber, D. Purdom, D. Butcher, G. Frechette, P. Duong, and L. Markson. 2000. Salvage therapy with twice daily indinavir (Crixivan®) 800mg plus ritonavir (Norvir®) 200mg based regimen in clinical practice. Antiviral Therapy 5(Suppl. 2):23, abstr. 27.

46. Grunfeld, C., D. P. Kotler, R. Hamadeh, A. Tierney, J. Wang, and R. N. Pierson. 1989. Hypertriglyceridemia in the acquired immunodeficiency syndrome. Am. J. Med. 86:27–31.

47. Grunfeld, C., M. Pang, W. Doerrler, J. K. Shigenaga, P. Jensen, and K. R. Feingold. 1992. Lipids, lipoproteins, triglyceride clearance, and cytokines in human immunodeficiency virus infection and the acquired immunodeficiency syndrome. J. Clin. Endocrinol. Metab. 74:1045–1052.

48. Gulick, R. M., J. W. Mellors, D. Havlir, J. J. Eron, C. Gonzalez, D. McMahon, L. Jonas, A. Meibohm, D. Holder, W. A. Schleif, J. H. Condra, E. A. Emini, R. Isaacs, J. A. Chodakewitz, and D. D. Richman. 1998. Simultaneous vs. sequential initiation of therapy with indinavir, zidovudine, and lamivudine for HIV-1 infection: 100-week follow-up. JAMA 280:35–41.

49. Gulick, R. M., J. W. Mellors, D. Havlir, J. J. Eron, C. Gonzalez, D. McMahon, D. D. Richman, F. T. Valentine, L. Jonas, A. Meibohm, E. A. Emini, P. Deutsch, D. Holder, W. A. Schleif, J. H. Condra, and J. A. Chodakewitz. 1997. Treatment with indinavir, zidovudine, and lamivudine in adults with human-immunodeficiency-virus infection and prior antiretroviral therapy. N. Engl. J. Med. 337:734–739.

50. Gulick, R. M., J. W. Mellors, D. Havlir, J. J. Eron, A. Meibohm, J. H. Condra, F. T. Valentine, D. McMahon, C. Gonzalez, L. Jonas, E. A. Emini, J. A. Chodakewitz, R. Isaacs, and D. D. Richman. 2000. 3-year suppression of HIV viremia with indinavir, zidovudine, and lamivudine. Ann. Intern. Med. 133:35–39.

51. Gunthard, H. F., J. K. Wong, C. C. Ignacio, J. C. Guatelli, N. L. Riggs, D. V. Havlir, and D. D. Richman. 1998. Human immunodeficiency virus replication and genotypic resistance in blood and lymph nodes after a year of potent antiretroviral therapy. J. Virol. 72:2422–2428.

52. Gutmann, H., G. Fricker, J. Drewe, M. Toeroek, and D. S. Miller. 1999. Interactions of HIV protease inhibitors with ATP-dependent drug export proteins. Mol. Pharmacol. 56:383–389.

53. Hadigan, C., K. Miller, C. Corcoran, E. Anderson, N. Basgoz, and S. Grinspoon. 1999. Fasting hyperinsulinemia and changes in regional body composition in human immunodeficiency virus-infected women. J. Clin. Endocrinol. Metab. 84:1932–1937.

54. Hall, C. S., C. P. Raines, S. H. Barnett, R. D. Moore, and J. E. Gallant. 1999. Efficacy of salvage therapy containing ritonavir and saquinavir after failure of single protease inhibitor-containing regimens. AIDS 13:1207–1212.

55. Hammer, S. M., K. E. Squires, M. D. Hughes, J. M. Grimes, L. M. Demeter, J. S. Currier, J. J. Eron, J. E. Feinberg, H. H. Balfour, L. R. Dayton, J. A. Chodakewitz, J. P. Phair, W. Spreen, L. Pedneault, B.-Y. Nguyen, J. C. Cook, and M. A. Fischl. 1997. A controlled trial of 2 nucleoside analogs plus indinavir in persons with human immunodeficiency virus infection and CD4 cell counts of 200 per cubic millimeter or less. N. Engl. J. Med. 337:725–733.

56. Harrigan, P. R., K. Hertogs, W. Verbiest, R. Pauwels, B. Larder, S. Kemp, S. Bloor, B. Yip, R. Hogg, C. Alexander, and J. S. G. Montaner. 1999. Baseline HIV drug resistance profile predicts response to ritonavir-saquinavir protease inhibitor therapy in a community setting. AIDS 13:1863–1871.

57. Haubrich, R., M. Thompson, R. Schooley, W. Lang, A. Stein, D. Sereni, M. E. van der Ende, F. Antunes, D. Richman, G. Pagano, L. Kahl, A. Fetter, D. J. Brown, and N. Clumeck. 1999. A phase II safety and efficacy study of amprenavir in combination with zidovudine and lamivudine in HIV-infected patients with limited antiretroviral experience. AIDS 13:2411–2420.

58. Hertogs, K., S. Bloor, S. Kemp, C. Van den Eynde, T. M. Alcorn, R. Pauwels, M. Van Houtte, S. Staszewski, V. Miller, and B. A. Larder. 2000. Phenotypic and genotypic analysis of clinical HIV-1 isolates reveals extensive protease inhibitor cross-resistance: a survey of over 6000 samples. AIDS 14:1203–1210.

59. Ho, D. D., T. Toyoshima, H. M. Mo, D. J. Kempf, D. Norbeck, C. M. Chen, N. E. Wideburg, S. K. Burt, J. W. Erickson, and M. K. Singh. 1994. Characterization of human immunodeficiency virus type-1 variants with increased resistance to a c2-symmetrical protease inhibitor. J. Virol. 68:2016–2020.

60. Hsu, A., G. R. Granneman, and R. J. Bertz. 1998. Ritonavir: clinical pharmacokinetics and interactions with other anti-HIV agents. Clin. Pharmacokinetics 35:275–291.

61. Hsu, A., G. R. Granneman, G. L. Cao, L. Carothers, A. Japour, T. El-Shourbagy, S. Dennis, J. Berg, K. Erdman, J. M. Leonard, and E. G. Sun. 1998. Pharmacokinetic interaction between ritonavir and indinavir in healthy volunteers. Antimicrob. Agents Chemother. 42:2784–2791.

62. Inaba, T., N. E. Fischer, D. S. Riddick, D. J. Stewart, and T. Hidaka. 1997. HIV protease inhibitors, saquinavir, indinavir and ritonavir: inhibition of CYP3A4-mediated metabolism of testosterone and benzoxazinorifamycin, KRM-1648, in human liver microsomes. Toxicol. Lett. 93:215–219.

63. Jacobsen, H., M. Hanggi, M. Ott, I. B. Duncan, S. Owen, M. Andreoni, S. Vella, and J. Mous. 1996. In vivo resistance to a human immunodeficiency virus type 1 proteinase inhibitor: mutations, kinetics, and frequencies. J. Infect. Dis. 173:1379–1387.

64. Jacobsen, H., K. Yasargil, D. L. Winslow, J. C. Craig, A. Krohn, I. B. Duncan, and J. Mous. 1995. Characterization of human immunodeficiency virus type 1 mutants with decreased sensitivity to proteinase inhibitor Ro 31-8959. Virology 206:527–534.

65. Johnson, M., M. Nelson, B. Peters, B. Clotet, A. Petersen, and Y. Chang. 1998. A comparison of bid and tid dosing of nelfinavir when given in combination with stavudine (d4T) and lamivudine (3TC) for up to 48 weeks. 38th Meeting of the Interscience Conference on Antimicrobial Agents and Chemotherapy, September 24–28, 1999, San Diego, abstr. and poster I-216.

66. Kaldor, S. W., V. J. Kalish, J. F. Davies, B. V. Shetty, J. E. Fritz, K. Appelt, J. A. Burgess, K. M. Campanale, N. Y. Chirgadze, D. K. Clawson, B. A. Dressman, S. D. Hatch, D. A. Khalil, M. B. Kosa, P. P. Lubbehusen, M. A. Muesing, A. K. Patick, S. H. Reich, K. S. Su, and J. H. Tatlock. 1997. Viracept (nelfinavir mesylate, AG1343)—a potent, orally bioavailable inhibitor of HIV-1 protease. J. Med. Chem. 40:3979–3985.

67. Kalish, V. J., J. H. Tatlock, J. F. Davies, S. W. Kaldor, B. A. Dressman, S. Reich, M. Pino, D. Nyugen, K. Appelt, L. Musick, and B. W. Wu. 1995. Structure-based drug design of nonpeptidic p-2 substituents for HIV-1 protease inhibitors. Bioorganic Med. Chem. Lett. 5:727–732.

68. Katzenstein, T. L., L. Kirk, C. Pedersen, J. D. Lundgren, H. Nielsen, N. Obel, C. Nielsen, L. R. Mathiesen, and J. Gerstoft. 2000. The Danish protease inhibitor study: a randomized study comparing the virological efficacy of 3 protease inhibitor-containing regimens for the treatment of human immunodeficiency virus type 1 infection. J. Infect. Dis. 182:744–750.

69. Kaufmann, G. R., C. Duncombe, P. Cunningham, A. Beveridge, A. Carr, D. Sayer, M. French, and D. A. Cooper. 1998. Treatment response and durability of a double protease inhibitor therapy with saquinavir and ritonavir in an observational cohort of HIV-1-infected individuals. AIDS 12:1625–1630.

70. Kemp, S. D., M. Salim, N. Field, P. Dehertogh, K. Hertogs, H. Azijn, M.-P. de Bethune, and B. Larder. 2000. Site-directed mutagenesis and in vitro drug selection studies have failed to reveal a consistent genotypic resistance pattern for tipranavir. Antiviral Therapy 5(Suppl. 3):31, abstr. 40.

71. Kempf, D., S. Brun, R. Rode, J. Isaacson, M. King, Y. Xu, K. Real, A. Hsu, R. Granneman, Y. Lie, N. Hellmann, B. Bernstein, and E. Sun. 2000. Identification of clinically relevant phenotypic and genotypic breakpoints for ABT-378/r in multiple PI-experienced, NNRTI-naive patients. Antiviral Therapy 5:70, abstr. 89.

72. Kempf, D., J. Isaacson, M. King, S. Brun, Y. Xu, K. Real, Y. Lie, N. Hellmann, K. Hertogs, B. Larder, B. Bernstein, A. Japour, E. Sun, and R. Rode. 2000. Genotypic correlates of reduced in vitro susceptibility to ABT-378 in HIV isolates from patients failing protease inhibitor therapy. Antiviral Therapy 5:29–30, abstr. 38.

73. Kempf, D. J., K. C. Marsh, J. F. Denissen, E. McDonald, S. Vasavanonda, C. A. Flentge, B. E. Green, L. Fino, C. H. Park, X. P. Kong, N. E. Wideburg, A. Sal-

divar, L. Ruiz, W. M. Kati, H. L. Sham, T. Robins, K. D. Stewart, A. Hsu, J. J. Plattner, J. M. Leonard, and D. W. Norbeck. 1995. ABT-538 is a potent inhibitor of human-immunodeficiency-virus protease and has high oral bioavailability in humans. Proc. Natl. Acad. Sci. USA 92:2484–2488.

74. Kempf, D. J., K. C. Marsh, D. A. Paul, M. F. Knigge, D. W. Norbeck, W. E. Kohlbrenner, L. Codacovi, S. Vasavanonda, P. Bryant, X. C. Wang, N. E. Wideburg, J. J. Clement, J. J. Plattner, and J. Erickson. 1991. Antiviral and pharmacokinetic properties of c2 symmetrical inhibitors of the human-immunodeficiency-virus type-1 protease. Antimicrob. Agents Chemother. 35:2209–2214.

75. Kempf, D. J., D. W. Norbeck, K. C. Marsh, and J. Erickson. 1993. Design and development of symmetry-based inhibitors of HIV protease. Abstracts of Papers of the American Chemical Society 206:119.

76. Kempf, D. J., R. A. Rode, Y. Xu, E. Sun, M. E. Heath-Chiozzi, J. Valdes, A. J. Japour, S. Danner, C. Boucher, A. Molla, and J. M. Leonard. 1998. The duration of viral suppression during protease inhibitor therapy for HIV-1 infection is predicted by plasma HIV-1 RNA at the nadir. AIDS 12:F9–14.

77. Kim, E. E., C. T. Baker, M. D. Dwyer, M. A. Murcko, B. G. Rao, R. D. Tung, and M. A. Navia. 1995. Crystal structure of HIV-1 protease in complex with VX-478, a potent and orally bioavailable inhibitor of the enzyme. J. Am. Chem. Soc. 117:1181–1182.

78. Kim, R. B., M. F. Fromm, C. Wandel, B. Leake, A. J. J. Wood, D. M. Roden, and G. R. Wilkinson. 1998. The drug transporter P-glycoprotein limits oral absorption and brain entry of HIV-1 protease inhibitors. J. Clin. Invest. 101:289–294.

79. Kitchen, V. S., C. Skinner, K. Ariyoshi, E. A. Lane, I. B. Duncan, J. Burckhardt, H. U. Burger, K. Bragman, A. J. Pinching, and J. N. Weber. 1995. Safety and activity of saquinavir in HIV-infection. Lancet 345:952–955.

80. Kohl, N. E., E. A. Emini, W. A. Schleif, L. J. Davis, J. C. Heimbach, R. Dixon, E. M. Scolnick, and I. S. Sigal. 1988. Active human immunodeficiency virus protease is required for viral infectivity. Proc. Natl. Acad. Sci. USA 85:4686–4690.

81. Kozal, M. J., N. Shah, N. P. Shen, R. Yang, R. Fucini, T. C. Merigan, D. D. Richman, D. Morris, E. R. Hubbell, M. Chee, and T. R. Gingeras. 1996. Extensive polymorphisms observed in HIV-1 clade-b protease gene using high-density oligonucleotide arrays. Nature Med. 2:753–759.

82. Kumar, G. N., A. D. Rodrigues, A. M. Buko, and J. F. Denissen. 1996. Cytochrome p450-mediated metabolism of the HIV-1 protease inhibitor ritonavir (ABT-538) in human liver-microsomes. J. Pharmacol. Exp. Therapeut. 277:423–431.

83. Lalezari, J., R. Haubrich, H. U. Burger, D. Beattie, L. Donatacci, M. P. Salgo, and the NVI4256 Study Team. 1996. Improved survival and decreased progression of HIV in patients treated with saquinavir (Invirase, SQV) plus HIVID (zalcitabine, ddC). Abstracts of XI International Conference on AIDS, Vancouver, B.C., no. LB.B.6033.

84. Lawrence, J., J. Schapiro, M. Winters, J. Montoya, A. Zolopa, R. Pesano, B. Efron, D. Winslow, and T. C. Merigan. 1999. Clinical resistance patterns and

responses to two sequential protease inhibitor regimens in saquinavir and reverse transcriptase inhibitor-experienced persons. J. Infect. Dis. 179:1356–1364.

85. Lech, W. J., G. Wang, Y. L. Yang, Y. Chee, K. Dorman, D. Mccrae, L. C. Lazzeroni, J. W. Erickson, J. S. Sinsheimer, and A. H. Kaplan. 1996. In-vivo sequence diversity of the protease of human immunodeficiency virus type-1—presence of protease inhibitor-resistant variants in untreated subjects. J. Virol. 70:2038–2043.

86. Lee, C. G., M. M. Gottesman, C. O. Cardarelli, M. Ramachandra, K. T. Jeang, S. V. Ambudkar, I. Pastan, and S. Dey. 1998. HIV-1 protease inhibitors are substrates for the MDR1 multidrug transporter. Biochemistry 37:3594–3601.

87. Lewi, D. S., J. M. Suleiman, D. E. Uip, R. J. Pedro, R. A. Souza, G. S. Suleiman, C. Accetturi, O. M. Leite, W. B. Abreu, A. O. Kalichman, J. P. Moraes-Filho, E. F. Motti, M. L. Pecoraro, M. R. Makurath, M. L. Nessly, and R. Y. Leavitt, for the Protocol 028 Study Group. 2000. Randomized, double-blind trial comparing indinavir alone, zidovudine alone and indinavir plus zidovudine in antiretroviral therapy-naive HIV-infected individuals with CD4 cell counts between 50 and 250/mm^3. Rev. Inst. Med. Trop. Sao Paulo 42:27–36.

88. Lorenzi, P., S. Yerly, K. Abderrakim, M. Fathi, O. T. Rutschmann, J. Vonoverbeck, D. Leduc, L. Perrin, B. Hirschel, M. Battegay, P. Burgisser, R. Doorly, M. Egger, P. Erb, W. Fierz, M. Flepp, P. Francioli, P. Grob, U. Gruninger, B. Ledergerber, R. Luthy, R. Malinverni, L. Matter, M. Opravil, F. Paccaud, W. Pichler, M. Rickenbach, O. Rutschmann, and P. Vernazza. 1997. Toxicity, efficacy, plasma drug concentrations and protease mutations in patients with advanced HIV-infection treated with ritonavir plus saquinavir. AIDS 11:99.

89. Mammano, F., V. Troupin, V. Zennou, and F. Clavel. 2000. Retracing the evolutionary pathways of human immunodeficiency virus type 1 resistance to protease inhibitors: virus fitness in the absence and in the presence of drug. J. Virol. 74:8524–8531.

90. Markland, W., L. Zuchowski, J. Black, B. G. Rao, J. D. Parsons, S. Pazhanisamy, J. Fulghum, J. P. Griffith, M. Tisdale, and R. Tung. 1998. Kinetic and structural analysis of HIV-1 protease mutations: amprenavir resistance, cross-resistance, and resensitization. Abstracts of the Second International Workshop on HIV Drug Resistance and Treatment Strategies, June 24–27, 1998, Lake Maggiore, Italy, no. 24.

91. Markowitz, M., M. Conant, A. Hurley, R. Schluger, M. Duran, J. Peterkin, S. Chapman, A. Patick, A. Hendricks, G. J. Yuen, W. Hoskins, N. Clendeninn, and D. D. Ho. 1998. A preliminary evaluation of nelfinavir mesylate, an inhibitor of human immunodeficiency virus (HIV)-1 protease, to treat HIV infection. J. Infect. Dis. 177:1533–1540.

92. Markowitz, M., H. M. Mo, D. J. Kempf, D. W. Norbeck, T. N. Bhat, J. W. Erickson, and D. D. Ho. 1995. Selection and analysis of human-immunodeficiency-virus type-I variants with increased resistance to ABT-538, a novel protease inhibitor. J. Virol. 69:701–706.

93. Markowitz, M., M. Saag, W. G. Powderly, A. M. Hurley, A. Hsu, J. M. Valdes, D. Henry, F. Sattler, A. Lamarca, J. M. Leonard, and D. D. Ho. 1995. A preliminary study of ritonavir, an inhibitor of HIV-1 protease, to treat HIV-1 infection. N. Engl. J. Med. 333:1534–1539.

94. Martinez-Picado, J., L. V. Savara, L. Sutton, and R. T. D'Aquila. 1999. Replicative fitness of protease inhibitor-resistant mutants of human immunodeficiency virus type 1. J. Virol. 73:3744–3752.

95. Maschera, B., M. Tisdale, G. Darby, R. Mayers, G. Pal, and E. D. Blair. 1996. In vitro growth characteristics of HIV-1 variants with reduced sensitivity to saquinavir explain the appearance of L90M escape mutants in vivo. Antiviral Therapy 1(Suppl. 1):53.

96. Mathez, D., P. Bagnarelli, I. Gorin, C. Katlama, G. Pialoux, G. Saimot, P. Tubiana, P. DeTruchis, J. P. Chauin, R. Mills, R. Rode, M. Clementi, and J. Leibowitch. 1997. Reductions in viral load and increases in T lymphocyte numbers in treatment-naive patients with advanced HIV-1 infection treated with ritonavir, zidovudine and zalcitabine triple therapy. Antiviral Therapy 2:175–183.

97. Mellors, J., R. Steigbigel, R. Gulick, I. Frank, P. Berry, D. McMahon, J. Fuhrer, C. Farthing, C. Hildebrand, W. Schleif, J. Condra, M. Nessly, G. Calandra, E. Emini, and J. Chodakewitz. 1995. A randomized, double-blind study of the oral HIV protease inhibitor, L-735,524 vs. Zidovudine (ZDV) in p24 antigenemic, HIV-1 infected patients with <500 CD4 cells/mm^3. 2nd National Conference on Human Retroviruses and Related Infections, abstr. 183.

98. Mellors, J. W., D. K. McMahon, J. A. Chodakewitz, W. A. Schleif, E. A. Emini, and J. H. Condra. 1995. Correlation between genotypic evidence of HIV-1 resistance to the protease inhibitor MK-639 and loss of antiretroviral effect in treated patients. J. Acquired Immune Defic. Syndr. Hum. Retrovirol. 10:71.

99. Mellors, J. W., C. R. Rinaldo, Jr., P. Gupta, R. M. White, J. A. Todd, and L. A. Kingsley. 1996. Prognosis in HIV-1 infection predicted by the quantity of virus in plasma. Science 272:1167–1170.

100. Mitsuyasu, R. T., P. R. Skolnik, S. R. Cohen, B. Conway, M. J. Gill, P. C. Jensen, J. J. Pulvirenti, L. N. Slater, R. T. Schooley, M. A. Thompson, R. A. Torres, and C. M. Tsoukas. 1998. Activity of the soft gelatin formulation of saquinavir in combination therapy in antiretroviral-naive patients. NV15355 Study Team. AIDS 12:F103–109.

101. Molla, A., S. Brun, H. Mo., K. Real, J. Poddig, B. Bernstein, K. Hertogs, B. Larder, Y. Lie, N. Hellmann, S. Vasavononda, T. Chernyavskiy, W. Freimuth, A. Japour, E. Sun, and D. Kempf. 2000. Genotypic and phenotypic analysis of viral isolates from subjects with detectable viral load on therapy with ABT-378/ritonavir (ABT-378/r). Antiviral Therapy 5:30, abstr. 39.

102. Molla, A., M. Korneyeva, Q. Gao, S. Vasavanonda, P. J. Schipper, H. M. Mo, M. Markowitz, T. Chernyavskiy, P. Niu, N. Lyons, A. Hsu, G. R. Granneman, D. D. Ho, C. Boucher, J. M. Leonard, D. W. Norbeck, and D. J. Kempf. 1996. Ordered accumulation of mutations in HIV protease confers resistance to ritonavir. Nature Med. 2:760–766.

103. Molla, A., S. Vasavanonda, G. Kumar, H. L. Sham, M. Johnson, B. Grabowski, J. F. Denissen, W. Kohlbrenner, J. J. Plattner, J. M. Leonard, D. W. Norbeck, and D. J. Kempf. 1998. Human serum attenuates the activity of protease inhibitors toward wild-type and mutant human immunodeficiency virus. Virology 250:255–262.

104. Mouton, Y., S. Alfandari, M. Valette, F. Cartier, P. Dellamonica, G. Humbert, J. M. Lang, P. Massip, D. Mechali, P. Leclercq, J. Modai, and H. Portier. 1997. Impact of protease inhibitors on AIDS-defining events and hospitalizations in 10 French AIDS reference centers. AIDS 11:105.

105. Murphy, R. L., R. M. Gulick, V. DeGruttola, R. T. D'Aquila, J. J. Eron, J. P. Sommadossi, J. S. Currier, L. Smeaton, I. Frank, A. M. Caliendo, J. G. Gerber, R. Tung, and D. R. Kuritzkes. 1999. Treatment with amprenavir alone or amprenavir with zidovudine and lamivudine in adults with human immunodeficiency virus infection. J. Infect. Dis. 179:808–816.

106. Myers, G., S. Wain-Hobson, L. E. Henderson, B. Korber, K.-T. Jeang, and G. N. Pavlakis. 1993. Human retroviruses and AIDS 1993. Los Alamos National Laboratory, Los Alamos, N.Mex.

107. O'Brien, W. A., P. M. Hartigan, D. Martin, J. Esinhart, A. Hill, S. Benoit, M. Rubin, M. S. Simberkoff, J. D. Hamilton, and the Veterans Affairs Cooperative Study Group on AIDS. 1996. Changes in plasma HIV-1 RNA and CD4$^+$ lymphocyte counts and the risk of progression to AIDS. N. Engl. J. Med. 334:426–431.

108. Para, M. F., A. Collier, R. Coombs, D. Glidden, R. Bassett, F. Duff, R. Y. Leavitt, C. Pettineilli, for the ACTG 333 Study Team. 1997. ACTG 333: antiviral effects of switching from saquinavir hard capsule (SQVhgc) to saquinavir soft gelatin capsule (SQVsgc) vs. switching to indinavir (IDV) after prior saquinavir. Infectious Disease Society of America 35th Annual Meeting, September 13–16, 1997, San Francisco, abstr. 21.

109. Para, M. F., D. V. Glidden, R. W. Coombs, A. C. Collier, J. H. Condra, C. Craig, R. Bassett, R. Leavitt, S. Snyder, V. McAuliffe, C. Boucher, for the AIDS Clinical Trials Protocol 333 Team. 2000. Baseline human immunodeficiency virus type 1 phenotype, genotype, and RNA response after switching from long-term hard-capsule saquinavir to indinavir or soft-gel-capsule saquinavir in AIDS Clinical Trials Group Protocol 333. J. Infect. Dis. 182:733–743.

110. Paredes, R., T. Puig, A. Arno, E. Negredo, M. Balague, A. Bonjoch, A. Jou, A. Tuldra, C. Tural, G. Sirera, A. Veny, J. Romeu, L. Ruiz, and B. Clotet. 1999. High-dose saquinavir plus ritonavir: long-term efficacy in HIV-positive protease inhibitor-experienced patients and predictors of virologic response. J. Acquired Immune Defic. Syndr. 22:132–138.

111. Partaledis, J. A., K. Yamaguchi, M. Tisdale, E. E. Blair, C. Falcione, B. Maschera, R. E. Myers, S. Pazhanisamy, O. Futer, A. B. Cullinan, C. M. Stuver, R. A. Byrn, and D. J. Livingston. 1995. In-vitro selection and characterization of human-immunodeficiency-virus type-1 (HIV-1) isolates with reduced sensitivity to hydroxyethylamino sulfonamide inhibitors of HIV-1 aspartyl protease. J. Virol. 69:5228–5235.

112. Patick, A. K., M. Duran, Y. Cao, T. Ho, Z. Pei, M. R. Keller, J. Peterkin, S. Chapman, B. Anderson, D. Ho, and M. Markowitz. 1996. Genotypic and phenotypic characterization of HIV-1 variants isolated from in vitro selection studies and from patients treated with the protease inhibitor, nelfinavir. Antiviral Therapy 1(Suppl. 1):17–18.

113. Patick, A. K., M. Duran, Y. Cao, T. Ho, P. Zhou, M. R. Keller, S. Chapman, R. Anderson, D. Kuritzkes, D. Shugarts, D. Ho, and M. Markowitz. 1997. Geno-

typic analysis of HIV-1 variants isolated from patients treated with the protease inhibitor nelfinavir, alone or in combination with d4T or AZT and 3TC. Abstracts of the Fourth Conference on Retroviruses and Opportunistic Infections, January 22–26, 1997, Washington, D.C., no. 10.

114. Patick, A. K., M. Duran, Y. Cao, D. Shugarts, M. R. Keller, E. Mazabel, M. Knowles, S. Chapman, D. R. Kuritzkes, and M. Markowitz. 1998. Genotypic and phenotypic characterization of human immunodeficiency virus type 1 variants isolated from patients treated with the protease inhibitor nelfinavir. Antimicrob. Agents Chemother. 42:2637–2644.

115. Patick, A. K., R. L. Jackson, Y. Chang, J. Mota, A. Marchese, J. A. Isaacson, and T. Nash-Alexander. 2000. Evaluation of D30N and L90M resistance profiles in patients treated with nelfinavir alone or in combination therapy. Antiviral Therapy 5(Suppl. 3):35, abstr. 46.

116. Patick, A. K., M. Markowitz, K. Appelt, B. Wu, L. Musick, V. Kalish, S. Kaldor, S. Reich, D. Ho, and S. Webber. 1996. Antiviral and resistance studies of AG1343, an orally bioavailable inhibitor of human immunodeficiency virus protease. Antimicrob. Agents Chemother. 40:292–297.

117. Patick, A. K., H. Mo, M. Markowitz, K. Appelt, B. Wu, L. Musick, V. Kalish, S. Kaldor, S. Reich, D. Ho, and S. Webber. 1996. Antiviral and resistance studies of AG1343, an orally bioavailable inhibitor of human-immunodeficiency-virus protease. Antimicrob. Agents Chemother. 40:1575.

118. Peng, C., B. K. Ho, T. W. Chang, and N. T. Chang. 1989. Role of human immunodeficiency virus type 1-specific protease in core protein maturation and viral infectivity. J. Virol. 63:2550–2556.

119. Petropoulos, C. J., N. T. Parkin, K. L. Limoli, Y. S. Lie, T. Wrin, W. Huang, H. Tian, D. Smith, G. A. Winslow, D. J. Capon, and J. M. Whitcomb. 2000. A novel phenotypic drug susceptibility assay for human immunodeficiency virus type 1. Antimicrob. Agents Chemother. 44:920–928.

120. Piketty, C., E. Race, P. Castiel, L. Belec, G. Peytavin, A. Si Mohamed, G. Gonzalez Canali, L. Weiss, F. Clavel, and M. D. Kazatchkine. 1999. Efficacy of a five-drug combination including ritonavir, saquinavir and efavirenz in patients who failed on a conventional triple-drug regimen: phenotypic resistance to protease inhibitors predicts outcome of therapy. AIDS 13:F71–77.

121. Piketty, C., E. Race, P. Castiel, L. Belec, G. Peytavin, A. Si Mohamed, G. Gonzalez Canali, L. Weiss, F. Clavel, and M. D. Kazatchkine. 2000. Phenotypic resistance to protease inhibitors in patients who fail on highly active antiretroviral therapy predicts the outcome at 48 weeks of a five-drug combination including ritonavir, saquinavir and efavirenz. AIDS 14:626–628.

122. Piscitelli, S., C. Bechtel, B. Sadler, and J. Falloon. 2000. The addition of a second protease inhibitor eliminates amprenavir-efavirenz drug interactions and increases plasma amprenavir concentrations. Abstracts of the Seventh Conference on Retroviruses and Opportunistic Infections, January 30–February 2, 2000, San Francisco, no. 78.

123. Poppe, S. M., D. E. Slade, K. T. Chong, R. R. Hinshaw, P. J. Pagano, M. Markowitz, D. D. Ho, H. Mo, R. R. Gorman, T. J. Dueweke, S. Thaisrivongs, and W. G. Tarpley. 1997. Antiviral activity of the dihydropyrone PNU-140690, a new nonpeptidic human-immunodeficiency-virus protease inhibitor. Antimicrob. Agents Chemother. 41:1058–1063.

124. Race, E., J. G. Sheldon, S. Kaye, S. M. Gilbert, A. R. Moffatt, and I. B. Duncan. 1997. Mutations associated with reduced sensitivity to saquinavir occur in a minority of patients treated in combination with ddC: results from a phase III clinical trial (NV14256). Abstracts of the Fourth Conference on Retroviruses and Opportunistic Infections, January 22–26, 1997, Washington, D.C., poster 600.

125. Rachlis, A. R., R. H. Palmer, M. Bast, G. Robinson, K. Logue, and A. Klein. 1997. Predictors of decreases in plasma HIV-1 RNA in patients treated with indinavir. Abstracts of 37th Interscience Conference on Antimicrobial Agents and Chemotherapy, Toronto, Ontario, no. A-17.

126. Roberts, N. A., J. A. Martin, D. Kinchington, A. V. Broadhurst, J. C. Craig, I. B. Duncan, S. A. Galpin, B. K. Handa, J. Kay, A. Krohn, R. W. Lambert, J. Merrett, J. S. Mills, K. E. B. Parkes, S. Redshaw, A. J. Ritchie, D. L. Taylor, G. J. Thomas, and P. J. Machin. 1990. Rational design of peptide-based HIV proteinase inhibitors. Science 248:358–361.

127. Robinson, B. S., K. A. Riccardi, Y. F. Gong, Q. Guo, D. A. Stock, W. S. Blair, B. J. Terry, C. A. Deminie, F. Djang, R. J. Colonno, and P. F. Lin. 2000. BMS-232632, a highly potent human immunodeficiency virus protease inhibitor that can be used in combination with other available antiretroviral agents. Antimicrob. Agents Chemother. 44:2093–2099.

128. Rockstroh, J. K., F. Bergmann, W. Wiesel, A. Rieke, A. Theisen, G. Fatkenheuer, M. Oette, H. Carls, S. Fenske, M. Nadler, and H. Knechten. 2000. Efficacy and safety of twice daily first-line ritonavir/indinavir plus double nucleoside combination therapy in HIV-infected individuals. AIDS 14:1181–1185.

129. Rusconi, S., S. L. A. Catamancio, P. Citterio, S. Kurtagic, M. Violin, C. Balotta, M. Moroni, M. Galli, and A. D'Arminio-Monforte. 2000. Susceptibility to PNU-140690 (Tipranavir) of human immunodeficiency virus type 1 isolates derived from patients with multidrug resistance to other protease inhibitors. Antimicrob. Agents Chemother. 44:1328–1332.

130. Saah, A., G. Winchell, M. Seniuk, D. Mehrota, and P. Deutsch. 1999. Multiple-dose pharmacokinetics (PK) and tolerability of indinavir (IDV) and ritonavir (RTV) combinations in healthy volunteers. Abstracts of the Sixth Conference on Retroviruses and Opportunistic Infections, January 31–February 4, 1999, Chicago, abstr. and poster 362.

131. Saah, A. J., D. W. Haas, R. Rhodes, M. Nessly, J. H. Condra, and D. Holder. 2000. Virologic response to indinavir (IDV), efavirenz (EFV) and adefovir (ADV) among patients failing nelfinavir (NFV). XIII International AIDS Conference, Durban, South Africa, abstr. WePeB4169.

132. Safrin, S., and C. Grunfeld. 1999. Fat distribution and metabolic changes in patients with HIV infection. AIDS 13:2493–2505.

133. Schapiro, J. M., M. A. Winters, J. Lawrence, and T. C. Merigan. 1999. Clinical cross-resistance between the HIV-1 protease inhibitors saquinavir and indinavir and correlations with genotypic mutations. AIDS 13:359–365.

134. Schapiro, J. M., M. A. Winters, F. Stewart, B. Efron, J. Norris, M. J. Kozal, and T. C. Merigan. 1996. The effect of high-dose saquinavir on viral load and CD4(+)T-cell counts in HIV-infected patients. Ann. Intern. Med. 124:1039–1050.

135. Schmit, J. C., L. Ruiz, B. Clotet, A. Raventos, J. Tor, J. Leonard, J. Desmyter, E. Declercq, and A. M. Vandamme. 1996. Resistance-related mutations in the HIV-1 protease gene of patients treated for 1 year with the protease inhibitor ritonavir (ABT-538). AIDS 10:995–999.

136. Schock, H. B., V. M. Garsky, and L. C. Kuo. 1996. Mutational anatomy of an HIV-1 protease variant conferring cross-resistance to protease inhibitors in clinical trials—compensatory modulations of binding and activity. J. Biol. Chem. 271:31957–31963.

137. Sham, H. L., D. J. Kempf, A. Molla, K. C. Marsh, G. N. Kumar, C. M. Chen, W. Kati, K. Stewart, R. Lal, A. Hsu, D. Betebenner, M. Korneyeva, S. Vasa-vanonda, E. McDonald, A. Saldivar, N. Wideburg, X. Chen, P. Niu, C. Park, V. Jayanti, B. Grabowski, G. R. Granneman, E. Sun, A. J. Japour, J. M. Leonard, J. J. Plattner, and D. W. Norbeck. 1998. ABT-378, a highly potent inhibitor of the human immunodeficiency virus protease. Antimicrob. Agents Chemother. 42:3218–3224.

138. Smith, T., and R. Swanstrom. 1996. Selection for high-level resistance to HIV-1 protease inhibitors used in pairs. Antiviral Therapy 1(Suppl. 1):12–13.

139. Smith, T., and R. Swanstrom. 1997. Biological cross-resistance to HIV-1 protease inhibitors. Abstracts of the International Workshop on HIV Drug Resistance, Treatment Strategies and Eradication, St. Petersburg, Fla., no. 15.

140. Swanstrom, R., and J. Eron. 2000. Human immunodeficiency virus type-1 protease inhibitors: therapeutic successes and failures, suppression and resistance. Pharmacology and Therapeutics 86:145–170.

141. Tebas, P., A. K. Patick, E. Kane, M. Klebert, J. Simpson, B. Atkinson, J. Isaac-son, W. G. Powderly, and K. Henry. 1999. 60-week virologic responses to a ritonavir/saquinavir containing regimen in patients who had previously failed nelfinavir. Abstracts of the Sixth Conference on Retroviruses and Opportunistic Infections, Chicago, no. 392.

142. Tebas, P., A. K. Patick, E. M. Kane, M. K. Klebert, J. H. Simpson, A. Erice, W. G. Powderly, and K. Henry. 1999. Virologic responses to a ritonavir–saquinavir-containing regimen in patients who had previously failed nelfinavir. AIDS 13:F23–28.

143. Thaisrivongs, S., and J. W. Strohbach. 1999. Structure-based discovery of tipranavir disodium (PNU-140690E): a potent, orally bioavailable, nonpeptidic HIV protease inhibitor. Biopolymers 51:51–58.

144. Tisdale, M., R. E. Myers, B. Maschera, N. R. Parry, N. M. Oliver, and E. D. Blair. 1995. Cross-resistance analysis of human immunodeficiency virus type-1 variants individually selected for resistance to 5 different protease inhibitors. Antimicrob. Agents Chemother. 39:1704–1710.

145. Tisdale, M., R. E. Myers, and W. Snowdon. 1998. Genotypic and phenotypic analysis of HIV from patients on ZDV/3TC/amprenavir combination therapy. Abstracts of the 12th World AIDS Conference, June 28–July 3, 1998, Geneva, no. 32312.

146. Toh, H., R. Kikuno, H. Hayashida, T. Miyata, W. Kugimiya, S. Inouye, S. Yuki, and K. Saigo. 1985. Close structural resemblance between putative polymerase of a Drosophila transposable genetic element 17.6 and pol gene product of Moloney murine leukaemia virus. EMBO J. 4:1267–1272.

147. Turner, S. R., J. W. Strohbach, R. A. Tommasi, P. A. Aristoff, P. D. Johnson, H. I. Skulnick, L. A. Dolak, E. P. Seest, P. K. Tomich, M. J. Bohanan, M. M. Horng, J. C. Lynn, K. T. Chong, R. R. Hinshaw, K. D. Watenpaugh, M. N. Janakiraman, and S. Thaisrivongs. 1998. Tipranavir (PNU-140690): a potent, orally bioavailable nonpeptidic HIV protease inhibitor of the 5,6-dihydro-4-hydroxy-2-pyrone sulfonamide class. J. Med. Chem. 41:3467–3476.

148. Vacca, J. P., B. D. Dorsey, W. A. Schleif, R. B. Levin, S. L. McDaniel, P. L. Darke, J. Zugay, J. C. Quintero, O. M. Blahy, E. Roth, V. V. Sardana, A. J. Schlabach, P. I. Graham, J. H. Condra, L. Gotlib, M. K. Holloway, J. Lin, I. W. Chen, K. Vastag, D. Ostovic, P. S. Anderson, E. A. Emini, and J. R. Huff. 1994. L-735,524—an orally bioavailable human immunodeficiency virus type-1 protease inhibitor. Proc. Natl. Acad. Sci. USA 91:4096–4100.

149. Vaillancourt, M., D. Irlbeck, T. Smith, R. W. Coombs, and R. Swanstrom. 1999. The HIV type 1 protease inhibitor saquinavir can select for multiple mutations that confer increasing resistance. AIDS Res. Hum. Retroviruses 15:355–363.

150. Vaillancourt, M., D. Irlbeck, and R. Swanstrom. 1995. Sequence analysis of viral RNA from patients on AZT-saquinavir double therapy (ACTG 229). Abstracts of the Fourth International Workshop on HIV Drug Resistance, July 6–9, 1995, Sardinia, Italy, no. 74.

151. Wang, Y., C. Daenzer, R. Wood, D. Nickens, M. Borin, W. Freimuth, J. Morales, S. Green, M. Mucci, and W. Decian. 2000. The safety, efficacy and viral dynamics analysis of tipranavir, a new-generation protease inhibitor, in a phase II study in antiretroviral-naive HIV-1-infected patients. Abstracts of the Seventh Conference on Retroviruses and Opportunistic Infections, San Francisco, no. 673.

152. Wang, Y., W. W. Freimuth, C. L. Daenzer, M. T. Borin, C. M. Tutton, A. A. Piergies, R. M. Wurtz, H. I. Li, J. W. Davis, D. J. Crampton, and the PNU-140690 Team. 1998. Safety and efficacy of PNU-140690, a new non-peptidic HIV protease inhibitor, and HIV genotypic changes in patients in a phase II study. Abstracts of the Second International Workshop on HIV Drug Resistance and Treatment Strategies, June 24–27, 1998, Lake Maggiore, Italy, no. 5.

153. Winters, M. A., J. M. Schapiro, J. Lawrence, and T. C. Merigan. 1998. Human immunodeficiency virus type 1 protease genotypes and in vitro protease inhibitor susceptibilities of isolates from individuals who were switched to other protease inhibitors after long-term saquinavir treatment. J. Virol. 72:5303–5306.

154. Workman, C., R. Musson, W. Dyer, and J. Sullivan. 1998. Novel double protease combinations combining indinavir (IDV) with ritonavir (RTV): results from first study. Abstracts of the 12th World AIDS Conference, June 28–July 3, 1998, Geneva, no. 22372.

155. Zhang, X. Q., R. T. Schooley, and J. G. Gerber. 1999. The effect of increasing alpha(1)-acid glycoprotein concentration on the antiviral efficacy of human immunodeficiency virus protease inhibitors. J. Infect. Dis. 180:1833–1837.

156. Zhang, Y. M., H. Imamichi, T. Imamichi, H. C. Lane, J. Falloon, M. B. Vasudevachari, and N. P. Salzman. 1997. Drug-resistance during indinavir therapy is caused by mutations in the protease gene and in its gag substrate cleavage sites. J. Virol. 71:6662–6670.

157. Ziermann, R., K. Limoli, K. Das, E. Arnold, C. J. Petropoulos, and N. T. Parkin. 2000. A mutation in human immunodeficiency virus type 1 protease, N88S, that causes in vitro hypersensitivity to amprenavir. J. Virol. 74:4414–4419.

158. Zolopa, A., P. Keiser, P. Tebas, J. Gallant, M. Sension, P. Smith, J. Gathe, J. Flamm, T. Hawkins, J. Nadler, R. Shafer, and K. Henry. 2000. Predictors of response to ritonavir (RTV)/saquinavir (SQV) antiretroviral therapy (ART) in patients for whom nelfinavir (NFV) failed: a multi-center clinical cohort study. XIII International AIDS Conference, Durban, South Africa, abstr. WePeB4173.

159. Zolopa, A. R., R. W. Shafer, A. Warford, J. G. Montoya, P. Hsu, D. Katzenstein, T. C. Merigan, and B. Efron. 1999. HIV-1 genotypic resistance patterns predict response to saquinavir-ritonavir therapy in patients in whom previous protease inhibitor therapy had failed. Ann. Intern. Med. 131:813–821.

The Biology and Biochemistry of Integration as a Target for Chemotherapeutic Intervention

6

DARIA J. HAZUDA

The development of chemotherapeutic agents for the treatment of human immunodeficiency virus type 1 (HIV-1) infection has to date focused primarily on the retroviral enzymes, reverse transcriptase (RT) and protease (PR). Treatment regimens that include agents directed at each of these biochemical targets are effective in reducing viral load and morbidity and mortality; however, the chronic nature of the infection and the genetic plasticity inherent to HIV-1 have made it apparent that new antiretroviral agents are required to deal with the appearance and spread of resistant variants (reviewed in reference 96). Integrase (IN) is the third of the virally encoded enzymes and the only one for which clinical agents have not yet been developed. IN catalyzes the insertion of the HIV-1 DNA into the genome of the host cell. Integration is a hallmark of retroviruses and is required for stable maintenance of the viral genome as well as efficient viral gene expression. As integration is essential for HIV-1 replication, it is an attractive target for novel antiretroviral agents (13, 35, 40, 67, 102, 112). Although many IN inhibitors have been described (reviewed in references 92, 93), it is only recently that bona fide inhibitors of integration have been identified (60). These compounds exhibit a unique and validated antiviral mechanism providing new insights into IN as a molecular target for drug discovery and a deeper appreciation of the complexities of the integration process (41, 57, 60).

The Requirement for IN in HIV-1 Infection

Together with the viral RT and PR, IN is synthesized as a product of the HIV-1 Gag-Pol polypeptide (Fig. 6.1). Proteolytic processing by the HIV-1 PR is necessary for IN to manifest activity appropriately during the course of viral replication (117). IN is a 33-kDa protein with three structurally discrete

223

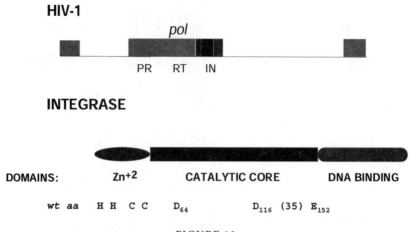

FIGURE 6.1

HIV-1 IN is synthesized as part of the HIV-1 Gag-Pol polypeptide

Processing by the HIV-1 PR generates the active 33-kDa IN protein. The three domains of IN are all required to express the complete enzymatic function of the protein. The HHCC motif in the N-terminal domain coordinates zinc. The catalytic core domain (amino acids 50–212) encompasses the highly conserved active-site residues Asp64, Asp116, and Glu152 (DD35E). The C-terminal domain is highly basic and will bind DNA nonspecifically.

domains: an N-terminal zinc binding domain (amino acids 1–50), a C-terminal DNA binding domain (amino acids 212–288), and the central catalytic core domain (amino acids 50–212) (Fig. 6.1) (reviewed in reference 113). In the core domain, three acidic residues, Asp64, Asp116, and Glu152, constitute the enzyme active site (30, 37, 65, 70). The DD35E motif is a conserved feature among all retroviral INs and retrotransposases and is involved in coordinating either Mg or Mn, the divalent cation cofactor required for catalysis (4, 28, 31, 61, 65, 81). Each of the residues in the DD35E motif is therefore essential for catalytic activity. The catalytic core domain, Zn binding domain, and C-terminal domain are all required to express the complete enzymatic function of IN in vitro and in infected cells (10, 16, 35, 36, 51, 106, 117). However, IN is active as a multimer, and proteins with inactivating mutations in a single domain can function when combined with proteins containing defects in a heterologous domain (35, 36, 51, 116). Although each of the three isolated domains is dimeric (12, 31, 32, 79), the intact enzyme will form higher-order multimers (2, 17, 18, 35, 36, 62, 64, 73, 90, 120); thus the exact nature of the active IN species has yet to be determined.

Together with the viral RT and PR, IN is packaged with the single-stranded viral RNA genome into HIV-1 virions. The incorporation of IN into virions is a prerequisite for establishing an integration-competent complex with the reverse transcribed viral DNA during the subsequent infection cycle. Although the incorporation of IN into viral particles is normally coincident with Gag-Pol assembly and processing, the process can be circumvented by using the HIV-1 Vpr protein to direct packaging of IN Vpr-fusion proteins into viral particles during virion assembly (51, 78, 116, 117). When incorporated into HIV-1 particles, IN Vpr-fusion proteins can complement defects in the endogenously expressed IN and restore infectivity to IN-deficient viruses (51, 116). Studies of IN complementation in *trans* using Vpr-fusion proteins have suggested a requirement for IN in HIV-1 replication in addition to integration (116). Mutations in the IN coding region have also been shown to affect multiple functions in the HIV-1 infection process, including virion morphology and reverse transcription and nuclear import of the viral DNA (8, 38, 68, 103, 112). Although a precise role for IN in any of these processes has not been defined, it appears to be separable from catalysis, as mutations that affect the latter functions can be distinct from those that affect integration. Remarkably, a variety of IN mutations that have no discernible effect in biochemical assays have a deleterious effect on HIV-1 replication when they are introduced into the virus.

In contrast to those mutations that have pleiotropic effects on HIV-1 replication, mutation of any of the three active-site residues, Asp64, Asp116, and Glu152, will diminish IN catalytic function and abrogate integration and viral replication without affecting virion structure, viral DNA synthesis, or nuclear import (40, 112). When integration is blocked, the viral DNA stalled in the nuclear compartment of the infected cell is a potential substrate for cellular recombination and repair enzymes, and within hours these cellular enzymes can convert the integration-competent linear HIV-1 genome into integration-incompetent circles (112). HIV-1 circles are not efficiently transcribed and, without an origin of replication, are not stably maintained in cells. The so-called 1 and 2 long terminal repeat (LTR) circles that result from these reactions are thus dead ends in the HIV-1 infection process. The presence of LTR circles can therefore be used as a signature of a recent HIV-1 infection event and as a hallmark for viral DNA blocked at a stage in the infection prior to the point of integration (99, 112).

The Integration Process in HIV-1 Infected Cells

IN is the only protein known to be required to catalyze each of the specific steps necessary for integration (9, 11, 33, 39, 100, 106). During HIV-1 infection, integration occurs as an ordered series of staged reactions that include (1) *assembly* of a stable complex with the viral DNA, (2) *3′ processing* of the viral DNA ends, (3) *strand transfer* or *joining* of the viral and cellular DNAs, and (4) *repair* (Fig. 6.2). Steps 1, 2, and 3 are accomplished by IN itself; step 4 may require cellular repair enzymes. IN assembles on specific sequences within the U3 and U5 region at each of the LTRs at either end of the HIV-1 genome (34, 61, 107, 115; reviewed in reference 53). The requirements for

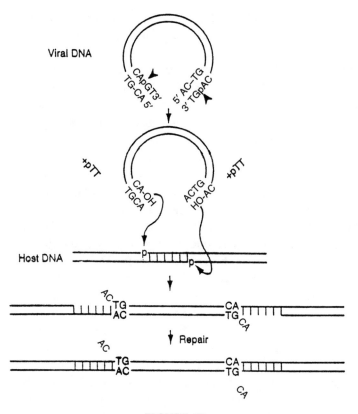

Viral DNA

Host DNA

Repair

FIGURE 6.2

Integration occurs as an ordered series of staged reactions

The series includes the following steps: Step 1, assembly. IN interacts with specific sequences in the LTR region at each end of the HIV-1 genome and forms a stable PIC. Step 2, 3′ processing. IN catalyzes the specific endonucleolytic removal of the terminal (GT) dinucleotide from each 3′ end of the viral DNA. Step 3, strand transfer. IN nicks the cellular or target DNA and joins the processed viral and cellular DNAs, resulting in insertion. Step 4, repair. The two-ended integration reaction generates a four- to six-base gap that is repaired, producing a small duplication of cellular DNA sequence at the site of the insertion event.

establishing a productive interaction between IN and the viral DNA are not entirely understood but involve recognition of a specific sequence (5′ XXCAGT 3′) as well as a unique structural component that in part appears to be defined by the conformation of the DNA end. The importance of sequence specificity in substrate recognition is evidenced by experiments demonstrating that mutation of any of the five residues at the 3′ terminus of the LTR will diminish both specific 3′ processing activity and strand transfer (20, 42, 66, 69, 104). Although IN will not utilize the HIV-1 LTR sequence when it is embedded into a region of DNA that is strictly double stranded, a nonterminal LTR sequence is recognized by IN in the context of a nicked DNA substrate in the process known as disintegration (see below and Fig. 6.3B) (20, 21, 52, 104). The ability to process appropriately disintegration substrates in which the HIV-1 LTR sequence is adjacent to a single-stranded nick suggests that a structural component inherent to partially denatured DNA may be a feature critical for specific substrate recognition by IN. This is consistent with the observation that LTR sequence oligonucleotides wherein the ends are disrupted by non-base-paired substitutions function more efficiently as substrates in 3' processing and strand transfer (98).

During HIV-1 replication, the specific interaction between IN and the viral DNA end results in the formation of a high molecular weight nucleoprotein complex known as the viral preintegration complex (PIC) (step 1, Fig. 6.2) (7, 33, 47, 48, 85, 111). Viral PICs are stable to biochemical isolation and can be prepared from infected cells in an integration-competent state. Stable complexes competent for catalysis can also be formed in vitro using synthetic oligonucleotides encoding HIV-1 LTR sequences and recombinantly expressed IN (34, 61, 107, 115). Analysis of complexes assembled on oligonucleotide substrates has shown that a precise interaction between IN and the terminal LTR DNA is a prerequisite for establishing a stable complex and defining the catalytically competent conformation of the enzyme. It is only in the context of this complex that IN will perform the specific catalytic reactions required for integration: 3' end processing and strand transfer.

In the first of these enzymatic reactions, 3' endonucleolytic processing, IN removes the dinucleotide from each of the 3' termini of the viral DNA (step 2, Fig. 6.2). The viral DNA ends in isolated HIV-1 PICs are fully processed, and it is therefore presumed that in the context of viral replication the 3' end processing reaction occurs coincident with or soon after assembly (85). The free 3' hydroxyls that are created as a consequence of the end processing reaction serve as nucleophiles in the subsequent strand transfer step, in which IN covalently links the viral DNA to the host cellular DNA (39, 105; reviewed in reference 6). In the strand transfer or joining reaction, IN nicks the cellular DNA once on each DNA strand, and the two 3' OH processed viral DNA ends are joined to the 5' phosphates of the nicked cellular DNA (step 3, Fig. 6.2). The nicking and joining activities of IN are concerted, and thus the strand transfer reaction is isoenergetic and ATP-independent.

In the infected cell, IN must insert each end of the viral DNA into the cellular genome without promoting large duplications or deletions deleterious to the host. Integration of the two ends of the HIV-1 DNA into each of the opposite strands of the host cell target DNA occurs within four to six base pairs. Repair of the gap that is generated subsequent to integration therefore results in four- to six-base-pair duplication of cellular DNA sequence at the site of insertion (step 4, Fig. 6.2) (108, 109; reviewed in refer-

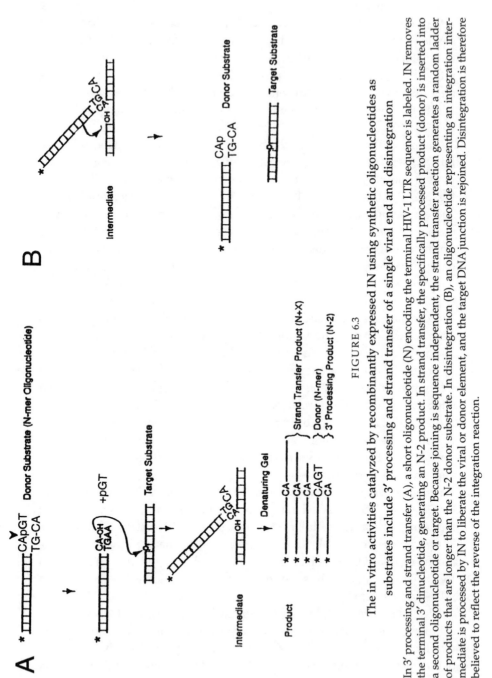

FIGURE 6.3

The in vitro activities catalyzed by recombinantly expressed IN using synthetic oligonucleotides as substrates include 3' processing and strand transfer of a single viral end and disintegration

In 3' processing and strand transfer (A), a short oligonucleotide (N) encoding the terminal HIV-1 LTR sequence is labeled. IN removes the terminal 3' dinucleotide, generating an N-2 product. In strand transfer, the specifically processed product (donor) is inserted into a second oligonucleotide or target. Because joining is sequence independent, the strand transfer reaction generates a random ladder of products that are longer than the N-2 donor substrate. In disintegration (B), an oligonucleotide representing an integration intermediate is processed by IN to liberate the viral or donor element, and the target DNA junction is rejoined. Disintegration is therefore believed to reflect the reverse of the integration reaction.

ences 22 and 53). Although the mechanism(s) responsible for the repair have yet to be elucidated, cellular enzymes such as the DNA-dependent protein kinase (DNA-PK) mediated DNA repair pathway are generally assumed to be involved in filling and sealing the gap as required to complete the integration process (25). It has also been suggested that gap repair may be facilitated by IN itself (1).

Although IN is the only protein known to be required to catalyze 3' processing and strand transfer, cellular proteins—for example, topoisomerase II and DNA-PK—may assist the integration process in vivo (5, 25). Viral or cellular proteins, or both, in addition to IN are associated with viral PICs and may also be required either to assemble or to maintain PICs during infection (85, 111). These factors can contribute to the efficiency of integration either directly by promoting integration or indirectly by preventing "autointegration" or self-insertion, or both. Several such putative auxiliary factors have been identified based on their ability to associate with or potentiate integration activity (or both) in vitro, including barrier-to-autointegration factor (BAF) HMGI Y and the HIV-1 nucleocapsid protein (NC) (14, 15, 46, 71, 72). Of these proteins, only the viral NC has been shown to have a moderate effect on in vitro reactions catalyzed by recombinantly expressed IN (14).

HIV-1 PICs can persist in the cytosolic compartment in an integration-competent state for several hours to several weeks depending on the activation state of the cell (101, 121). When isolated and provided with a cellular DNA surrogate, PICs can be used to perform integration reactions in vitro (7, 33, 47, 48, 111). PICs isolated from cells infected with Moloney murine leukemia virus (Mo-MuLV), HIV-1, and Rous sarcoma virus (RSV) catalyze efficient two-ended or full-site integration reactions in vitro when provided with a heterologous target DNA substrate. Although recombinantly expressed INs are generally inefficient at catalyzing full-site integration, 3' end processing and strand transfer of a single viral DNA end (half-site reactions) can be reproduced using recombinantly derived INs from a wide variety of retroviruses. Efficient full-site integration activity has recently been demonstrated using the isolated enzyme from two distinct sources: IN purified from avian myeloblastosis virus (AMV) and recombinantly expressed simian immunodeficiency virus (SIV) IN (56, 108, 109). The observation that purified INs can faithfully recapitulate the full-site reaction suggests that IN is itself sufficient to catalyze full-site integration, although auxiliary factors such as those described above may be required to facilitate the process in the context of viral infection.

Assays for IN Activity in Vitro

In vitro assays that use PICs isolated from HIV-1-infected cells or recombinantly expressed IN have proven useful in the biochemical characterization of the integration reaction and in the identification and evaluation of IN inhibitors (16, 50, 58, 111; reviewed in references 92, 94). The 3' end processing and strand transfer reactions can be reproduced using recombinant IN and synthetic oligonucleotides to represent both the viral and cellular DNA substrates (Fig. 6.3A) (9, 11, 33, 39, 100, 106). In these assays the sequence-specific oligonucleotide representing the U3 or U5 LTR end of HIV-1 is referred to as the viral end or donor substrate, and the nonspecific oligonucleotide that acts as a surrogate for the cellular DNA is termed the target substrate. In addition to 3' end processing and strand transfer, the recombinant enzyme will use model integration intermediates as substrates and catalyze a family of reactions known as disintegration (Fig. 6.3B) (20, 21, 52, 104). In disintegration, IN excises the viral DNA element and joins adjacent target sequences from a branched oligonucleotide containing both donor and target DNA sequences. As the oligonucleotide substrate in disintegration mimics an integration intermediate, disintegration is often referred to as the reverse of integration (21). Assays monitoring 3' end processing, strand transfer, or disintegration are routinely analyzed by polyacrylamide gel electrophoresis but can be adapted to a microtiter plate format for high throughput screening of chemicals and natural product extracts (reviewed in reference 22). To date, IN inhibitors have been identified using assays that employ recombinant IN; however, HIV-1 PICs have proven useful in the subsequent evaluation of these compounds.

When compared with many of the standard biochemical methods that use recombinant IN, assays that use authentic viral PICs are less suscepti-

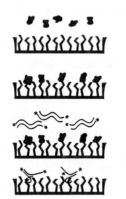

1) Add integrase to preprocessed donor (30' @ 37° C)

2) Remove unbound integrase
   Wash

3) Add target substrate (30' @ 37° C)
   → Titrate compound

4) Assay strand transfer products

FIGURE 6.4

Inhibition of strand transfer

Immobilized LTR-sequence oligonucleotides can be used to uncouple assembly and catalysis. IN complexes assembled on viral sequence donor substrates are stable and can be used to perform strand transfer assays with an exogenously added labeled target DNA substrate as illustrated. This assay format can be adapted to microtiter plates and used as a surrogate for authentic viral PICs to screen for inhibitors of strand transfer (60).

ble to the effects of many IN inhibitors (50, 58). When PICs are isolated from HIV-1-infected cells, assembly and processing are complete; thus, PICs are sensitive only to those compounds that can inhibit the final step in the process, strand transfer (85). Purified recombinant IN will form stable complexes with HIV-1 LTR sequence oligonucleotides (34, 61, 107, 115). The stability of the interaction between IN and the HIV-1 LTR has been exploited to uncouple assembly and catalysis and stage the reaction in vitro (61). Assays using immobilized donor substrate oligonucleotides and recombinant IN that are configured to uncouple assembly and 3' processing from strand transfer thus can reflect the PIC reaction with respect to IN inhibitors (Fig. 6.4). A comparative analysis of inhibitors using PICs and recombinant IN has demonstrated that staged strand transfer assays can be predictive of activity in integration reactions using viral PICs (59, 60, 61). Staged assays are also useful in the analysis of inhibitor mechanism and have been exploited to target specifically the identification of compounds that inhibit strand transfer (60).

IN Inhibitors: Biochemical versus Biological Activity

Although a variety of small molecules have been shown to inhibit the activity of IN in various biochemical assays, identifying compounds that block integration in HIV-1-infected cells has been more difficult (reviewed in references 92, 93, 94). Discounting those compounds that affect the substrate itself, compounds that inhibit the activity of IN in vitro include (i) modified nucleotides and nucleic acid mimetics, (ii) bis-catechols and polyhydroxylated aromatics, (iii) bis-sulfonamides, (iv) hydrazides, and (v) diketo acids (DKAs) and DKA homologs (Fig. 6.5). Several of these compounds also inhibit HIV-1 replication; however, only a subset of compounds belonging to the last class, the DKAs, have been shown to be bona fide inhibitors of integration (60).

Because integration is a complex process, for any novel inhibitor it is not easy to assign mechanism of action in the infected cell. Thus, there are several examples wherein antiviral activity has been mistakenly attributed to IN (26). L-chicoric acid (dicaffeoyltartaric acid), a symmetrical bis-catechol, and AR177 (Zintevir), a guanosine quartet forming 17-mer oligonucleotide, are two such examples of IN inhibitors that inhibit HIV-1 replication as a result of their effect on viral fusion and entry (19, 44, 89, 91, 97, 118). AR177 is also the first (and only) compound claimed to be an IN inhibitor to reach clinical evaluation. Although each of these compounds is an effective inhibitor both of IN and of HIV-1 replication, resistance mutations map to the HIV-1 envelope, specifically the V2, V3, and V4 loop regions of gp120 (44, 84, 91). The identification of resistance mutations in the HIV-1 envelope gene is consistent with rigorous time-of-addition analyses demonstrating that the inhibitor must be present at the time of infection to

1. Modified nucleotides

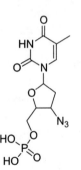

2. Polyhydroxylated aromatics

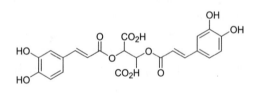

3. Sulfonamides

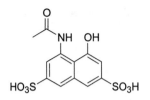

4. Hydrazides

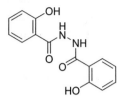

5. Diketo acids (DKAs)

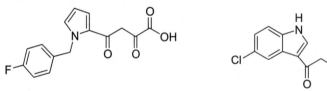

FIGURE 6.5

Representative structures of common inhibitors of HIV-1 IN

(1) 5-N$_3$-AZTMP (29); (2) L-chicoric acid (97); (3) Y3, 4-acetylamino-5-hydroxynaptha-lene-2,7-disulfonic acid (82); (4) salicylhydrazide (87); (5) the diketo acid, L-731,988 (60), and the diketo tetrazole, 5CITEP (54).

elicit an antiviral effect. Polyanions such as the bis-sulfonamides also have an extensive history as inhibitors of both IN activity in vitro and viral fusion (23, 24, 27, 45, 63, 74, 75, 76, 77, 88). Given that most inhibitors of IN fall into one of the three structural classes in which compounds have been shown to have entry-associated effects, antiviral activity claimed for any related structures must be interpreted with extreme caution. Many of these inhibitors will also affect retroviral INs and other DNA-modifying enzymes without specificity (49) and/or have little or no inhibitory activity when assayed in the presence of the biologically relevant divalent metal cofactor, Mg (59). The latter observation diminishes interest in such compounds as mechanistically relevant inhibitors of IN and as reasonable lead structures for this target.

Despite an apparent diversity of structure, IN inhibitors that include representative modified nucleotides, catechols, and sulfonamides have been shown to express a common mechanism of action. As inhibitors of IN in in vitro biochemical assays, these compounds prevent the interaction between IN and DNA oligonucleotides. Because these compounds inhibit assembly, they appear to inhibit all the enzymatic functions of IN without discrimination but are generally ineffective in integration assays using PICs and in staged strand transfer reactions (50, 58, 59). To date, inhibitors of assembly have proven to be inactive as inhibitors of integration in the context of HIV-1 infection. In the course of HIV-1 replication, the effective local concentration of IN and the viral DNA may drive the assembly process and thus preclude inhibition by compounds with this specific mode of action.

The DKAs are the first biologically active IN inhibitors validated by both careful analysis of mechanism in infected cells and resistance (60). It is intriguing to speculate that the DKAs are more effective as antiviral agents than assembly inhibitors owing to their unique mechanism of action. In biochemical assays, the DKAs have little or no effect on assembly, 3' end processing, or disintegration (41, 60). The DKAs are selective inhibitors of strand transfer in vitro and exert their effect on HIV-1 replication exclusively as a result of inhibiting the strand transfer reaction in the infected cell (60). At inhibitor concentrations sufficient to block HIV-1 infection by more than 95%, the DKAs have no effect on viral DNA synthesis or 3' processing of the U5 and U3 LTRs by IN. The DKAs inhibit the strand transfer activity of IN in the context of the viral PIC and prevent integration resulting in the accumulation of 1 and 2 LTR circles in the nucleus of the infected cell. Circles are dead ends in the HIV-1 infection process; thus the consequence of inhibiting strand transfer in the cell is both an effective and irreversible block of viral replication.

Viruses selected for DKA resistance harbor specific mutations in the IN active site (Thr 66 Iso, Ser 153 Tyr, and Met 154 Iso) (60). These IN mutations engender resistance to the DKAs in both biological and biochemical assays when introduced into either the virus or the recombinantly expressed enzyme, respectively. Any of the single DKA resistance–associated mutations in IN confers a modest loss of susceptibility to the inhibitor (two- to fivefold) and appear to be tolerated in the virus. Although the combination of two mutations, specifically T66I/S153Y or T66I/M154I, results in increased resistance (10- to 15-fold), this also results in impaired enzymatic activity and virological fitness. The decreased replicative capacity associated with viruses that display increased resistance to the DKAs is almost certainly responsible for the observation that resistance selection in cell culture requires many months of continual passage (60).

Although mutagenesis studies have suggested that the same active-site residues in IN are required for 3' end processing and strand transfer (30, 37, 65), the DKAs have provided the first evidence that the catalytic activities of IN can differ markedly in their ability to be affected by active-site-directed inhibitors. These results suggest that screening assays that focus exclusively on a subset of the enzymatic activities of IN (e.g., 3' processing) may miss mechanistically interesting and biologically relevant inhibitors. The DKAs were identified in assays specifically biased to identify inhibitors of strand transfer using recombinant IN assembled onto immobilized oligonucleotides as a surrogate for HIV-1 PICs (60). It is interesting to note that the structurally related diketo tetrazole 1-(5-chloroindol-3-yl)-3-hydroxy-3-(2H-tetrazol-5-yl)-pro-penone (5CITEP) (Fig. 6.5) was identified using a similar assay strategy (54, 60). Notably, the intrinsic activity that the DKAs exhibit in strand transfer assay is nearly identical to the activity they express in assays using viral PICs, providing the first validation of the use of an assay using recombinantly expressed IN as a means of identifying biologically relevant inhibitors (60). Given the selectivity that the DKAs exhibit for strand transfer, it is not surprising that screens for 3' end processing and disintegration have failed to identify compounds that are effective inhibitors of isolated HIV-1 PICs. It is questionable whether biological screening assays that attempt to exploit the nonspecific endonucleolytic activities of IN would be sensitive to inhibitors that exhibit this specific mechanism.

Mechanism of the DKAs as Inhibitors of Strand Transfer

The mechanistic basis underlying the unique activity of the DKAs as strand transfer inhibitors has recently been explored using two prototype inhibitors, including L-731,988 (41, 57, 110). Understanding this activity has enabled the identification of several differences that distinguish these compounds from inhibitors of assembly. The interaction between IN and the DKAs requires assembly of an active complex on the HIV-1 LTR. There is an approximately three-order-of-magnitude difference between the affinity of the DKAs for the isolated enzyme and IN in the context of the assembled strand transfer complex (20 µM versus 20 nM) (41). The high-affinity DKA interaction is completely restrictive for IN associated with the HIV-1-specific LTR sequence. The DKAs will not associate with complexes assembled on non-LTR-sequence oligonucleotides, and mutations in the LTR sequence that affect the activity of the donor substrate in enzymatic assays affect DKA binding to a similar degree (41, 57).

The DKA binding site is therefore defined by a conformation of IN that is adopted only after proper assembly with the viral DNA. In the context of this complex, competition between the target DNA substrate and the inhibitor leads to the observed selectivity for strand transfer. The interaction of target DNA substrates with the strand transfer complex has been shown to reduce the efficacy of the DKAs in strand transfer assays and has a direct effect on inhibitor binding (41). Function as a target DNA substrate in strand transfer correlates with the ability to compete with the DKAs. Single-stranded DNAs that do not function as target substrates do not affect inhibitor binding, and target DNAs that are better substrates in strand transfer reaction owing to differences in length or sequence are better competitors in direct DKA binding assays. Competition for the target substrate binding site is consistent with the observation that the DKAs are poorly active in disintegration assays wherein the substrate simultaneously occupies both the donor and target substrate sites in the complex. Disintegration substrates also fail to promote the high-affinity interaction between the DKAs and IN that is observed in the presence of viral ends.

Therefore, in direct contrast to assembly inhibitors that prevent the interaction between IN and the donor substrate, the DKAs require assembly on the viral DNA and are competitive with the target substrate. These fundamental differences thus define two distinct classes of inhibitors that differ with respect to both their mechanism of action and their ability to recognize structurally unique enzyme states as determined by either the presence or absence of the viral DNA end (Fig. 6.6). Available structural information for two inhibitors, 5CITEP and the napthalene disulfate Y3, is consistent with the recognition of distinct binding sites on the enzyme. The assembly inhibitor Y3 binds outside the IN active site in a region that has been implicated in establishing interdomain contacts required in the stabilized complex and/or forming part of the interaction surface for the viral DNA (82). In contrast, strand transfer inhibitors bind within the IN active site itself. Resistance to several DKAs has consistently mapped to residues within the IN active site that are adjacent to the catalytic residues Asp64 and Glu152 (Fig. 6.7) (60). The DKA resistance mutations as well as the mutation of the catalytic residues themselves have been shown to abrogate DKA binding (41, 57). DKA resistance mutations also affect binding and inhibition of the diketo tetrazole 5CITEP (57) and are consistent with several of the active-site contacts observed for 5CITEP in the X-ray structure with the catalytic core domain of HIV-1 IN (54).

Within the IN active site, Asp64, Asp116, and Glu152 bind the divalent metal ion cofactors required for catalysis (reviewed in reference 114). Several lines of evidence have suggested that the interaction of the DKAs with one or both of the divalent metals in the active site may be an essential component of the inhibitory mechanism (57). The DKAs exhibit comparable binding affinity and inhibitory activity when assayed in the presence of Mn or Mg. In contrast, compounds with certain acid replacements such as the tetrazole in the 5CITEP structure are dependent on the nature of the divalent cation cofactor used in the assay and exhibit higher affinity and greater potency in the presence of Mn as compared with the biologically

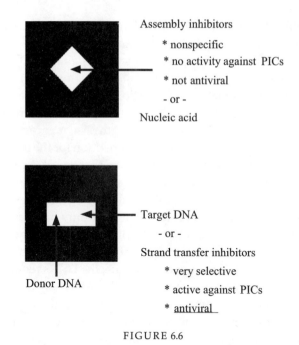

Assembly inhibitors
* nonspecific
* no activity against PICs
* not antiviral
- or -
Nucleic acid

Target DNA
- or -
Strand transfer inhibitors
* very selective
* active against PICs
* antiviral

Donor DNA

FIGURE 6.6

Inhibitors of IN exhibit two different mechanisms of action and recognize distinct enzyme conformations as defined by the presence or absence of the viral donor substrate

Assembly inhibitors bind to the unliganded enzyme and prevent the interaction with the donor substrate; strand transfer inhibitors bind only to the IN/donor substrate complex and selectively inhibit strand transfer by competing with the target DNA substrate.

relevant Mg (57). In addition, simple esters of compounds that are potent inhibitors as DKAs bind IN with submicromolar affinity but are inactive as inhibitors of IN-catalyzed strand transfer (>100 μM versus 100 nM for the corresponding acid). These results indicate that the interaction between the acid moiety in these inhibitors and the metal factor may have a direct role in inhibition and illustrate the importance of evaluating IN activity and inhibition in the context of the relevant metal cofactor.

The acid moiety is thus a critical component of the inhibitory mechanism of the DKAs; however, the entirety of structure has been shown to contribute to both the selectivity and intrinsic potency of this class of compounds. Unlike many previously described inhibitors of IN that can accommodate substantial structural changes, small modifications to the DKAs can have a dramatic effect on potency in strand transfer assays and HIV-1 replication (110). Modifications to the original lead compounds have led to the elucidation of IN inhibitors that exhibit antiviral activities in vitro

INTEGRASE

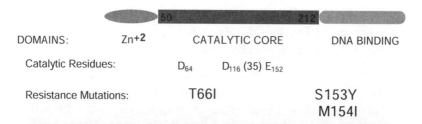

DOMAINS:	Zn^{+2}	CATALYTIC CORE	DNA BINDING
Catalytic Residues:		D_{64} D_{116} (35) E_{152}	
Resistance Mutations:		T66I	S153Y M154I

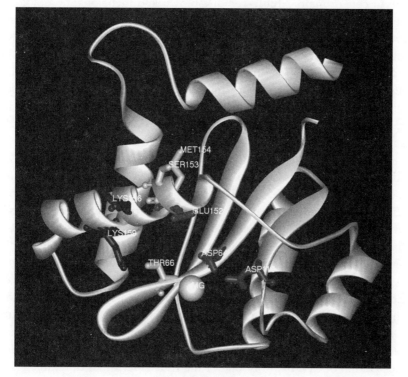

FIGURE 6.7

Resistance to the DKA inhibitors maps to the IN active site

Mutations responsible for resistance to the DKA include Thr 66 Ile, Ser 153 Tyr, and Met 154 Val (60), residues that are adjacent to the catalytic residues Asp64 and Glu152 in the crystal structure of IN (55). The catalytic residues, Asp64, Asp 116, and Glu152, coordinate the divalent metal ion cofactors essential for catalysis.

that are 100-fold more potent and thus comparable to many of the current clinically effective antiretroviral agents.

The Structure of IN: Implications for Inhibitor Binding and Mechanism

The X-ray structure of the catalytic core domain (amino acids 50–212) has been solved for INs from several different retroviruses (31, 55, 80, 83; reviewed in reference 114). Despite little or no sequence conservation, the IN catalytic core domain exhibits remarkable three-dimensional homology to several unrelated phosphotransferase enzymes including RNase H and RuvC (3, 31, 86, 95, 119; reviewed in reference 43). This is particularly evident when comparing the relative positioning of the conserved catalytic residues and the juxtaposition of the divalent metal ions in the active site. Structures of the IN catalytic core domain with either one or two active-site bound divalent metals are available, as are co-crystal structures of the IN core domain with two inhibitors, 4-acetylamino-5-hydroxynapthalene-2,7-disulfonic acid (Y3) (82) and the diketo tetrazole 5CITEP (54).

More recently, the structures for the extended two-domain (the catalytic core domain plus C-terminal domain) enzyme have been solved for three retroviral INs: HIV-1, SIV-1, and RSV (17, 18, 120). Although the catalytic core domain dimer in each of the extended two-domain structures is nearly identical and virtually indistinguishable from that observed in the isolated core domain, the three extended structures are substantially different in the architecture of their respective interdomain interactions (Fig. 6.8). In the HIV-1 structure, the molecule is a Y-shaped structure in which the two C-terminal domains are independent and each is linked to the catalytic core domain dimer by a 26-amino-acid linker (17). The RSV structure is L-shaped with the two C-terminal domains dimerized; in the RSV structure the C-domain dimer is connected to the core dimer via a six-residue tether (120). For SIV IN, only one of the four C-terminal domains in the asymmetric unit was sufficiently defined as to be resolved. In contrast to the ASV and HIV-1 structures, the SIV structure is the only one in which the C-domain is observed to make extensive interdomain contacts with the core dimer (18). It should also be noted that the positioning of the resolved C-terminal domain relative to the core dimer in the SIV structure cannot accommodate an additional C-domain if dimerized as in either of the dimeric structures observed for the isolated C-domain or in the extended RSV IN.

Beyond the gross differences observed for each of the IN two-domain structures, subtle but nonetheless significant differences have been noted within the active site itself. IN crystal structures can be strikingly different in the positioning of the active-site residues, in particular Glu152 (114).

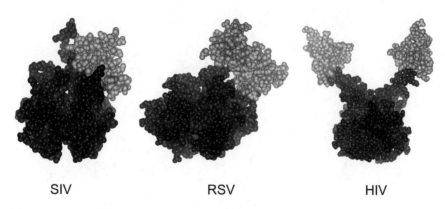

SIV   RSV   HIV

FIGURE 6.8

The X-ray structures of the three two-domain INs
suggest a remarkably flexible molecule

The structures for the catalytic core domain plus C-terminal domain of SIV IN (18), RSV
IN (120), and HIV-1 IN (17) highlight differences in their respective interdomain interactions.

This conformational flexibility is also evident when comparing the active
sites of individual monomers within a single structure as in the structure
of the extended SIV-1 core plus C-terminal domain (Fig. 6.9) (18). The observation that the active site may not be appropriately configured until IN
has assembled on the viral end is consistent with the observation that the
DKAs that are active-site-directed strand transfer inhibitors do not bind
with high affinity in the absence of the donor substrate. The striking differences in the orientations of the catalytic core and C-terminal domains
among the RSV, SIV, and HIV-1 IN structures also support the notion of a
flexible molecule in which the ultimate juxtaposition of the domains is determined by and required to stabilize a functional complex with the viral
DNA during the course of integration.

Because the IN active site can exist in multiple conformations and IN
does not adopt a conformation that is appropriate for binding the DKA in
the absence of the donor DNA substrate, attempts to model and refine
active-site-directed strand transfer inhibitors based on any of the non-
liganded structures of the IN core domain or N-terminally truncated enzymes are problematic and in fact may not prove relevant. Recognition of
the active IN conformation by L-731,988 and related compounds suggests
that this class of inhibitors may provide a valuable tool to probe the active-
site structure itself and address many of the difficult questions in the field
of IN biochemistry, including the stoichiometry of the minimal catalytically active IN/DNA complex and the number of active sites required for
catalysis.

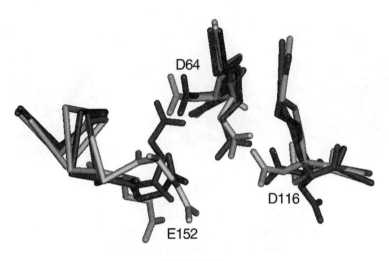

FIGURE 6.9

The active-site residues in the extended SIV IN
structure adopt distinct conformations in each
of the four monomers in the asymmetric unit

The conformational flexibility of the active site is particularly evident in the
region including Glu152, which is at or near the binding site implicated for
the DKA inhibitors of IN and the related compound 5CITEP (18).

Summary

HIV-1 IN presents a potential opportunity for the development of novel
antiretroviral agents. Although many compounds identified as inhibitors
of IN activity in vitro have failed as inhibitors of HIV-1 replication, the
recent discovery of the DKAs as bona fide integration inhibitors and the
elucidation of their distinct mechanism of action as inhibitors of strand
transfer have validated a new approach for exploiting this important
chemotherapeutic target. The observation that inhibition of strand transfer in the infected cell leads to an accumulation of dead-end circular products and an irreversible block of the infection process is consistent with
previous results with integration-defective viruses and may be an intrinsic feature critical to the biological efficacy of IN inhibitors that exhibit this
mechanism of action.

Strand transfer inhibitors can be both highly selective and potent as
inhibitors of IN activity in vitro and as inhibitors of HIV-1 replication in
cell culture. Although HIV-1 can overcome the activity of these agents by
acquiring specific mutations in IN, the observation that (i) resistance requires multiple mutations in the IN active site and (ii) viruses with these
multiple mutations display reduced replicative capacity is consistent with
the observation that resistance is relatively difficult to achieve in cell cul-

ture and suggests that strand transfer inhibitors may present a fairly high genetic barrier to resistance selection in vivo. The development of clinically useful IN inhibitors with this unique mechanism of action should therefore provide a valuable addition to current antiretroviral therapy choices.

REFERENCES

1. Acel, A., B. E. Udashkin, M. A. Wainberg, and E. A. Faust. 1998. Efficient gap repair catalyzed in vitro by an intrinsic DNA polymerase activity of human immunodeficiency virus type 1 integrase. J. Virol. 72:2062–2071.

2. Andrake, M. D., and A. M. Skalka. 1995. Multimerization determinants reside in both the catalytic core and C terminus of avian sarcoma virus integrase. J. Biol. Chem. 270:29299–29306.

3. Andrake, M. D., and A. M. Skalka. 1996. Retroviral integrase, putting the pieces together. J. Biol. Chem. 271:19633–19636.

4. Asante-Appiah, E., and A. M. Skalka. 1997. A metal-induced conformational change and activation of HIV-1 integrase. J. Biol. Chem. 272:16196–16205.

5. Bouille, P., F. Subra, J. F. Mouscadet, and C. Auclair. 1999. Antisense-mediated repression of DNA topoisomerase II expression leads to an impairment of HIV-1 replicative cycle. J. Mol. Biol. 285:945–954.

6. Brown, P. O. 1998. Retroviruses, p. 161–203. *In* J. M. Coffin, S. H. Hughes, and H. E. Varmus (ed.), Retroviruses. Cold Spring Harbor Laboratory Press, Cold Spring Harbor, N.Y.

7. Brown, P. O., B. Bowerman, H. E. Varmus, and J. M. Bishop. 1987. Correct integration of retroviral DNA in vitro. Cell 49:347–356.

8. Bukovsky, A., and H. Gottlinger. 1996. Lack of integrase can markedly affect human immunodeficiency virus type 1 particle production in the presence of an active viral protease. J. Virol. 70:6820–6825.

9. Bushman, F. D., and R. Craigie. 1991. Activities of human immunodeficiency virus (HIV) integration protein in vitro: specific cleavage and integration of HIV DNA. Proc. Natl. Acad. Sci. USA 88:1339–1343.

10. Bushman, F. D., A. Engelman, I. Palmer, P. Wingfield, and R. Craigie. 1993. Domains of the integrase protein of human immunodeficiency virus type 1 responsible for polynucleotidyl transfer and zinc binding. Proc. Natl. Acad. Sci. USA 90:3428–3432.

11. Bushman, F. D., T. Fujiwara, and R. Craigie. 1990. Retroviral DNA integration directed by HIV integration protein in vitro. Science 249:1555–1558.

12. Cai, M., R. Zheng, M. Caffrey, R. Craigie, G. M. Clore, and A. M. Gronenborn. 1997. Solution structure of the N-terminal zinc binding domain of HIV-1 integrase. Nat. Struct. Biol. 4:567–577. (Erratum, 4(10):839–840.)

13. Cannon, P. M., W. Wilson, E. Byles, S. M. Kingsman, and A. J. Kingsman. 1994. Human immunodeficiency virus type 1 integrase: effect on viral replication of mutations at highly conserved residues. J. Virol. 68:4768–4775.

14. Carteau, S., R. J. Gorelick, and F. D. Bushman. 1999. Coupled integration of human immunodeficiency virus type 1 cDNA ends by purified integrase in vitro: stimulation by the viral nucleocapsid protein. J. Virol. 73:6670–6679.

15. Chen, H., and A. Engelman. 1998. The barrier-to-autointegration protein is a host factor for HIV type 1 integration. Proc. Natl. Acad. Sci. USA 95: 15270–15274.

16. Chen, H., S. Q. Wei, and A. Engelman. 1999. Multiple integrase functions are required to form the native structure of the human immunodeficiency virus type I intasome. J. Biol. Chem. 274:17358–17364.

17. Chen, J. C., J. Krucinski, L. J. Miercke, J. S. Finer-Moore, A. H. Tang, A. D. Leavitt, and R. M. Stroud. 2000. Crystal structure of the HIV-1 integrase catalytic core and C-terminal domains: a model for viral DNA binding. Proc. Natl. Acad. Sci. USA 97:8233–8238.

18. Chen, Z., Y. Yan, S. Munshi, Y. Li, J. Zugay-Murphy, B. Xu, M. Witmer, P. Felock, A. Wolfe, V. Sardana, E. A. Emini, D. Hazuda, and L. C. Kuo. 2000. X-ray structure of simian immunodeficiency virus integrase containing the core and C-terminal domain (residues 50–293)—an initial glance of the viral DNA binding platform. J. Mol. Biol. 296:521–533.

19. Cherepanov, P., J. A. Este, R. F. Rando, J. O. Ojwang, G. Reekmans, R. Steinfeld, G. David, E. De Clercq, and Z. Debyser. 1997. Mode of interaction of G-quartets with the integrase of human immunodeficiency virus type 1. Mol. Pharmacol. 52:771–780.

20. Chow, S. A., and P. O. Brown. 1994. Substrate features important for recognition and catalysis by human immunodeficiency virus type 1 integrase identified by using novel DNA substrates. J. Virol. 68:3896–3907.

21. Chow, S. A., K. A. Vincent, V. Ellison, and P. O. Brown. 1992. Reversal of integration and DNA splicing mediated by integrase of human immunodeficiency virus. Science 255:723–726.

22. Craigie, R., A. B. Hickman, and A. Engelman. 1995. Integrase, p. 53–71. In J. Karn (ed.), HIV. A practical approach, vol. II. Oxford University Press, Oxford, England.

23. Cushman, M., W. M. Golebiewski, Y. Pommier, A. Mazumder, D. Reymen, E. De Clercq, L. Graham, and W. G. Rice. 1995. Cosalane analogues with enhanced potencies as inhibitors of HIV-1 protease and integrase. J. Med. Chem. 38:443–452.

24. Cushman, M., and P. Sherman. 1992. Inhibition of HIV-1 integration protein by aurintricarboxylic acid monomers, monomer analogs, and polymer fractions. Biochem. Biophys. Res. Commun. 185:85–90.

25. Daniel, R., R. A. Katz, and A. M. Skalka. 1999. A role for DNA-PK in retroviral DNA integration. Science 284:644–647.

26. De Clercq, E. 2000. Novel compounds in preclinical/early clinical development for the treatment of HIV infections. Rev. Med. Virol. 10:255–277.

27. Degols, G., C. Devaux, and B. Lebleu. 1994. Oligonucleotide-poly(L-lysine)-heparin complexes: potent sequence-specific inhibitors of HIV-1 infection. Bioconjugate Chem. 5:8–13.

28. Doak, T. G., F. P. Doerder, C. L. Jahn, and G. Herrick. 1994. A proposed superfamily of transposase genes: transposon-like elements in ciliated protozoa and a common "D35E" motif. Proc. Natl. Acad. Sci. USA 91:942–946.

29. Drake, R. R., N. Neamati, H. Hong, A. A. Pilon, P. Sunthankar, S. D. Hume, G. W. Milne, and Y. Pommier. 1998. Identification of a nucleotide binding site in HIV-1 integrase. Proc. Natl. Acad. Sci. USA 95:4170–4175.

30. Drelich, M., R. Wilhelm, and J. Mous. 1992. Identification of amino acid residues critical for endonuclease and integration activities of HIV-1 IN protein in vitro. Virology 188:459–468.

31. Dyda, F., A. B. Hickman, T. M. Jenkins, A. Engelman, R. Craigie, and D. R. Davies. 1994. Crystal structure of the catalytic domain of HIV-1 integrase: similarity to other polynucleotidyl transferases [see comments]. Science 266:1981–1986.

32. Eijkelenboom, A. P., R. A. Lutzke, R. Boelens, R. H. Plasterk, R. Kaptein, and K. Hard. 1995. The DNA-binding domain of HIV-1 integrase has an SH3-like fold. Nat. Struct. Biol. 2:807–810.

33. Ellison, V., H. Abrams, T. Roe, J. Lifson, and P. Brown. 1990. Human immunodeficiency virus integration in a cell-free system. J. Virol. 64:2711–2715.

34. Ellison, V., and P. O. Brown. 1994. A stable complex between integrase and viral DNA ends mediates human immunodeficiency virus integration in vitro. Proc. Natl. Acad. Sci. USA 91:7316–7320.

35. Ellison, V., J. Gerton, K. A. Vincent, and P. O. Brown. 1995. An essential interaction between distinct domains of HIV-1 integrase mediates assembly of the active multimer. J. Biol. Chem. 270:3320–3326.

36. Engelman, A., F. D. Bushman, and R. Craigie. 1993. Identification of discrete functional domains of HIV-1 integrase and their organization within an active multimeric complex. EMBO J. 12:3269–3275.

37. Engelman, A., and R. Craigie. 1992. Identification of conserved amino acid residues critical for human immunodeficiency virus type 1 integrase function in vitro. J. Virol. 66:6361–6369.

38. Engelman, A., G. Englund, J. M. Orenstein, M. A. Martin, and R. Craigie. 1995. Multiple effects of mutations in human immunodeficiency virus type 1 integrase on viral replication. J. Virol. 69:2729–2736.

39. Engelman, A., K. Mizuuchi, and R. Craigie. 1991. HIV-1 DNA integration: mechanism of viral DNA cleavage and DNA strand transfer. Cell 67:1211–1221.

40. Englund, G., T. S. Theodore, E. O. Freed, A. Engleman, and M. A. Martin. 1995. Integration is required for productive infection of monocyte-derived macrophages by human immunodeficiency virus type 1. J. Virol. 69:3216–3219.

41. Espeseth, A. S., P. Felock, A. Wolfe, M. Witmer, J. Grobler, N. Anthony, M. Egbertson, J. Y. Melamed, S. Young, T. Hamill, J. L. Cole, and D. J. Hazuda. 2000. HIV-1 integrase inhibitors that compete with the target DNA substrate define a unique strand transfer conformation for integrase. Proc. Natl. Acad. Sci. USA 97:11244–11249.

42. Esposito, D., and R. Craigie. 1998. Sequence specificity of viral end DNA binding by HIV-1 integrase reveals critical regions for protein-DNA interaction. EMBO J. 17:5832–5843.

43. Esposito, D., and R. Craigie. 1999. HIV integrase structure and function. Adv. Virus Res. 52:319–333.

44. Este, J. A., C. Cabrera, D. Schols, P. Cherepanov, A. Gutierrez, M. Witvrouw, C. Pannecouque, Z. Debyser, R. F. Rando, B. Clotet, J. Desmyter, and E. De Clercq. 1998. Human immunodeficiency virus glycoprotein gp120 as the primary target for the antiviral action of AR177 (Zintevir). Mol. Pharmacol. 53:340–345.

45. Este, J. A., D. Schols, K. De Vreese, K. Van Laethem, A. M. Vandamme, J. Desmyter, and E. De Clercq. 1997. Development of resistance of human immunodeficiency virus type 1 to dextran sulfate associated with the emergence of specific mutations in the envelope gp120 glycoprotein. Mol. Pharmacol. 52:98–104.

46. Farnet, C. M., and F. D. Bushman. 1997. HIV-1 cDNA integration: requirement of HMG I(Y) protein for function of preintegration complexes in vitro. Cell 88:483–492.

47. Farnet, C. M., and W. A. Haseltine. 1990. Integration of human immunodeficiency virus type 1 DNA in vitro. Proc. Natl. Acad. Sci. USA 87:4164–4168.

48. Farnet, C. M., and W. A. Haseltine. 1991. Determination of viral proteins present in the human immunodeficiency virus type 1 preintegration complex. J. Virol. 65:1910–1915.

49. Farnet, C. M., B. Wang, M. Hansen, J. R. Lipford, L. Zalkow, W. E. Robinson, Jr., J. Siegel, and F. Bushman. 1998. Human immunodeficiency virus type 1 cDNA integration: new aromatic hydroxylated inhibitors and studies of the inhibition mechanism. Antimicrob. Agents Chemother. 42:2245–2253.

50. Farnet, C. M., B. Wang, J. R. Lipford, and F. D. Bushman. 1996. Differential inhibition of HIV-1 preintegration complexes and purified integrase protein by small molecules. Proc. Natl. Acad. Sci. USA 93:9742–9747.

51. Fletcher, T. M., III, M. A. Soares, S. McPhearson, H. Hui, M. Wiskerchen, M. A. Muesing, G. M. Shaw, A. D. Leavitt, J. D. Boeke, and B. H. Hahn. 1997. Complementation of integrase function in HIV-1 virions. EMBO J. 16:5123–5138.

52. Gerton, J. L., and P. O. Brown. 1997. The core domain of HIV-1 integrase recognizes key features of its DNA substrates. J. Biol. Chem. 272:25809–25815.

53. Goff, S. P. 1992. Genetics of retroviral integration. Annu. Rev. Genet. 26:527–544.

54. Goldgur, Y., R. Craigie, G. H. Cohen, T. Fujiwara, T. Yoshinaga, T. Fujishita, H. Sugimoto, T. Endo, H. Murai, and D. R. Davies. 1999. Structure of the HIV-1 integrase catalytic domain complexed with an inhibitor: a platform for antiviral drug design. Proc. Natl. Acad. Sci. USA 96:13040–13043.

55. Goldgur, Y., F. Dyda, A. B. Hickman, T. M. Jenkins, R. Craigie, and D. R. Davies. 1998. Three new structures of the core domain of HIV-1 integrase: an active site that binds magnesium. Proc. Natl. Acad. Sci. USA 95:9150–9154.

56. Goodarzi, G., M. Pursley, P. Felock, M. Witmer, D. Hazuda, K. Brackmann, and D. Grandgenett. 1999. Efficiency and fidelity of full-site integration reactions using recombinant simian immunodeficiency virus integrase. J. Virol. 73:8104–8111.

57. Grobler, J., K. Stillmock, B. Hu, M. Witmer, P. Felock, A. Espeseth, M. Egbertson, H. Selnick, M. Bpurgois, J. Malemed, J. Medina, T. Hamill, and D. Hazuda. The effect of divalent metals on active site inhibitors of HIV-1 integrase: a model for two metals in the active site. Submitted for publication.

58. Hansen, M. S., and F. D. Bushman. 1997. Human immunodeficiency virus type 2 preintegration complexes: activities in vitro and response to inhibitors. J. Virol. 71:3351–3356.

59. Hazuda, D., P. J. Felock, J. C. Hastings, B. Pramanik, and A. L. Wolfe. 1997. Discovery and analysis of inhibitors of the human immunodeficiency integrase. Drug Design and Discovery 15:17–24.

60. Hazuda, D. J., P. Felock, M. Witmer, A. Wolfe, K. Stillmock, J. Grobler, A. Espeseth, L. Gabryelski, W. Schleif, C. Blau, and M. D. Miller. 2000. Inhibitors of strand transfer that prevent integration and inhibit HIV-1 replication in cells. Science 287:646–650.

61. Hazuda, D. J., P. J. Felock, J. C. Hastings, B. Pramanik, and A. L. Wolfe. 1997. Differential divalent cation requirements uncouple the assembly and catalytic reactions of human immunodeficiency virus type 1 integrase. J. Virol. 71:7005–7011.

62. Heuer, T. S., and P. O. Brown. 1998. Photo-cross-linking studies suggest a model for the architecture of an active human immunodeficiency virus type 1 integrase-DNA complex. Biochemistry 37:6667–6678.

63. Jansen, R. W., D. Schols, R. Pauwels, E. De Clercq, and D. K. Meijer. 1993. Novel, negatively charged, human serum albumins display potent and selective in vitro anti-human immunodeficiency virus type 1 activity. Mol. Pharmacol. 44:1003–1007.

64. Jones, K. S., J. Coleman, G. W. Merkel, T. M. Laue, and A. M. Skalka. 1992. Retroviral integrase functions as a multimer and can turn over catalytically. J. Biol. Chem. 267:16037–16040.

65. Kulkosky, J., K. S. Jones, R. A. Katz, J. P. Mack, and A. M. Skalka. 1992. Residues critical for retroviral integrative recombination in a region that is highly conserved among retroviral/retrotransposon integrases and bacterial insertion sequence transposases. Mol. Cell. Biol. 12:2331–2338.

66. LaFemina, R. L., P. L. Callahan, and M. G. Cordingley. 1991. Substrate specificity of recombinant human immunodeficiency virus integrase protein. J. Virol. 65:5624–5630.

67. LaFemina, R. L., C. L. Schneider, H. L. Robbins, P. L. Callahan, K. LeGrow, E. Roth, W. A. Schleif, and E. A. Emini. 1992. Requirement of active human immunodeficiency virus type 1 integrase enzyme for productive infection of human T-lymphoid cells. J. Virol. 66:7414–7419.

68. Leavitt, A. D., G. Robles, N. Alesandro, and H. E. Varmus. 1996. Human immunodeficiency virus type 1 integrase mutants retain in vitro integrase activity yet fail to integrate viral DNA efficiently during infection. J. Virol. 70:721–728.

69. Leavitt, A. D., R. B. Rose, and H. E. Varmus. 1992. Both substrate and target oligonucleotide sequences affect in vitro integration mediated by human immunodeficiency virus type 1 integrase protein produced in Saccharomyces cerevisiae. J. Virol. 66:2359–2368.

70. Leavitt, A. D., L. Shiue, and H. E. Varmus. 1993. Site-directed mutagenesis of HIV-1 integrase demonstrates differential effects on integrase functions in vitro. J. Biol. Chem. 268:2113–2119.

71. Lee, M. S., and R. Craigie. 1994. Protection of retroviral DNA from auto-integration: involvement of a cellular factor. Proc. Natl. Acad. Sci. USA 91:9823–9827.

72. Lee, M. S., and R. Craigie. 1998. A previously unidentified host protein pro-

tects retroviral DNA from autointegration. Proc. Natl. Acad. Sci. USA 95: 1528–1533.

73. Leh, H., P. Brodin, J. Bischerour, E. Deprez, P. Tauc, J. C. Brochon, E. LeCam, D. Coulaud, C. Auclair, and J. F. Mouscadet. 2000. Determinants of Mg(2+)-dependent activities of recombinant human immunodeficiency virus type 1 integrase. Biochemistry 39:9285–9294.

74. Leydet, A., V. Barragan, B. Boyer, J. L. Montero, J. P. Roque, M. Witvrouw, J. Este, R. Snoeck, G. Andrei, and E. De Clercq. 1997. Polyanion inhibitors of human immunodeficiency virus and other viruses. 5. Telomerized anionic surfactants derived from amino acids. J. Med. Chem. 40:342–349.

75. Leydet, A., P. Barthelemy, B. Boyer, G. Lamaty, J. P. Roque, A. Bousseau, M. Evers, Y. Henin, R. Snoeck, G. Andrei, et al. 1995. Polyanion inhibitors of human immunodeficiency virus and other viruses. 1. Polymerized anionic surfactants. J. Med. Chem. 38:2433–2440.

76. Leydet, A., H. El Hachemi, B. Boyer, G. Lamaty, J. P. Roque, D. Schols, R. Snoeck, G. Andrei, S. Ikeda, J. Neyts, D. Reymen, J. Este, M. Witvrouw, and E. De Clercq. 1996. Polyanion inhibitors of human immunodeficiency virus and other viruses. Part 2. Polymerized anionic surfactants derived from amino acids and dipeptides. J. Med. Chem. 39:1626–1634.

77. Leydet, A., C. Moullet, J. P. Roque, M. Witvrouw, C. Pannecouque, G. Andrei, R. Snoeck, J. Neyts, D. Schols, and E. De Clercq. 1998. Polyanion inhibitors of HIV and other viruses. 7. Polyanionic compounds and polyzwitterionic compounds derived from cyclodextrins as inhibitors of HIV transmission. J. Med. Chem. 41:4927–4932.

78. Liu, H., X. Wu, H. Xiao, J. A. Conway, and J. C. Kappes. 1997. Incorporation of functional human immunodeficiency virus type 1 integrase into virions independent of the Gag-Pol precursor protein. J. Virol. 71:7704–7710.

79. Lodi, P. J., J. A. Ernst, J. Kuszewski, A. B. Hickman, A. Engelman, R. Craigie, G. M. Clore, and A. M. Gronenborn. 1995. Solution structure of the DNA binding domain of HIV-1 integrase. Biochemistry 34:9826–9833.

80. Lubkowski, J., Z. Dauter, F. Yang, J. Alexandratos, G. Merkel, A. M. Skalka, and A. Wlodawer. 1999. Atomic resolution structures of the core domain of avian sarcoma virus integrase and its D64N mutant. Biochemistry 38: 13512–13522. (Erratum, 38 (45):15060.)

81. Lubkowski, J., F. Yang, J. Alexandratos, G. Merkel, R. A. Katz, K. Gravuer, A. M. Skalka, and A. Wlodawer. 1998. Structural basis for inactivating mutations and pH-dependent activity of avian sarcoma virus integrase. J. Biol. Chem. 273:32685–32689.

82. Lubkowski, J., F. Yang, J. Alexandratos, A. Wlodawer, H. Zhao, T. R. Burke, Jr., N. Neamati, Y. Pommier, G. Merkel, and A. M. Skalka. 1998. Structure of the catalytic domain of avian sarcoma virus integrase with a bound HIV-1 integrase-targeted inhibitor. Proc. Natl. Acad. Sci. USA 95:4831–4836.

83. Maignan, S., J. P. Guilloteau, Q. Zhou-Liu, C. Clement-Mella, and V. Mikol. 1998. Crystal structures of the catalytic domain of HIV-1 integrase free and complexed with its metal cofactor: high level of similarity of the active site with other viral integrases. J. Mol. Biol. 282:359–368.

84. Meylan, P. R., R. S. Kornbluth, I. Zbinden, and D. D. Richman. 1994. Influence of host cell type and V3 loop of the surface glycoprotein on susceptibil-

ity of human immunodeficiency virus type 1 to polyanion compounds. Antimicrob. Agents Chemother. 38:2910–2916.

85. Miller, M. D., C. M. Farnet, and F. D. Bushman. 1997. Human immunodeficiency virus type 1 preintegration complexes: studies of organization and composition. J. Virol. 71:5382–5390.

86. Mizuuchi, K. 1997. Polynucleotidyl transfer reactions in site-specific DNA recombination. Genes Cells 2:1–12.

87. Neamati, N., H. Hong, J. M. Owen, S. Sunder, H. E. Winslow, J. L. Christensen, H. Zhao, T. R. Burke, Jr., G. W. Milne, and Y. Pommier. 1998. Salicylhydrazine-containing inhibitors of HIV-1 integrase: implication for a selective chelation in the integrase active site. J. Med. Chem. 41:3202–3209.

88. Neamati, N., A. Mazumder, S. Sunder, J. M. Owen, R. J. Schultz, and Y. Pommier. 1997. 2-Mercaptobenzenesulfonamides as novel inhibitors of human immunodeficiency virus type I integrase and replication. Antiviral Chem. Chemother. 8:485–495.

89. Ojwang, J. O., R. W. Buckheit, Y. Pommier, A. Mazumder, K. De Vreese, J. A. Este, D. Reymen, L. A. Pallansch, C. Lackman-Smith, T. L. Wallace, et al. 1995. T30177, an oligonucleotide stabilized by an intramolecular guanosine octet, is a potent inhibitor of laboratory strains and clinical isolates of human immunodeficiency virus type 1. Antimicrob. Agents Chemother. 39:2426–2435.

90. Petit, C., O. Schwartz, and F. Mammano. 1999. Oligomerization within virions and subcellular localization of human immunodeficiency virus type 1 integrase. J. Virol. 73:5079–5088.

91. Pluymers, W., N. Neamati, C. Pannecouque, V. Fikkert, C. Marchand, T. R. Burke, Jr., Y. Pommier, D. Schols, E. De Clercq, Z. Debyser, and M. Witvrouw. 2000. Viral entry as the primary target for the anti-HIV activity of chicoric acid and its tetra-acetyl esters. Mol. Pharmacol. 58:641–648.

92. Pommier, Y., C. Marchand, and N. Neamati. 2000. Retroviral integrase inhibitors year 2000: update and perspectives. Antiviral Res. 47:139–148.

93. Pommier, Y., and N. Neamati. 1999. Inhibitors of human immunodeficiency virus integrase, p. 427. In K. Maramorosch, F. Murphy, and A. Shatkin (ed.), Advances in virus research, vol. 52. Academic Press, New York.

94. Pommier, Y., A. Pilon, K. Bajaj, A. Mazumder, and N. Neamati. 1997. HIV-1 integrase as a target for antiviral drugs. Antiviral Chem. Chemother. 8:463–483.

95. Rice, P., R. Craigie, and D. R. Davies. 1996. Retroviral integrases and their cousins. Curr. Opin. Struct. Biol. 6:76–83.

96. Richman, D. D. 1996. Antiviral drug resistance. Wiley, New York.

97. Robinson, W. E., Jr., M. G. Reinecke, S. Abdel-Malek, Q. Jia, and S. A. Chow. 1996. Inhibitors of HIV-1 replication that inhibit HIV integrase. Proc. Natl. Acad. Sci. USA 93:6326–6331.

98. Scottoline, B. P., S. Chow, V. Ellison, and P. O. Brown. 1997. Disruption of the terminal base pairs of retroviral DNA during integration. Genes Dev. 11:371–382.

99. Sharkey, M. E., I. Teo, T. Greenough, N. Sharova, K. Luzuriaga, J. L. Sullivan, R. P. Bucy, L. G. Kostrikis, A. Haase, C. Veryard, R. E. Davaro, S. H. Cheeseman, J. S. Daly, C. Bova, R. T. Ellison III, B. Mady, K. K. Lai, G. Moyle, M. Nelson, B. Gazzard, S. Shaunak, and M. Stevenson. 2000. Persistence of epi-

somal HIV-1 infection intermediates in patients on highly active anti-retroviral therapy. Nature Med. 6:76–81.

100. Sherman, P. A., and J. A. Fyfe. 1990. Human immunodeficiency virus integration protein expressed in Escherichia coli possesses selective DNA cleaving activity. Proc. Natl. Acad. Sci. USA 87:5119–5123.

101. Stevenson, M., T. L. Stanwick, M. P. Dempsey, and C. A. Lamonica. 1990. HIV-1 replication is controlled at the level of T cell activation and proviral integration. EMBO J. 9:1551–1560.

102. Taddeo, B., W. A. Haseltine, and C. M. Farnet. 1994. Integrase mutants of human immunodeficiency virus type 1 with a specific defect in integration. J. Virol. 68:8401–8405.

103. Tsurutani, N., M. Kubo, Y. Maeda, T. Ohashi, N. Yamamoto, M. Kannagi, and T. Masuda. 2000. Identification of critical amino acid residues in human immunodeficiency virus type 1 IN required for efficient proviral DNA formation at steps prior to integration in dividing and nondividing cells. J. Virol. 74:4795–4806.

104. van den Ent, F. M., C. Vink, and R. H. Plasterk. 1994. DNA substrate requirements for different activities of the human immunodeficiency virus type 1 integrase protein. J. Virol. 68:7825–7832.

105. van Gent, D. C., A. A. Oude Groeneger, and R. H. Plasterk. 1993. Identification of amino acids in HIV-2 integrase involved in site-specific hydrolysis and alcoholysis of viral DNA termini. Nucleic Acids Res. 21:3373–3377.

106. Vincent, K. A., V. Ellison, S. A. Chow, and P. O. Brown. 1993. Characterization of human immunodeficiency virus type 1 integrase expressed in Escherichia coli and analysis of variants with amino-terminal mutations. J. Virol. 67:425–437.

107. Vink, C., R. A. Lutzke, and R. H. Plasterk. 1994. Formation of a stable complex between the human immunodeficiency virus integrase protein and viral DNA. Nucleic Acids Res. 22:4103–4110.

108. Vora, A. C., and D. P. Grandgenett. 1995. Assembly and catalytic properties of retrovirus integrase-DNA complexes capable of efficiently performing concerted integration. J. Virol. 69:7483–7488.

109. Vora, A. C., M. McCord, M. L. Fitzgerald, R. B. Inman, and D. P. Grandgenett. 1994. Efficient concerted integration of retrovirus-like DNA in vitro by avian myeloblastosis virus integrase. Nucleic Acids Res. 22:4454–4461.

110. Wai, J. S., M. S. Egbertson, L. S. Payne, T. E. Fisher, M. W. Embrey, L. O. Tran, J. Y. Melamed, H. M. Langford, J. P. Guare, Jr., L. Zhuang, V. E. Grey, J. P. Vacca, M. K. Holloway, A. M. Naylor-Olsen, D. J. Hazuda, P. J. Felock, A. L. Wolfe, K. A. Stillmock, W. A. Schleif, L. J. Gabryelski, and S. D. Young. 2000. 4-Aryl-2,4-dioxobutanoic acid inhibitors of HIV-1 integrase and viral replication in cells. J. Med. Chem. 43:4923–4926.

111. Wei, S. Q., K. Mizuuchi, and R. Craigie. 1997. A large nucleoprotein assembly at the ends of the viral DNA mediates retroviral DNA integration. EMBO J. 16:7511–7520.

112. Wiskerchen, M., and M. A. Muesing. 1995. Human immunodeficiency virus type 1 integrase: effects of mutations on viral ability to integrate, direct viral gene expression from unintegrated viral DNA templates, and sustain viral propagation in primary cells. J. Virol. 69:376–386.

113. Wlodawer, A. 1999. Crystal structures of catalytic core domains of retroviral integrases and role of divalent cations in enzymatic activity. Adv. Virus Res. 52:335–350.

114. Wlodawer, A. 1999. Crystal structures of the catalytic core domains of retroviral integrases and the role of divalent cations in enzymatic activity, p. 335–350. *In* K. Maramorosch, F. A. Murphy, and A. J. Shatkin (ed.), Advances in virus research, vol. 52. Academic Press, New York.

115. Wolfe, A. L., P. J. Felock, J. C. Hastings, C. U. Blau, and D. J. Hazuda. 1996. The role of manganese in promoting multimerization and assembly of human immunodeficiency virus type 1 integrase as a catalytically active complex on immobilized long terminal repeat substrates. J. Virol. 70:1424–1432.

116. Wu, X., H. Liu, H. Xiao, J. A. Conway, E. Hehl, G. V. Kalpana, V. Prasad, and J. C. Kappes. 1999. Human immunodeficiency virus type 1 integrase protein promotes reverse transcription through specific interactions with the nucleoprotein reverse transcription complex. J. Virol. 73:2126–2135.

117. Wu, X., H. Liu, H. Xiao, J. A. Conway, E. Hunter, and J. C. Kappes. 1997. Functional RT and IN incorporated into HIV-1 particles independently of the Gag/Pol precursor protein. EMBO J. 16:5113–5122.

118. Wyatt, J. R., T. A. Vickers, J. L. Roberson, R. W. Buckheit, Jr., T. Klimkait, E. De-Baets, P. W. Davis, B. Rayner, J. L. Imbach, and D. J. Ecker. 1994. Combinatorially selected guanosine-quartet structure is a potent inhibitor of human immunodeficiency virus envelope-mediated cell fusion. Proc. Natl. Acad. Sci. USA 91:1356–1360.

119. Yang, W., and T. A. Steitz. 1995. Recombining the structures of HIV integrase, RuvC and RNase H. Structure 3:131–134.

120. Yang, Z. N., T. C. Mueser, F. D. Bushman, and C. C. Hyde. 2000. Crystal structure of an active two-domain derivative of Rous sarcoma virus integrase. J. Mol. Biol. 296:535–548.

121. Zack, J. A., A. M. Haislip, P. Krogstad, and I. S. Chen. 1992. Incompletely reverse-transcribed human immunodeficiency virus type 1 genomes in quiescent cells can function as intermediates in the retroviral life cycle. J. Virol. 66:1717–1725.

Chemokine Receptors in HIV Infection and AIDS

7

NATHANIEL R. LANDAU

Historical Perspectives

Identification of CD4 as a Receptor

One of the first hallmarks of AIDS to be recognized was the striking loss of circulating CD4$^+$ T cells that was associated with disease progression. The identification of CD4 as the receptor for HIV-1 entry in 1984 provided a straightforward explanation for HIV pathogenicity: the virus infects and then kills CD4$^+$ cells, gradually depleting Th cells. As a result, the protective function provided by the cellular arm of the immune system is lost. CD4 was identified as the HIV-1 receptor based on the findings that (i) transfecting HeLa cells with CD4 expression vector rendered them permissive to HIV-1 replication (116); (ii) HIV-1 infection could be inhibited with some anti-CD4 MAbs (44, 99); (iii) soluble recombinant gp120 bound with nanomolar affinity to cell surface CD4; and (iv) gp120 coimmunoprecipitated with CD4 in lysates of infected cells (125). Later, recombinant soluble CD4 (rsCD4) was found to be a potent inhibitor of laboratory HIV-1 isolates (reviewed in reference 209). These findings, taken together, clearly implicated CD4 as critically important for HIV-1 entry and strongly suggested that it serves as a required receptor for entry of the virus.

Hints of a Coreceptor

Resistance of Murine Cells to Infection. If CD4 were necessary and sufficient for HIV-1 entry, expressing it in nonhuman cells should cause them to become permissive for virus replication, or at least entry. Puzzlingly, murine 3T3 cells expressing transfected CD4 remained nonpermissive for both replication and virus entry (116). In fact, most nonhuman mammalian cells fail to support HIV-1 entry following the introduction of human CD4

250

vectors (141). Experiments with HIV-1 Env pseudotypes of vesicular stoma-
titus virus (VSV[HIV]) were particularly useful for demonstrating the
block to entry in nonhuman mammalian cells (116). Such pseudotypes entered human cells through CD4 but were unable to infect murine CD4+
cells. The block to HIV-1 entry in human CD4-expressing murine cells was
further demonstrated by pseudotyping HIV-1 virions with the amphotropic murine leukemia virus (A-MLV) Env (105, 114, 148). The A-MLV Env
allowed the virus to circumvent the entry block by using the amphotropic
receptor. Upon infection of murine cells, the pseudotyped virus proceeded
through entry and postentry steps including uncoating, reverse transcription, and integration. Studies using rodent/human heterokaryons provided evidence for a human-specific entry cofactor (59). While the virus
failed to enter hu-CD4+ rodent cells, fusing them to human cells complemented the defect. The most direct explanation of these findings was that
a cell surface cofactor in addition to CD4 had been provided in *trans* to
facilitate virus entry.

HIV-1 Isolates with Altered Tropism. By characterizing many independent virus isolates from different infected patients or from individual patients over time, it became apparent that there were differences in the properties of independent isolates. Viruses isolated in the asymptomatic phase
of the disease usually replicated slowly and were restricted in tropism.
They replicated in activated primary CD4+ T cells and monocyte-derived
macrophages (MDMs) but failed to infect transformed T-cell lines (M-
tropic) (31, 71, 74). In contrast, viruses isolated later, during the symptomatic phase of the disease, replicated efficiently on transformed cell lines
(reviewed in reference 129) and activated primary T cells but failed to
replicate on MDMs (T-tropic). A small proportion of clinical isolates had a
combined phenotype and could infect MDMs and transformed T-cell lines
(dual tropic). Interestingly, T-tropic viruses tended to appear in patients at
or just preceding the appearance of symptoms, a phenomenon termed the
"phenotypic switch" (129, 180). Virus tropism was typically defined on the
basis of whether isolates replicated and formed syncytia (SI) or not (NSI)
in the transformed T-cell line MT4. The association of T-tropic or SI virus
with CD4+ T-cell depletion suggested that these viruses might represent
the pathogenic form of the virus. However, it is important to note that phenotypic switching is detected in only about 50% of patients and thus is not
necessarily required for disease progression (81).

The cellular determinants of HIV-1 tropism were unknown, but the
major viral determinant controlling virus tropism mapped to the viral *env*
gene (82, 92, 144, 183, 184, 204). As might be expected considering the role
of Env in virus entry, tropism was found to be controlled prior to reverse
transcription of the incoming virus (144). Tropism was mapped to *env* by
swapping portions of *env* between viruses of different phenotypes and an-

alyzing the properties of the resulting chimeras. Virus phenotype was found to map largely to the region of Env containing the third variable loop (V3), and in some cases could be mapped to particular amino acids in the loop (82). V3 did not appear to be involved in CD4 binding but was the primary epitope bound by neutralizing antibodies. The finding that Env could control tropism without altering CD4 recognition was difficult to explain. It implied the existence of an entry cofactor that was either differentially expressed or present in different forms on the various target cell types.

Inhibitory Cytokines. The search for biological regulatory molecules that influence AIDS progression has been a central focus in the field as a whole. Such factors could be potent therapeutic tools and would also provide insight into AIDS pathogenesis. However, there was no suspicion that this field might provide a key to identifying the elusive entry cofactor.

In the late 1980s Jay Levy's group at the University of California, San Francisco, detected an activity in the culture supernatants of activated primary CD8$^+$ T cells that could inhibit HIV-1 replication in activated primary CD4$^+$ T cells in culture (201). They suggested that the unidentified factor, termed "CD8$^+$ T-cell antiviral factor" (CAF), might influence disease progression in patients (reviewed in reference 108) and that such a factor could have important therapeutic use. The factor appeared to be produced by CD8$^+$ T cells but did not correspond to any of the known interleukins.

Although the identity of that factor remains obscure to date, Cocchi et al. (37) detected potent inhibitory activity in the culture supernatants of immortalized CD8$^+$ T cells. Purification and sequencing of the activity revealed that it corresponded to three separate cytokines, each belonging to the chemokine family of chemotactic cytokines: RANTES (regulated on activation, normal T cell expressed and secreted), MIP-1α, and MIP-1β (macrophage inflammatory protein 1α and 1β). Interestingly, the chemokines inhibited M-tropic HIV-1 isolates but had no effect on T-tropic virus. RANTES was the most potent inhibitor of primary isolates; at 3 ng/ml it effectively shut down virus replication. MIP-1α and MIP-1β were only slightly less active. Data demonstrating the block to HIV-1 entry are illustrated in Fig. 7.1.

Identification of Chemokine Receptors as Coreceptors

The Chemokine/Chemokine Receptor System

Chemotactic cytokines, or chemokines, are secreted proteins, 70–100 amino acids in length, that regulate diverse physiological processes including leukocyte trafficking, angiogenesis, hematopoiesis, and organogenesis (for recent reviews, see references 12, 137). They are involved in

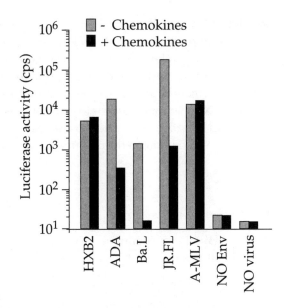

FIGURE 7.1

Detecting the chemokine-mediated
block to HIV-1 entry

PM1, a CD4+/CCR5+ human T-cell line, was treated with a mixture of
RANTES, MIP-1α, and MIP-1β. The treated cells were then infected with luciferase reporter viruses pseudotyped with M-tropic Envs (Ba.L, JR.FL, or
ADA), T-tropic Env (HXB2), or A-MLV Env. Virus lacking Env is also shown.
These viruses contain a luciferase reporter gene that is expressed in the infected
cells, and the amount of luciferase activity in the culture is shown. The
chemokines inhibited entry of M-tropic pseudotypes about 50- to 200-fold but
did not block entry of T-tropic or amphotropic virus.

acute inflammatory responses such as bacterial infection and sepsis and
also in chronic inflammatory conditions such as arthritis, inflammatory
bowel disease, asthma, and psoriasis. Their activity is most frequently
measured by their ability to induce the chemotaxis of specific subsets of
leukocytes, to activate intracellular second messengers such as inositol
phosphates, or to increase intracellular calcium concentration of target
cells. The chemokines fall into four classes (α, β, γ, δ) based on conserved
N-terminal cysteine residues. The majority of chemokines fall into the α
and β classes, which are defined by their respective CXC and CC motifs.
The other two classes, γ and δ, are defined by their C and CX_3C motifs, respectively, and each consists of a single member. The CXC chemokines, the
prototype for which is IL-8, act primarily on neutrophils; the CC
chemokines act on T and B lymphocytes and monocytes.

The chemokines exert their effects by binding to seven-transmembrane (7TM) G protein–coupled receptors (GPCRs) expressed on the responding cells. Typically, chemokine receptors are named according to their ligand binding specificity and are later subsequently renamed according to a systematic nomenclature. There are currently five receptors for the CC chemokines (CXCR1-5) and nine for the CC chemokines (CCR1-9). At least 50 chemokines have been described to date, and it is likely that additional ligands and receptors exist in the mammalian genome yet to be discovered.

Identification of the T-Tropic Virus Coreceptor

The first coreceptor for HIV-1 was identified in Edward Berger's laboratory at the National Institutes of Health using a gene transfer screening strategy (70). A human cDNA expression library was screened for the ability to render an hu-CD4$^+$ murine cell line permissive for fusion with a T-tropic Env. A single clone was isolated and found to encode a 7TM GPCR that had been earlier identified as the orphan receptor LESTR (leukocyte-derived 7TM domain receptor) (111) or HUMSTR. Berger termed this molecule "fusin" on the basis of its activity (70). Fusin was about 34% identical to the IL-8 receptor, a CXC chemokine receptor. It did not facilitate infection of M-tropic virus, suggesting the existence of at least one other coreceptor.

The ligands for fusin were later found to be the CXC chemokines stromal derived factor-1α (SDF-1α) and SDF-1β (alternatively spliced transcripts from the same gene) (23, 142). On the basis of its homology to CXCR1 and its ligand binding specificity, fusin was renamed CXCR4, in accordance with the systematic nomenclature. SDF1 had been defined as an activity produced by marrow stromal cells that promoted the growth of pre–B cell progenitors (139). It was a potent blocker of T-tropic HIV-1 entry but had no effect on M-tropic virus (23, 142).

Identification of the M-Tropic Virus Coreceptor

The identification of CXCR4 as a coreceptor for T-tropic HIV-1, combined with the identification of the inhibitory activity of the three CC chemokines, pointed to the existence of an M-tropic coreceptor whose ligands would be RANTES, MIP-1α, and MIP-1β. Just such a receptor was identified and, being the fifth CC receptor, was assigned the name CCR5 (39, 162, 173). It was activated by RANTES, MIP-1α, and MIP-1β (MCP-2 [macrophage chemoattractant protein-2] was later found to activate CCR5 also and inhibit HIV-1 infection) (80, 172). Shortly after its description, five groups reported within a few weeks that it functioned in transfected cells as a coreceptor for M-tropic isolates (1, 35, 48, 58, 60). In cells expressing a transfected CCR5 vector, infection with M-tropic virus could be inhibited by adding physiological concentrations of RANTES, MIP-1α, or MIP-1β. These findings tied together the earlier results: M- and T-tropism could be attributed to differential coreceptor use by the different viruses; CC and CXC chemokines inhibited M-tropic and T-tropic virus by interfering with the availability of the coreceptors to the viral Env; tropism was controlled by V3 sequences that altered the ability of Env to recognize CCR5 or CXCR4.

If the inhibitory activity of the chemokines was due to their ability to interfere with the Env-coreceptor interaction, then chemokines would be predicted to block HIV-1 entry but not to affect subsequent steps in the virus replication cycle. Studies using single-cycle pseudotyped reporter viruses demonstrated this to be the case. Pseudotypes containing the Env of M-tropic viruses JR.FL, ADA, or Ba.L were blocked by chemokine at an IC_{50} around 1 ng/ml (48); pseudotypes bearing T-tropic Env or A-MLV that enters cells using an unrelated receptor were not inhibited by 1,000-fold-higher concentrations of chemokine. Moreover, the chemokines specifically blocked entry based on their receptor binding activity. RANTES, MIP-1α, and MIP-1β blocked entry of M-tropic virus; SDF1 blocked entry of T-tropic virus.

Another prediction derived from these findings was that the murine homologs of the two chemokine receptors would not function as coreceptors. For CCR5, this is true. The murine protein differs from human by 18% and does not allow entry of any known HIV-1 isolates (10). For CXCR4, the prediction is not correct; mu-CXCR4 in transfected cell assays has considerable coreceptor activity, at least for some T-tropic isolates (18, 150, 194). Apparently, the lack of HIV-1 entry into murine cells expressing hu-CD4 was due to the absence of expression of the gene, not to a species-specific block as had been assumed over several years.

A Simple Model for HIV Tropism

These findings suggest a simple explanation for HIV-1 tropism in which coreceptor usage and cell-type expression determine target cell susceptibility to infection (diagrammed in Fig. 7.2). M-tropic virus uses CCR5 (Fig. 7.3), which is expressed on CD4+ T cells and monocytes/macrophages; T-tropic isolates use CXCR4, which is expressed on primary CD4+ cells and transformed T-cell lines. The "phenotypic switch" from M- to T-tropism (or more accurately "phenotypic expansion") that precedes the onset of disease symptoms would result from the appearance of viruses with additional coreceptor specificity.

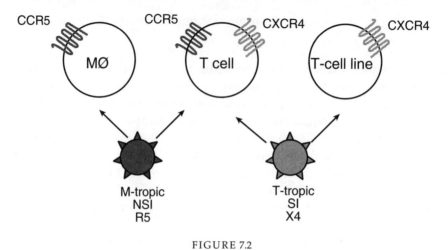

FIGURE 7.2

A simple model of HIV-1 tropism

In the model, CCR5 is expressed on MDMs and primary T cells but not on transformed T-cell lines. CXCR4 is expressed on primary T cells and transformed T-cell lines.

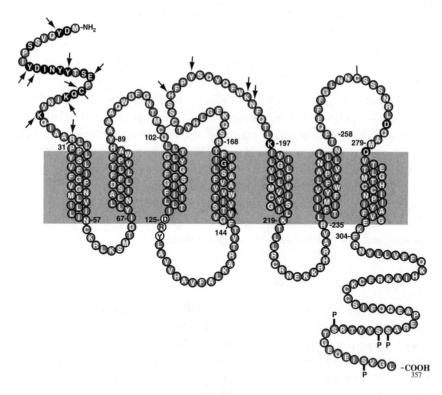

FIGURE 7.3

Schematic of CCR5

Functionally important amino acid residues are indicated. Arrows indicate residues required for chemokine binding. Phosphorylation sites in the cytoplasmic tail are indicated.

The model is for the most part supported by the evidence. All primary isolates to date replicate in activated CD4$^+$ T cells, and CCR5 and CXCR4 are both expressed at high levels in these cell types. In T cells, CCR5 is expressed at levels detectable by fluorescence-activated cell sorter (FACS) mainly on the CD45 RO$^+$ memory subset (24, 208), and these cells are efficient targets for HIV-1 replication (208). CCR5 is also expressed on MDMs, as predicted, and not expressed on the large majority of transformed T-cell lines (48, 208). PM1, a derivative of the transformed T-cell line HUT78 that had been reported to support replication of M-tropic isolates (113), is the only laboratory cell line to express CCR5 at readily detectable levels (48). CCR5 expression levels can be influenced by several cytokines, notably IL-2, which causes about a twofold increase in its cell surface levels (24).

The model has been somewhat problematic with respect to monocytes and MDMs. CCR5 is barely detectable on the immature monocytes that circulate in the blood but is induced upon differentiation into MDMs in culture and supports entry of M-tropic isolates (41, 140, 161, 188). However, some isolates use CCR5 but fail to infect MDMs, suggesting that CCR5 usage is not sufficient to allow infection of these cells (31, 54). An additional complexity is that MDMs express low to intermediate levels of CXCR4 (15, 53, 177, 200, 211) and mediate signal transduction in response to SDF-1α. Thus, these cells should be infected by CXCR4-specific viruses. Although they are classically not susceptible to infection by SI viruses, some such viruses do infect MDMs (187). The basis of these differences is not clear, but it could have to do with requirements for sufficient coreceptor and CD4 expression levels, culture conditions, and differences in virus isolates. MDMs may also have postentry-related restrictions to virus replication (132, 177).

MDMs present another complexity: chemokines seem to inhibit their infection by M-tropic viruses less efficiently than they inhibit T-cell infection. For some investigators, chemokines, especially RANTES (27, 38), effectively inhibit infection of MDMs, although generally at higher concentration than that required for T cells; for others, chemokines inhibit weakly even at mg/ml concentrations (60, 133, 146). Some differences may be attributed to different methods for isolating and culturing MDMs, as these can influence CD4 and coreceptor expression levels. In addition, chemokine inhibition appears to be augmented by cell surface heparin sulfate, which is not present on MDMs (146). The timing of chemokine addition may also be important. In contrast to expectation, adding chemokines before infection enhanced instead of inhibited infection; adding them postinfection was inhibitory (96).

The model further predicts that the NSI-to-SI switch that precedes AIDS-defining symptoms results from the diversification in coreceptor usage to encompass CXCR4 in addition to CCR5. This finding has been borne out in studies that have examined the coreceptor usage of viruses over the course of infection (15, 21, 42, 175). In one study, viruses isolated from rapid progressors during the asymptomatic phase were found to be restricted to CCR5 usage (42). Later, the majority of virus isolates efficiently used CXCR4 and to a lesser extent CCR2 and CCR3. Long-term nonprogressor isolates remained restricted to CCR5 over time.

To simplify HIV-1 nomenclature, it has been suggested that viruses be classified according to coreceptor usage rather than on the basis of tropism or phenotype. Thus, viruses that use CXCR4 are X4 viruses; those that use CCR5 are R5 viruses; dual-tropic viruses are R5X4 (16).

Identification of Minor Coreceptors

While CXCR4 and CCR5 support efficient entry of HIV-1 isolates, several 7TM GPCRs have been shown to have moderate to weak coreceptor activity for particular HIV-1, HIV-2, and simian immunodeficiency virus (SIV) isolates. CCR2B (58) and CCR3 (35, 58) have coreceptor activity for some M-tropic and dual-tropic isolates. CCR3 has coreceptor activity for some HIV-1 isolates and has been implicated in infection of microglial cells of the brain (83). Eotaxin, the primary ligand for CCR3, blocks infection of these cells in culture. STRL33/ Bonzo/TYMSTR and GPR15/BOB mediate efficient entry of the rhesus macaque virus, SIV_{mac} (49, 69). GPR1 is also active but to a lesser extent. Whether these are used in vivo is not clear, since all SIV_{mac} isolates to date also use CCR5 with high efficiency. Occasional HIV-1 isolates have been shown to use these in vitro (213).

CCR2B is the most similar to CCR5 (85% amino acid sequence identity), and thus its use might be expected. However, HIV-1 isolates that use it do so inefficiently, and the majority of primary isolates do not use it at detectable levels. An interesting exception to this rule is SIV-RCM (30, 76), a subtype of SIV derived from a red-capped mangeby in Gabon. The virus efficiently uses CCR2 for replication in cultured cells and presumably uses it in vivo as its major coreceptor. This seems to be an adaptation of the virus for growth in this species, for which a common allele of the CCR5 gene contains a 24-base-pair deletion.

Several other GPCRs have been shown to have at least some ability to support HIV-1 entry in laboratory infections or in syncytium assays. These molecules include CCR8 (88, 94, 171), CCR9 (34), V28/CX_3CR1/CMK-BRL1 (40, 171), APJ (34, 63), US28, a CC chemokine receptor encoded by human cytomegalovirus (156, 171), and the nonchemokine receptor molecule ChemR23, which is related to the formyl peptide receptor. BLTR, the leukotriene B_4 receptor, has also been reported to have coreceptor activity (147). Table 7.1 lists the major and minor HIV/SIV coreceptors.

It is also worth noting that chemokines in addition to MIP-1α, MIP-1β, and RANTES block entry of some HIV-1 isolates. Monocyte chemo-attractant protein-2 (MCP-2), which is a ligand for CCR5, blocks entry of

TABLE 7.1

Major and minor HIV/SIV coreceptors

	Receptor	Also known as	Ligands	Coreceptor activity	Expression
Major	CCR5	CC CKR5	MIP-1α, MIP-1β, RANTES	M-tropic and dual-tropic HIV-1, HIV-2, SIV	Monocytes, Th1 cells, memory (CD45RO) cells, stem cells, DCs, microglia
	CXCR4	LESTR, HUMSTR, FUSIN	SDF-1α, SDF-1β	T-tropic and dual-tropic HIV-1, HIV-2	T cells, B cells, fibroblasts, thymocytes, stem cells, monocytes, microglia, neutrophils
Minor	CCR2B	MCP-1RB	MCP-1, MCP-2, MCP-3, MCP-4	Some HIV-1	Monocytes, Th1 and Th2 cells, stem cells
	CCR3	EotaxinR, CC CKR3	Eotaxin, RANTES, MCP-2, MCP-3, MCP-4	Some HIV-1 and HIV-2	Eosinophils, microglia, Th2 cells, DCs, basophils
	CCR8	ChemR1	I-309, MIP-1β	HIV-1, HIV-2, SIV	Monocytes, thymocytes
	CCR9			Some HIV-1 and SIV	Thymocytes
	CX₃CR1	CMKBRL1, V28	Fractalkine	HIV-2, some HIV-1	Neutrophils, monocytes, T lymphocytes, brain
	GPR15	BOB	Orphan	SIV, some HIV-1, and HIV-2	T cells, colon
	STRL33	BONZO	Orphan	SIV	T cells, monocytes, placenta
	APJ		Orphan	T-tropic and dual-tropic HIV-1, SIV	Brain, activated PBMCs
	US28		Orphan	Some HIV-1 (i.e., ADA and Ba.L)	Encoded by cytomegalovirus

M-tropic isolates (78, 172), and eotaxin (83), the primary ligand for CCR3, blocks infection of brain microglial cells. MDC (monocyte-derived chemokine) was reported to block M- and T-tropic isolates (149), a finding that is surprising because its receptor is CCR4 (93), which does not have co-receptor activity. Initially this finding could not be independently confirmed (9, 13, 170); however, a recent report suggested that MDC inhibits HIV replication in MDM and that it acts after entry (43a).

Are the Minor Coreceptors Physiologically Relevant?

The importance of CCR5 and CXCR4 as coreceptors in vivo is clear (as discussed in later sections). Their use by nearly all primary HIV-1 isolates regardless of clade or geographic origin supports this conclusion. This finding is striking given the considerable variability in Env primary sequence between these diverse virus isolates. Furthermore, SIV_{mac} isolates nearly always use CCR5, although STRL33 and GPR15 can substitute (2, 49).

The physiological importance of the minor coreceptors in vivo is less clear. These chemokine receptors facilitate entry of only a small minority of HIV isolates and then usually only with reduced efficiency. Moreover, viruses that are able to use a minor coreceptor seem to prefer to use either of the majors. A survey of a large number of primary isolates for ability to infect $CCR5\Delta32/CCR5\Delta32$ T cells (cells lacking cell surface CCR5) showed that most failed to infect these cells and that those that did could be blocked by SDF-1α (212). Another analysis of coreceptor usage of various primary isolates showed that nearly all used either CCR5 or CXCR4, although occasional SI viruses that used CXCR4 could also efficiently use V28, APJ and CCR8 (213). Moreover, viruses that can use STRL33/Bonzo on transfected cell lines fail to replicate in T cells lacking CCR5. Similarly, a series of SI primary viruses used a broad range of coreceptors on transfected cell lines but were inefficient at infecting CCR5⁻ MDMs, suggesting that they preferred to use CCR5. Adding a CXCR4 antagonist completely blocked their infection, demonstrating that the viruses entered only through CCR5 or CXCR4 (187). For SIV, usage of BOB/GPR15 in vitro is clear, but a recent study showed that SIV_{mac} containing a Pro321 → Ser alteration in Env could not use this coreceptor but maintained its pathogenicity in infected macaques (157).

Of the minor coreceptors, only CCR3 has been implicated as being used in vivo. CCR3 has been found in some studies to mediate efficient entry of several HIV-1 isolates (15, 35, 171) but not in others (21, 41, 48, 60, 212), and supporting its physiological relevance, its coreceptor activity is blocked by eotaxin in microglial cells of the brain (35, 83).

One caveat concerning in vivo coreceptor usage involves the requirement that cells coexpress CD4 to be infectable. Chemokine receptors such as CCR2 are expressed on T cells and MDMs and therefore have the potential to serve as coreceptors on primary cells. For potential coreceptors such as CCR3, Apj, and ChemR23, this is less clear.

Another caveat concerning the relevance of the minor coreceptors lies in the methods that are used to detect their activity. Some of the laboratory methods to detect coreceptor activity are very sensitive and thus can overestimate the ability of virus isolate to use a particular coreceptor. For example, syncytium-formation assays are frequently used in which an Env expression vector and chemokine receptor expression vector are introduced into two different cell populations that are then cocultivated. Fusion of two cells involves a much larger surface area and a much greater number of molecular interactions than that which occurs during virus-cell interaction. Moreover, expression vectors generally overexpress both the Env and the coreceptor. Other methods involve infecting CD4/coreceptor transfected cell lines. Such cells are also likely to overexpress the transfected gene products. Thus, a surface protein that has coreceptor activity in a laboratory assay may not be used for virus entry at a meaningful frequency in vivo. A more accurate method of judging coreceptor usage is to monitor virus entry on primary cells using antibody or chemical inhibitors of the chemokine receptor in question.

Coreceptor Polymorphisms in AIDS Pathogenesis

A central question in understanding HIV pathogenesis is why disease progression rates vary so much from person to person. Explanations fall into two broad categories: the virus or the host. In "the virus" explanation, progression rates are influenced by infection of the subject with viruses of differing pathogenicity. Rapid progressors would be infected with highly cytopathic, rapidly replicating virus; slow progressors would have received naturally occurring attenuated virus variants. Two examples of infection with attenuated viruses have been reported; in both, the individuals harbored viruses that contained deletions in Nef (98). In the Sydney blood bank cohort, prior to 1985, a donor transmitted to eight recipients an attenuated virus harboring a deletion in Nef and in the long terminal repeats. These individuals maintained low virus loads and experienced little disease progression. In the majority of long-term nonprogressors, however, no attenuation of the virus is discerned by DNA sequence analysis (90). Thus "the virus" explanation is probably very rare, and host differences are likely to be at work in the vast majority of cases.

Differences in the susceptibility of individuals to HIV-1 infection had been suggested in several early epidemiological studies. Discordant couples have been identified in which one partner is infected and the other, although repeatedly exposed to the virus through unprotected sex, remains uninfected (36). The most dramatic example of this phenomenon involves commercial sex workers in Africa (73, 168). In a cohort of Nairobi prostitutes who were subjected to daily multiple exposures through unprotected intercourse but were uninfected at the start of the study, about 10% remained uninfected over several years (73). Statistical analysis of the likelihood of infection of an individual in the cohort over a year showed that the uninfected individuals were truly resistant and not simply statistical outliers. According to "the host" theory, resistance could have been caused by an immune mechanism in which the host develops a protective immunity in response to frequent exposure to viral antigen (17, 36, 168), or, alternatively, host genes could provide innate resistance to infection.

Initial analysis of virus susceptibility and disease progression focused on the influence of the major histocompatibility complex (MHC). The MHC is highly polymorphic, and susceptibility to a number of infectious diseases in humans and laboratory mice has been linked to specific MHC haplotypes. HLA and TAP alleles have recently been confirmed as influencing AIDS progression beneficially (119) or negatively (29). With the advent of HIV coreceptors and their inhibitory ligands, the genes encoding these proteins became prime suspects as the source of disease-controlling polymorphisms. Epidemiological studies coupled with genetic analyses have since implicated polymorphisms in both the receptors and their ligands as key factors influencing AIDS progression rates and transmission susceptibility.

CCR5Δ32/CCR5Δ32 *Protects against HIV-1 Transmission*

Evidence for genetic resistance to HIV-1 infection was first demonstrated in Richard Koup's laboratory at the Aaron Diamond AIDS Research Center in a cohort of multiply exposed uninfected (EU) individuals. Laboratory infection of the activated primary CD4+ T cells from 26 EU donors showed that two donors' primary cells failed to support M-tropic virus replication (153). The cells readily supported T-tropic virus replication, suggesting that the defect was at virus entry. In two of the donors, and then later in a third (R. Liu and N. Landau, unpublished observations), this was found to be due to a homozygous 32-base-pair deletion in the region of the coding sequence corresponding to the second extracellular loop of the receptor (110, 174). The encoded protein failed to be expressed on the surface of the donor T cells or of cell lines transfected with expression vectors containing the deleted CCR5 allele. Not surprisingly, the encoded protein lacked detectable coreceptor activity.

The deleted allele, termed *CCR5Δ32*, is present at a frequency of about 0.1 in American and European Caucasians and is present at Hardy-Weinberg equilibrium (++ 83%, +/− 14%, and −/− 1–3%) (110, 123, 174), indicating an absence of pronounced selection pressure in the general population. Analysis of the allele frequency in infected populations showed a very different frequency. Homozygous wild types and heterozygotes were represented at control levels, but the homozygous *CCR5Δ32/CCR5Δ32* genotype was virtually absent (47, 89, 174), a finding that has been confirmed in several studies using a total of several thousand individuals (67, 126, 151, 215).

Initially, *CCR5Δ32/CCR5Δ32* homozygotes appeared to be completely protected from HIV-1 infection because none was found to be infected; however, subsequent studies have to date identified a total of eight infected homozygotes (14, 20, 84, 102, 143, 195). With what viruses were these individuals infected? Where it has been studied, virus isolated from infected *CCR5Δ32/CCR5Δ32* homozygotes exclusively used CXCR4 (128). Thus, entry through CCR5 is not absolutely required for transmission (although it is highly preferred). The failure of the homozygous *CCR5Δ32/CCR5Δ32* genotype to provide absolute protection means that individuals with the genotype are at risk of infection upon high-risk behavior and do not benefit from knowing their genetic status. It is also worth noting that the remainder of the original EU cohort was *CCR5⁺/CCR5⁺*, as are the Kenyan prostitutes (169), suggesting that other, less clear-cut mechanisms, possibly involving T-cell-mediated immunity (17, 36), exist that lead to resistance to infection (77).

Taken together, these findings link the laboratory identification of the HIV-1 coreceptors to their function "in the field." They establish a critical role for CCR5 in transmission of the virus and demonstrate the in vivo importance of CXCR4. The findings argue against the hypothesis that it is the CXCR4-specific virus that is solely responsible for AIDS pathogenesis. The rare infected *CCR5Δ32/CCR5Δ32* individuals do not appear to experience particularly rapid disease progression as would be predicted by this hypothesis. Thus, the phenotypic switch is not the cause of AIDS; it is more likely the result of a deteriorating immune response that previously held virus replication in check.

CCR5⁺/CCR5Δ32 *Genotype Delays Disease Progression*

Unlike homozygotes, *CCR5⁺/CCR5Δ32* heterozygotes are fully susceptible to HIV-1 transmission. This conclusion is derived from comparing the frequency of infected versus uninfected heterozygotes. In most studies, the frequency of infected heterozygotes is not significantly different from that of the uninfected control groups, both for adults (47, 89, 126) and for maternal-infant transmission (62, 118, 130, 167, 182). A few studies have noted a small decrease in the frequency of infected heterozygotes; however, it is not clear that these differences are statistically significant. Samson et al. (174) found in a study of discordant couples that a weak protection was associated with heterozygosity (10.8%, compared with 16.2% infected:noninfected [n = 1,427]). A protective effect of heterozygosity on maternal-fetal transmission was reported by Mandl et al. (117), who found

5.9% compared with 17.8% transmission rates for heterozygous versus wild-type infected mothers.

Although *CCR5Δ32* heterozygosity has modest effects on transmissibility, it has a clear influence on AIDS progression (47, 67, 89, 95, 126, 151, 163, 215). Overall, it is associated with a delay of about two years in time to progression of disease and time to death and is associated with significant decreases in viral load throughout the disease course (25, 50, 89, 95, 127). The effect of the mutant allele becomes more pronounced when subjects are classified according to their virus phenotype in addition to *CCR5* genotype. Heterozygotes whose virus is restricted to CCR5 showed a marked delay in disease progression; subjects with CXCR4-specific virus are not protected by *CCR5Δ32* heterozygosity. This finding makes sense because once viruses have emerged that use CXCR4, the influence of CCR5 expression level becomes less critical. The effect of *CCR5Δ32* heterozygosity can be modeled using the SCID-hu mouse model (155). In mice reconstituted with heterozygous as compared with wild-type peripheral blood lymphocytes, T-cell depletion was delayed, and virus loads were significantly reduced. In a few studies, *CCR5Δ32* heterozygotes were not found to delay disease progression (131, 135, 176, 205). Such apparent discrepancies are likely to be due to differences in the effect of the allele at different stages of the disease. Late in infection, disease progression may appear to accelerate as the *CCR5Δ32* heterozygotes catch up with the homozygotes.

It seems likely that the *CCR5Δ32*-associated delay in disease progression results from the effective twofold decrease in CCR5 gene dosage. On average, heterozygous primary CD4$^+$ T cells have half as much cell surface CCR5 as do those of homozygous wild types (120, 152, 208). The decrease in CCR5 abundance presumably results in less efficient virus entry, causing the observed reduction in virus load and reduced rate of T-cell depletion. Taken together, these findings point out how dependent disease progression is on relatively small differences in CCR5 expression level. They also demonstrate that CCR5 not only is critical for virus transmission in most cases but also serves as a key rate-limiting factor in AIDS pathogenesis. This conclusion leads to the suspicion that in addition to coding region polymorphisms that affect the primary structure of CCR5, there may be regulatory mechanisms that control coreceptor cell surface levels that also influence disease progression.

The findings described above highlight the rich source of information that has been provided by the evolutionary quirk of *CCR5Δ32*. The allele appears to have arisen around 700 years ago in northern Europe, most likely from a single individual (192). In parts of Scandinavia and Russia, 1–3% of individuals are homozygous *CCR5Δ32/CCR5Δ32*, while about 14% are heterozygous (123). The allele is not present at significant frequency in Asian or African populations. Assuming a single individual as its source, the allele frequency increased rapidly in northern Europe to achieve the current-day frequency of 0.1. The rapid rise in allele frequency suggests that some sort of selective pressure was at work, perhaps, analogous to the selection for mutant hemoglobin alleles that provide resistance to malaria in regions of Africa. What sort of selective pressure could have selected for *CCR5Δ32* 700 years ago in northern Europe? It seems highly unlikely that an early unrecorded AIDS epidemic could have been the source. It has been speculated that *CCR5Δ32* provided resistance to bubonic plague, which swept through Europe in the fourteenth century (192). However, there is no evidence supporting this possibility, and it seems unlikely that the pathogen Yersinia pestis uses CCR5 as a receptor.

The *CCR5Δ32/CCR5Δ32* genotype has no known clinical manifestation. This is perhaps not surprising given the amount of redundancy in the chemokine/chemokine receptor system. Most chemokines bind multiple receptors, and most of the receptors bind multiple ligands (216). Moreover, single cells typically express several chemokine receptors, some with overlapping binding specificities. As is the case in humans, CCR5 is dispensable in mice (214). *CCR5* knockout mice are viable and healthy, but a modest reduction compared with wild-type littermates has been noted in their ability to clear Listeria infection, probably due to a defect in MDM function. The mice also have increased B- and T-cell responses to antigenic challenge, suggesting a potential negative regulatory role for CCR5.

Rare Coding Region Polymorphisms

Additional polymorphisms in the CCR5 coding region have been found, although these are present at much lower frequency than *CCR5Δ32*. *CCR5m303*, identified in French blood donors, contains a single nucleotide mutation that introduces an in-frame stop codon in the first extracellular loop of the receptor (159). A single, multiply exposed uninfected individual was identified with the genotype *CCR5Δ32/CCR5m303*, and the individual's T cells were resistant to M-tropic HIV-1 infection. Additional rare alleles have been found containing single amino acid substitutions or deletions (28) or a one-base-pair deletion causing a C-terminal 54 amino acid truncation of the cytoplasmic tail present at an allelic frequency of 4% in Japanese and Chinese populations (5). Whether these alleles affect resistance or pathogenicity is not known.

In contrast to CCR5, allelic variants of CXCR4 are much rarer. In a study of more than 200 individuals, only a single synonymous nucleotide substitution was found (121). This probably reflects an essential physiological role for this receptor. Supporting this possibility is the finding that knockout mice for either CXCR4 or its ligand, SDF-1α, are lethal, leading to brain and heart formation defects and suggesting a critical role for the receptor in development (138, 217). In addition, the reciprocally exclusive binding of SDF-1α with CXCR4 suggests a lack of redundancy for this receptor-ligand pair. In contrast, CCR5 binds at least four CC chemokines.

CCR5 Promoter Polymorphisms

As discussed above, HIV-1 replication in vivo seems to be sensitive to small differences in CCR5 expression level. Analysis of the infectability of donor T cells and CCR5 cell surface density shows wide donor-to-donor variability in CCR5 expression level. These differences correlated with how well M-tropic virus replicated on the donor T cells (208). Thus, it seems likely that polymorphisms in the genome that control CCR5 expression help determine virus transmissibility and disease progression rates. Polymorphisms in genomic sequences that regulate *CCR5* transcription are likely candidates. In addition, polymorphisms in the genes that encode the inhibitory chemokines or genes that control intracellular trafficking and stability of chemokine receptors could also be important. Much attention has been devoted to associations between disease progression rates and various polymorphisms in potential chemokine receptor and chemokine transcriptional regulatory regions; however, few experimental data have been reported on possible mechanism.

The CCR2-64I *Allele*

The gene in the genome most similar to CCR5 is CCR2. CCR2, which is produced as two spliced variants, CCR2A and CCR2B, is about 82% identical to CCR5 and is encoded on a gene lying 15 kb 5′ of *CCR5*. CCR2B has weak coreceptor activity for only a few HIV-1 isolates but is not generally considered a physiologically important coreceptor. A polymorphic allele for CCR2, *CCR2-64I* (189), is present in various populations at relatively high frequency (Caucasians, 10%; African Americans, 15%; Asians, 25%; and Hispanics, 17%). The allele encodes a variant CCR2B molecule containing a Val64 → Ile substitution in the first transmembrane domain of the receptor. The allele is associated with a delay in disease progression comparable to that in *CCR5Δ32* heterozygotes (189), a finding that has been confirmed in some cohorts (100, 135, 165) but not in others (66, 127, 176). Its effect seems more pronounced in African Americans (135) and Africans (6) than in Caucasians. The effect is more noticeable in seroincident than in seroprevalent subjects in study groups (100). This could be because the delaying effect occurs early in the disease course. Over time, disease progression in the *CCR2-64I* individuals catches up, obscuring the effect.

Identifying a mechanism by which the *CCR2-64I* allele exerts its effect on disease progression has been difficult. CCR2 is not used by the vast majority of HIV-1 isolates. The mutation does not affect CCR2 ligand binding or signaling (107, 120). It has been suggested that the mutant allele may dimerize with CXCR4, inducing its endocytosis and thereby reducing its coreceptor activity, although evidence supporting this mechanism is lacking. It seems more likely that the *CCR2-64I* effect is due not to CCR2 itself but rather to a marker that is in linkage disequilibrium with it. The best candidate for such a polymorphism would be one that affects *CCR5*, which is physically linked on chromosome 3 (47, 110).

Potential Regulatory Polymorphisms

Mutations in the CCR5 coding region are not found in association with *CCR2-64I*; however, a complex constellation of polymorphisms has been described in sequences corresponding to potential regulatory regions flanking the gene (122, 135). Kostrikis et al. (100) identified a mutation in the first intron of CCR5 that was tightly linked to *CCR2-64I*, and Martin et al. (122) identified 10 different alleles of *CCR5* designated P1–P10. The P1 allele was associated with an acceleration in disease progression rate of about four years. In addition, an A $\rightarrow$ G substitution at nt 59029 is associated with a four-year delay in progression to AIDS (124). In promoter reporter assays, the mutant allele was about twofold less active than wild type, a finding that has not yet been independently confirmed but that could provide the first mechanistic explanation of the effect. Whether the endogenous allele affects *CCR5* mRNA levels or CCR5 protein levels in primary T cells has not been reported.

SDF1-3'A

In light of the inhibitory activities of the coreceptor ligands, alterations in their coding sequences or regulatory regions could have effects on AIDS progression analogous to those in *CCR5*. A G $\rightarrow$ A transition at nt 801 in the region corresponding to the 3'-untranslated region of SDF-1α, called SDF-1-3'A, is the first example of this (206). Homozygosity for SDF-1 3'A was found in the initial report to delay disease progression to an extent at least as great as *CCR5Δ32* heterozygosity. Similar findings were reported for the French GRIV cohort (85), but in others (135, 198), the allele was found to be associated with accelerated rather than delayed AIDS progression. With regard to mechanism, Winkler et al. (206) speculated that the polymorphism increases SDF-1α mRNA half-life. This would increase systemic levels of the ligand, inhibiting HIV entry and decreasing virus loads. Mechanistic studies have not yet been reported on whether the genotype is associated with increased SDF-1α levels.

Disease association with a second chemokine polymorphism was recently reported (109). A C $\rightarrow$ G mutation at nt–28 in the RANTES promoter appears to associate with AIDS pathogenesis. The allele is present in the Japanese population with a frequency of 0.17. Infected individuals with the allele show a reduced rate of $CD4^+$ T-cell depletion. In reporter assays, the −28G promoter was slightly more active than the wild-type RANTES promoter. It was speculated that the more active RANTES promoter could increase systemic levels of this inhibitory chemokine.

A Caveat Concerning Mechanism

Much attention has been given to the association of chemokine and chemokine receptor polymorphisms with AIDS, yet little attention has been paid to the mechanism by which these mutations might act. Without evidence that the polymorphisms themselves have a cellular phenotype, it is not possible to know whether they cause the observed effects on AIDS pathogenesis or serve as markers for other yet unidentified linked genes. To date, the different genotypes have not been correlated with CCR5 mRNA and protein levels or chemokine levels. Moreover, promoter activities have not been reported for most of the *CCR5* promoter polymorphisms. In addition, the SDF-1 3′-A polymorphism has not yet been tested for effects on mRNA stability or SDF-1α protein level.

Coreceptor-Mediated Entry Mechanisms

Mechanism of Coreceptor-Mediated Entry

The HIV-1 Env is a trimer (68) of noncovalently linked gp120:gp41 subunits; gp120 contains the CD4 and coreceptor binding sites, and gp41 is the transmembrane component that mediates virus-cell membrane fusion. Gp120 consists of five variable loops (V1–V5) and five conserved regions (C1–C5). The importance of V3 has been described in a large body of literature, predating the identification of coreceptors (209). V3 serves as a binding site for many neutralizing antibodies against the virus and is the most critical determinant of HIV-1 tropism and coreceptor specificity. Structural analysis suggests that the coreceptor binding site is composed of the stems of V1/V2, which form a sheet, and C4.

For viruses such as influenza, entry occurs in a two-step mechanism in which the hemagglutinin binds cell surface carbohydrate and subsequently, upon exposure to low-pH endosomes, fusion is initiated (202). HIV-1 entry can be thought of as a similar process but one that is pH independent and requires an additional step. Virus attachment is initiated by binding of gp120 to CD4. This induces a conformational change in gp120 that exposes its coreceptor binding site. Following interaction with the coreceptor, the gp41 hydrophobic peptide, which is effectively spring-loaded in the native trimer state, is triggered. This causes it to extend into the lipid bilayer of the target cell, inducing fusion of the virus and cell membranes.

This sequence of events has not been observed in real time but can be inferred from a large body of supporting data (for a review, see reference 209). Initial binding to CD4 followed by binding to the coreceptor is suggested by the ability of soluble gp120 to bind CD4 with high affinity but only weakly to the coreceptor (106, 196, 207). Treating gp120 with soluble CD4 (sCD4) allows it to bind CCR5 with affinity sufficient to compete with MIP-1α or MIP-1β (86, 196, 207) and to form a ternary complex that can be immunoprecipitated (106). Changes in gp120 conformation following CD4 binding can be detected by the ability of various gp120–specific MAbs to bind more readily following sCD4 binding. Changes in gp120 conformation following CD4 binding are also suggested by the crystal structure of the ternary complex of gp120:CD4:anti–gp120 solved by Kwong et al. (103). The existence of HIV-2 and SIV Envs that are able to mediate fusion in the absence of CD4 is of interest in this regard (64, 65, 164). These Envs interact with the coreceptor in the absence of CD4, allowing infection of CD4⁻ cells. Such Envs are predicted to exist in the partially triggered state in which the coreceptor binding site is constitutively exposed.

Binding Domains on CCR5 and CXCR4

Chemokine receptors are oriented in the cell membrane with the N-terminus outside and the C-terminus inside the cell. The 7TM regions span the membrane in an antiparallel arrangement, supporting three extracellular loops and three intracellular loops. The intracellular loops and C-tail serve as interaction sites for the trimeric G proteins, while the extracellular loops and N-terminus serve as sites for ligand binding. Functional domains on the coreceptors were initially analyzed by generating chimeric receptors and then testing their ability to support HIV-1 infection, ligand binding, or MAb recognition. Testing chimeric mouse/human CCR5 (10, 19, 101, 154), CCR5/CCR2 (10, 57), or CXCR4/CXCR2 and CXCR4/CCR5 (112) for ability to support entry of M-tropic and T-tropic viruses provided a complex picture of gp120 interaction domains. Overall, the N-terminus and the second extracellular loop appeared to be critical. However, these analyses were complicated by several examples of nonreciprocal binding specificities in which both chimeras either failed to support virus entry or were both active. These complexities probably reflect interaction of Env with multiple regions of the coreceptor.

Point mutagenesis has also implicated the N-terminus and the extracellular loops as important, although precise binding sites have yet to be defined. Mapping has been difficult because most single amino acid changes have no altered phenotype (57). As might be expected, the two pairs of disulfide-bonded extracellular loop Cys residues are important for chemokine binding but surprisingly are not critical for HIV-1 entry (22), suggesting flexibility in the Env-coreceptor interaction. Amino acid residues that have been shown to be important for entry of some HIV-1 isolates are clustered in the extracellular N-terminal domain. Ala substitutions at positions 2, 11, and 18 and substitution of Tyr residues, particularly Tyr15, were found to be critical for entry of CCR5-specific isolates (57, 61, 160). Gly163, which lies at the border of the fourth transmembrane segment and ECL-2, has been shown to be important (185). In the African green monkey, CCR5, Gly163 contains an Arg substitute. As a result it has little coreceptor activity. Changing it back to Gly restores its coreceptor activity for M-tropic HIV-1 Envs.

Env Determinants of Coreceptor Recognition

Early studies using viruses with chimeric Env showed that the V3 loop, and to a lesser extent V1 and V2 (81), were critical for determining HIV-1 tropism. Revisiting this topic following identification of the coreceptors showed that mutations in V3 could determine coreceptor specificity (91, 190). Moreover, clinical isolates that changed from CCR5 to CXCR4 usage during disease progression altered their V3 loop sequence to change coreceptor specificity (175). Analysis of the sequences of primary isolates with differing tropisms showed that V3 loops with a negative charge or no charge tend to be M-tropic or NSI, whereas those with a positive charge tend to be T-tropic or SI (32, 72, 210). The N-terminus of CXCR4 is rich in negative charges, and thus the trend toward increasingly positive V3 loops may be an adaptation of Env to fit the coreceptor. It therefore seems likely that V3 forms at least a part of the interaction site with the coreceptor. In addition to V3, studies using chimeric Envs have implicated V1 and V2 as influencing coreceptor recognition (87, 166). Introducing V1/V2 or V3 from a dual-tropic virus into AD8, a CCR5-specific virus, was sufficient to allow it to use CXCR4 (33).

Inhibition of Infection by Chemokines

Inhibition of HIV-1 entry by chemokines appears to be mediated by a combination of competitive binding of chemokines to the coreceptor and to ligand-induced endocytosis of the receptor (4, 8, 86, 196). Removing the cytoplasmic tail of CXCR4 (4) or CCR5 (3) prevented its endocytosis in response to ligand and reduced the potency of the chemokine in blocking HIV-1 entry. Ligand binding to CCR5 results in the rapid phosphorylation of Ser and Thr residues in the cytoplasmic tail (145). Phosphorylation may be mediated by G protein kinases 2 or 3. Following phosphorylation the receptor is internalized, in a β-arrestin-mediated process (8).

Role of Signaling through the Coreceptor

The possibility that gp120 binding to CD4 and coreceptor induces intracellular signals is attractive. Signaling could conceivably play a role in entry or in enhancing virus replication. The natural ligands induce signal transduction through the associated G proteins upon binding to chemokine receptors, and HIV-1 may have evolved to mimic ligand binding. Such a scenario would provide a rationale for the use of the chemokine receptors as coreceptors. However, this possibility appears not to be the case. Mutant CCR5 molecules that are defective in signaling owing to truncation of the cytoplasmic tail or to alteration of the highly conserved DRY G-protein interaction site or Phe293 are functional coreceptors (3, 8, 79). In addition, pertussis toxin, which inhibits G_i signaling, does not interfere with virus entry (3, 15). Thus, signaling through the coreceptor is not required for virus entry.

The finding that signaling is not required for entry should not be taken to mean that Env-induced signaling plays no role in infection. Signaling could act postentry. It might, for example, prime target T cells for efficient infection, could increase their ability to produce new virions following proviral formation, or could induce chemotaxis of uninfected target cells toward infected cells, increasing the efficiency of virus spread. Evidence for enhanced virus replication as a result of chemokine binding has been reported (97, 197).

Two types of Env-induced signals have been detected. Recombinant soluble gp160 truncated before the membrane-spanning domain induced transient calcium fluxes and chemotaxis in a T-cell line and in activated primary $CD4^+$ T cells. M-tropic HIV-1 gp160s and $SIV_{mac}239$ gp160, applied at physiological concentration, were active; T-tropic HIV-1 was not (203). Gp160 also induces tyrosine phosphorylation of pyk2 (46), a nonreceptor tyrosine kinase that is involved in transducing intracellular signals from GPCRs and is activated by intracellular calcium (52). In contrast to calcium flux, both M- and T-tropic Envs were active.

Therapeutic Strategies

Chemokine Analogs and Small-Molecule
Inhibitors of CXCR4 and CCR5

Several companies have developed chemokine receptor antagonists (reviewed in reference 181). Given the success with which 7TM GPCRs have been targeted in the past (e.g., adrenaline, dopamine, serotonin, histamine), it seems likely that additional antagonists of CCR5 and CXCR4 will be identified and that at least some of these will find therapeutic application. Small-molecule antagonists have already been identified for several of the chemokine receptors, including CCR1, CCR2, CCR3, CXCR4, and CCR5.

The first CCR5 antagonists described were chemokine derivatives that, as a result of modification to their N-termini, failed to transduce signals yet maintained the ability to bind their receptor. AOP-RANTES, in which the N-terminal Ser residue is replaced with aminooxypentane, inhibits M-tropic virus replication at about 10-fold lower IC_{50} as compared with native RANTES (186) yet does not induce a chemotactic response in target cells. It does this by a threefold mechanism. It blocks the interaction of gp120 with CCR5, stimulates CCR5 internalization, and prevents its recycling to the surface (115). AOP-RANTES is not completely inactive in inducing signal transduction and therefore is not a true antagonist (145). RANTES has also been modified by adding a methionine residue to its N-terminus. Met-RANTES is a potent HIV-1 entry inhibitor and is much reduced in agonist activity (158). A small-molecule antagonist of CCR5, TAK-779, has recently been described (11). The molecule blocks RANTES binding to CCR5 with an IC_{50} of 1.4 nM and inhibits M-tropic HIV-1 replication at 2 nM.

Small-molecule antagonists that inhibit T-tropic virus replication have also been identified. A family of bicyclic small molecules, the bicyclams, the prototype of which is AMD3100, bind CXCR4, inhibiting entry of T-tropic virus at an ID_{50} of about 1 ng/ml (55, 179). The compound appears to interact specifically with ECL2 on CXCR4 (104). In the SCID-hu Thy/Liv model, bicyclams have been shown to reduce virus loads and prevent CD4$^+$ cell depletion (45). Another compound, ALX40-4C, blocks T-tropic HIV-1 entry, blocks SDF1-α-induced signaling, and prevents the binding of the anti-CXCR4 MAb 12G5 to cells (56). A peptide CXCR4 antagonist with similar properties has also been identified (7, 136). The peptide, T134, and its variant are 14 amino and 18 amino acids, respectively, and are analogs of a peptide isolated from horseshoe crab hemocytes.

Mechanisms of Resistance to Chemokine Receptor Inhibitors

One of the shortcomings of current antiviral drugs lies in the ability of the virus to become resistant to their inhibitory effects. Current drugs target the viral reverse transcriptase or protease, both of which are relatively tolerant of amino acid sequence alterations and mutate at high frequency during virus replication. In contrast, the coreceptor genes are cellular and not viral, and thus their mutation rate is negligible. This leads to the possibility that coreceptor antagonists will be less susceptible to the generation of resistant virus. Moreover, the absence of clinical effect due to the lack of CCR5 in CCR5Δ32 homozygotes is encouraging with respect to the potential therapeutic use of chemokine receptor inhibitors, since this suggests that blocking the coreceptor with a small-molecule antagonist would not have adverse side effects.

However, the issue of resistance is still critical. Although the coreceptor cannot mutate, its recognition is mediated by the virus, and it is therefore susceptible to alteration by mutagenesis. Two mechanisms of resistance are possible: Env could escape inhibition by using an alternative coreceptor, or it could alter its interaction site on the coreceptor. Both scenarios have been observed in the laboratory. SDF-1α- or AMD3100-resistant variants can be readily selected in vitro (51, 178). The resistant virus maintained its restriction to CXCR4 usage but may have altered its recognition of its coreceptor by altering gp120, since it contained several amino acid substitutions.

SCID mice reconstituted with human peripheral blood lymphocytes and then infected with HIV and treated with CCR5 antagonists serve as a useful model for understanding what might happen in treated humans (134). The mice were infected with a CCR5-specific virus that had earlier been shown to be capable of switching to CXCR4 usage. They were treated with AOP-RANTES or NNY-RANTES (N-nonanoyol RANTES [2-68]). The drugs were effective at blocking infection but in some cases selected a virus that could use CXCR4. It is important to keep in mind that in this model immune selection mechanisms present in humans are not fully recapitulated. Thus, selective pressure to interfere with the emergence of CXCR4 virus may be absent and may give a more pessimistic picture of the effectiveness of CCR5 antagonists. The findings also suggest that it may be necessary to block two of the coreceptors to achieve a reduction in virus load in vivo.

Implications for HIV Pathogenesis

The findings reviewed earlier in this chapter point to the importance of CCR5 in HIV transmission and pathogenesis. The data implicating CCR5 regulatory polymorphisms and the data on CCR5Δ32 both support this. CCR5-specific virus is present in infected individuals even when the transmitting partner can be shown to harbor CXCR4-specific virus (43).

Why is HIV-1 transmission and replication in vivo CCR5-dependent? A straightforward explanation is that of the accessibility of $CCR5^+$ cells at sites of initial virus exposure. In this model, the genital mucosal surfaces where exposure occurs during sexual transmission would be rich in $CD4^+/CCR5^+$ but not $CD4^+/CXCR4^+$ cells. In support of this, MDMs and dendritic cells (DCs) are present in these tissues and have been shown to transmit virus to T cells very efficiently (26). DCs appear to be the initial target of the virus in the vaginal mucosa (191). Accessibility, however, does not fully account for the phenomenon, since transmission by parenteral exposure, in which the virus is injected into blood vessels where it has access to the $CD4^+/CXCR4^+$ primary T cells of the peripheral immune system, is also CCR5-dependent (199).

An attractive explanation for CCR5 dependence is that it reflects a requirement of the virus to infect MDMs and DCs. Although MDMs do express some CXCR4, infection of these cells is largely mediated by CCR5. The majority of peripheral T cells are resting and thus are resistant to infection. MDMs, in contrast to T cells, do not need to be activated to support productive infection and once infected become long-lived virus producers (74, 75). Thus, CCR5 dependence could reflect the requirement of the virus to infect MDMs. MDMs, whose physiological function involves interacting with and sending activating signals to T cells, would then efficiently transfer the virus to CD4+ T cells. Recent findings by Swingler et al. (193) provide a rationale for this sort of model. They found that the Nef accessory protein of HIV-1 induces MDMs to secrete CCR5 ligands. The chemokines caused chemotaxis of CCR5+ T cells to infected MDMs. Nef also induced MDMs to produce a yet unidentified potent T-cell-activating activity that renders the cells highly infectable. Thus, infected MDMs provide virus to T cells and then, diabolically, make them permissive to HIV-1 replication. The expansion of coreceptor usage late in the disease course to CXCR4 might reflect the loss of a requirement for virus-induced activation. At this stage in the disease, an increase in the proportion of replicating T cells that are produced in response to the requirement for immune system homeostasis provides a pool of target cells, and the requirement for CCR5 use would be diminished as a result.

Conclusion

Our increasing understanding of HIV/AIDS is an impressive testament to the ability of molecular biology and modern medicine to cope with a major medical crisis. Effective treatments for AIDS that were direct products of basic research are in widespread use (at least in the countries that can afford them). Current best hopes lie in the development of new, less expensive drugs and in a vaccine. Our rapidly growing understanding of the HIV coreceptors may provide the next breakthroughs on both fronts.

ACKNOWLEDGMENTS

The author thanks Stephanie Brandt and Beth Rasala for their editorial assistance.

REFERENCES

1. Alkhatib, G., C. Combadiere, C. C. Broder, Y. Feng, P. E. Kennedy, P. M. Murphy, and E. A. Berger. 1996. CC CKR5: a RANTES, MIP-1alpha, MIP-1beta receptor as a fusion cofactor for macrophage-tropic HIV-1. Science 272:1955–1958.

2. Alkhatib, G., F. Liao, E. A. Berger, J. M. Farber, and K. W. Peden. 1997. A new SIV co-receptor, STRL33 [letter] [see comments]. Nature 388:238.

3. Alkhatib, G., M. Locati, P. E. Kennedy, P. M. Murphy, and E. A. Berger. 1997. HIV-1 coreceptor activity of CCR5 and its inhibition by chemokines: independence from G protein signaling and importance of coreceptor down-modulation. Virology 234:340–348.

4. Amara, A., S. L. Gall, O. Schwartz, J. Salamero, M. Montes, P. Loetscher, M. Baggiolini, J. L. Virelizier, and F. Arenzana-Seisdedos. 1997. HIV coreceptor downregulation as antiviral principle: SDF-1alpha-dependent internalization of the chemokine receptor CXCR4 contributes to inhibition of HIV replication. J. Exp. Med. 186:139–146.

5. Ansari-Lari, M. A., X. M. Liu, M. L. Metzker, A. R. Rut, and R. A. Gibbs. 1997. The extent of genetic variation in the CCR5 gene [letter]. Nat. Genet. 16: 221–222.

6. Anzala, A. O., T. B. Ball, T. Rostron, S. J. O'Brien, F. A. Plummer, and S. L. Rowland-Jones. 1998. CCR2-64I allele and genotype association with delayed AIDS progression in African women. University of Nairobi Collaboration for HIV Research [letter]. Lancet 351:1632–1633.

7. Arakaki, R., H. Tamamura, M. Premanathan, K. Kanbara, S. Ramanan, K. Mochizuki, M. Baba, N. Fujii, and H. Nakashima. 1999. T134, a small-molecule CXCR4 inhibitor, has no cross-drug resistance with AMD3100, a CXCR4 antagonist with a different structure. J. Virol. 73:1719–1723.

8. Aramori, I., S. S. Ferguson, P. D. Bieniasz, J. Zhang, B. Cullen, and M. G. Cullen. 1997. Molecular mechanism of desensitization of the chemokine receptor CCR-5: receptor signaling and internalization are dissociable from its role as an HIV-1 co-receptor. EMBO J. 16:4606–4616. (Erratum, 16 (19):6055.)

9. Arenzana-Seisdedos, F., A. Amara, D. Thomas, and J. L. Virelizier. 1998. Beta-chemokine MDC and HIV-1 infection. Science 281:487a.

10. Atchison, R. E., J. Gosling, F. S. Monteclaro, C. Franci, L. Digilio, I. F. Charo, and M. A. Goldsmith. 1996. Multiple extracellular elements of CCR5 and HIV-1 entry: dissociation from response to chemokines. Science 274:1924–1926.

11. Baba, M., O. Nishimura, N. Kanzaki, M. Okamoto, H. Sawada, Y. Iizawa, M. Shiraishi, Y. Aramaki, K. Okonogi, Y. Ogawa, K. Meguro, and M. Fujino. 1999. A small-molecule, nonpeptide CCR5 antagonist with highly potent and selective anti-HIV-1 activity. Proc. Natl. Acad. Sci. USA 96:5698–5703.

12. Baggiolini, M., B. Dewald, and B. Moser. 1997. Human chemokines: an update. Annu. Rev. Immunol. 15:675–705.

13. Baleux, F., I. Clark-Lewis, D. F. Legler, B. Moser, and M. Baggiolini. 1998. Beta-chemokine MDC and HIV-1 infection. Science 281:487a.

14. Balotta, C., P. Bagnarelli, M. Violin, A. L. Ridolfo, D. Zhou, A. Berlusconi, S. Corvasce, M. Corbellino, M. Clementi, M. Clerici, M. Moroni, and M. Galli. 1997. Homozygous delta 32 deletion of the CCR-5 chemokine receptor gene in an HIV-1-infected patient. AIDS 11:F67–71.

15. Bazan, H. A., G. Alkhatib, C. C. Broder, and E. A. Berger. 1998. Patterns of CCR5, CXCR4, and CCR3 usage by envelope glycoproteins from human immunodeficiency virus type 1 primary isolates. J. Virol. 72:4485–4491.

16. Berger, E. A., R. W. Doms, E. M. Fenyö, B. T. Korber, D. R. Littman, J. P. Moore, Q. J. Sattentau, H. Schuitemaker, J. Sodroski, and R. A. Weiss. 1998. A new classification for HIV-1 [letter]. Nature 391:240.

17. Bernard, N. F., C. M. Yannakis, J. S. Lee, and C. M. Tsoukas. 1999. Human immunodeficiency virus (HIV)-specific cytotoxic T lymphocyte activity in HIV-exposed seronegative persons. J. Infect. Dis. 179:538–547.

18. Bieniasz, P. D., R. A. Fridell, K. Anthony, and B. R. Cullen. 1997. Murine CXCR-4 is a functional coreceptor for T-cell-tropic and dual-tropic strains of human immunodeficiency virus type 1. J. Virol. 71:7097–7100.

19. Bieniasz, P. D., R. A. Fridell, I. Aramori, S. S. Ferguson, M. G. Caron, and B. R. Cullen. 1997. HIV-1-induced cell fusion is mediated by multiple regions within both the viral envelope and the CCR-5 co-receptor. EMBO J. 16:2599–2609.

20. Biti, R., R. French, J. Young, B. Bennetts, G. Stewart, and T. Liang. 1997. HIV-1 infection in an individual homozygous for the CCR5 deletion allele [letter; comment]. Nature Med. 3:252–253.

21. Björndal, A., H. Deng, M. Jansson, J. R. Fiore, C. Colognesi, A. Karlsson, J. Albert, G. Scarlatti, D. R. Littman, and E. M. Fenyö. 1997. Coreceptor usage of primary human immunodeficiency virus type 1 isolates varies according to biological phenotype. J. Virol. 71:7478–7487.

22. Blanpain, C., B. Lee, J. Vakili, B. J. Doranz, C. Govaerts, I. Migeotte, M. Sharron, V. Dupriez, G. Vassart, R. W. Doms, and M. Parmentier. 1999. Extracellular cysteines of CCR5 are required for chemokine binding, but dispensable for HIV-1 coreceptor activity. J. Biol. Chem. 274:18902–18908.

23. Bleul, C. C., M. Farzan, H. Choe, C. Parolin, I. Clark-Lewis, J. Sodroski, and T. A. Springer. 1996. The lymphocyte chemoattractant SDF-1 is a ligand for LESTR/fusin and blocks HIV-1 entry. Nature 382:829–833.

24. Bleul, C. C., L. Wu, J. A. Hoxie, T. A. Springer, and C. R. Mackay. 1997. The HIV coreceptors CXCR4 and CCR5 are differentially expressed and regulated on human T lymphocytes. Proc. Natl. Acad. Sci. USA 94:1925–1930.

25. Bratt, G., A. C. Leandersson, J. Albert, E. Sandström, and B. Wahren. 1998. MT-2 tropism and CCR-5 genotype strongly influence disease progression in HIV-1-infected individuals. AIDS 12:729–736.

26. Cameron, P. U., P. S. Freudenthal, J. M. Barker, S. Gezelter, K. Inaba, and R. M. Steinman. 1992. Dendritic cells exposed to human immunodeficiency virus type-1 transmit a vigorous cytopathic infection to CD4+ T cells. Science 257:383–387. (Erratum, 257(5078):1848.)

27. Capobianchi, M. R., I. Abbate, G. Antonelli, O. Turriziani, A. Dolei, and F. Dianzani. 1998. Inhibition of HIV type 1 BaL replication by MIP-1alpha, MIP-1beta, and RANTES in macrophages. AIDS Res. Hum. Retroviruses 14:233–240.

28. Carrington, M., T. Kissner, B. Gerrard, S. Ivanov, S. J. O'Brien, and M. Dean. 1997. Novel alleles of the chemokine-receptor gene CCR5. Am. J. Hum. Genet. 61:1261–1267.

29. Carrington, M., G. W. Nelson, M. P. Martin, T. Kissner, D. Vlahov, J. J. Goedert, R. Kaslow, S. Buchbinder, K. Hoots, and S. J. O'Brien. 1999. HLA and HIV-1: heterozygote advantage and B*35-Cw*04 disadvantage. Science 283:1748–1752.

30. Chen, Z., D. Kwon, Z. Jin, S. Monard, P. Telfer, M. S. Jones, C. Y. Lu, R. F. Aguilar, D. D. Ho, and P. A. Marx. 1998. Natural infection of a homozygous delta24 CCR5 red-capped mangabey with an R2b-tropic simian immuno-deficiency virus. J. Exp. Med. 188:2057–2065.

31. Cheng-Mayer, C., R. Liu, N. R. Landau, and L. Stamatatos. 1997. Macrophage tropism of human immunodeficiency virus type 1 and utilization of the CC-CKR5 coreceptor. J. Virol. 71:1657–1661.

32. Chesebro, B., K. Wehrly, J. Nishio, and S. Perryman. 1996. Mapping of inde-pendent V3 envelope determinants of human immunodeficiency virus type 1 macrophage tropism and syncytium formation in lymphocytes. J. Virol. 70:9055–9059.

33. Cho, M. W., M. K. Lee, M. C. Carney, J. F. Berson, R. W. Doms, and M. A. Mar-tin. 1998. Identification of determinants on a dualtropic human immuno-deficiency virus type 1 envelope glycoprotein that confer usage of CXCR4. J. Virol. 72:2509–2515.

34. Choe, H., M. Farzan, M. Konkel, K. Martin, Y. Sun, L. Marcon, M. Cayabyab, M. Berman, M. E. Dorf, N. Gerard, C. Gerard, and J. Sodroski. 1998. The or-phan seven-transmembrane receptor apj supports the entry of primary T-cell-line-tropic and dualtropic human immunodeficiency virus type 1. J. Virol. 72:6113–6118.

35. Choe, H., M. Farzan, Y. Sun, N. Sullivan, B. Rollins, P. D. Ponath, L. Wu, C. R. Mackay, G. LaRosa, W. Newman, N. Gerard, C. Gerard, and J. Sodroski. 1996. The beta-chemokine receptors CCR3 and CCR5 facilitate infection by primary HIV-1 isolates. Cell 85:1135–1148.

36. Clerici, M., J. V. Giorgi, C. C. Chou, V. K. Gudeman, J. A. Zack, P. Gupta, H. N. Ho, P. G. Nishanian, J. A. Berzofsky, and G. M. Shearer. 1992. Cell-mediated immune response to human immunodeficiency virus (HIV) type 1 in seronegative homosexual men with recent sexual exposure to HIV-1. J. Infect. Dis. 165:1012–1019.

37. Cocchi, F., A. L. DeVico, A. Garzino-Demo, S. K. Arya, R. C. Gallo, and P. Lusso. 1995. Identification of RANTES, MIP-1 alpha, and MIP-1 beta as the major HIV-suppressive factors produced by CD8+ T cells [see comments]. Science 270:1811–1815.

38. Coffey, M. J., C. Woffendin, S. M. Phare, R. M. Strieter, and D. M. Markovitz. 1997. RANTES inhibits HIV-1 replication in human peripheral blood mono-cytes and alveolar macrophages. Am. J. Physiol. 272:L1025–1029.

39. Combadiere, C., S. K. Ahuja, H. L. Tiffany, and P. M. Murphy. 1996. Cloning and functional expression of CC CKR5, a human monocyte CC chemokine re-ceptor selective for MIP-1(alpha), MIP-1(beta), and RANTES. J. Leukocyte Biol. 60:147–152.

40. Combadiere, C., K. Salzwedel, E. D. Smith, H. L. Tiffany, E. A. Berger, and P. M. Murphy. 1998. Identification of CX3CR1. A chemotactic receptor for the human CX3C chemokine fractalkine and a fusion coreceptor for HIV-1. J. Biol. Chem. 273:23799–23804.

41. Connor, R. I., W. A. Paxton, K. E. Sheridan, and R. A. Koup. 1996. Macrophages and CD4+ T lymphocytes from two multiply exposed, unin-fected individuals resist infection with primary non-syncytium-inducing iso-lates of human immunodeficiency virus type 1. J. Virol. 70:8758–8764.

42. Connor, R. I., K. E. Sheridan, D. Ceradini, S. Choe, and N. R. Landau. 1997. Change in coreceptor use correlates with disease progression in HIV-1-infected individuals. J. Exp. Med. 185:621–628.

43. Cornelissen, M., G. Mulder-Kampinga, J. Veenstra, F. Zorgdrager, C. Kuiken, S. Hartman, J. Dekker, L. van der Hoek, C. Sol, and R. Coutinho. 1995. Syncytium-inducing (SI) phenotype suppression at seroconversion after intramuscular inoculation of a non-syncytium-inducing/SI phenotypically mixed human immunodeficiency virus population. J. Virol. 69:1810–1818.

43a. Cota, M., M. Mengozzi, E. Vicenzi, P. Panina-Bordignon, F. Sinigaglia, P. Transidico, S. Sozzani, A. Mantovani, and G. Poli. 2000. Selective inhibition of HIV replication in primary macrophages but not T lymphocytes by macrophage-derived chemokine. Proc. Natl. Acad. Sci. USA 97:9162–9167.

44. Dalgleish, A. G., P. C. Beverley, P. R. Clapham, D. H. Crawford, M. F. Greaves, and R. A. Weiss. 1984. The CD4 (T4) antigen is an essential component of the receptor for the AIDS retrovirus. Nature 312:763–767.

45. Datema, R., L. Rabin, M. Hincenbergs, M. B. Moreno, S. Warren, V. Linquist, B. Rosenwirth, J. Seifert, and J. M. McCune. 1996. Antiviral efficacy in vivo of the anti-human immunodeficiency virus bicyclam SDZ SID 791 (JM 3100), an inhibitor of infectious cell entry. Antimicrob. Agents Chemother. 40: 750–754.

46. Davis, C. B., I. Dikic, D. Unutmaz, C. M. Hill, J. Arthos, M. A. Siani, D. A. Thompson, J. Schlessinger, and D. R. Littman. 1997. Signal transduction due to HIV-1 envelope interactions with chemokine receptors CXCR4 or CCR5. J. Exp. Med. 186:1793–1798.

47. Dean, M., M. Carrington, C. Winkler, G. A. Huttley, M. W. Smith, R. Allikmets, J. J. Goedert, S. P. Buchbinder, E. Vittinghoff, E. Gomperts, S. Donfield, D. Vlahov, R. Kaslow, A. Saah, C. Rinaldo, R. Detels, and S. J. O'Brien. 1996. Genetic restriction of HIV-1 infection and progression to AIDS by a deletion allele of the CKR5 structural gene. Hemophilia Growth and Development Study, Multicenter AIDS Cohort Study, Multicenter Hemophilia Cohort Study, San Francisco City Cohort, ALIVE Study [see comments]. Science 273:1856–1862. (Erratum, 274 (5290):1069.)

48. Deng, H., R. Liu, W. Ellmeier, S. Choe, D. Unutmaz, M. Burkhart, P. Di Marzio, S. Marmon, R. E. Sutton, C. M. Hill, C. B. Davis, S. C. Peiper, T. J. Schall, D. R. Littman, and N. R. Landau. 1996. Identification of a major coreceptor for primary isolates of HIV-1 [see comments]. Nature 381:661–666.

49. Deng, H. K., D. Unutmaz, V. N. Kewal-Ramani, and D. R. Littman. 1997. Expression cloning of new receptors used by simian and human immunodeficiency viruses [see comments]. Nature 388:296–300.

50. de Roda Husman, A. M., M. Koot, M. Cornelissen, I. P. Keet, M. Brouwer, S. M. Broersen, M. Bakker, M. T. Roos, M. Prins, F. de Wolf, R. A. Coutinho, F. Miedema, J. Goudsmit, and H. Schuitemaker. 1997. Association between CCR5 genotype and the clinical course of HIV-1 infection [see comments]. Ann. Intern. Med. 127:882–890.

51. de Vreese, K., V. Kofler-Mongold, C. Leutgeb, V. Weber, K. Vermeire, S. Schacht, J. Anné, E. de Clercq, R. Datema, and G. Werner. 1996. The molecular target of bicyclams, potent inhibitors of human immunodeficiency virus replication. J. Virol. 70:689–696.

52. Dikic, I., G. Tokiwa, S. Lev, S. A. Courtneidge, and J. Schlessinger. 1996. A role for Pyk2 and Src in linking G-protein-coupled receptors with MAP kinase activation. Nature 383:547–550.

53. Di Marzio, P., J. Tse, and N. R. Landau. 1998. Chemokine receptor regulation and HIV-1 tropism in monocytes/macrophages. Submitted for publication. AIDS Res. Hum. Retroviruses 14:129–138.

54. Dittmar, M. T., A. McKnight, G. Simmons, P. R. Clapham, R. A. Weiss, and P. Simmonds. 1997. HIV-1 tropism and co-receptor use [letter]. Nature 385: 495–496.

55. Donzella, G. A., D. Schols, S. W. Lin, J. A. Esté, K. A. Nagashima, P. J. Maddon, G. P. Allaway, T. P. Sakmar, G. Henson, E. De Clercq, and J. P. Moore. 1998. AMD3100, a small molecule inhibitor of HIV-1 entry via the CXCR4 coreceptor. Nature Med. 4:72–77.

56. Doranz, B. J., K. Grovit-Ferbas, M. P. Sharron, S. H. Mao, M. B. Goetz, E. S. Daar, R. W. Doms, and W. A. O'Brien. 1997. A small-molecule inhibitor directed against the chemokine receptor CXCR4 prevents its use as an HIV-1 coreceptor. J. Exp. Med. 186:1395–1400.

57. Doranz, B. J., Z. H. Lu, J. Rucker, T. Y. Zhang, M. Sharron, Y. H. Cen, Z. X. Wang, H. H. Guo, J. G. Du, M. A. Accavitti, R. W. Doms, and S. C. Peiper. 1997. Two distinct CCR5 domains can mediate coreceptor usage by human immunodeficiency virus type 1. J. Virol. 71:6305–6314.

58. Doranz, B. J., J. Rucker, Y. Yi, R. J. Smyth, M. Samson, S. C. Peiper, M. Parmentier, R. G. Collman, and R. W. Doms. 1996. A dual-tropic primary HIV-1 isolate that uses fusin and the beta-chemokine receptors CKR-5, CKR-3, and CKR-2b as fusion cofactors. Cell 85:1149–1158.

59. Dragic, T., P. Charneau, F. Clavel, and M. Alizon. 1992. Complementation of murine cells for human immunodeficiency virus envelope/CD4-mediated fusion in human/murine heterokaryons. J. Virol. 66:4794–4802.

60. Dragic, T., V. Litwin, G. P. Allaway, S. R. Martin, Y. Huang, K. A. Nagashima, C. Cayanan, P. J. Maddon, R. A. Koup, J. P. Moore, and W. A. Paxton. 1996. HIV-1 entry into CD4+ cells is mediated by the chemokine receptor CC-CKR-5 [see comments]. Nature 381:667–673.

61. Dragic, T., A. Trkola, S. W. Lin, K. A. Nagashima, F. Kajumo, L. Zhao, W. C. Olson, L. Wu, C. R. Mackay, G. P. Allaway, T. P. Sakmar, J. P. Moore, and P. J. Maddon. 1998. Amino-terminal substitutions in the CCR5 coreceptor impair gp120 binding and human immunodeficiency virus type 1 entry. J. Virol. 72:279–285.

62. Edelstein, R. E., L. A. Arcuino, J. P. Hughes, A. J. Melvin, K. M. Mohan, P. D. King, C. L. McLellan, B. L. Murante, B. P. Kassman, and L. M. Frenkel. 1997. Risk of mother-to-infant transmission of HIV-1 is not reduced in CCR5/delta32ccr5 heterozygotes. J. Acquired Immune Defic. Syndr. Hum. Retrovirol. 16:243–246.

63. Edinger, A. L., T. L. Hoffman, M. Sharron, B. Lee, Y. Yi, W. Choe, D. L. Kolson, B. Mitrovic, Y. Zhou, D. Faulds, R. G. Collman, J. Hesselgesser, R. Horuk, and R. W. Doms. 1998. An orphan seven-transmembrane domain receptor expressed widely in the brain functions as a coreceptor for human immunodeficiency virus type 1 and simian immunodeficiency virus. J. Virol. 72: 7934–7940.

64. Edinger, A. L., J. L. Mankowski, B. J. Doranz, B. J. Margulies, B. Lee, J. Rucker, M. Sharron, T. L. Hoffman, J. F. Berson, M. C. Zink, V. M. Hirsch, J. E. Clements, and R. W. Doms. 1997. CD4-independent, CCR5-dependent infection of brain capillary endothelial cells by a neurovirulent simian immunodeficiency virus strain. Proc. Natl. Acad. Sci. USA 94:14742–14747.

65. Endres, M. J., P. R. Clapham, M. Marsh, M. Ahuja, J. D. Turner, A. McKnight, J. F. Thomas, B. Stoebenau-Haggarty, S. Choe, P. J. Vance, T. N. Wells, C. A. Power, S. S. Sutterwala, R. W. Doms, N. R. Landau, and J. A. Hoxie. 1996. CD4-independent infection by HIV-2 is mediated by fusin/CXCR4. Cell 87:745–756.

66. Eugen-Olsen, J., A. K. Iversen, T. L. Benfield, U. Koppelhus, and P. Garred. 1998. Chemokine receptor CCR2b 64I polymorphism and its relation to CD4 T-cell counts and disease progression in a Danish cohort of HIV-infected individuals. Copenhagen AIDS cohort. J. Acquired Immune Defic. Syndr. Hum. Retrovirol. 18:110–116.

67. Eugen-Olsen, J., A. K. Iversen, P. Garred, U. Koppelhus, C. Pedersen, T. L. Benfield, A. M. Sorensen, T. Katzenstein, E. Dickmeiss, J. Gerstoft, P. Skinhøj, A. Svejgaard, J. O. Nielsen, and B. Hofmann. 1997. Heterozygosity for a deletion in the CKR-5 gene leads to prolonged AIDS-free survival and slower CD4 T-cell decline in a cohort of HIV-seropositive individuals. AIDS 11:305–310.

68. Farzan, M., H. Choe, E. Desjardins, Y. Sun, J. Kuhn, J. Cao, D. Archambault, P. Kolchinsky, M. Koch, R. Wyatt, and J. Sodroski. 1998. Stabilization of human immunodeficiency virus type 1 envelope glycoprotein trimers by disulfide bonds introduced into the gp41 glycoprotein ectodomain. J. Virol. 72:7620–7625.

69. Farzan, M., H. Choe, K. Martin, L. Marcon, W. Hofmann, G. Karlsson, Y. Sun, P. Barrett, N. Marchand, N. Sullivan, N. Gerard, C. Gerard, and J. Sodroski. 1997. Two orphan seven-transmembrane segment receptors which are expressed in CD4-positive cells support simian immunodeficiency virus infection. J. Exp. Med. 186:405–411.

70. Feng, Y., C. C. Broder, P. E. Kennedy, and E. A. Berger. 1996. HIV-1 entry cofactor: functional cDNA cloning of a seven-transmembrane, G protein-coupled receptor [see comments]. Science 272:872–877.

71. Fenyö, E. M., L. Morfeldt-Månson, F. Chiodi, B. Lind, A. von Gegerfelt, J. Albert, E. Olausson, and B. Asjö. 1988. Distinct replicative and cytopathic characteristics of human immunodeficiency virus isolates. J. Virol. 62:4414–4419.

72. Fouchier, R. A., M. Groenink, N. A. Kootstra, M. Tersmette, H. G. Huisman, F. Miedema, and H. Schuitemaker. 1992. Phenotype-associated sequence variation in the third variable domain of the human immunodeficiency virus type 1 gp120 molecule. J. Virol. 66:3183–3187.

73. Fowke, K. R., T. Dong, S. L. Rowland-Jones, J. Oyugi, W. J. Rutherford, J. Kimani, P. Krausa, J. Bwayo, J. N. Simonsen, G. M. Shearer, and F. A. Plummer. 1998. HIV type 1 resistance in Kenyan sex workers is not associated with altered cellular susceptibility to HIV type 1 infection or enhanced beta-chemokine production. AIDS Res. Hum. Retroviruses 14:1521–1530.

74. Gartner, S., P. Markovits, D. M. Markovitz, M. H. Kaplan, R. C. Gallo, and M.

Popovic. 1986. The role of mononuclear phagocytes in HTLV-III/LAV infection. Science 233:215–219.

75. Gendelman, H. E., J. M. Orenstein, L. Baca, B. Weiser, H. Burger, D. C. Kalter, and M. Meltzer. 1989. The macrophage in the persistence and pathogenesis of HIV infection. AIDS 3:475–495.

76. Georges-Courbot, M. C., C. Y. Lu, M. Makuwa, P. Telfer, R. Onanga, G. Dubreuil, Z. Chen, S. M. Smith, A. Georges, F. Gao, B. H. Hahn, and P. A. Marx. 1998. Natural infection of a household pet red-capped mangabey (Cercocebus torquatus torquatus) with a new simian immunodeficiency virus. J. Virol. 72:600–608.

77. Goh, W. C., J. Markee, R. E. Akridge, M. Meldorf, L. Musey, T. Karchmer, M. Krone, A. Collier, L. Corey, M. Emerman, and M. J. McElrath. 1999. Protection against human immunodeficiency virus type 1 infection in persons with repeated exposure: evidence for T cell immunity in the absence of inherited CCR5 coreceptor defects. J. Infect. Dis. 179:548–557.

78. Gong, W., O. M. Howard, J. A. Turpin, M. C. Grimm, H. Ueda, P. W. Gray, C. J. Raport, J. J. Oppenheim, and J. M. Wang. 1998. Monocyte chemotactic protein-2 activates CCR5 and blocks CD4/CCR5-mediated HIV-1 entry/replication. J. Biol. Chem. 273:4289–4292.

79. Gosling, J., F. S. Monteclaro, R. E. Atchison, H. Arai, C. L. Tsou, M. A. Goldsmith, and I. F. Charo. 1997. Molecular uncoupling of C-C chemokine receptor 5-induced chemotaxis and signal transduction from HIV-1 coreceptor activity. Proc. Natl. Acad. Sci. USA 94:5061–5066.

80. Greco, G., C. Mackewicz, and J. A. Levy. 1999. Sensitivity of human immunodeficiency virus infection to various alpha, beta and gamma chemokines. J. Gen. Virol. 80:2369–2373.

81. Groenink, M., R. A. Fouchier, S. Broersen, C. H. Baker, M. Koot, A. B. van't Wout, H. G. Huisman, F. Miedema, M. Tersmette, and H. Schuitemaker. 1993. Relation of phenotype evolution of HIV-1 to envelope V2 configuration [see comments]. Science 260:1513–1516.

82. Harrowe, G., and C. Cheng-Mayer. 1995. Amino acid substitutions in the V3 loop are responsible for adaptation to growth in transformed T-cell lines of a primary human immunodeficiency virus type 1. Virology 210:490–494.

83. He, J., Y. Chen, M. Farzan, H. Choe, A. Ohagen, S. Gartner, J. Busciglio, X. Yang, W. Hofmann, W. Newman, C. R. Mackay, J. Sodroski, and D. Gabuzda. 1997. CCR3 and CCR5 are co-receptors for HIV-1 infection of microglia. Nature 385:645–649.

84. Heiken, H., S. Becker, I. Bastisch, and R. E. Schmidt. 1999. HIV-1 infection in a heterosexual man homozygous for CCR-5 delta32 [letter]. AIDS 13:529–530.

85. Hendel, H., N. Hénon, H. Lebuanec, A. Lachgar, H. Poncelet, S. Caillat-Zucman, C. A. Winkler, M. W. Smith, L. Kenefic, S. O'Brien, W. Lu, J. M. Andrieu, D. Zagury, F. Schächter, J. Rappaport, and J. F. Zagury. 1998. Distinctive effects of CCR5, CCR2, and SDF1 genetic polymorphisms in AIDS progression. J. Acquired Immune Defic. Syndr. Hum. Retrovirol. 19:381–386.

86. Hill, C. M., H. Deng, D. Unutmaz, V. N. Kewal-Ramani, L. Bastiani, M. K. Gorny, S. Zolla-Pazner, and D. R. Littman. 1997. Envelope glycoproteins from

human immunodeficiency virus types 1 and 2 and simian immunodeficiency virus can use human CCR5 as a coreceptor for viral entry and make direct CD4-dependent interactions with this chemokine receptor. J. Virol. 71: 6296–6304.

87. Hoffman, T. L., E. B. Stephens, O. Narayan, and R. W. Doms. 1998. HIV type I envelope determinants for use of the CCR2b, CCR3, STRL33, and APJ co-receptors. Proc. Natl. Acad. Sci. USA 95:11360–11365.

88. Horuk, R., J. Hesselgesser, Y. Zhou, D. Faulds, M. Halks-Miller, S. Harvey, D. Taub, M. Samson, M. Parmentier, J. Rucker, B. J. Doranz, and R. W. Doms. 1998. The CC chemokine I-309 inhibits CCR8-dependent infection by diverse HIV-1 strains. J. Biol. Chem. 273:386–391.

89. Huang, Y., W. A. Paxton, S. M. Wolinsky, A. U. Neumann, L. Zhang, T. He, S. Kang, D. Ceradini, Z. Jin, K. Yazdanbakhsh, K. Kunstman, D. Erickson, E. Dragon, N. R. Landau, J. Phair, D. D. Ho, and R. A. Koup. 1996. The role of a mutant CCR5 allele in HIV-1 transmission and disease progression [see comments]. Nature Med. 2:1240–1243.

90. Huang, Y., L. Zhang, and D. D. Ho. 1995. Characterization of nef sequences in long-term survivors of human immunodeficiency virus type 1 infection. J. Virol. 69:93–100.

91. Hung, C. S., N. Vander Heyden, and L. Ratner. 1999. Analysis of the critical domain in the V3 loop of human immunodeficiency virus type 1 gp120 involved in CCR5 utilization. J. Virol. 73:8216–8226.

92. Hwang, S. S., T. J. Boyle, H. K. Lyerly, and B. R. Cullen. 1992. Identification of envelope V3 loop as the major determinant of CD4 neutralization sensitivity of HIV-1. Science 257:535–537.

93. Imai, T., D. Chantry, C. J. Raport, C. L. Wood, M. Nishimura, R. Godiska, O. Yoshie, and P. W. Gray. 1998. Macrophage-derived chemokine is a functional ligand for the CC chemokine receptor 4. J. Biol. Chem. 273:1764–1768.

94. Jinno, A., N. Shimizu, Y. Soda, Y. Haraguchi, T. Kitamura, and H. Hoshino. 1998. Identification of the chemokine receptor TER1/CCR8 expressed in brain-derived cells and T cells as a new coreceptor for HIV-1 infection. Biochem. Biophys. Res. Commun. 243:497–502.

95. Katzenstein, T. L., J. Eugen-Olsen, B. Hofmann, T. Benfield, C. Pedersen, A. K. Iversen, A. M. Sørensen, P. Garred, U. Koppelhus, A. Svejgaard, and J. Gerstoft. 1997. HIV-infected individuals with the CCR delta32/CCR5 genotype have lower HIV RNA levels and higher CD4 cell counts in the early years of the infection than do patients with the wild type. Copenhagen AIDS Cohort Study Group. J. Acquired Immune Defic. Syndr. Hum. Retrovirol. 16: 10–14.

96. Kelly, M. D., H. M. Naif, S. L. Adams, A. L. Cunningham, and A. R. Lloyd. 1998. Dichotomous effects of beta-chemokines on HIV replication in monocytes and monocyte-derived macrophages. J. Immunol. 160:3091–3095.

97. Kinter, A., A. Catanzaro, J. Monaco, M. Ruiz, J. Justement, S. Moir, J. Arthos, A. Oliva, L. Ehler, S. Mizell, R. Jackson, M. Ostrowski, J. Hoxie, R. Offord, and A. S. Fauci. 1998. CC-chemokines enhance the replication of T-tropic strains of HIV-1 in CD4(+) T cells: role of signal transduction. Proc. Natl. Acad. Sci. USA 95:11880–11885.

98. Kirchhoff, F., T. C. Greenough, D. B. Brettler, J. L. Sullivan, and R. C. Desrosiers. 1995. Brief report: absence of intact nef sequences in a long-term survivor with nonprogressive HIV-1 infection. N. Engl. J. Med. 332:228–232.

99. Klatzmann, D., E. Champagne, S. Chamaret, J. Gruest, D. Guetard, T. Hercend, J. C. Gluckman, and L. Montagnier. 1984. T-lymphocyte T4 molecule behaves as the receptor for human retrovirus LAV. Nature 312: 767–768.

100. Kostrikis, L. G., Y. Huang, J. P. Moore, S. M. Wolinsky, L. Zhang, Y. Guo, L. Deutsch, J. Phair, A. U. Neumann, and D. D. Ho. 1998. A chemokine receptor CCR2 allele delays HIV-1 disease progression and is associated with a CCR5 promoter mutation [see comments]. Nature Med. 4:350–353.

101. Kuhmann, S. E., E. J. Platt, S. L. Kozak, and D. Kabat. 1997. Polymorphisms in the CCR5 genes of African green monkeys and mice implicate specific amino acids in infections by simian and human immunodeficiency viruses. J. Virol. 71:8642–8656.

102. Kuipers, H., C. Workman, W. Dyer, A. Geczy, J. Sullivan, and R. Oelrichs. 1999. An HIV-1-infected individual homozygous for the CCR-5 delta32 allele and the SDF-1 3'A allele [letter]. AIDS 13:433–434.

103. Kwong, P. D., R. Wyatt, J. Robinson, R. W. Sweet, J. Sodroski, and W. A. Hendrickson. 1998. Structure of an HIV gp120 envelope glycoprotein in complex with the CD4 receptor and a neutralizing human antibody [see comments]. Nature 393:648–659.

104. Labrosse, B., A. Brelot, N. Heveker, N. Sol, D. Schols, E. De Clercq, and M. Alizon. 1998. Determinants for sensitivity of human immunodeficiency virus coreceptor CXCR4 to the bicyclam AMD3100. J. Virol. 72:6381–6388.

105. Landau, N. R., K. A. Page, and D. R. Littman. 1991. Pseudotyping with human T-cell leukemia virus type I broadens the human immunodeficiency virus host range. J. Virol. 65:162–169.

106. Lapham, C. K., J. Ouyang, B. Chandrasekhar, N. Y. Nguyen, D. S. Dimitrov, and H. Golding. 1996. Evidence for cell-surface association between fusin and the CD4-gp120 complex in human cell lines [see comments]. Science 274:602–605.

107. Lee, B., B. J. Doranz, S. Rana, Y. Yi, M. Mellado, J. M. Frade, C. Martinez-A, S. J. O'Brien, M. Dean, R. G. Collman, and R. W. Doms. 1998. Influence of the CCR2-V64I polymorphism on human immunodeficiency virus type 1 coreceptor activity and on chemokine receptor function of CCR2b, CCR3, CCR5, and CXCR4. J. Virol. 72:7450–7458.

108. Levy, J. A., C. E. Mackewicz, and E. Barker. 1996. Controlling HIV pathogenesis: the role of the noncytotoxic anti-HIV response of CD8+ T cells. Immunol. Today 17:217–224.

109. Liu, H., D. Chao, E. E. Nakayama, H. Taguchi, M. Goto, X. Xin, J. K. Takamatsu, H. Saito, Y. Ishikawa, T. Akaza, T. Juji, Y. Takebe, T. Ohishi, K. Fukutake, Y. Maruyama, S. Yashiki, S. Sonoda, T. Nakamura, Y. Nagai, A. Iwamoto, and T. Shioda. 1999. Polymorphism in RANTES chemokine promoter affects HIV-1 disease progression. Proc. Natl. Acad. Sci. USA 96:4581–4585.

110. Liu, R., W. A. Paxton, S. Choe, D. Ceradini, S. R. Martin, R. Horuk, M. E. MacDonald, H. Stuhlmann, R. A. Koup, and N. R. Landau. 1996. Homozygous

defect in HIV-1 coreceptor accounts for resistance of some multiply-exposed individuals to HIV-1 infection. Cell 86:367–377.

111. Loetscher, M., T. Geiser, T. O'Reilly, R. Zwahlen, M. Baggiolini, and B. Moser. 1994. Cloning of a human seven-transmembrane domain receptor, LESTR, that is highly expressed in leukocytes. J. Biol. Chem. 269:232–237.

112. Lu, Z., J. F. Berson, Y. Chen, J. D. Turner, T. Zhang, M. Sharron, M. H. Jenks, Z. Wang, J. Kim, J. Rucker, J. A. Hoxie, S. C. Peiper, and R. W. Doms. 1997. Evolution of HIV-1 coreceptor usage through interactions with distinct CCR5 and CXCR4 domains. Proc. Natl. Acad. Sci. USA 94:6426–6431.

113. Lusso, P., F. Cocchi, C. Balotta, P. D. Markham, A. Louie, P. Farci, R. Pal, R. C. Gallo, and M. S. J. Reitz. 1995. Growth of macrophage-tropic and primary human immunodeficiency virus type 1 (HIV-1) isolates in a unique CD4+ T-cell clone (PM1): failure to downregulate CD4 and to interfere with cell-line-tropic HIV-1. J. Virol. 69:3712–3720.

114. Lusso, P., F. di Marzo Veronese, B. Ensoli, G. Franchini, C. Jemma, S. E. De-Rocco, V. S. Kalyanaraman, and R. C. Gallo. 1990. Expanded HIV-1 cellular tropism by phenotypic mixing with murine endogenous retroviruses [see comments]. Science 247:848–852.

115. Mack, M., B. Luckow, P. J. Nelson, J. Cihak, G. Simmons, P. R. Clapham, N. Signoret, M. Marsh, M. Stangassinger, F. Borlat, T. N. Wells, D. Schlöndorff, and A. E. Proudfoot. 1998. Aminooxypentane-RANTES induces CCR5 internalization but inhibits recycling: a novel inhibitory mechanism of HIV infectivity. J. Exp. Med. 187:1215–1224.

116. Maddon, P. J., A. G. Dalgleish, J. S. McDougal, P. R. Clapham, R. A. Weiss, and R. Axel. 1986. The T4 gene encodes the AIDS virus receptor and is expressed in the immune system and the brain. Cell 47:333–348.

117. Mandl, C. W., S. W. Aberle, J. H. Henkel, E. Puchhammer-Stöckl, and F. X. Heinz. 1998. Possible influence of the mutant CCR5 allele on vertical transmission of HIV-1. J. Med. Virol. 55:51–55.

118. Mangano, A., F. Prada, A. Roldán, G. Picchio, R. Bologna, and L. Sen. 1998. Distribution of CCR-5 delta32 allele in Argentinian children at risk of HIV-1 infection: its role in vertical transmission [letter]. AIDS 12:109–110.

119. Mann, D. L., R. P. Garner, D. E. Dayhoff, K. Cao, M. A. Fernández-Viña, C. Davis, N. Aronson, N. Ruiz, D. L. Birx, and N. L. Michael. 1998. Major histocompatibility complex genotype is associated with disease progression and virus load levels in a cohort of human immunodeficiency virus type 1-infected Caucasians and African Americans. J. Infect. Dis. 178:1799–1802.

120. Mariani, R., S. Wong, L. C. Mulder, D. A. Wilkinson, A. L. Reinhart, G. LaRosa, R. Nibbs, T. R. O'Brien, N. L. Michael, R. I. Connor, M. Macdonald, M. Busch, R. A. Koup, and N. R. Landau. 1999. CCR2-64I polymorphism is not associated with altered CCR5 expression or coreceptor function. J. Virol. 73:2450–2459.

121. Martin, M. P., M. Carrington, M. Dean, S. J. O'Brien, H. W. Sheppard, S. A. Wegner, and N. L. Michael. 1998. CXCR4 polymorphisms and HIV-1 pathogenesis [letter]. J. Acquired Immune Defic. Syndr. Hum. Retrovirol. 19:430.

122. Martin, M. P., M. Dean, M. W. Smith, C. Winkler, B. Gerrard, N. L. Michael, B. Lee, R. W. Doms, J. Margolick, S. Buchbinder, J. J. Goedert, T. R. O'Brien,

M. W. Hilgartner, D. Vlahov, S. J. O'Brien, and M. Carrington. 1998. Genetic acceleration of AIDS progression by a promoter variant of CCR5. Science 282:1907–1911.

123. Martinson, J. J., N. H. Chapman, D. C. Rees, Y. T. Liu, and J. B. Clegg. 1997. Global distribution of the CCR5 gene 32-basepair deletion. Nat. Genet. 16:100–103.

124. McDermott, D. H., P. A. Zimmerman, F. Guignard, C. A. Kleeberger, S. F. Leitman, and P. M. Murphy. 1998. CCR5 promoter polymorphism and HIV-1 disease progression. Multicenter AIDS Cohort Study (MACS). Lancet 352:866–870.

125. McDougal, J. S., M. S. Kennedy, J. M. Sligh, S. P. Cort, A. Mawle, and J. K. Nicholson. 1986. Binding of HTLV-III/LAV to T4+ T cells by a complex of the 110K viral protein and the T4 molecule. Science 231:382–385.

126. Michael, N. L., G. Chang, L. G. Louie, J. R. Mascola, D. Dondero, D. L. Birx, and H. W. Sheppard. 1997. The role of viral phenotype and CCR-5 gene defects in HIV-1 transmission and disease progression. Nature Med. 3:338–340.

127. Michael, N. L., L. G. Louie, A. L. Rohrbaugh, K. A. Schultz, D. E. Dayhoff, C. E. Wang, and H. W. Sheppard. 1997. The role of CCR5 and CCR2 polymorphisms in HIV-1 transmission and disease progression [see comments]. Nature Med. 3:1160–1162.

128. Michael, N. L., J. A. Nelson, V. N. Kewal-Ramani, G. Chang, S. J. O'Brien, J. R. Mascola, B. Volsky, M. Louder, G. C. White II, D. R. Littman, R. Swanstrom, and T. R. O'Brien. 1998. Exclusive and persistent use of the entry coreceptor CXCR4 by human immunodeficiency virus type 1 from a subject homozygous for CCR5 delta32. J. Virol. 72:6040–6047.

129. Miedema, F., L. Meyaard, M. Koot, M. R. Klein, M. T. Roos, M. Groenink, R. A. Fouchier, A. B. Van't Wout, M. Tersmette, P. T. Schellekens, et al. 1994. Changing virus-host interactions in the course of HIV-1 infection. Immunol. Rev. 140:35–72.

130. Misrahi, M., J. P. Teglas, N. N'Go, M. Burgard, M. J. Mayaux, C. Rouzioux, J. F. Delfraissy, and S. Blanche. 1998. CCR5 chemokine receptor variant in HIV-1 mother-to-child transmission and disease progression in children. French Pediatric HIV Infection Study Group [see comments]. JAMA 279:277–280.

131. Morawetz, R. A., G. P. Rizzardi, D. Glauser, O. Rutschmann, B. Hirschel, L. Perrin, M. Opravil, M. Flepp, J. von Overbeck, M. P. Glauser, S. Ghezzi, E. Vicenzi, G. Poli, A. Lazzarin, and G. Pantaleo. 1997. Genetic polymorphism of CCR5 gene and HIV disease: the heterozygous (CCR5/delta ccr5) genotype is neither essential nor sufficient for protection against disease progression. Swiss HIV Cohort. Eur. J. Immunol. 27:3223–3227.

132. Mori, K., D. J. Ringler, and R. C. Desrosiers. 1993. Restricted replication of simian immunodeficiency virus strain 239 in macrophages is determined by env but is not due to restricted entry. J. Virol. 67:2807–2814.

133. Moriuchi, H., M. Moriuchi, C. Combadiere, P. M. Murphy, and A. S. Fauci. 1996. CD8+ T-cell-derived soluble factor(s), but not beta-chemokines RANTES, MIP-1 alpha, and MIP-1 beta, suppress HIV-1 replication in monocyte/macrophages. Proc. Natl. Acad. Sci. USA 93:15341–15345.

134. Mosier, D. E., G. R. Picchio, R. J. Gulizia, R. Sabbe, P. Poignard, L. Picard, R. E. Offord, D. A. Thompson, and J. Wilken. 1999. Highly potent RANTES analogues either prevent CCR5-using human immunodeficiency virus type 1 infection in vivo or rapidly select for CXCR4-using variants. J. Virol. 73: 3544–3550.

135. Mummidi, S., S. S. Ahuja, E. Gonzalez, S. A. Anderson, E. N. Santiago, K. T. Stephan, F. E. Craig, P. O'Connell, V. Tryon, R. A. Clark, M. J. Dolan, and S. K. Ahuja. 1998. Genealogy of the CCR5 locus and chemokine system gene variants associated with altered rates of HIV-1 disease progression. Nature Med. 4:786–793.

136. Murakami, T., T. Nakajima, Y. Koyanagi, K. Tachibana, N. Fujii, H. Tamamura, N. Yoshida, M. Waki, A. Matsumoto, O. Yoshie, T. Kishimoto, N. Yamamoto, and T. Nagasawa. 1997. A small molecule CXCR4 inhibitor that blocks T cell line-tropic HIV-1 infection. J. Exp. Med. 186:1389–1393.

137. Murphy, P. M. 1996. Chemokine receptors: structure, function and role in microbial pathogenesis. Cytokine Growth Factor Rev. 7:47–64.

138. Nagasawa, T., S. Hirota, K. Tachibana, N. Takakura, S. Nishikawa, Y. Kitamura, N. Yoshida, H. Kikutani, and T. Kishimoto. 1996. Defects of B-cell lymphopoiesis and bone-marrow myelopoiesis in mice lacking the CXC chemokine PBSF/SDF-1. Nature 382:635–638.

139. Nagasawa, T., H. Kikutani, and T. Kishimoto. 1994. Molecular cloning and structure of a pre-B-cell growth-stimulating factor. Proc. Natl. Acad. Sci. USA 91:2305–2309.

140. Naif, H. M., S. Li, M. Alali, A. Sloane, L. Wu, M. Kelly, G. Lynch, A. Lloyd, and A. L. Cunningham. 1998. CCR5 expression correlates with susceptibility of maturing monocytes to human immunodeficiency virus type 1 infection. J. Virol. 72:830–836.

141. Nussbaum, O., C. C. Broder, and E. A. Berger. 1994. Fusogenic mechanisms of enveloped-virus glycoproteins analyzed by a novel recombinant vaccinia virus-based assay quantitating cell fusion-dependent reporter gene activation. J. Virol. 68:5411–5422.

142. Oberlin, E., A. Amara, F. Bachelerie, C. Bessia, J. L. Virelizier, F. Arenzana-Seisdedos, O. Schwartz, J. M. Heard, I. Clark-Lewis, D. F. Legler, M. Loetscher, M. Baggiolini, and B. Moser. 1996. The CXC chemokine SDF-1 is the ligand for LESTR/fusin and prevents infection by T-cell-line-adapted HIV-1. Nature 382:833–835. (Erratum, 384(6606):288.)

143. O'Brien, T. R., C. Winkler, M. Dean, J. A. Nelson, M. Carrington, N. L. Michael, and G. C. White II. 1997. HIV-1 infection in a man homozygous for CCR5 delta 32 [letter] [see comments]. Lancet 349:1219.

144. O'Brien, W. A., Y. Koyanagi, A. Namazie, J. Q. Zhao, A. Diagne, K. Idler, J. A. Zack, and I. S. Chen. 1990. HIV-1 tropism for mononuclear phagocytes can be determined by regions of gp120 outside the CD4-binding domain. Nature 348:69–73.

145. Oppermann, M., M. Mack, A. E. Proudfoot, and H. Olbrich. 1999. Differential effects of CC chemokines on CC chemokine receptor 5 (CCR5) phosphorylation and identification of phosphorylation sites on the CCR5 carboxyl terminus. J. Biol. Chem. 274:8875–8885.

146. Oravecz, T., M. Pall, J. Wang, G. Roderiquez, M. Ditto, and M. A. Norcross. 1997. Regulation of anti-HIV-1 activity of RANTES by heparan sulfate proteoglycans. J. Immunol. 159:4587–4592.

147. Owman, C., A. Garzino-Demo, F. Cocchi, M. Popovic, A. Sabirsh, and R. C. Gallo. 1998. The leukotriene B4 receptor functions as a novel type of co-receptor mediating entry of primary HIV-1 isolates into CD4-positive cells. Proc. Natl. Acad. Sci. USA 95:9530–9534.

148. Page, K. A., N. R. Landau, and D. R. Littman. 1990. Construction and use of a human immunodeficiency virus vector for analysis of virus infectivity. J. Virol. 64:5270–5276.

149. Pal, R., A. Garzino-Demo, P. D. Markham, J. Burns, M. Brown, R. C. Gallo, and A. L. DeVico. 1997. Inhibition of HIV-1 infection by the beta-chemokine MDC. Science 278:695–698.

150. Parolin, C., A. Borsetti, H. Choe, M. Farzan, P. Kolchinsky, M. Heesen, Q. Ma, C. Gerard, G. Palú, M. E. Dorf, T. Springer, and J. Sodroski. 1998. Use of murine CXCR-4 as a second receptor by some T-cell-tropic human immunodeficiency viruses. J. Virol. 72:1652–1656.

151. Paxton, W. A., S. Kang, and R. A. Koup. 1998. The HIV type 1 coreceptor CCR5 and its role in viral transmission and disease progression. AIDS Res. Hum. Retroviruses 14(Suppl. 1):S89–92.

152. Paxton, W. A., R. Liu, S. Kang, L. Wu, T. R. Gingeras, N. R. Landau, C. R. Mackay, and R. A. Koup. 1998. Reduced HIV-1 infectability of CD4+ lymphocytes from exposed-uninfected individuals: association with low expression of CCR5 and high production of beta-chemokines. Virology 244:66–73.

153. Paxton, W. A., S. R. Martin, D. Tse, T. R. O'Brien, J. Skurnick, N. L. Van Devanter, N. Padian, J. F. Braun, D. P. Kotler, S. M. Wolinsky, and R. A. Koup. 1996. Relative resistance to HIV-1 infection of CD4 lymphocytes from persons who remain uninfected despite multiple high-risk sexual exposure. Nature Med. 2:412–417.

154. Picard, L., G. Simmons, C. A. Power, A. Meyer, R. A. Weiss, and P. R. Clapham. 1997. Multiple extracellular domains of CCR-5 contribute to human immunodeficiency virus type 1 entry and fusion. J. Virol. 71:5003–5011.

155. Picchio, G. R., R. J. Gulizia, and D. E. Mosier. 1997. Chemokine receptor CCR5 genotype influences the kinetics of human immunodeficiency virus type 1 infection in human PBL-SCID mice. J. Virol. 71:7124–7127.

156. Pleskoff, O., C. Tréboute, A. Brelot, N. Heveker, M. Seman, and M. Alizon. 1997. Identification of a chemokine receptor encoded by human cytomegalovirus as a cofactor for HIV-1 entry [see comments]. Science 276:1874–1878.

157. Pohlmann, S., N. Stolte, J. Munch, P. Ten Haaft, J. L. Heeney, C. Stahl-Hennig, and F. Kirchhoff. 1999. Co-receptor usage of BOB/GPR15 in addition to CCR5 has no significant effect on replication of simian immunodeficiency virus in vivo. J. Infect. Dis. 180:1494–1502.

158. Proudfoot, A. E., C. A. Power, A. J. Hoogewerf, M. O. Montjovent, F. Borlat, R. E. Offord, and T. N. Wells. 1996. Extension of recombinant human RANTES by the retention of the initiating methionine produces a potent antagonist. J. Biol. Chem. 271:2599–2603.

159. Quillent, C., E. Oberlin, J. Braun, D. Rousset, G. Gonzalez-Canali, P. Métais, L. Montagnier, J. L. Virelizier, F. Arenzana-Seisdedos, and A. Beretta. 1998. HIV-1-resistance phenotype conferred by combination of two separate inherited mutations of CCR5 gene [see comments]. Lancet 351:14–18.

160. Rabut, G. E., J. A. Konner, F. Kajumo, J. P. Moore, and T. Dragic. 1998. Alanine substitutions of polar and nonpolar residues in the amino-terminal domain of CCR5 differently impair entry of macrophage- and dualtropic isolates of human immunodeficiency virus type 1. J. Virol. 72:3464–3468.

161. Rana, S., G. Besson, D. G. Cook, J. Rucker, R. J. Smyth, Y. Yi, J. D. Turner, H. H. Guo, J. G. Du, S. C. Peiper, E. Lavi, M. Samson, F. Libert, C. Liesnard, G. Vassart, R. W. Doms, M. Parmentier, and R. G. Collman. 1997. Role of CCR5 in infection of primary macrophages and lymphocytes by macrophage-tropic strains of human immunodeficiency virus: resistance to patient-derived and prototype isolates resulting from the delta ccr5 mutation. J. Virol. 71:3219–3227.

162. Raport, C. J., J. Gosling, V. L. Schweickart, P. W. Gray, and I. F. Charo. 1996. Molecular cloning and functional characterization of a novel human CC chemokine receptor (CCR5) for RANTES, MIP-1beta, and MIP-1alpha. J. Biol. Chem. 271:17161–17166.

163. Rappaport, J., Y. Y. Cho, H. Hendel, E. J. Schwartz, F. Schachter, and J. F. Zagury. 1997. 32 bp CCR-5 gene deletion and resistance to fast progression in HIV-1 infected heterozygotes [letter]. Lancet 349:922–923.

164. Reeves, J. D., and T. F. Schulz. 1997. The CD4-independent tropism of human immunodeficiency virus type 2 involves several regions of the envelope protein and correlates with a reduced activation threshold for envelope-mediated fusion. J. Virol. 71:1453–1465.

165. Rizzardi, G. P., R. A. Morawetz, E. Vicenzi, S. Ghezzi, G. Poli, A. Lazzarin, and G. Pantaleo. 1998. CCR2 polymorphism and HIV disease. Swiss HIV Cohort [letter]. Nature Med. 4:252–253.

166. Ross, T. M., and B. R. Cullen. 1998. The ability of HIV type 1 to use CCR-3 as a coreceptor is controlled by envelope V1/V2 sequences acting in conjunction with a CCR-5 tropic V3 loop. Proc. Natl. Acad. Sci. USA 95:7682–7686.

167. Rousseau, C. M., J. J. Just, E. J. Abrams, J. Casabona, Z. Stein, and M. C. King. 1997. CCR5del32 in perinatal HIV-1 infection. J. Acquired Immune Defic. Syndr. Hum. Retrovirol. 16:239–242.

168. Rowland-Jones, S., J. Sutton, K. Ariyoshi, T. Dong, F. Gotch, S. McAdam, D. Whitby, S. Sabally, A. Gallimore, T. Corrah, et al. 1995. HIV-specific cytotoxic T-cells in HIV-exposed but uninfected Gambian women. Nature Med. 1:59–64. (Erratum, 1(6):598.)

169. Rowland-Jones, S. L., T. Dong, K. R. Fowke, J. Kimani, P. Krausa, H. Newell, T. Blanchard, K. Ariyoshi, J. Oyugi, E. Ngugi, J. Bwayo, K. S. MacDonald, A. J. McMichael, and F. A. Plummer. 1998. Cytotoxic T cell responses to multiple conserved HIV epitopes in HIV-resistant prostitutes in Nairobi [see comments]. J. Clin. Invest. 102:1758–1765.

170. Rucker, J., R. W. Doms, M. Tsang, X. Hu, M. Dietz, R. Bailer, L. J. Montaner, C. Gerard, N. Sullivan, J. Sodroski, T. S. Stantchev, and C. C. Broder. 1998. Beta-chemokine MDC and HIV-1 infection. Science 281:487a.

171. Rucker, J., A. L. Edinger, M. Sharron, M. Samson, B. Lee, J. F. Berson, Y. Yi, B. Margulies, R. G. Collman, B. J. Doranz, M. Parmentier, and R. W. Doms. 1997. Utilization of chemokine receptors, orphan receptors, and herpesvirus-encoded receptors by diverse human and simian immunodeficiency viruses. J. Virol. 71:8999–9007.

172. Ruffing, N., N. Sullivan, L. Sharmeen, J. Sodroski, and L. Wu. 1998. CCR5 has an expanded ligand-binding repertoire and is the primary receptor used by MCP-2 on activated T cells. Cell Immunol. 189:160–168.

173. Samson, M., O. Labbe, C. Mollereau, G. Vassart, and M. Parmentier. 1996. Molecular cloning and functional expression of a new human CC-chemokine receptor gene. Biochemistry 35:3362–3367.

174. Samson, M., F. Libert, B. J. Doranz, J. Rucker, C. Liesnard, C. M. Farber, S. Saragosti, C. Lapoumeroulie, J. Cognaux, C. Forceille, G. Muyldermans, C. Verhofstede, G. Burtonboy, M. Georges, T. Imai, S. Rana, Y. Yi, R. J. Smyth, R. G. Collman, R. W. Doms, G. Vassart, and M. Parmentier. 1996. Resistance to HIV-1 infection in Caucasian individuals bearing mutant alleles of the CCR-5 chemokine receptor gene [see comments]. Nature 382:722–725.

175. Scarlatti, G., E. Tresoldi, A. Björndal, R. Fredriksson, C. Colognesi, H. K. Deng, M. S. Malnati, A. Plebani, A. G. Siccardi, D. R. Littman, E. M. Fenyö, and P. Lusso. 1997. In vivo evolution of HIV-1 co-receptor usage and sensitivity to chemokine-mediated suppression. Nature Med. 3:1259–1265.

176. Schinkel, J., M. W. Langendam, R. A. Coutinho, A. Krol, M. Brouwer, and H. Schuitemaker. 1999. No evidence for an effect of the CCR5 delta32/+ and CCR2b 64I/+ mutations on human immunodeficiency virus (HIV)-1 disease progression among HIV-1-infected injecting drug users. J. Infect. Dis. 179: 825–831.

177. Schmidtmayerova, H., M. Alfano, G. Nuovo, and M. Bukrinsky. 1998. Human immunodeficiency virus type 1 T-lymphotropic strains enter macrophages via a CD4- and CXCR4-mediated pathway: replication is restricted at a postentry level. J. Virol. 72:4633–4642.

178. Schols, D., J. A. Esté, C. Cabrera, and E. De Clercq. 1998. T-cell-line-tropic human immunodeficiency virus type 1 that is made resistant to stromal cell-derived factor 1alpha contains mutations in the envelope gp120 but does not show a switch in coreceptor use. J. Virol. 72:4032–4037.

179. Schols, D., S. Struyf, J. Van Damme, J. A. Esté, G. Henson, and E. De Clercq. 1997. Inhibition of T-tropic HIV strains by selective antagonization of the chemokine receptor CXCR4. J. Exp. Med. 186:1383–1388.

180. Schuitemaker, H., M. Koot, N. A. Kootstra, M. W. Dercksen, R. E. de Goede, R. P. van Steenwijk, J. M. Lange, J. K. Schattenkerk, F. Miedema, and M. Tersmette. 1992. Biological phenotype of human immunodeficiency virus type 1 clones at different stages of infection: progression of disease is associated with a shift from monocytotropic to T-cell-tropic virus population. J. Virol. 66:1354–1360.

181. Schwarz, M. K., and T. Wells. 1999. Interfering with chemokine networks—the hope for new therapeutics. Curr. Opin. Chem. Biol. 3:407–417.

182. Shearer, W. T., L. A. Kalish, and P. A. Zimmerman. 1998. CCR5 HIV-1 verti-

cal transmission. Women and Infants Transmission Study Group [letter]. J. Acquired Immune Defic. Syndr. Hum. Retrovirol. 17:180–181.

183. Shioda, T., J. A. Levy, and C. Cheng-Mayer. 1991. Macrophage and T cell-line tropisms of HIV-1 are determined by specific regions of the envelope gp120 gene. Nature 349:167–169.

184. Shioda, T., J. A. Levy, and C. Cheng-Mayer. 1992. Small amino acid changes in the V3 hypervariable region of gp120 can affect the T-cell-line and macrophage tropism of human immunodeficiency virus type 1. Proc. Natl. Acad. Sci. USA 89:9434–9438.

185. Siciliano, S. J., S. E. Kuhmann, Y. Weng, N. Madani, M. S. Springer, J. E. Lineberger, R. Danzeisen, M. D. Miller, M. P. Kavanaugh, J. A. DeMartino, and D. Kabat. 1999. A critical site in the core of the CCR5 chemokine receptor required for binding and infectivity of human immunodeficiency virus type 1. J. Biol. Chem. 274:1905–1913.

186. Simmons, G., P. R. Clapham, L. Picard, R. E. Offord, M. M. Rosenkilde, T. W. Schwartz, R. Buser, T. N. C. Wells, and A. E. Proudfoot. 1997. Potent inhibition of HIV-1 infectivity in macrophages and lymphocytes by a novel CCR5 antagonist. Science 276:276–279.

187. Simmons, G., J. D. Reeves, A. McKnight, N. Dejucq, S. Hibbitts, C. A. Power, E. Aarons, D. Schols, E. De Clercq, A. E. Proudfoot, and P. R. Clapham. 1998. CXCR4 as a functional coreceptor for human immunodeficiency virus type 1 infection of primary macrophages. J. Virol. 72:8453–8457.

188. Simmons, G., D. Wilkinson, J. D. Reeves, M. T. Dittmar, S. Beddows, J. Weber, G. Carnegie, U. Desselberger, P. W. Gray, R. A. Weiss, and P. R. Clapham. 1996. Primary, syncytium-inducing human immunodeficiency virus type 1 isolates are dual-tropic and most can use either Lestr or CCR5 as coreceptors for virus entry. J. Virol. 70:8355–8360.

189. Smith, M. W., M. Dean, M. Carrington, C. Winkler, G. A. Huttley, D. A. Lomb, J. J. Goedert, T. R. O'Brien, L. P. Jacobson, R. Kaslow, S. Buchbinder, E. Vittinghoff, D. Vlahov, K. Hoots, M. W. Hilgartner, and S. J. O'Brien. 1997. Contrasting genetic influence of CCR2 and CCR5 variants on HIV-1 infection and disease progression. Hemophilia Growth and Development Study (HGDS), Multicenter AIDS Cohort Study (MACS), Multicenter Hemophilia Cohort Study (MHCS), San Francisco City Cohort (SFCC), ALIVE Study. Science 277:959–965.

190. Speck, R. F., K. Wehrly, E. J. Platt, R. E. Atchison, I. F. Charo, D. Kabat, B. Chesebro, and M. A. Goldsmith. 1997. Selective employment of chemokine receptors as human immunodeficiency virus type 1 coreceptors determined by individual amino acids within the envelope V3 loop. J. Virol. 71:7136–7139.

191. Spira, A. I., P. A. Marx, B. K. Patterson, J. Mahoney, R. A. Koup, S. M. Wolinsky, and D. D. Ho. 1996. Cellular targets of infection and route of viral dissemination after an intravaginal inoculation of simian immunodeficiency virus into rhesus macaques. J. Exp. Med. 183:215–225.

192. Stephens, J. C., D. E. Reich, D. B. Goldstein, H. D. Shin, M. W. Smith, M. Carrington, C. Winkler, G. A. Huttley, R. Allikmets, L. Schriml, B. Gerrard, M. Malasky, M. D. Ramos, S. Morlot, M. Tzetis, C. Oddoux, F. S. di Giovine, G. Nasioulas, D. Chandler, M. Aseev, M. Hanson, L. Kalaydjieva, D. Glavac, P.

Gasparini, M. Dean, et al. 1998. Dating the origin of the CCR5-delta32 AIDS-resistance allele by the coalescence of haplotypes. Am. J. Hum. Genet. 62:1507–1515.

193. Swingler, S., A. Mann, J. Jacqué, B. Brichacek, V. G. Sasseville, K. Williams, A. A. Lackner, E. N. Janoff, R. Wang, D. Fisher, and M. Stevenson. 1999. HIV-1 Nef mediates lymphocyte chemotaxis and activation by infected macrophages. Nature Med. 5:997–1003.

194. Tachibana, K., T. Nakajima, A. Sato, K. Igarashi, H. Shida, H. Iizasa, N. Yoshida, O. Yoshie, T. Kishimoto, and T. Nagasawa. 1997. CXCR4/fusin is not a species-specific barrier in murine cells for HIV-1 entry. J. Exp. Med. 185:1865–1870.

195. Theodorou, I., L. Meyer, M. Magierowska, C. Katlama, and C. Rouzioux. 1997. HIV-1 infection in an individual homozygous for CCR5 delta 32. Seroco Study Group [letter] [see comments]. Lancet 349:1219–1220.

196. Trkola, A., T. Dragic, J. Arthos, J. M. Binley, W. C. Olson, G. P. Allaway, C. Cheng-Mayer, J. Robinson, P. J. Maddon, and J. P. Moore. 1996. CD4-dependent, antibody-sensitive interactions between HIV-1 and its co-receptor CCR-5 [see comments]. Nature 384:184–187.

197. Trkola, A., C. Gordon, J. Matthews, E. Maxwell, T. Ketas, L. Czaplewski, A. E. Proudfoot, and J. P. Moore. 1999. The CC-chemokine RANTES increases the attachment of human immunodeficiency virus type 1 to target cells via glycosaminoglycans and also activates a signal transduction pathway that enhances viral infectivity. J. Virol. 73:6370–6379.

198. van Rij, R. P., S. Broersen, J. Goudsmit, R. A. Coutinho, and H. Schuitemaker. 1998. The role of a stromal cell-derived factor-1 chemokine gene variant in the clinical course of HIV-1 infection. AIDS 12:F85–90.

199. van't Wout, A. B., N. A. Kootstra, G. A. Mulder-Kampinga, N. Albrecht-van Lent, H. J. Scherpbier, J. Veenstra, K. Boer, R. A. Coutinho, F. Miedema, and H. Schuitemaker. 1994. Macrophage-tropic variants initiate human immunodeficiency virus type 1 infection after sexual, parenteral, and vertical transmission. J. Clin. Invest. 94:2060–2067.

200. Verani, A., E. Pesenti, S. Polo, E. Tresoldi, G. Scarlatti, P. Lusso, A. G. Siccardi, and D. Vercelli. 1998. CXCR4 is a functional coreceptor for infection of human macrophages by CXCR4-dependent primary HIV-1 isolates. J. Immunol. 161:2084–2088.

201. Walker, C. M., D. J. Moody, D. P. Stites, and J. A. Levy. 1986. CD8+ lymphocytes can control HIV infection in vitro by suppressing virus replication. Science 234:1563–1566.

202. Weissenhorn, W., A. Dessen, L. J. Calder, S. C. Harrison, J. J. Skehel, and D. C. Wiley. 1999. Structural basis for membrane fusion by enveloped viruses. Mol. Membr. Biol. 16:3–9.

203. Weissman, D., R. L. Rabin, J. Arthos, A. Rubbert, M. Dybul, R. Swofford, S. Venkatesan, J. M. Farber, and A. S. Fauci. 1997. Macrophage-tropic HIV and SIV envelope proteins induce a signal through the CCR5 chemokine receptor. Nature 389:981–985.

204. Westervelt, P., H. E. Gendelman, and L. Ratner. 1991. Identification of a determinant within the human immunodeficiency virus 1 surface envelope gly-

coprotein critical for productive infection of primary monocytes. Proc. Natl. Acad. Sci. USA 88:3097–3101.

205. Wilkinson, D. A., E. A. Operskalski, M. P. Busch, J. W. Mosley, and R. A. Koup. 1998. A 32-bp deletion within the CCR5 locus protects against transmission of parenterally acquired human immunodeficiency virus but does not affect progression to AIDS-defining illness. J. Infect. Dis. 178:1163–1166.

206. Winkler, C., W. Modi, M. W. Smith, G. W. Nelson, X. Wu, M. Carrington, M. Dean, T. Honjo, K. Tashiro, D. Yabe, S. Buchbinder, E. Vittinghoff, J. J. Goedert, T. R. O'Brien, L. P. Jacobson, R. Detels, S. Donfield, A. Willoughby, E. Gomperts, D. Vlahov, J. Phair, and S. J. O'Brien. 1998. Genetic restriction of AIDS pathogenesis by an SDF-1 chemokine gene variant. ALIVE Study, Hemophilia Growth and Development Study (HGDS), Multicenter AIDS Cohort Study (MACS), Multicenter Hemophilia Cohort Study (MHCS), San Francisco City Cohort (SFCC) [see comments]. Science 279:389–393.

207. Wu, L., N. P. Gerard, R. Wyatt, H. Choe, C. Parolin, N. Ruffing, A. Borsetti, A. A. Cardoso, E. Desjardin, W. Newman, C. Gerard, and J. Sodroski. 1996. CD4-induced interaction of primary HIV-1 gp120 glycoproteins with the chemokine receptor CCR-5 [see comments]. Nature 384:179–183.

208. Wu, L., W. A. Paxton, N. Kassam, N. Ruffing, J. B. Rottman, N. Sullivan, H. Choe, J. Sodroski, W. Newman, R. A. Koup, and C. R. Mackay. 1997. CCR5 levels and expression pattern correlate with infectability by macrophage-tropic HIV-1, in vitro. J. Exp. Med. 185:1681–1691.

209. Wyatt, R., and J. Sodroski. 1998. The HIV-1 envelope glycoproteins: fusogens, antigens, and immunogens. Science 280:1884–1888.

210. Xiao, L., S. M. Owen, I. Goldman, A. A. Lal, J. J. deJong, J. Goudsmit, and R. B. Lal. 1998. CCR5 coreceptor usage of non-syncytium-inducing primary HIV-1 is independent of phylogenetically distinct global HIV-1 isolates: delineation of consensus motif in the V3 domain that predicts CCR-5 usage. Virology 240:83–92.

211. Yi, Y., S. Rana, J. D. Turner, N. Gaddis, and R. G. Collman. 1998. CXCR-4 is expressed by primary macrophages and supports CCR5-independent infection by dual-tropic but not T-tropic isolates of human immunodeficiency virus type 1. J. Virol. 72:772–777.

212. Zhang, L., Y. Huang, T. He, Y. Cao, and D. D. Ho. 1996. HIV-1 subtype and second-receptor use [letter]. Nature 383:768.

213. Zhang, Y. J., T. Dragic, Y. Cao, L. Kostrikis, D. S. Kwon, D. R. Littman, V. N. Kewal-Ramani, and J. P. Moore. 1998. Use of coreceptors other than CCR5 by non-syncytium-inducing adult and pediatric isolates of human immunodeficiency virus type 1 is rare in vitro. J. Virol. 72:9337–9344.

214. Zhou, Y., T. Kurihara, R. P. Ryseck, Y. Yang, C. Ryan, J. Loy, G. Warr, and R. Bravo. 1998. Impaired macrophage function and enhanced T cell-dependent immune response in mice lacking CCR5, the mouse homologue of the major HIV-1 coreceptor. J. Immunol. 160:4018–4025.

215. Zimmerman, P. A., A. Buckler-White, G. Alkhatib, T. Spalding, J. Kubofcik, C. Combadiere, D. Weissman, O. Cohen, A. Rubbert, G. Lam, M. Vaccarezza, P. E. Kennedy, V. Kumaraswami, J. V. Giorgi, R. Detels, J. Hunter, M. Chopek, E. A. Berger, A. S. Fauci, T. B. Nutman, and P. M. Murphy. 1997. Inherited re-

sistance to HIV-1 conferred by an inactivating mutation in CC chemokine receptor 5: studies in populations with contrasting clinical phenotypes, defined racial background, and quantified risk. Mol. Med. 3:23–36.

216. Zlotnik, A., J. Morales, and J. A. Hedrick. 1999. Recent advances in chemokines and chemokine receptors. Critical Rev. Immunol. 19:1–47.

217. Zou, Y. R., A. H. Kottmann, M. Kuroda, I. Taniuchi, and D. R. Littman. 1998. Function of the chemokine receptor CXCR4 in haematopoiesis and in cerebellar development [see comments]. Nature 393:595–599.

Novel HIV-1 Therapeutic Targets: Regulatory Functions

8

CATHERINE ULICH
RICHARD B. GAYNOR

The HIV-1 genome is composed of approximately 9.0 kb of DNA flanked by two long terminal repeats (LTRs) (5, 68, 109). Fifteen gene products are encoded by this relatively compact genome structure including the critical regulatory proteins Tat and Rev; the accessory proteins Nef, Vif, Vpu, and Vpr; the structural proteins Gag (p24, p17, and p6) and Env (gp120 and gp41); and enzymes including reverse transcriptase, protease, and integrase (55). The regulation of HIV-1 gene expression depends on the efficient production of each of these gene products. A variety of unique mechanisms have evolved to permit HIV-1 gene expression to be regulated in a temporal manner.

Two essential proteins involved in this regulation are the HIV-1 Tat (36, 51, 155) and Rev proteins (48, 101, 160). Both proteins, in addition to the Nef protein, are the products of a 2.0-kb multiply spliced RNA that is expressed early after HIV-1 infection (93). The Tat protein is essential for the expression of other HIV-1 gene products. It is the ability of Tat to bind to an RNA element known as TAR in conjunction with a cellular kinase complex positive-acting transcription elongation factor (P-TEFb) that increases the processivity of RNA polymerase II (RNAPII) as it transverses the HIV-1 genome (2, 115, 117–119, 196, 198). Therefore, Tat expression is critical for expression of the Rev protein.

Rev is critical for the nuclear-cytoplasmic transport of incompletely spliced or unspliced HIV-1 RNA that encodes viral structural proteins or serves as genomic RNA (42, 113). Thus, Rev plays an important role in the differential splicing of HIV-1 transcripts to regulate its gene expression temporally. Since both Tat and Rev are essential proteins required for HIV-1 replication, they provide potential therapeutic targets to inhibit HIV-1 replication. This review provides a summary of the mechanisms by which Tat and Rev regulate HIV-1 replication and suggests potential ways to inhibit their function.

The Tat Transactivator Protein

Tat is an essential viral protein of 101 amino acids and is encoded by two exons. The first exon of Tat is essential for its ability to activate HIV-1 gene expression (147). Tat strongly activates gene expression of the HIV-1 LTR and, in addition, has been shown to activate weakly some cellular genes involved in signal transduction (22, 124, 128) and apoptosis (11, 22, 103, 180). The significance of Tat activation of cellular gene expression remains unclear at this time. In addition to its effects on viral gene expression, Tat has been demonstrated to be required for efficient HIV-1 reverse transcription (72, 172). Thus, Tat likely has multiple functions that are important in the pathogenesis of HIV-1 infection.

Structure of Tat and TAR RNA

The *tat* gene has been extensively mutagenized (60, 97, 130, 161). Four domains within the first exon have been identified: acidic, cysteine-rich, core, and basic domains. The first three regions are grouped together functionally as an activation domain that has been shown to interact with cellular proteins (149) (Fig. 8.1). The Tat activation domain is required for both efficient HIV-1 gene expression and reverse transcription. Mutations in the Tat activation domain severely impair HIV-1 replication. The basic domain, also referred to as the arginine-rich motif (ARM), contains a nuclear localization signal (NLS) and also facilitates the binding of Tat to TAR RNA that is crucial for Tat-mediated transactivation of transcription (39, 49).

The second exon of Tat is not required for activation of HIV-1 gene expression, although it has been reported to have effects on an integrated HIV-1 provirus (87). However, the second exon of Tat has been shown to have effects on the expression of other cellular genes. For example, the second exon of Tat leads to increases in IL-2 gene expression by effects on factors that bind to the CD28-response element in the IL-2 promoter (138). The second exon of Tat was also found to increase the expression of caspase 8, which is a critical protease involved in the induction of apoptosis (11). Finally, the second exon of Tat has been shown to function in the repression of major histocompatibility complex (MHC) class I gene transcription, which potentially contributes to viral persistence (80). These results suggest that the second exon of Tat may play a role in modulating the expression of diverse cellular genes.

TAR RNA forms a stable stem-loop structure that extends from +1 to +60 (131, 136). This structure contains a trinucleotide bulge (+21/+24) and a six-nucleotide loop (+30/+35), each of which is essential for its function (Fig. 8.2). Tat binds to a three-nucleotide bulge of TAR RNA (31, 40, 75, 164, 165). This interaction induces a conformational change in TAR that exposes critical groups on the RNA that lead to enhanced Tat binding to TAR

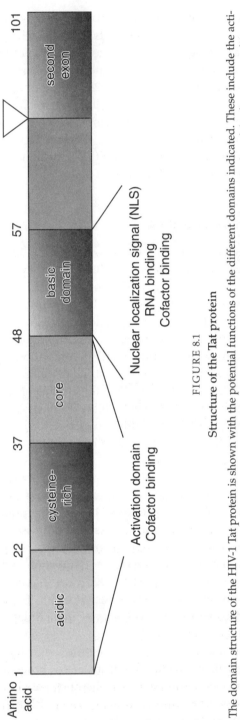

FIGURE 8.1

Structure of the Tat protein

The domain structure of the HIV-1 Tat protein is shown with the potential functions of the different domains indicated. These include the activation domain, which comprises the acidic, cysteine-rich, and core domains; the basic domain; and the remainder of the first exon coding sequences and the second exon coding sequences.

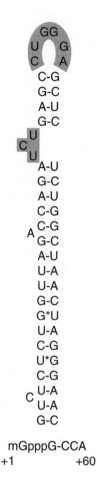

FIGURE 8.2
Schematic of TAR RNA

The structure of HIV-1 TAR from residues +1 to +60 is indicated with the positions of critical regulatory elements shaded, including the bulge and loop sequences.

RNA (1). The minimal TAR domain required for Tat activation has been mapped from +19/+44, although sequences that make up the lower TAR RNA stem (49, 61, 158) may also influence Tat activation (176). There have also been reports of a lower-stem binding protein, p140, which has been proposed to stabilize Tat-TAR interactions during virus replication (152, 153). It has been suggested, therefore, that an extended HIV-1 TAR hairpin structure is required for efficient gene expression in T cells.

Preservation of the upper-stem base pairing in TAR RNA as well as correct spacing between the loop and bulge elements (86) must be maintained for efficient viral transcription and replication. The selective pressure to maintain each of these TAR RNA structural elements has been shown in vivo. Viruses with mutant TAR elements introduced into the 5′ and 3′ LTRs either reverted to wild-type sequence or developed compensatory mutations that were able to confer *tat* responsiveness to these viruses upon prolonged culture (13, 71). An intact TAR RNA secondary structure is important for Tat function, although it may also be important at other steps in the HIV-l life cycle.

Functions of Tat

The HIV-1 Tat protein is essential for the regulation of HIV-1 gene expression (reviewed in reference 89). Although the HIV-1 LTR contains binding sites for a variety of transcription factors including NF-κB, SP-1, and TBP, gene expression from the HIV-1 LTR is relatively inefficient because RNAPII does not efficiently elongate through its genome (90). The reason that RNAPII elongation is relatively inefficient as it transverses the HIV-1 genome remains to be determined. The Tat protein in conjunction with TAR RNA overcomes the structural constraints of the HIV-1 LTR to allow efficient transcriptional elongation through the 9.0-kb HIV-1 genome. Tat expression leads to 100- to 1,000-fold increases of HIV-1 gene expression and viral replication (36, 51, 155). As mentioned previously, Tat is also required for efficient reverse transcription (72, 172). In the absence of a functional *tat* gene, defects in reverse transcription are found at very early steps of this process and within the virion particle itself. This suggests a role for Tat in the reverse transcription process during viral assembly at a stage prior to receptor binding.

Tat has also been demonstrated to have a variety of other effects. For example, it has been proposed that Tat modulates the phosphorylation of SP-1 by DNA-PK (30), which may result in effects on cellular growth as well as HIV-1 transcription. Other groups have studied effects of Tat on T-cell activation and apoptosis (11, 103, 180). The addition of exogenous Tat has also been demonstrated to increase NF-κB binding (32, 181), to upregulate viral gene expression from latently infected cell lines (24), and to stimulate T-cell activation (104). It has been reported that Tat may actually potentiate the effects of cytokines such as TNF-α by altering the redox states of the HIV-1-infected or bystander cells (181). Tat has also been shown to increase the expression of some cellular genes, for example IL-8 (139), IL-6 (150, 191), and the IL-4 receptor (83), likely through activation of the NF-κB pathway and increasing the transcription of these genes. Tat may act as a cellular growth factor (3, 4, 38, 99, 129, 137), such as its involvement in the development of Kaposi's sarcoma (43, 44) to increase angiogenesis. In addition to its role in activating gene expression, Tat has also been shown to repress gene expression of the class I MHC gene (80). This effect, which is mediated by the second exon of Tat, is potentially related to the ability of Tat to repress the histone acetylase activity of TAF250 (179).

Identification of Cellular Cofactors Involved in Tat Function

Tat has been reported to increase both transcription initiation (35, 101) and elongation (47, 64, 91, 101, 102, 116). However, more recent data suggest that the primary effect of Tat is to stimulate the degree of promoter clearance or the formation of more processive elongation complexes or both. Tat associates with preinitiation complexes assembled on the HIV-1 LTR template, and this association requires an intact TATA element and functional TBP (62). Given the fact that Tat has been shown to interact with SP1 (88) and RNAPII (121), it is possible that these or other factors may also be involved in the functional association of Tat with HIV-1 transcription complexes.

Since the major effect of Tat is to increase the processivity of RNAPII, polymerase is likely a major target for Tat effects. RNAPII contains 10 subunits, and the largest subunit is regulated by its phosphorylation state (193). This subunit of RNAPII contains a C-terminal domain (CTD) composed of 52 conserved heptad repeats that can be phosphorylated by cellular kinases to stimulate promoter clearance or elongation or both (29, 134). It was demonstrated that an intact RNAPII CTD is essential for Tat transactivation in vivo (29, 135, 187). Furthermore, the nucleoside inhibitor DRB can abrogate the effects of Tat stimulation of HIV-1 gene expression by preventing phosphorylation of the CTD (116). Thus, it was hypothesized that Tat might interact with a cellular kinase that could hyperphosphorylate the CTD to increase HIV-1 transcriptional elongation. Several groups subsequently reported the identification of kinases that bound to Tat, hyperphosphorylated the CTD, and increased in vitro transcription (34, 63, 78, 115, 140, 178, 198).

Transcription factor IIH (TFIIH) was independently identified by three groups as a potential CTD kinase that binds to the activation domain of Tat and can stimulate transcription (34, 63, 140). The kinase activity of TFIIH resides in the kinase CDK7 (cyclin-dependent kinase 7) (2), which associates with cyclin H and MAT1 to form a CDK-activating kinase complex (CAK) that phosphorylates the RNAPII CTP and is associated with increases in promoter clearance. The addition of Tat to purified cellular fractions of TFIIH increased its ability to phosphorylate the CTD, confirming that the interactions between TFIIH, Tat, and RNAPII are functionally significant. Tat was also demonstrated to associate with the RNAPII holoenzyme, which includes TFIIH (33). Another group also identified TFIIH as the Tat-associated kinase by specifically defining Tat/TFIIH interactions (34). It demonstrated that recombinant CDK7 interacted specifically with wild-type Tat, leading to the association of CAK with other components of the multisubunit TFIIH complex (34).

A novel kinase that functions in a Tat-dependent manner to hyperphosphorylate the RNAPII CTD was also identified. This kinase was first identified as a nuclear serine/threonine kinase that was part of a larger complex called TAK (Tat-associated kinase), and its properties were characterized in biochemical assays (78). The interaction between Tat and TAK appeared to correlate with both the ability of Tat to stimulate transcription in vivo and the ability of Tat to stimulate CTD phosphorylation in vitro. However, the identity of this kinase was unknown until work on transcriptional elongation in *Drosophila* resulted in important insights into the mechanisms of Tat activation (117–119). Biochemical studies of RNAPII transcriptional elongation complexes in *Drosophila* extracts resulted in the isolation of a two-subunit complex called P-TEFb that is required for transcriptional elongation. P-TEFb stimulates the transcriptional elongation properties of a variety of cellular genes and contains a kinase activity capable of hyperphosphorylating the CTD (117). It likely associates with the HIV-1 preinitiation complex prior to transcriptional elongation (144). The catalytic subunit of this complex was purified, and amino acid sequencing demonstrated that it had a high degree of sequence homology with a human CDC2-related kinase named PITALRE (66, 198).

PITALRE was found to be a component of TAK, and depletion of this kinase from nuclear extracts abolished Tat stimulation of the HIV-1 LTR in in vitro transcription assays (198). Further evidence that PITALRE/P-TEFb is involved in Tat-activated transcription came from another group screening for inhibitors of Tat function (115). Characterization of compounds that block Tat-dependent stimulation of transcriptional elongation from the HIV-1 LTR indicated that the PITALRE was the likely target for these kinase inhibitors.

PITALRE was renamed CDK9 after it was shown to associate with a novel 87-kDa cyclin named cyclin T1 (59, 142, 143, 178). Cyclin T1 was isolated from purified TAK complexes and shown to bind strongly to the activation domain of Tat. It was demonstrated that interactions between Tat and cyclin T1 increased the affinity of Tat binding to TAR RNA (15, 27, 57, 59, 84, 178, 182, 195). This interaction required intact TAR RNA loop and bulge sequences. RNA binding studies suggested that Tat binds to the TAR RNA bulge region while cyclin T1 likely makes direct contact with TAR RNA loop sequences. Cyclin T1 itself does not bind TAR RNA in the absence of Tat, while CDK9 does not bind to TAR RNA unless it is associated with the complex composed of Tat, cyclin T1, and TAR RNA (59, 84, 98, 178, 182). Mutagenesis studies of human and murine cyclin T1 and the related cyclins T2a and T2b, which also bind to CDK9 (142, 143), demonstrate that the interaction between Tat and human cyclin T1 is highly specific (58, 59, 84, 98, 182).

Tat can specifically interact with human cyclin T1 but not human cyclin T2a or T2b or murine cyclin T1 (15, 27, 58, 59, 84, 98, 182). The inability of Tat to activate HIV-1 gene expression efficiently in rodent cells is due to the differential binding of Tat to human cyclin T1 but not murine cyclin T1. For example, the introduction of human chromosome 12 into rodent cells can rescue Tat activation of the HIV-1 LTR (6, 74). Human cyclin T1 is present on chromosome 12, and transfection of a human cyclin T1 cDNA clone into rodent cells results in Tat activation of the HIV-1 LTR (59, 178).

These data suggest that cyclin T1 is the human-specific factor required for Tat activation in rodent cells. The question of how transfection of the human but not the murine cyclin T1 gene can restore Tat activation in rodent cells remained. Mutagenesis studies identified a single cysteine residue at position 261 within human cyclin T1 that, when substituted for a tyrosine residue normally present in the murine cyclin T1 protein, can confer Tat responsiveness of the HIV-1 LTR in murine cells (15, 27, 58, 59, 84, 98, 182). These studies could potentially aid in the development of murine models of HIV-1 infection.

Additional factors have been isolated that increase Tat-mediated transcription, including Tat-SF1 (105, 197) and SPT5 (184). These factors do not directly interact with either Tat or TAR RNA and likely play a more indirect role in stimulating transcriptional elongation by interacting with RNAPII directly or modulating the activity of other cellular factors that mediate Tat function. Most of the studies outlined have analyzed the role of Tat on HIV-1 LTR templates in the absence of chromatin. However, Tat has also been shown to activate HIV-1 gene expression assembled with chromatin (41). In fact, Tat can bind the transcription coactivators CBP and p300, which both have histone acetyltransferase activity (12, 79, 120). This activity likely plays a role in removing the inhibition of nucleosome arrangement downstream of the HIV-1 transcription initiation site (174, 175).

Finally, a cellular protein that interacts with the basic region (ARM) of Tat has recently been identified (171). This protein, importin-β, binds to the NLS of Tat to direct it through the nuclear pore complex (NPC) to the nucleus, where it can activate transcription. Interestingly, this is the same cellular protein that has been shown to associate with Rev during nuclear import. These results indicate that Tat likely associates with a number of cellular proteins that are involved in the regulation of HIV-1 replication.

Model for Tat Stimulation of HIV-1 Gene Expression

Although there are still some questions as to the specificity and importance of different cellular factors involved in HIV-1 gene expression, a reasonable model can be proposed that includes many of the previously described observations (Fig. 8.3). Tat is associated with HIV-1 preinitiation complexes prior to the synthesis of TAR RNA and may facilitate interactions between SP-1, TBP, TFIIH, and RNAPII or other components of the basal transcription apparatus (62, 88, 121). Tat interactions with TFIIH may function at the initial stage of promoter clearance (34, 63, 140). Once TAR RNA is synthesized, the transcription complex may pause as a result of binding of RNAPII to TAR RNA. This pausing may facilitate Tat binding to the TAR RNA bulge and subsequently recruit the CDK9/cyclin T1 complex to TAR RNA (178). CDK9/cyclin T1, together with other stimulatory factors, functions to hyperphosphorylate the CTD and stimulate the elon-

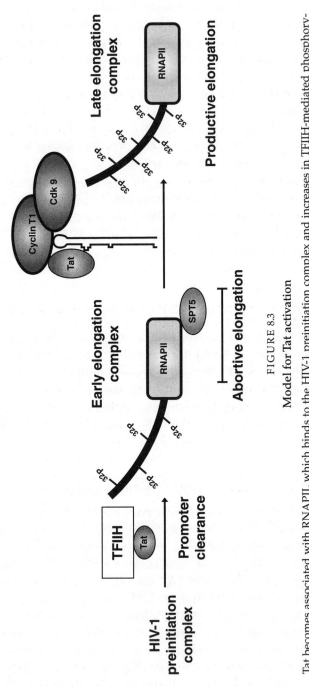

FIGURE 8.3

Model for Tat activation

Tat becomes associated with RNAPII, which binds to the HIV-1 preinitiation complex and increases in TFIIH-mediated phosphorylation of the RNAPII CTD to result in the early phase of promoter clearance. RNAPII stalls as a result of the binding of SPT5 and binding to TAR RNA. Tat, in conjunction with P-TEFb, binds to the TAR RNA bulge and loop elements, respectively, to enhance phosphorylation of the RNAPII CTD with resultant increases in its processivity.

gation properties of RNAPII. As the hypophosphorylated form of the polymerase binds more efficiently to TAR RNA (121), the hyperphosphorylated RNAPII is preferentially released from TAR RNA and proceeds to transcribe the proviral DNA efficiently. It has been proposed that Tat remains associated with the HIV-1 transcriptional elongation complex to maintain the hyperphosphorylated state of the RNAPII CTD as it transcribes the HIV-1 genome (92).

The activation state of the cell and cell-type specificity are likely to be important determinants of the type of transcription complexes that are formed on the HIV-1 LTR. For example, CDK9/cyclin T1 complex expression is markedly increased upon activation of T cells by agents such as phorbol esters (65, 77, 186). It is quite possible that additional factors, including as yet uncharacterized kinases, are involved in regulating Tat function. It is likely that not all the factors described in this section will be required for transcription reactions in all cells relevant for HIV-1 replication. However, the specificity of the transcription process suggests that the basic mechanisms of Tat function will be conserved in most sites of HIV-1 replication.

A Role for *tat* and TAR RNA in HIV-1 Reverse Transcription

HIV-1 replication is markedly decreased by mutations in the *tat* gene (36, 51, 81, 155). This effect was attributed to the failure of Tat to activate HIV-1 gene expression. However, the effects of Tat on modulating the HIV-1 reverse transcription process are likely also responsible for these replication defects. HIV-1 either lacking the *tat* gene or containing mutations in TAR RNA that disrupt its secondary structure are both very defective in the initiation of reverse transcription (72, 73, 172). This defect results in decreases in both the synthesis of minus-strand strong-stop DNA and full-length DNA. HIV-1 virions lacking *tat* can also exhibit defects in natural endogenous reverse transcription assays (72, 192). These results suggest that the processivity of the reverse transcriptase might be altered in HIV-1 virions lacking Tat. Although Tat has not been demonstrated to be a virion-associated protein, Tat may be incorporated into HIV-1 virion particles via binding to TAR RNA (23, 39, 177). Tat binding to TAR RNA within the virion could potentially modify TAR structure to enhance both the initiation and the processivity of reverse transcriptase.

By using a variety of *tat* mutants, the defects in reverse transcription seen with viruses lacking *tat* could be separable from the effects of these *tat* mutants on transcriptional activation (172). It is possible that intravirion Tat can facilitate interactions between TAR RNA and other RNA elements such as tRNA^{Lys3} or U5 RNA that are involved in the reverse transcription process. Whether Tat association with these RNAs can result in the direct association of Tat with either reverse transcriptase or other proteins in the reverse transcription complex remains to be determined. Although a favorable reverse transcription complex may be formed during virus assembly and involve recruitment of Tat, indirect effects such as activation of cellular kinases that can phosphorylate HIV-1 proteins involved in the reverse transcription are also possible. A potential model for the role of Tat on HIV-1 reverse transcription is diagrammed in Fig. 8.4.

Inhibition of Tat Function

A number of studies have attempted to inhibit Tat directly or prevent Tat/TAR RNA interactions. For example, antisense RNA strategies (106), polymeric TAR elements as decoys (19, 20, 185), anti-Tat single-chain intrabodies (126, 127), anti-Tat ribozymes (108, 194), and peptides that block formation of the Tat/TAR complex (70, 82) have all been used in attempts to inhibit Tat function. Dominant-negative Tat mutants have also

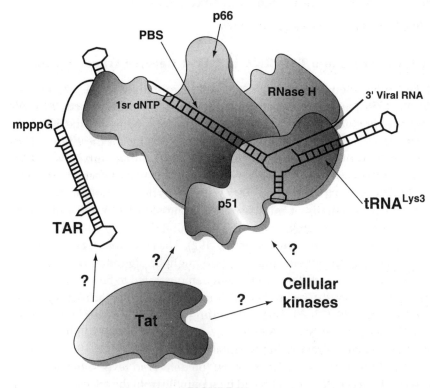

FIGURE 8.4

Potential roles for Tat on HIV-1 reverse transcription

The structure of HIV-1 reverse transcriptase with the p66 and p51 subunits, tRNA^{Lys3}, and HIV-1 RNA from the U5 and R regions are shown. Potential sites of Tat modulation of reverse transcription including direct or indirect interactions with either reverse transcriptase or TAR RNA or activation of cellular kinase pathways are shown.

been used in a number of studies to inhibit HIV-1 gene expression and replication (28, 130, 141, 173). Specifically, the substitution of the basic domain of Tat with neutral amino acids gives rise to the transdominant phenotype. Although these molecules were able to inhibit HIV-1 gene expression markedly, they were only able to delay HIV-1 replication, likely because of the relatively high levels of wild-type Tat synthesized during HIV-1 infection. The mechanism of dominant-negative Tat inhibition most likely involves the cytoplasmic sequestration of cellular factors such as CDK9 or cyclin T1 that are necessary for efficient viral transcription.

Finally, synthetic compounds have been screened for their ability to inhibit Tat function (8, 115, 159). In fact, it was the identification of compounds that inhibit Tat function that led to the identification of P-TEFb as a Tat-associated kinase. These compounds markedly decrease P-TEFb kinase activity but are not specific for Tat function. Compounds that show the most specificity in inhibiting Tat function prevent the formation of the Tat/TAR RNA complex (69, 70, 122, 123).

The Rev Transactivator Protein

Rev is an essential HIV-1 regulatory protein of 116 amino acids that is critical for the temporal expression of HIV-1 structural proteins (93). Specifically, Rev functions posttranscriptionally to mediate the cytoplasmic export of unspliced and singly spliced HIV-1 RNAs where they are either utilized to encode viral proteins expressed or packaged into virion particles (48, 160). This function is accomplished by the active shuttling of Rev between the nucleus and the cytoplasm (125), by virtue of both its NLS and nuclear export signal (NES). It has also been proposed that Rev prevents complete splicing of HIV-1 RNAs by interfering with the splicing machinery in the nucleus (25, 146), although this activity is believed to play a minor role in Rev function.

Structure of Rev and Rev-Responsive Element (RRE)

The domain organization of Rev has been determined through extensive mutagenesis and functional studies (110, 114, 189) (Fig. 8.5). There are three major domains in Rev: arginine- and leucine-rich domains and a region that flanks the ARM that is important for oligomerization (189). The structure of the native Rev protein has proven difficult to determine, and thus far the majority of information comes from modeling studies.

The amino terminus of Rev contains an ARM that is required for RNA binding and nuclear/nucleolar localization (110, 189). Rev binds to a highly ordered RNA stem-loop structure that is termed the RRE, which encompasses a 234-nucleotide region situated within the intron of *env*-containing transcripts (37, 67, 110, 151, 188) (Fig. 8.6). It contains preferred

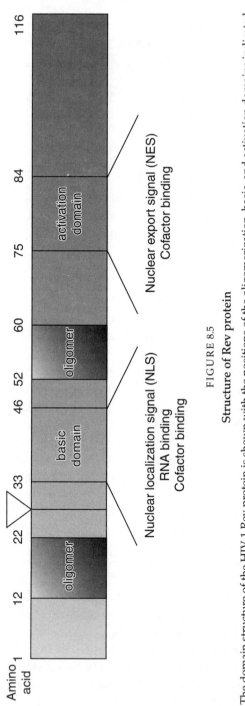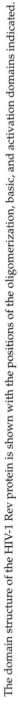

FIGURE 8.5

Structure of Rev protein

The domain structure of the HIV-1 Rev protein is shown with the positions of the oligomerization, basic, and activation domains indicated.

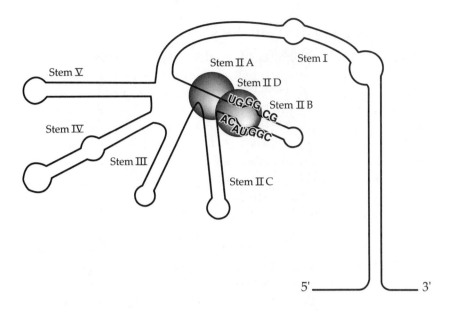

FIGURE 8.6

Structure of RRE

The 230+ nucleotide RRE RNA stem-loop structure, which is found within all *env*-containing transcripts, is shown. Important sequences required for initial Rev monomer and sequential Rev oligomerization are indicated.

binding sites for Rev, specifically within stem-loop IIB of the RRE (189). However, after the initial Rev interaction with this site, additional Rev proteins bind cooperatively to lower affinity sites on the RRE (111).

Rev also contains a leucine-rich domain in the carboxy terminus of the protein, which is referred to as the effector or activation domain (114). This domain contains an NES (50) that, when fused to heterologous proteins, mediates their rapid export from the nucleus of *Xenopus* oocytes (52). Specific mutations within this region of Rev, such as the Rev M10 mutant, result in a Rev/RRE complex that is nonfunctional. In fact, Rev mutants in this domain function as dominant-negative inhibitors of wild-type Rev function (110). The leucine-rich domain of Rev interacts with cellular proteins that facilitate Rev-mediated nuclear export of HIV-1 RNAs (52). Thus, Rev serves as an adapter protein to mediate the utilization of a conserved cellular protein export pathway (45, 56).

Rev also contains two multimerization domains flanking the ARM. Functional analysis of these multimerization domains indicates that they are components of an exposed hydrophobic patch that forms a potential oligomerization surface (169, 170). This domain contains residues, which upon phosphorylation have been suggested to induce a conformational change that results in more efficient RNA binding (54).

Rev-Mediated Export of HIV-1 RNA

In the past few years, a variety of cellular proteins that interact with the Rev NES were identified using both protein cross-linking studies and the yeast two-hybrid system (18, 56, 154). The function of these proteins in Rev modulation of nuclear import/export pathways was characterized. The first of the potential Rev cellular cofactors that was identified was the translation initiation factor eIF-5A (154). This protein is important for the translocation of 5S rRNA from the nucleus to the cytoplasm and associates with ribosomal protein L5, which is a key protein involved in the 5S rRNA export pathway (157). The second potential Rev cofactor that was identified was hRIP/Rab (18, 56). This protein, which contains FG repeat domains that are characteristic of many nucleoporins, was shown to interact with the NES of Rev in yeast two-hybrid analysis (18, 56, 162). However, as no direct in vitro interactions between Rev and hRIP/Rab could be demonstrated, it was postulated that their interaction was indirect. Thus, hRIP/Rab was thought potentially to serve as a bridging factor that contributes to the transport of Rev through the NPC (162).

Several independent lines of evidence indicate that the major cellular target for the Rev-NES is exportin 1 (XPO-1). This protein, which was formerly designated CRM 1, is a member of the importin-β family of shuttling transport receptors (53, 133, 183). The finding that XPO-1 is a target for Rev-mediated nuclear export resulted from data using the compound leptomycin B (LMB), which inhibits Rev shuttling activity, blocks export of viral mRNAs, and suppresses HIV-1 replication in primary cells (183). LMB is also a specific inhibitor of UsnRNA export in mammalian cells, which suggests that Rev exploits a conserved cellular RNA transport pathway. As CRM 1/XPO-1 is also the target for LMB inhibition of nuclear export in the yeast *Saccharomyces pombe,* and since it resembles importin-β, the human homolog of CRM 1/XPO-1 was tested for its ability to complex with Rev and to support its shuttling activity (53). These studies demonstrated that XPO-1 specifically and cooperatively binds to both the NES of Rev and Ran-GTP in an LMB-sensitive complex. LMB is able to inhibit the formation of this complex by directly binding to CRM 1/XPO-1 and competing with Ran-GTP (7, 96). The importance of Ran-GTP binding suggests directionality in the export process, that is, the converse of importin-β activity. In this latter model, XPO-1 cooperatively binds Ran-GTP and Rev in the nucleus and dissociates upon GTP hydrolysis to Ran-GDP in the cytoplasm, releasing Rev and RRE-containing RNAs. Finally, XPO-1 was shown to bridge the interaction between the Rev NES and the previously identified Rev-interacting protein hRIP1/Rab (133). Thus, hRIP1/Rab may facilitate association of the Rev/XPO-1/Ran-GTP complex with the NPC.

Additional factors that play a role in the nuclear export of Rev via an XPO-1 pathway have been identified. Not surprisingly, these factors are nucleoporins and contain FG repeat motifs, previously found to interact with the Rev NES in two-hybrid screens (18, 56, 154). Specifically, the nucleoporins Nup98 and Nup214 have been suggested to act as soluble targeting factors acting on the preassembled Rev/XPO-1 complex to direct it to the NPC for cytoplasmic transport (199).

It has also been suggested that Rev uses alternative trafficking pathways, for example, a pathway used by 5S rRNA (Pol III transcripts) through its interaction with eIF-5A (154, 157). Other studies have suggested that Rev might cooperatively interact with hnRNP A1, a splicing factor reported to shuttle between the nucleus and the cytoplasm (132). Although these other pathways may play a role in Rev function in specific cell types, they likely play a more minor role in overall Rev function.

Rev-Mediated Nuclear Import

In a series of experiments to address interactions between Rev and candidate nuclear import and export factors, Rev, through its NLS, was also shown to directly interact with importin-β (76, 171). This was unexpected, as importin-α was presumed to be the active nuclear transporter. The NLS of Rev is required for RRE binding; therefore, the RRE-containing RNAs must first be displaced from Rev to unmask its NLS. It was also demonstrated that Ran-GTP could dissociate the Rev/importin-β complex while its GDP-bound form had no significant effect. This is important because there is an asymmetric distribution of Ran-GTP and Ran-GDP across the nuclear membrane, with higher concentration of Ran-GTP in the nucleus. These results provide a model for the nuclear import and release of Rev.

Another cellular protein has also been implicated in the nuclear import of Rev. The nucleolar protein B23 has been reported to form a specific complex and stimulate nuclear import of HIV-1 Rev, an activity that is enhanced by its phosphorylation (167). However, this interaction is not absolutely required, although it may function to enhance the nuclear transport of Rev.

Rev Inhibition of Splicing

Rev is also thought to exert an inhibitory effect on the process of HIV-1 RNA splicing to stimulate late HIV-1 gene expression (94). Studies have demonstrated an in vitro interaction between the basic domain of Rev and the cellular splicing factor p32 (168). This factor co-purifies with the alternative SR-protein-splicing factor SF2/ASF, which has been shown to interact with the RRE (146). This latter interaction was found to be Rev dependent and likely requires a conformational change in the RRE stem-loop structure that occurs after Rev nucleation (26, 100). Together these studies suggest that splicing factors may assemble together with Rev in such a way as to occlude the binding of additional splicing factors and therefore form incomplete spliceosomes.

Other studies demonstrate that unspliced HIV-1 RNA co-localizes with SC-35-containing granules within the nucleolus only in the presence of Rev (16, 46), although there have been no reports of Rev or the RRE directly interacting with SC-35. These granules, however, are distinct from those in which active splicing occurs, and this further suggests that the Rev/RRE complex may be able to promote the formation of incomplete splicing complexes. Although Rev may play a role in inhibiting the splicing of HIV-1 RNA, its facilitation of the nuclear export of HIV-1 RNAs is probably the critical mechanism involved in cytoplasmic accumulation of unspliced transcripts.

Model for Rev Function

From the studies presented, a plausible model for Rev activity can be proposed (Fig. 8.7). First, Rev is synthesized early in infection from the multiply spliced HIV-1 transcripts and is transported to the nucleus by virtue of interactions of its NLS with importin-β and Ran-GDP (76, 171). Once inside the nucleus, a single Rev monomer binds to a high-affinity site on newly synthesized RRE-containing viral transcripts (189). At least seven other Rev molecules then oligomerize onto the RRE. The binding of Rev to the RRE may facilitate the recruitment of incomplete spliceosomes to prevent splicing of HIV-1 RNAs. The Rev/RRE complex then forms a higher-order complex with XPO-1 and Ran-GTP via their interaction with the Rev leucine-rich NES (53). This complex migrates to the nuclear envelope through interactions with the nucleoporins Nup98 and Nup214 to facilitate entry and transport through the NPC(199). This is an energy-requiring process that likely requires other proteins situated within the NPC. Once this complex enters the cytoplasm, it disassembles as a result of the hydrolysis of Ran-GTP to Ran-GDP, which may require other proteins that modulate Ran-G binding, including RanGAP and RanBP1 (85). XPO-1 is transported back to the nucleus through a conventional import pathway while Rev and HIV-1 RNA are released into the cytoplasm. HIV-1 RNA encoding the late viral proteins is translated while a portion of the full-length HIV-1 RNA transcripts are directed to the cell membrane for packaging into virion particles. Rev then interacts with importin-β and Ran-GDP for transport back into the nucleus (76, 171). This complex is disrupted when Ran-GDP is converted to its Ran-GTP form and free Rev monomers repeat this cycle.

Inhibition of Rev Function

A variety of methods have been utilized to inhibit Rev function. Dominant-negative inhibitors of Rev function can inhibit wild-type Rev function. Specifically, a mutation within the leucine-rich domain of Rev, called Rev

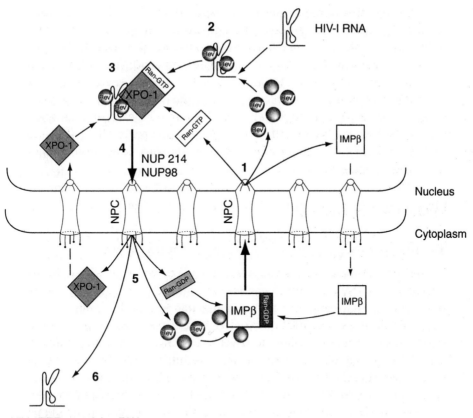

FIGURE 8.7

Mechanism of HIV-1 RNA export

Importin-β associated with Rev and Ran-GDP translocates from the cytoplasm to the nucleus (1); Rev binds to HIV-1 transcripts containing the RRE (2); XPO-1 and Ran-GTP then bind to Rev in a step that is sensitive to LMB inhibition (3); the binding of Rev to these proteins leads to nuclear export of this complex through the NPC(4); Rev dissociates from XPO-1 in the cytoplasm (5); and finally Rev dissociates from the RRE (6).

M10 (110, 112), has been used to inhibit wild-type Rev function and shows promise in gene-therapy studies. The Rev M10 protein is a potent inhibitor of HIV-1 replication in both T-cell lines and primary cells (10, 14, 110, 112). The level of Rev M10 expression is a critical feature for optimal inhibition of HIV-1 replication (21, 107, 145, 148, 163). Other Rev mutants, such as oligomerization mutants, have also been shown to exert transdominant inhibition, although they do not compare to the levels of inhibition seen with the Rev M10 protein (17).

RNA-based therapies, specifically RRE-like decoys, have also been shown to inhibit Rev function. Earlier studies investigated the use of RRE molecules that bound a single Rev molecule (95), but this strategy has been improved by the development of polyvalent artificial RRE molecules that contain multimerized Rev-binding sites (166). This type of approach has also been studied in primary cells and was shown to have similar efficacy, as seen in in vitro studies (9). Small molecules such as aminoglycosides can prevent Rev binding to the RRE and inhibit Rev function (190). Ribozymes can also inhibit Rev function and HIV-1 replication (156, 194). Finally, dominant-negative inhibitors of cellular Rev-associated proteins, for example, Nup214/ΔCAN, are able to effectively block late HIV-1 protein expression and replication but were less effective than Rev M10 (17).

Tat and Rev as Targets for Therapeutic Intervention

Tat and Rev proteins are adapter proteins that mediate the interactions between HIV-1 RNA and cellular regulatory proteins. These proteins share a number of similarities. First, both Tat and Rev require the unique RNA structures TAR and the RRE, respectively, for their function and bind to these RNA elements via arginine-rich domains. Second, the NLSs of both Tat and Rev interact with importin-β to facilitate nuclear localization. Finally, both Tat and Rev interact with critical cellular regulatory proteins. Tat interaction with cyclin T1 and the CDK9 kinase is required for its ability to stimulate RNAPII processivity, while Rev interaction with XPO-1 and Ran-GTP is required for nuclear-cytoplasmic export of RRE-containing RNAs. In addition, other proteins that do not directly interact with Tat or Rev, including SPT5 and the nucleoporins Nup98 and Nup214, are critical for Tat and Rev function, respectively. Recent insights into the mechanisms regulating Tat and Rev function have provided us with potential therapeutic targets to inhibit the function of these HIV-1 regulatory proteins. Potential sites to interrupt Tat and Rev function in the HIV-1 replication cycle are outlined in Fig. 8.8.

A potential target to inhibit Tat function is to prevent the interaction of Tat and cyclin T1 with TAR RNA so that subsequent CDK9 phosphorylation of RNAPII is impaired. Chemical inhibitors that bind to TAR RNA in either the bulge or the loop structures could prevent the interaction of Tat and cyclin T1 with TAR RNA. A second potential site of inhibition of Tat function would be compounds that might disrupt direct Tat interactions with cyclin T1. Third, inhibitors of P-TEFb kinase activity such as DRB prevent Tat-induced activation of HIV-1 gene expression. Since Tat increases P-TEFb kinase activity, it is possible that inhibitors of P-TEFb kinase activity may have a role in preventing Tat activation. Such kinase inhibitors have been identified, but since P-TEFb is required for other cellular processes, the toxicity of such compounds is problematic. Finally, Tat is required for efficient HIV-1 reverse transcription. This provides another

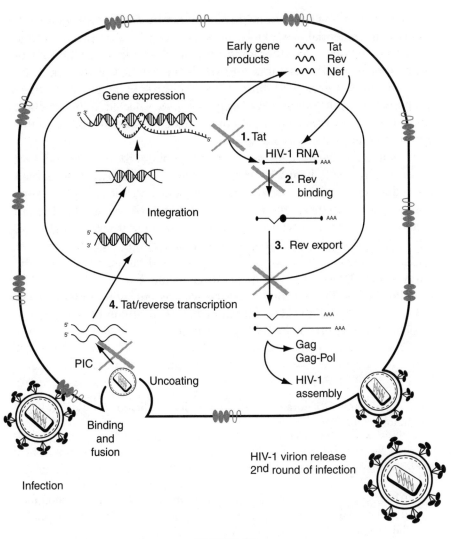

FIGURE 8.8

Potential sites to inhibit Tat and Rev function

The life cycle of HIV-1 is schematically represented. Potential blocks in this cycle caused by inhibiting Tat activation of HIV-1 gene expression (1); Rev binding to the RRE (2); Rev-mediated cytoplasmic transport (3); and Tat-mediated effects on reverse transcription (4) are shown.

potential site for inhibiting Tat function. However, it will be critical to determine the mechanism by which Tat activates HIV-1 reverse transcription in order to define appropriate cellular or viral targets.

A variety of potential targets are available to inhibit Rev function. Agents that bind to the RRE and thus prevent Rev binding are obvious agents to inhibit Rev function. Since Rev multimerizes following its binding to the RRE, inhibition of Rev multimerization could also be a potential target for preventing Rev action. Preventing Rev nuclear-cytoplasmic shutting is also a potential way to inhibit its function. For example, inhibition of Rev interactions with either importin-β (nuclear import) or XPO-1 (nuclear export) could be useful in inhibiting Rev function. However, it has been difficult to develop inhibitors of protein-protein interactions. Direct inhibition of importin-β or XPO-1 is possible, as reflected in the effects of LMB on XPO-1 function, but unacceptable toxicity due to inhibition of this critical cellular pathway is likely.

In summary, we have learned a great deal about the cellular and viral factors that regulate Tat and Rev function. However, more must be learned about the regulation of transcriptional elongation and nuclear-cytoplasmic transport to understand the functions of Tat and Rev better. In addition, there will need to be advances in drug design so that targets including HIV-1 RNA, disruption of protein-protein interactions, and disruption of nuclear-cytoplasmic transport can serve as useful targets for therapeutic intervention. Thus, although great progress has been made in understanding Tat and Rev function, further developments will be necessary in order to develop Tat and Rev inhibitors that are useful in therapeutic approaches for the treatment of HIV-1 infection.

ACKNOWLEDGMENTS

The authors thank Alejandra Herrerra for artwork and Sharon Johnson and Gail Wright for manuscript preparation.

REFERENCES

1. Aboul-ela, F., J. Karn, and G. Varani. The structure of the human immunodeficiency virus type-1 TAR RNA reveals principles of RNA recognition by Tat protein. J. Mol. Biol. 253:313–332.
2. Akoulitchev, S., T. P. Makela, R. A. Weinberg, and D. Reinberg. 1995. Requirement for TFIIH kinase activity in transcription by RNA polymerase II. Nature 377:557–560.
3. Albini, A., R. Benelli, M. Presta, M. Rusnati, M. Ziche, A. Rubartelli, G. Paglialunga, F. Bussolino, and D. Noonan. 1996. HIV-tat protein is a heparin-binding angiogenic growth factor. Oncogene 12:289–297.
4. Albini, A., R. Soldi, D. Giunciuglio, E. Giraudo, R. Benelli, L. Primo, D. Noonan, M. Salio, G. Camussi, W. Rockl, and F. Bussolino. 1996. The angiogenesis induced by HIV-1 tat protein is mediated by the Flk-1/KDR receptor on vascular endothelial cells. Nature Med. 2:1371–1375.
5. Alizon, M., P. Sonigo, S. F. Barre, J. C. Chermann, P. Tiollais, L. Montagnier, and H. S. Wain. 1984. Molecular cloning of lymphadenopathy-associated virus. Nature 312:757–760.
6. Alonso, A., T. P. Cujec, and B. M. Peterlin. 1994. Effects of human chromosome 12 on interactions between tat and TAR of human immunodeficiency virus type 1. J. Virol. 68:6505–6513.

7. Askjaer, P., T. H. Jensen, J. Nilsson, L. Englmeier, and J. Kjems. 1998. The specificity of the CRM1-Rev nuclear export signal interaction is mediated by RanGTP. J. Biol. Chem. 273:33414–33422.

8. Baba, M., M. Okamoto, M. Kawamura, M. Makino, T. Higashida, T. Takashi, Y. Kimura, T. Ikeuchi, T. Tetsuka, and T. Okamoto. 1998. Inhibition of human immunodeficiency virus type 1 replication and cytokine production by fluoroquinoline derivatives. Mol. Pharmacol. 53:1097–1103.

9. Bahner, I., K. Kearns, Q.-L. Hao, E. M. Smogorzewska, and D. B. Kohn. 1996. Transduction of human CD34+ hematopoietic progenitor cells by a retroviral vector expressing an RRE decoy inhibits human immunodeficiency virus type 1 replication in myelomonocytic cells produced in long-term culture. J. Virol. 70:4352–4360.

10. Bahner, I., C. Zhou, X.-J. Yu, Q.-L. Hao, J. C. Guatelli, and D. B. Kohn. 1993. Comparison of transdominant inhibitory mutant human immunodeficiency virus type 1 genes expressed by retroviral vectors in human T-lymphocytes. J. Virol. 67:3199–3207.

11. Bartz, S. R., and M. Emerman. 1999. Human immunodeficiency virus type 1 Tat induced apoptosis and increases sensitivity to apoptotic signals by up-regulating FLICE/Caspase-8. J. Virol. 73:1956–1963.

12. Benkirane, M., R. F. Chun, H. Xiao, V. V. Ogryzko, B. H. Howard, Y. Nakatani, and K. T. Jeang. 1998. Activation of integrated provirus requires histone acetyltransferase. p300 and P/CAF are coactivators for HIV-1 Tat. J. Biol. Chem. 273:24898–24905.

13. Berkhout, B., and B. Klaver. 1995. Revertants and pseudo-revertants of human immunodeficiency virus type 1 viruses mutated in the long terminal repeat promoter region. J. Gen. Virol. 76:845–853.

14. Bevec, D., M. Dobrovnik, J. Hauber, and E. Bohnlein. 1992. Inhibition of human immunodeficiency virus type 1 replication in human T cells by retroviral-mediated gene transfer of a dominant-negative Rev trans-activator. Proc. Natl. Acad. Sci. USA 89:9870–9874.

15. Bieniasz, P. D., T. A. Grdina, H. P. Bogerd, and B. R. Cullen. 1998. Recruitment of a protein complex containing Tat and cyclin T1 to TAR governs the species specificity of HIV-1 Tat. EMBO J. 17:7056–7065.

16. Boe, S. O., B. Bjorndal, B. Rosok, A. M. Szilvay, and K. H. Kalland. 1998. Subcellular localization of human immunodeficiency virus type 1 RNAs, Rev, and the splicing factor SC-35. Virology 244:473–482.

17. Bogerd, H. P., A. Echarri, T. M. Ross, and B. R. Cullen. 1998. Inhibition of human immunodeficiency virus Rev and human T-cell leukemia virus Rex function, but not Mason-Pfizer monkey virus constitutive transport element activity, by a mutant human nucleoporin targeted to Crm1. J. Virol. 72:8627–8635.

18. Bogerd, H. P., R. A. Fridell, S. Madore, and B. R. Cullen. 1995. Identification of a novel cellular cofactor for the Rev/Rex class of retroviral regulatory proteins. Cell 82:485–494.

19. Bohjanen, P. R., R. A. Colvin, M. Puttaraju, M. D. Been, and M. A. Garcia-Blanco. 1996. A small circular TAR RNA decoy specifically inhibits Tat-activated HIV-1 transcription. Nucleic Acids Res. 24:3733–3738.

20. Bohjanen, P. R., Y. Liu, and M. A. Garcia-Blanco. 1997. TAR RNA decoys inhibit Tat-activated HIV-1 transcription after preinitiation complex formation. Nucleic Acids Res. 25:4481–4486.

21. Bonyhadi, M. L., K. Moss, A. Voytovich, J. Auten, C. Kalfoglou, I. Plavec, S. Forestell, L. Su, E. Bohnlein, and H. Kaneshima. 1997. RevM10-expressing T cells derived in vivo from transduced human hematopoietic stem-progenitor cells inhibit human immunodeficiency virus replication. J. Virol. 71:4707–4716.

22. Borgatti, P., G. Zauli, M. L. Colamussi, D. Gibellini, M. Previati, L. L. Cantley, and S. Capitani. 1997. Extracellular HIV-1 Tat protein activates phosphatidylinositol 3- and Akt/PKB kinases in CD4+ T lymphoblastoid Jurkat cells. Eur. J. Immunol. 27:2805–2811.

23. Calnan, B. J., B. Tidor, S. Biancalana, D. Hudson, and A. D. Frankel. 1991. Arginine-mediated RNA recognition: the arginine fork. Science 252:1167–1171.

24. Cannon, P., S. H. Kim, C. Ulich, and S. Kim. 1994. Analysis of Tat function in human immunodeficiency virus type 1-infected low-level-expression cell lines U1 and ACH-2. J. Virol. 68:1993–1997.

25. Chang, D. D., and P. A. Sharp. 1989. Regulation by HIV Rev depends upon recognition of splice sites. Cell 59:789–795.

26. Charpentier, B., F. Stutz, and M. Rosbash. 1997. A dynamic in vivo view of the HIV-I Rev-RRE interaction. J. Mol. Biol. 266:950–962.

27. Chen, D., Y. Fong, and Q. Zhou. 1999. Specific interaction of Tat with the human but not rodent P-TEFb complex mediates the species-specific Tat activation of HIV-1 transcription. Proc. Natl. Acad. Sci. USA 96:2728–2733.

28. Chinen, J., E. Aguilar-Cordova, D. Ng-Tang, D. E. Lewis, and J. W. Belmont. 1997. Protection of primary human T cells from HIV infection by Trev: a transdominant fusion gene. Hum. Gene Ther. 8:861–868.

29. Chun, R. F., and K. T. Jeang. 1996. Requirements for RNA polymerase II carboxyl-terminal domain for activated transcription of human retroviruses human T-cell lymphotropic virus I and HIV-1. J. Biol. Chem. 271:27888–27894.

30. Chun, R. F., O. J. Semmes, C. Neuveut, and K. T. Jeang. 1998. Modulation of Sp1 phosphorylation by human immunodeficiency virus type 1 Tat. J. Virol. 72:2615–2629.

31. Churcher, M. J., C. Lamont, F. Hamy, C. Dingwall, S. M. Green, A. D. Lowe, J. G. Butler, M. J. Gait, and J. Karn. 1993. High affinity binding of TAR RNA by the human immunodeficiency virus type-1 tat protein requires base-pairs in the RNA stem and amino acid residues flanking the basic region. J. Mol. Biol. 230:90–110.

32. Conant, K., M. Ma, A. Nath, and E. O. Major. 1996. Extracellular human immunodeficiency virus type 1 Tat protein is associated with an increase in both NF-kappa B binding and protein kinase C activity in primary human astrocytes. J. Virol. 70:1384–1389.

33. Cujec, T. P., H. Cho, E. Maldonado, J. Meyer, D. Reinberg, and B. M. Peterlin. 1997. The human immunodeficiency virus transactivator Tat interacts with the RNA polymerase II holoenzyme. Mol. Cell. Biol. 17:1817–1823.

34. Cujec, T. P., H. Okamoto, K. Fujinaga, J. Meyer, H. Chamberlin, D. O. Morgan, and B. M. Peterlin. 1997. The HIV transactivator TAT binds to the CDK-activating kinase and activates the phosphorylation of the carboxy-terminal domain of RNA polymerase II. Genes Dev. 11:2645–2657.

35. Cullen, B. R. 1993. Does HIV-1 Tat induce a change in viral initiation rights? Cell 73:417–420.

36. Dayton, A. I., J. G. Sodroski, C. A. Rosen, W. C. Goh, and W. A. Haseltine. 1986. The trans-activator gene of the human T cell lymphotropic virus type III is required for replication. Cell 44:941–947.

37. Dayton, E. T., D. M. Powell, and A. I. Dayton. 1989. Functional analysis of CAR, the target sequence for the Rev protein of HIV-1. Science 246:1625–1629.

38. Dhawan, S., R. K. Puri, A. Kumar, H. Duplan, J. M. Masson, and B. B. Aggarwal. 1997. Human immunodeficiency virus-1-tat protein induces the cell surface expression of endothelial leukocyte adhesion molecule-1, vascular cell adhesion molecule-1, and intercellular adhesion molecule-1 in human endothelial cells. Blood 90:1535–1544.

39. Dingwall, C., I. Ernberg, M. J. Gait, S. M. Green, S. Heaphy, J. Karn, A. D. Lowe, M. Singh, and M. A. Skinner. 1990. HIV-1 Tat protein stimulates transcription by binding to a U-rich bulge in the stem of the TAR RNA structure. EMBO J. 9:4145–4153.

40. Elangovan, B., T. Subramanian, and G. Chinnadurai. 1992. Functional comparison of the basic domains of the Tat proteins of human immunodeficiency virus types 1 and 2 in *trans* activation. J. Virol. 66:2031–2036.

41. El Kharroubi, A., G. Piras, R. Zensen, and M. A. Martin. 1998. Transcriptional activation of the integrated chromatin-associated human immunodeficiency virus type 1 promoter. Mol. Cell. Biol. 18:2535–2544.

42. Emerman, M., R. Vazeux, and K. Peden. 1989. The rev gene product of the human immunodeficiency virus affects envelope-specific RNA localization. Cell 57:1155–1165.

43. Ensoli, B., G. Barillari, S. Z. Salahuddin, R. C. Gallo, and S. F. Wong. 1990. Tat protein of HIV-1 stimulates growth of cells derived from Kaposi's sarcoma lesions of AIDS patients. Nature 345:84–86.

44. Ensoli, B., R. Gendelman, P. Markham, V. Fiorelli, S. Colombini, M. Raffeld, A. Cafaro, H. K. Chang, J. N. Brady, and R. C. Gallo. 1994. Synergy between basic fibroblast growth factor and HIV-1 Tat protein in induction of Kaposi's sarcoma. Nature 371:674–680.

45. Farjot, G., A. Sergeant, and I. Mikaelian. 1999. A new nucleoporin-like protein interacts with both HIV-1 Rev nuclear export signal and CRM-1. J. Biol. Chem. 274:17309–17317.

46. Favaro, J. P., K. T. Borg, S. J. Arrigo, and M. G. Schmidt. 1998. Effect of Rev on the intranuclear localization of HIV-1 unspliced RNA. Virology 249:286–296.

47. Feinberg, M. B., D. Baltimore, and A. D. Frankel. 1991. The role of Tat in the human immunodeficiency virus life cycle indicates a primary effect on transcriptional elongation. Proc. Natl. Acad. Sci. USA 88:4045–4049.

48. Feinberg, M. B., R. F. Jarrett, A. Aldovini, R. C. Gallo, and F. Wong-Staal. 1986. HTLV-III expression and production involve complex regulation at the levels of splicing and translation of viral RNA. Cell 46:807–817.

49. Feng, S., and E. C. Holland. 1988. HIV-1 Tat trans-activation requires the loop sequence within TAR. Nature 334:165–167.

50. Fischer, U., S. Meyer, M. Teufel, C. Heckel, R. Luhrmann, and G. Rautmann. 1994. Evidence that HIV-1 Rev directly promotes the nuclear export of unspliced RNA. EMBO J. 13:4105–4112.

51. Fisher, A. G., M. B. Feinberg, S. F. Josephs, M. E. Harper, L. M. Marselle, G. Reyes, M. A. Gonda, A. Aldovini, C. Debouk, R. C. Gallo, and F. Wong-Staal.

1986. The trans-activator gene of HTLV-III is essential for virus replication. Nature 320:367–371.

52. Fisher, A. G., J. Huber, W. C. Boeiens, I. W. Mattaj, and R. Luhrmann. 1995. The HIV-1 Rev activation domain is a nuclear export signal that accesses an export pathway used by specific cellular RNAs. Cell 82:475–483.

53. Fornerod, M., M. Ohno, M. Yoshida, and I. W. Mattaj. 1997. CRM1 is an export receptor for leucine-rich nuclear export signals. Cell 90:1051–1060.

54. Fouts, D. E., H. L. True, K. A. Cengel, and D. W. Celander. 1997. Site-specific phosphorylation of the human immunodeficiency virus type-1 Rev protein accelerates formation of an efficient RNA-binding conformation. Biochemistry 36:13256–13262.

55. Frankel, A. D., and J. A. Young. 1998. HIV-1: fifteen proteins and an RNA. Annu. Rev. Biochem. 67:1–25.

56. Fritz, C. C., M. L. Zapp, and M. R. Green. 1995. A human nucleoporin-like protein that specifically interacts with HIV Rev. Nature 376:530–533.

57. Fujinaga, K., T. P. Cujec, J. Peng, J. Garriga, D. H. Price, X. Grana, and B. M. Peterlin. 1998. The ability of positive transcription elongation factor B to transactivate human immunodeficiency virus transcription depends on a functional kinase domain, cyclin T1, and Tat. J. Virol. 72:7154–7159.

58. Fujinaga, K., R. Taube, J. Wimmer, T. P. Cujec, and B. M. Peterlin. 1999. Interactions between human cyclin T, Tat, and the transactivation response element (TAR) are disrupted by a cysteine to tyrosine substitution found in mouse cyclin T. Proc. Natl. Acad. Sci. USA 96:1285–1290.

59. Garber, M. E., P. Wei, V. N. Kewal-Ramani, T. P. Mayall, C. H. Herrmann, A. P. Rice, D. R. Littman, and K. A. Jones. 1998. The interaction between HIV-1 Tat and human cyclin T1 requires zinc and a critical cysteine residue that is not conserved in the murine CycT1 protein. Genes Dev. 12:3512–3527.

60. Garcia, J. A., D. Harrich, L. Pearson, R. Mitsuyasu, and R. B. Gaynor. 1988. Functional domains required for *tat*-induced transcriptional activation of the HIV-1 long terminal repeat. EMBO J. 7:3143–3147.

61. Garcia, J. A., D. Harrich, E. Soultanakis, F. Wu, R. Mitsuyasu, and R. B. Gaynor. 1989. Human immunodeficiency virus type 1 LTR TATA and TAR region sequences required for transcriptional regulation. EMBO J. 8:765–778.

62. García-Martínez, L. F., D. Ivanov, and R. B. Gaynor. 1997. Association of Tat with purified HIV-1 and HIV-2 transcription preinitiation complexes. J. Biol. Chem. 272:6951–6958.

63. García-Martínez, L. F., G. Mavankal, J. Neveu, W. Lane, D. Sigman, D. Ivanov, and R. B. Gaynor. 1997. Purification of a Tat associated kinase reveals a TFIIH complex that modulates HIV-1 transcription. EMBO J. 16:2836–2850.

64. García-Martínez, L. F., G. Mavankal, P. Peters, F. Wu-Baer, and R. B. Gaynor. 1995. Tat functions to stimulate the elongation properties of transcription complexes paused by the duplicated TAR RNA element of human immunodeficiency virus 2. J. Mol. Biol. 254:350–363.

65. Garriga, J., J. Peng, M. Parreno, D. H. Price, E. E. Henderson, and X. Grana. 1998. Upregulation of cyclin T1/CDK9 complexes during T cell activation. Oncogene 17:3093–3102.

66. Grana, X., A. De Luca, N. Sang, Y. Fu, P. P. Claudio, J. Rosenblatt, D. O. Morgan, and A. Giordano. 1994. PITALRE, a nuclear CDC2-related protein kinase

that phosphorylates the retinoblastoma protein in vitro. Proc. Natl. Acad. Sci. USA 91:3834–3838.

67. Hadzopoulou-Cladaras, M., B. K. Felber, C. Cladaras, A. Athanassopoulos, A.Tse, and G. N. Pavlakis. 1989. The rev (trs/art) protein of human immuno-deficiency virus type 1 affects viral mRNA and protein expression via a cis-acting sequence in the env region. J. Virol. 63:1265–1274.

68. Hahn, B. H., G. M. Shaw, S. K. Arya, M. Popovic, R. C. Gallo, and S. F. Wong. 1984. Molecular cloning and characterization of the HTLV-III virus associated with AIDS. Nature 312:166–169.

69. Hamy, F., V. Brondani, A. Florsheimer, W. Stark, M. J. Blommers, and T. Klimkait. 1998. A new class of HIV-1 Tat antagonist acting through Tat-TAR inhibition. Biochemistry 37:5086–5095.

70. Hamy, F., E. R. Felder, G. Heizmann, J. Lazdins, F. Aboul-ela, G. Varani, J. Karn, andT. Klimkait. 1997. An inhibitor of the Tat/TAR RNA interaction that effectively suppresses HIV-1 replication. Proc. Natl. Acad. Sci. USA 94:3548–3553.

71. Harrich, D., G. Mavankal, A. Mette-Snider, and R. B. Gaynor. 1995. Human immunodeficiency virus type 1 TAR element revertant viruses define RNA structures required for efficient viral gene expression and replication. J. Virol. 69:4906–4913.

72. Harrich, D., C. Ulich, L. F. García-Martínez, and R. B. Gaynor. 1997. Tat is re-quired for efficient HIV-1 reverse transcription. EMBO J. 16:1224–1235.

73. Harrich, D., C. Ulich, and R. B. Gaynor. 1996. A novel role for the HIV-1 TAR element: a critical regulator of viral reverse transcription. J. Virol. 70:4017–4027.

74. Hart, C. E., J. C. Galphin, M. A. Westhafer, and G. Schochetman. 1993. TAR loop-dependent HIV-1 trans activation requires factors encoded on human chromosome 12. J. Virol. 67:5020–5024.

75. Hauber, J., M. Malim, and B. C. Cullen. 1989. Mutational analysis of the con-served basic domain of human immunodeficiency virus *tat* protein. J. Virol. 63:1181–1187.

76. Henderson, B. R., and P. Percipalle. 1997. Interactions between HIV Rev and nuclear import and export factors: the Rev nuclear localisation signal medi-ates specific binding to human importin-beta. J. Mol. Biol. 274:693–707.

77. Herrmann, C. H., R. G. Carroll, P. Wei, K. A. Jones, and A. P. Rice. 1998. Tat-associated kinase, TAK, activity is regulated by distinct mechanisms in pe-ripheral blood lymphocytes and promonocytic cell lines. J. Virol. 72:9881–9888.

78. Herrmann, C. H., and A. P. Rice. 1995. Lentivirus Tat proteins specifically as-sociate with a cellular protein kinase, TAK, that hyperphosphorylates the carboxyl-terminal domain of the large subunit of RNA polymerase II: candi-date for a Tat cofactor. J. Virol. 69:1612–1620.

79. Hottiger, M. O., and G. J. Nabel. 1998. Interaction of human immunodefi-ciency virus type 1 Tat with the transcriptional coactivators p300 and CREB binding protein. J. Virol. 72:8252–8256.

80. Howcroft, T. K., K. Strebel, M. A. Martin, and D. S. Singer. 1993. Repression of MHC class I gene promoter activity by two-exon tat of HIV. Science 260:1320–1322.

81. Huang, L., A. Joshi, R. Willey, J. Orenstein, and K. T. Jeang. 1994. Human immunodeficiency viruses regulated by alternative trans-activators: genetic evidence for a novel non-transcriptional function of Tat in virion infectivity. EMBO J. 13:2886–2896.

82. Huq, I., Y. H. Ping, N. Tamilarasu, and T. M. Rana. 1999. Controlling human immunodeficiency virus type 1 gene expression by unnatural peptides. Biochemistry 38:5172–5177.

83. Husain, S. R., P. Leland, B. B. Aggarwal, and R. K. Puri. 1996. Transcriptional up-regulation of interleukin 4 receptors by human immunodeficiency virus type 1 tat gene. AIDS Res. Hum. Retroviruses 12:1349–1359.

84. Ivanov, D., Y. T. Kwak, E. Nee, J. Guo, L. F. García-Martínez, and R. B. Gaynor. 1999. Cyclin T1 domains involved in complex formation with Tat and TAR RNA are critical for tat-activation. J. Mol. Biol. 288:41–56.

85. Izaurralde, E., U. Kutay, C. von Kobbe, I. W. Mattaj, and D. Gorlich. 1997. The asymmetric distribution of the constituents of the Ran system is essential for transport into and out of the nucleus. EMBO J. 16:6535–6547.

86. Jeang, K. T., and B. Berkhout. 1991. Detailed mutational analysis of TAR RNA: critical spacing between the bulge and loop recognition domains. Nucleic Acids Res. 19:6169–6176.

87. Jeang, K. T., B. Berkhout, and B. Dropulic. 1993. Effects of integration and replication on transcription of the HIV-1 long terminal repeat. J. Biol. Chem. 268:24940–24949.

88. Jeang, K. T., R. Chun, N. H. Lin, A. Gatignol, C. G. Glabe, and H. Fan. 1993. In vitro and in vivo binding of human immunodeficiency virus type 1 tat protein and Sp1 transcription factor. J. Virol. 67:6224–6233.

89. Jones, K. A., and B. M. Peterlin. 1994. Control of RNA initiation and elongation at the HIV-1 promoter. Annu. Rev. Biochem. 63:717–743.

90. Kao, S. Y., A. F. Calnan, P. A. Luciw, and B. M. Peterlin. 1987. Anti-termination of transcription within the long terminal repeat of HIV-1 by tat gene product. Nature 330:489–493.

91. Kato, H., H. Sumimoto, P. Pognonec, C. H. Chen, C. A. Rosen, and R. G. Roeder. 1992. HIV-1 Tat acts as a processivity factor *in vitro* in conjunction with cellular elongation factors. Genes Dev. 6:655–666.

92. Keen, N. J., M. J. Churcher, and J. Karn. 1997. Transfer of Tat and release of TAR RNA during the activation of the human immunodeficiency virus type-1 transcription elongation complex. EMBO J. 16:5260–5272.

93. Kim, S. Y., R. Byrn, J. Groopman, and D. Baltimore. 1989. Temporal aspects of DNA and RNA synthesis during human immunodeficiency virus infection: evidence for differential gene expression. J. Virol. 63:3708–3713.

94. Kjems, J., A. D. Frankel, and P. A. Sharp. 1991. Specific regulation of mRNA splicing in vitro by a peptide from HIV-1 Rev. Cell 67:169–178.

95. Kjems, J., and P. A. Sharp. 1993. The basic domain of Rev from human immunodeficiency virus-1 specifically blocks the entry of U4/U6.U5 small nuclear ribonucleoprotein in spliceosome asssembly. J. Virol. 67:4769–4776.

96. Kudo, N., B. Wolff, T. Sekimoto, E. P. Schreiner, Y. Yoneda, M. Yanagida, S. Horinouchi, and M. Yoshida. 1998. Leptomycin B inhibition of signal-mediated nuclear export by direct binding to CRM1. Exp. Cell Res. 242: 540–547.

97. Kuppuswamy, M., T. Subramanian, A. Srinivasan, and G. Chinnadurai. 1989. Multiple functional domains of Tat, the *trans*-activator of HIV-1, defined by mutational analysis. Nucleic Acids Res. 17:3551–3561.

98. Kwak, Y. T., D. Ivanov, J. Guo, E. Nee, and R. B. Gaynor. 1999. Role of the human and murine cyclin T proteins in regulating HIV-1 tat-activation. J. Mol. Biol. 288:57–69.

99. Lafrenie, R. M., L. M. Wahl, J. S. Epstein, K. M. Yamada, and S. Dhawan. 1997. Activation of monocytes by HIV-Tat treatment is mediated by cytokine expression. J. Immunol. 159:4077–4083.

100. Lam, W. C., J. M. Seifert, F. Amberger, C. Graf, M. Auer, and D. P. Millar. 1998. Structural dynamics of HIV-1 Rev and its complexes with RRE and 5S RNA. Biochemistry 37:1800–1809.

101. Laspia, M. F., A. P. Rice, and M. B. Mathews. 1989. HIV-1 Tat protein increases transcriptional initiation and stabilizes elongation. Cell 59:283–292.

102. Laspia, M. F., P. Wendel, and M. B. Mathews. 1993. HIV-1 Tat overcomes inefficient transcriptional elongation *in vitro*. J. Mol. Biol. 232:732–746.

103. Li, C. J., D. J. Friendman, C. Wang, V. Meteleve, and A. B. Pardee. 1995. Induction of apoptosis in uninfected lymphocytes by HIV-1 Tat protein. Science 268:429–431.

104. Li, C. J., Y. Ueda, B. Shi, L. Borodyansky, L. Huang, Y. Z. Li, and A. B. Pardee. 1997. Tat protein induces self-perpetuating permissivity for productive HIV-1 infection. Proc. Natl. Acad. Sci. USA 94:8116–8120.

105. Li, X.-Y., and M. R. Green. 1998. The HIV-1 Tat cellular coactivator Tat-SF1 is a general transcription elongation factor. Genes Dev. 12:2992–2996.

106. Lisziewicz, J., D. Sun, B. Trapnell, M. Thomson, H.-K. Chang, B. Ensoli, and B. Peng. 1995. An autoregulated dual-function *antitat* gene for human immunodeficiency virus type 1 gene therapy. J. Virol. 69:206–212.

107. Liu, J., C. Woffendin, Y. Zhi-yong, and G. J. Nabel. 1994. Regulated expression of a dominant negative form of Rev improves resistance to HIV replication in T-cells. Gene Ther. 1:32–37.

108. Lo, K. M. S., M. A. Biasolo, G. Dehni, G. Palu, and W. A. Haseltine. 1992. Inhibition of replication of HIV-1 by retroviral vectors expressing *tat*-antisense and anti-*tat* ribozyme RNA. Virology 190:176–183.

109. Luciw, P. A., S. J. Potter, K. Steimer, D. Dina, and J. A. Levy. 1984. Molecular cloning of AIDS-associated retrovirus. Nature 312:760–763.

110. Malim, M. H., S. Bohnlein, J. Hauber, and B. R. Cullen. 1989. Functional dissection of the HIV-1 Rev trans-activator—derivation of a trans-dominant repressor of Rev function. Cell 58:205–214.

111. Malim, M. H., and B. R. Cullen. 1991. HIV-1 structural gene expression requires the binding of multiple Rev monomers to the viral RRE: implications for HIV-1 latency. Cell 65:241–248.

112. Malim, M. H., W. W. Freimuth, J. Liu, T. J. Boyle, H. K. Lyerly, B. R. Cullen, and G. J. Nabel. 1992. Stable expression of transdominant Rev protein in human T-cells inhibits human immunodeficiency virus replication. J. Exp. Med. 176:1197–1201.

113. Malim, M. H., J. Hauber, S. Y. Le, J. V. Maizel, and B. R. Cullen. 1989. The HIV-1 rev trans-activator acts through a structured target sequence to activate nuclear export of unspliced viral mRNA. Nature 338:254–257.

114. Malim, M. H., D. F. McCarn, L. S. Tiley, and B. R. Cullen. 1991. Mutational definition of the human immunodeficiency virus type 1 Rev activation domain. J. Virol. 65:4248–4254.

115. Mancebo, H. S.Y., G. Lee, J. Flygare, J.Tomassini, P. Luu,Y. Zhu, J. Peng, C. Blau, D. Hazuda, D. Price, and O. Flores. 1997. P-TEFb kinase is required for HIV Tat transcriptional activation *in vivo* and *in vitro*. Genes Dev. 11:2633–2644.

116. Marciniak, R. A., and P. A. Sharp. 1991. HIV-1 Tat protein promotes formation of more-processive elongation complexes. EMBO J. 10:4189–4196.

117. Marshall, N. F., J. Peng, P. Xie, and D. H. Price. 1996. Control of RNA polymerase II elongation potential by a novel carboxyl-terminal domain kinase. J. Biol. Chem. 271:27176–27183.

118. Marshall, N. F., and D. H. Price. 1992. Control of formation of two district classes of RNA polymerase II elongation complexes. Mol. Cell. Biol. 12:2078–2090.

119. Marshall, N. F., and D. H. Price. 1995. Purification of P-TEFb, a transcription factor required for the transition into productive elongation. J. Biol. Chem. 270:12335–12338.

120. Marzio, G., M.Tyagi, M. I. Gutierrez, and M. Giacca. 1998. HIV-1 tat transactivator recruits p300 and CREB-binding protein histone acetyltransferases to the viral promoter. Proc. Natl. Acad. Sci. USA 95:13519–13524.

121. Mavankal, G., S. H. I. Ou, H. Oliver, D. Sigman, and R. B. Gaynor. 1996. HIV-1 and HIV-2 Tat proteins specifically interact with RNA polymerase II. Proc. Natl. Acad. Sci. USA 93:2089–2094.

122. Mei, H.Y., M. Cui, A. Heldsinger, S. M. Lemrow, J. A. Loo, K. A. Sannes-Lowery, L. Sharmeen, and A. W. Czarnik. 1998. Inhibitors of protein-RNA complexation that target the RNA: specific recognition of human immunodeficiency virus type 1 TAR RNA by small organic molecules. Biochemistry 37:14204–14212.

123. Mei, H.Y., D. P. Mack, A. A. Galan, N. S. Halim, A. Heldsinger, J. A. Loo, D. W. Moreland, K. A. Sannes-Lowery, L. Sharmeen, H. N. Truong, and A. W. Czarnik. 1997. Discovery of selective, small-molecule inhibitors of RNA complexes—I. The Tat protein/TAR RNA complexes required for HIV-1 transcription. Bioorganic Med. Chem. 5:1173–1184.

124. Menegon, A., C. Leoni, F. Benfenati, and F. Valtorta. 1997. Tat protein from HIV-1 activates MAP kinase in granular neurons and glial cells from rat cerebellum. Biochem. Biophys. Res. Commun. 238:800–805.

125. Meyer, B. E., and M. H. Malim. 1994. The HIV-1 Rev trans-activator shuttles between the nucleus and the cytoplasm. Genes Dev. 8:1538–1547.

126. Mhashilkar, A. M., J. Bagley, S.Y. Chen, A. M. Szilvay, D. G. Helland, and W. A. Marasco. 1995. Inhibition of HIV-1 Tat-mediated LTR transactivation and HIV-1 infection by anti-Tat single chain intrabodies. EMBO J. 14:1542–1551.

127. Mhashilkar, A. M., D. K. Biswas, J. LaVecchio, A. B. Pardee, and W. A. Marasco. 1997. Inhibition of human immunodeficiency virus type 1 replication in vitro by a novel combination of anti-Tat single-chain intrabodies and NF-kappa B antagonists. J. Virol. 71:6486–6494.

128. Milani, D., M. Mazzoni, P. Borgatti, G. Zauli, L. Cantley, and S. Capitani. 1996. Extracellular human immunodeficiency virus type-1 Tat protein acti-

vates phosphatidylinositol 3-kinase in PC12 neuronal cells. J. Biol. Chem. 271:22961–22964.

129. Mitola, S., S. Sozzani, W. Luini, L. Primo, A. Borsatti, H. Weich, and F. Bussolino. 1997. Tat-human immunodeficiency virus-1 induces human monocyte chemotaxis by activation of vascular endothelial growth factor receptor-1. Blood 90:1365–1372.

130. Modesti, N., J. Garcia, C. Debouck, M. Peterlin, and R. Gaynor. 1991. Transdominant Tat mutants with alterations in the basic domain inhibit HIV-1 gene expression. New Biologist 3:759–768.

131. Muesing, M. A., D. H. Smith, and D. J. Capon. 1987. Regulation of mRNA accumulation by a human immunodeficiency virus trans-activator protein. Cell 48:691–701.

132. Najera, I., M. Krieg, and J. Karn. 1999. Synergistic stimulation of HIV-1 rev-dependent export of unspliced mRNA to the cytoplasm by hnRNP A1. J. Mol. Biol. 285:1951–1964.

133. Neville, M., F. Stutz, L. Lee, L. I. Davis, and M. Rosbash. 1997. The importin-beta family member Crm1p bridges the interaction between Rev and the nuclear pore complex during nuclear export. Curr. Biol. 7:767–775.

134. O'Brien, T., S. Hardin, A. Greenleaf, and J. T. Lis. 1994. Phosphorylation of RNA polymerase II C-terminal domain and transcriptional elongation. Nature 370:75–77.

135. Okamoto, H., C. T. Sheline, J. L. Corden, K. A. Jones, and B. M. Peterlin. 1996. Trans-activation by human immunodeficiency virus Tat protein requires the C-terminal domain of RNA polymerase II. Proc. Natl. Acad. Sci. USA 93: 11575–11579.

136. Okamoto, T., and F. Wong-Staal. 1986. Demonstration of virus-specific transcriptional activator(s) in cells infected with HTLV-III by an *in vitro* cell-free system. Cell 47:29–35.

137. Opalenik, S. R., J. T. Shin, J. N. Wehby, V. K. Mahesh, and J. A. Thompson. 1995. The HIV-1 TAT protein induces the expression and extracellular appearance of acidic fibroblast growth factor. J. Biol. Chem. 270:17457–17467.

138. Ott, M., S. Emiliani, C. Van Lint, G. Herbein, J. Lovett, N. Chirmule, T. McCloskey, S. Pahwa, and E. Verdin. 1997. Immune hyperactivation of HIV-1-infected T cells mediated by Tat and the CD28 pathway. Science 275:1481–1485.

139. Ott, M., J. L. Lovett, L. Mueller, and E. Verdin. 1998. Superinduction of IL-8 in T cells by HIV-1 Tat protein is mediated through NF-kappaB factors. J. Immunol. 160:2872–2880.

140. Parada, C. A., and R. G. Roeder. 1996. Enhanced processivity of RNA polymerase II triggered by Tat-induced phosphorylation of its carboxy-terminal domain. Nature 384:375–378.

141. Pearson, L., J. Garcia, F. Wu, N. Modesti, J. Nelson, and R. Gaynor. 1990. A transdominant tat mutant that inhibits tat-induced gene expression from the human immunodeficiency virus long terminal repeat. Proc. Natl. Acad. Sci. USA 87:5079–5083.

142. Peng, J., N. F. Marshall, and D. H. Price. 1998. Identification of a cyclin subunit required for the function of Drosophila P-TEFb. J. Biol. Chem. 273: 13855–13860.

143. Peng, J., Y. Zhu, J. T. Milton, and D. H. Price. 1998. Identification of multiple cyclin subunits of human P-TEFb. Genes Dev. 12:755–762.

144. Ping, Y. H., and T. M. Rana. 1999. Tat-associated kinase (P-TEFb): a component of transcription preinitiation and elongation complexes. J. Biol. Chem. 274:7399–7404.

145. Plavec, I., M. Agarwal, K. E. Ho, M. Pineda, J. Auten, J. Baker, H. Matsuzaki, S. Escaich, M. Bonyhadi, and E. Bohnlein. 1997. High transdominant RevM10 protein levels are required to inhibit HIV-1 replication in cell lines and primary T cells: implication for gene therapy of AIDS. Gene Ther. 4:128–139.

146. Powell, D. M., M. C. Amaral, J. Y. Wu, T. Maniatis, and W. C. Greene. 1997. HIV Rev-dependent binding of SF2/ASF to the Rev response element: possible role in Rev-mediated inhibition of HIV RNA splicing. Proc. Natl. Acad. Sci. USA 94:973–978.

147. Rana, T. M., and K. T. Jeang. 1999. Biochemical and functional interactions between HIV-1 Tat protein and TAR RNA. Arch. Biochem. Biophys. 365:175–185.

148. Ranga, U., C. Woffendin, Z. Y. Yang, L. Xu, S. Verma, D. R. Littman, and G. J. Nabel. 1997. Cell and viral regulatory elements enhance the expression and function of a human immunodeficiency virus inhibitory gene. J. Virol. 71:7020–7029.

149. Rappaport, J., S. J. Lee, K. Khalili, and S. F. Wong. 1989. The acidic amino-terminal region of the HIV-1 Tat protein constitutes an essential activating domain. New Biologist 1:101–110.

150. Rautonen, J., N. Rautonen, N. L. Martin, and D. W. Wara. 1994. HIV type 1 Tat protein induces immunoglobulin and interleukin 6 synthesis by uninfected peripheral blood mononuclear cells. AIDS Res. Hum. Retroviruses 10:781–785.

151. Rosen, C. A., E. Terwilliger, A. Dayton, J. G. Sodroski, and W. A. Haseltine. 1988. Intragenic cis-acting art gene-responsive sequences of the human immunodeficiency virus. Proc. Natl. Acad. Sci. USA 85:2071–2075.

152. Rounseville, M. P., and A. Kumar. 1992. Binding of a host cell nuclear protein to the stem region of human immunodeficiency virus type 1 *trans*-activation-responsive RNA. J. Virol. 66:1688–1694.

153. Rounseville, M. P., H. C. Lin, E. Agbottah, R. R. Shukla, A. B. Rabson, and A. Kumar. 1996. Inhibition of HIV-1 replication in viral mutants with altered TAR RNA stem structures. Virology 216:411–417.

154. Ruhl, M., M. Himmelspach, G. Bahr, F. Hammerschmid, H. Jaksche, B. Wolff, H. Ashauer, G. Farrington, H. Probst, and D. Bevec. 1993. Eukaryotic initiation factor 5A is a cellular target of the human immunodeficiency virus type 1 Rev activation domain mediating trans-activation. J. Cell Biol. 123:1309–1320.

155. Sadaie, M. R., T. Benter, and S. F. Wong. 1988. Site-directed mutagenesis of two trans-regulatory genes (tat-III, trs) of HIV-1. Science 239:910–913.

156. Sarver, N., E. M. Cantin, P. S. Chang, J. A. Zaia, P. A. Landne, D. A. Stephens, and J. J. Rossi. 1990. Ribozymes as potential anti-HIV-1 therapeutic agents. Science 247:1222–1225.

157. Schatz, O., M. Oft, C. Dascher, M. Schebesta, O. Rosorius, H. Jaksche, M. Dobrovnik, D. Bevec, and J. Hauber. 1998. Interaction of the HIV-1 rev cofactor

eukaryotic initiation factor 5A with ribosomal protein L5. Proc. Natl. Acad. Sci. USA 95:1607–1612.

158. Selby, M. J., E. S. Bain, P. A. Luciw, and B. M. Peterlin. 1989. Structure, sequence, and position of the stem-loop in TAR determine transcriptional elongation by Tat through the HIV-1 long terminal repeat. Genes Dev. 3:547–558.

159. Shoji, S., K. Furuishi, A. Ogata, K. Yamataka, K. Tachibana, R. Mukai, A. Uda, K. Harano, S. Matsushita, and S. Misumi. 1998. An allosteric drug, o,o'-bis-myristoyl thiamine disulfide, suppresses HIV-1 replication through prevention of nuclear translocation of both HIV-1 Tat and NF-kappa B. Biochem. Biophys. Res. Commun. 249:745–753.

160. Sodroski, J. G., W. C. Rosen, C. Dayton, A. Terwilliger, and W. Haseltine. 1986. A second post-transcriptional trans-activator gene required for HTLV-III replication. Nature 321:412–417.

161. Southgate, C. D., and M. R. Green. 1995. Delineating minimal protein domains and promoter elements for transcriptional activation by lentivirus Tat proteins. J. Virol. 69:2605–2610.

162. Stutz, F., J. Kantor, D. Zhang, T. McCarthy, M. Neville, and M. Rosbash. 1997. The yeast nucleoporin rip1p contributes to multiple export pathways with no essential role for its FG-repeat region. Genes Dev. 11:2857–2868.

163. Su, L., R. Lee, M. Bonyhadi, H. Matsuzaki, S. Forestell, S. Escaich, E. Bohn-lein, and H. Kaneshima. 1997. Hematopoietic stem cell-based gene therapy for acquired immunodeficiency syndrome: efficient transduction and expression of Rev M10 in myeloid cells in vivo and in vitro. Blood 89: 2283–2290.

164. Subramanian, T., R. Govindarajan, and G. Chinnadurai. 1991. Heterologous basic domain substitutions in the HIV-1 Tat protein reveal an arginine-rich motif required for transactivation. EMBO J. 10:2311–2318.

165. Subramanian, T., M. Kuppuswamy, L. Venkatesh, A. Srinivasan, and G. Chinnadurai. 1990. Functional substitution of the basic domain of the HIV-1 *trans*-activator, Tat, with the basic domain of the functionally heterologous Rev. Virology 176:178–183.

166. Symensma, T. L., S. Baskerville, A. Yan, and A. D. Ellington. 1999. Polyvalent Rev decoys act as artificial Rev-responsive elements. J. Virol. 73:4341–4349.

167. Szebeni, A., B. Mehrotra, A. Baumann, S. A. Adam, P. T. Wingfield, and M. O. J. Olson. 1997. Nucleolar protein B23 stimulates nuclear import of the HIV-1 Rev protein and NLS-conjugated albumin. Biochemistry 36:3941–3949.

168. Tange, T. O., T. H. Jensen, and J. Kjems. 1996. In vitro interaction between human immunodeficiency virus type 1 Rev protein and splicing factor ASF/SF2-associated protein, p32. J. Biol. Chem. 271:10066–10072.

169. Thomas, S. L., J. Hauber, and G. Casari. 1997. Probing the structure of the HIV-1 Rev trans-activator protein by functional analysis. Protein Eng. 10:103–107.

170. Thomas, S. L., M. Oft, H. Jaksche, G. Casari, P. Heger, M. Dobrovnik, D. Bevec, and J. Hauber. 1998. Functional analysis of the human immunodeficiency virus type 1 Rev protein oligomerization interface. J. Virol. 72:2935–2944.

171. Truant, R., and B. R. Cullen. 1999. The arginine-rich domains present in human immunodeficiency virus type 1 Tat and Rev function as direct importin b-dependent nuclear localization signals. J. Virol. 19:1210–1217.

172. Ulich, C., A. Dunne, E. Parry, C. W. Hooker, R. B. Gaynor, and D. Harrich. 1999. Functional domains of Tat required for efficient human immunodeficiency virus type 1 reverse transcription. J. Virol. 73:2499–2508.

173. Ulich, C., D. Harrich, P. Estes, and R. B. Gaynor. 1996. Inhibition of human immunodeficiency virus type 1 replication is enhanced by a combination of transdominant Tat and Rev proteins. J. Virol. 70:4871–4876.

174. Van Lint, C., S. Emiliani, M. Ott, and E. Verdin. 1996. Transcriptional activation and chromatin remodeling of the HIV-1 promoter in response to histone acetylation. EMBO J. 15:1112–1120.

175. Verdin, E., P. Paras, and C. Van Lint. 1993. Chromatin disruption in the promoter of human immunodeficiency virus type 1 during transcriptional activation. EMBO J. 12:3249–3259.

176. Verhoef, K., M. Tijms, and B. Berkhout. 1997. Optimal Tat-mediated activation of the HIV-1 LTR promoter requires a full-length TAR RNA hairpin. Nucleic Acids Res. 25:496–502.

177. Weeks, K. M., and D. M. Crothers. 1991. RNA recognition by Tat-derived peptides: interaction in the major groove? Cell 66:577–588.

178. Wei, P., M. E. Garber, S. M. Fang, W. H. Fischer, and K. A. Jones. 1998. A novel CDK9-associated C-type cyclin interacts directly with HIV-1 Tat and mediates its high-affinity, loop-specific binding to TAR RNA. Cell 92:451–462.

179. Weissman, J. D., J. A. Brown, T. K. Howcroft, J. Hwang, A. Chawla, P. A. Roche, L. Schiltz, Y. Nakatani, and D. S. Singer. 1998. HIV-1 tat binds TAFII250 and represses TAFII250-dependent transcription of major histocompatibility class I genes. Proc. Natl. Acad. Sci. USA 95:11601–11606.

180. Westendorp, M. O., R. Frank, C. Ochsenbauer, K. Stricker, J. Dhein, H. Walczak, K.-M. Debatin, and P. H. Krammer. 1995. Sensitization of T-cells to CD95-mediated apoptosis by HIV-1 Tat and gp120. Nature 375:497–500.

181. Westendorp, M. O., V. A. Shatrov, K. Schulze-Osthoff, R. Frank, M. Kraft, M. Los, P. H. Krammer, W. Droge, and V. Lehmann. 1995. HIV-1 Tat potentiates TNF-induced NF-kappa B activation and cytotoxicity by altering the cellular redox state. EMBO J. 14:546–554.

182. Wimmer, J., K. Fujinaga, R. Taube, T. P. Cujec, Y. Zhu, J. Peng, D. H. Price, and B. M. Peterlin. 1999. Interactions between Tat and TAR and human immunodeficiency virus replication are facilitated by human cyclin T1 but not cyclins T2a or T2b. Virology 255:182–189.

183. Wolff, B., J. J. Sanglier, and Y. Wang. 1997. Leptomycin B is an inhibitor of nuclear export: inhibition of nucleo-cytoplasmic translocation of the human immunodeficiency virus type 1 (HIV-1) Rev protein and Rev-dependent mRNA. Chem. Biol. 4:139–147.

184. Wu-Baer, F., W. S. Lane, and R. B. Gaynor. 1998. Role of the human homolog of the yeast transcription factor SPT5 in HIV-1 Tat-activation. J. Mol. Biol. 277:179–197.

185. Yamamoto, R., S. Koseki, J. Ohkawa, K. Murakami, S. Nishikawa, K. Taira, and P. K. Kumar. 1997. Inhibition of transcription by the TAR RNA of HIV-1 in a nuclear extract of HeLa cells. Nucleic Acids Res. 25:3445–3450.

186. Yang, X., M. O. Gold, D. N. Tang, D. E. Lewis, E. Aguilar-Cordova, A. P. Rice, and C. H. Herrmann. 1997. TAK, an HIV Tat-associated kinase, is a member of the cyclin-dependent family of protein kinases and is induced by activation of peripheral blood lymphocytes and differentiation of promonocytic cell lines. Proc. Natl. Acad. Sci. USA 94:12331–12336.

187. Yang, X., C. H. Herrmann, and A. P. Rice. 1996. The human immunodeficiency virus Tat proteins specifically associate with TAK *in vivo* and require the carboxyl-terminal domain of RNA polymerase II for function. J. Virol. 70:4576–4584.

188. Zapp, M. L., and M. R. Green. 1989. Sequence-specific RNA binding by the HIV-1 Rev protein. Nature 342:714–716.

189. Zapp, M. L., T. J. Hope, T. G. Parslow, and M. R. Green. 1991. Oligomerization and RNA binding domains of the type 1 human immunodeficiency virus Rev protein: a dual function for an arginine-rich binding motif. Proc. Natl. Acad. Sci. USA 88:7734–7738.

190. Zapp, M. L., S. Stern, and M. R. Green. 1993. Small molecules that selectively block RNA binding of HIV-1 Rev protein inhibit Rev function and viral production. Cell 74:969–978.

191. Zauli, G., G. Furlini, M. C. Re, D. Milani, S. Capitani, and M. La Placa. 1993. Human immunodeficiency virus type 1 (HIV-1) tat-protein stimulates the production of interleukin-6 (IL-6) by peripheral blood monocytes. New Microbiol. 16:115–120.

192. Zhang, H., G. Dornadula, and R. J. Pomerantz. 1996. Endogenous reverse transcription of human immunodeficiency virus type 1 in physiological microenvironments: an important stage for viral infection of nondividing cells. J. Virol. 70:2809–2824.

193. Zhang, J., and J. L. Corden. 1991. Identification of phosphorylation sites in the repetitive carboxyl-terminal domain of the mouse RNA polymerase II largest subunit. J. Biol. Chem. 226:2290–2296.

194. Zhou, C., I. Bahmer, G. Larson, J. Zaia, J. Rossi, and D. Koh. 1994. Inhibition of HIV-1 in human T-lymphocytes by retrovirally transduced anti-tat and rev hammerhead ribozymes. Gene 149:33–39.

195. Zhou, Q., D. Chen, E. Pierstorff, and K. Luo. 1998. Transcription elongation factor P-TEFb mediates Tat activation of HIV-1 transcription at multiple stages. EMBO J. 17:3681–3691.

196. Zhou, Q., and P. A. Sharp. 1995. Novel mechanism and factor for regulation by HIV-1 Tat. EMBO J. 14:321–328.

197. Zhou, Q., and P. A. Sharp. 1996. Tat-SF1: cofactor for stimulation of transcriptional elongation by HIV-1 Tat. Science 274:605–610.

198. Zhu, Y., T. Peery, J. Peng, Y. Ramanathan, N. Marshall, T. Marshall, B. Amendt, M. B. Mathews, and D. H. Price. 1997. Transcription elongation factor P-TEFb is required for HIV-1 Tat transactivation *in vitro*. Genes Dev. 11:2622–2632.

199. Zolotukhin, A. S., and B. K. Felber. 1999. Nucleoporins nup98 and nup214 participate in nuclear export of human immunodeficiency virus type 1 Rev. J. Virol. 73:120–127.

9

Novel HIV-1 Therapeutic Targets: Accessory Functions

MARIO STEVENSON

Accessory Proteins: Essential or Auxiliary?

The Nef, Vpu, Vpr, Vpx, and Vif proteins of primate lentiviruses (see Fig. 9.1) earned the designation "accessory" because, for the most part, they are dispensable for virus replication in tissue culture systems. Desrosiers and colleagues (61) made a systematic analysis of the relative replication defect of single and combined accessory gene disruptions on SIV_{mac} replication in vivo. That study allowed a rank ordering of the relative virulence (a reflection of replication capacity and pathogenicity phenotypes), from least attenuated to most attenuated, as follows: $\Delta Vpr > \Delta Vpx > \Delta Nef > \Delta Vif$ (the relative virulence of a ΔVpu virus could not be assessed because SIV_{mac} lacks a Vpu allele). This rank ordering appears to reflect the degree of impairment imposed on virus replication in primary cells in vitro in that ΔVif mutants exhibit the greatest replication defect in primary cells followed by ΔVpx and then ΔVpr. Nef is an exception to this general rule in that the markedly impaired virulence of ΔNef viruses is not reflected by a similar impairment in tissue culture systems (61, 252). Are accessory proteins required for pathogenicity? The answer appears to be no. For example, although mutations in Nef markedly impair the virulence of HIV (60, 134) and SIV (127), disease progression is observed in humans infected with ΔNef HIV-1 (91, 144), neonatal macaques infected with ΔNef SIV variants (13), and infant and adult macaques infected with SIV variants lacking Nef, Vpr, and the long terminal repeat (LTR)–negative regulatory element (14). Progression to disease in the absence of a functional *nef* gene can be interpreted as suggesting that accessory proteins such as Nef are facilitators of viral replication and pathogenicity but are otherwise dispensable for disease induction. Such studies are important to the understanding of the determinants in the genomes of primate lentiviruses

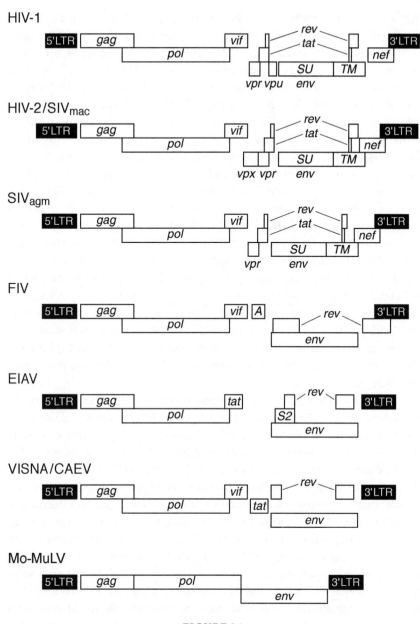

FIGURE 9.1

Genomic organization of primate and nonprimate lentiviruses

The major primate lentivirus lineages are represented together with several nonprimate lentiviruses and Mo-MuLV, an animal onco-retrovirus, for comparison. *vif* is common to the primate and nonprimate lentiviruses with the exception of EIAV. *vpr* is encoded by HIV-1 and HIV-2 and some strains of SIV. *vpx* is encoded by HIV-2/SIV$_{mac}$, and *vpu* is present only in HIV-1. Although the genomes of simple onco-retroviruses such as Mo-MuLV appear to lack open-reading frames for accessory proteins, it is possible that functions resembling certain accessory proteins (e.g., Vif) are contained within Mo-MuLV *gag, pol,* or *env* genes.

that lead to immunodeficiency. However, they are less relevant to the understanding of why primate lentiviruses have acquired these novel open-reading frames, and in this regard, the impact of accessory gene mutations on "viral fitness" may be a more informative indicator of how "essential" a viral gene product may be. The studies by Holland and colleagues (for review, see reference 240) demonstrated that the extremely high mutation rate associated with replication of RNA genomes of vesicular stomatitis virus (VSV) leads to the emergence of quasi-species virus populations that are genetically distinguishable. Changes in environmental conditions allow for the rapid emergence of individual variants that have a greater replication capacity in that environment to the extent that they can outcompete other variants in the quasi-species population. This paradigm reflects the situation in HIV-1 infection in which seropositive individuals harbor many different variants within a quasi-species population (268). Presumably, variants within these quasi-species populations exhibit varying degrees of fitness owing, for example, to their replication rate, ability to evade immune responses, or tropism for particular cell types that may afford some replication advantage. The upshot is that those variants better adapted to the environment will predominate and may ultimately have a greater chance of being transmitted to the next host. Therefore, the fittest viruses are those that persist and spread within the population (Fig. 9.2).

The fact that the accessory gene products have been acquired and are evolutionarily conserved across primate lentiviral lineages (221) suggests that viruses with a full complement of those accessory proteins exhibit the greatest degree of fitness within the host individual and ultimately within the host population. Thus, the impact of a particular accessory gene inactivation on virus replication may only be fully appreciated when that virus is examined in a competitive situation with its wild-type counterpart. To illustrate this, Hirsch and colleagues (106) compared the replicative capacity of pigtailed macaques infected with the highly pathogenic SIV_{sm} PBj virus containing an inactivated Vpr allele and demonstrated that the ΔVPR variant was fully pathogenic. However, in animals coinfected with wild-type and ΔVPR viruses, the wild-type variant rapidly predominated. If variants within a population of viruses are otherwise identical in terms of transmissibility properties, then the most abundant variant, that is, the fittest, has the greatest chance of being transmitted to a new host, and low-abundance variants would ultimately be lost from the population (Fig. 9.2). In this regard, Vpr may be considered essential to the maintenance of the virus in the population. In evolutionary terms, the acquisition of accessory genes would be predicted to confer a fitness advantage. The primate lentiviruses that we know today are probably the result of those evolutionary gene acquisition events that enhanced viral fitness.

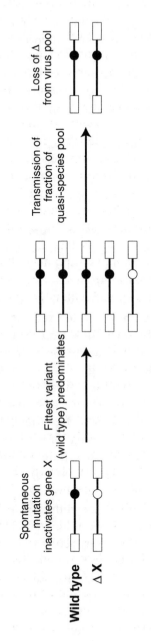

FIGURE 9.2

Negative selection of accessory gene mutants due to loss of competitive fitness

A spontaneous mutation in an accessory protein (ΔX) either inactivates the open-reading frame or results in attenuation of accessory gene function. This could affect several aspects of viral fitness, such as replicative capacity, dissemination, or evasion of immune responses. Over multiple rounds of replication, the greater replication capacity of the wild-type virus allows it to outcompete ΔX variants, and as a result the wild-type variant predominates in the quasi-species pool. A fraction of the quasi-species pool will be transmitted to the new host. Assuming that the accessory gene mutation does not influence transmission per se, wild-type and ΔX viruses will be transmitted with equal efficiency. However, because of the higher frequency of wild-type viruses in the donor pool, there is a higher probability that they will be transmitted. As a result, the ΔX mutation will eventually be lost from the virus pool and from the host population. A caveat to this is that highly pathogenic variants that induce acute disease onset will also be subject to negative selective pressure because disease in the host presumably reduces the frequency of potential transmission events.

The Vif Protein

All lentiviruses with the exception of equine infectious anemia virus (EIAV) possess a *vif* gene (Fig. 9.1). Vif was originally reported to be phosphorylated by protein kinase C (97), although the functional role of that modification is unclear. More recently, Vif has been shown to be phosphorylated both in vitro and in vivo. S^{144}, T^{155}, and T^{188} were identified as phosphate acceptor sites on Vif, and mutation of S^{144} resulted in 90% inhibition of HIV-1 replication (285). Vif is also phosphorylated by the mitogen-activated protein kinase ERK/MAPK (284) on T^{96} and S^{165}. Mutagenesis of T^{96}, which is highly conserved among Vif alleles of HIV-1, HIV-2, and SIV, results in a marked impairment of HIV-1 replication. Noteworthy is that phosphorylation of Vif by ERK/MAPK does not involve a consensus ERK/MAPK recognition sequence (PX S/T P). ERK/MAPK phosphorylates HIV-1 Gag, which also lacks an ERK/MAPK consensus sequence (114).

Vif consists of 192 amino acids and is highly basic in nature. Studies on the subcellular localization of Vif have failed to reach a consensus. Initially, Vif was demonstrated to associate with the Golgi complex in infected cells (96). When expressed in transfected COS cells, Vif exists in both cytosolic and membrane-associated forms (87). Vif co-localizes with the intermediate filament protein, vimentin, in both acutely infected cells and transfected cells (123). The C-terminal basic domain of Vif is required for membrane association, and mutations in Vif that disrupt this membrane association impair HIV-1 replication (88). Several groups have presented evidence to suggest that Vif co-localizes with structural Gag proteins in vitro and in vivo. Interaction between Vif and Pr55^{gag} can be detected in vitro and in infected cells (30), and deletion of the C-terminal 22 amino acids of *vif* abolishes this interaction. In cells in which Vif is essential for virus replication (nonpermissive cells), double-label immunofluorescence analysis indicates co-localization of Vif and Gag proteins (225). The majority of Vif in these cells is associated with cellular membranes, raising the possibility that Vif and Gag proteins may co-localize at the plasma membrane during the process of virus assembly and budding. Vif and Gag are independently targeted to membrane-free cytoplasmic complexes that co-purify in sucrose density gradients (224). However, there does not appear to be any specific interaction between Vif and Gag in gradient-purified cytoplasmic complexes. Thus, the functional significance of Vif/Gag interaction is as yet undefined. In an attempt to define an effector domain, *vif* has been subjected to extensive mutagenesis and deletional analysis, and these Vif mutants have been examined with respect to Vif subcellular localization and virus infectivity after expression of Vif in *trans* (230). Substitution of amino acids dispersed throughout the linear sequence of Vif is important for infectivity; however, these mutations also alter the subcellular distribution of Vif. Several mutations that inactivate Vif infectivity function without influencing Vif localization are located in a region spanning residues 114–146 and as such best adhere to the criterion for an "effector" domain. Interestingly, this region contains a motif (S^{144} LQYL) that is highly conserved in *vif* alleles from primate and nonprimate lentiviruses (176). Furthermore, S^{144} appears to be phosphorylated (at least in the case of HIV-1) and is important for viral infectivity (285).

A number of groups have suggested that Vif is incorporated into virions (26, 41, 74, 123, 151, 228). Vif co-sediments with sucrose-density-gradient-purified virions even after detergent treatment of virions, suggesting that Vif associates with virion cores (123, 151). The stoichiometry of Vif in virions is in the order of 1 molecule of Vif to 30 molecules of Gag, or around 30–100 molecules of Vif per virion (74, 151). Determinants in the HIV-1 genome that mediate packaging of Vif are not yet defined, and it is likely that virion incorporation of Vif is not mediated through a specific packaging signal. Envelope (Env), Nef, Vpr, Vpu, protease, reverse transcriptase, integrase, nucleocapsid, and p6 proteins as well as genomic viral RNA are dispensable for Vif packaging (41). Substitutions at highly conserved amino acids in Vif or deletion of the C-terminal 80 amino acids of Vif, which are critical for Vif function, do not impair incorporation of Vif into virions (41). Furthermore, HIV-1 Vif can be packaged in Moloney murine leukemia virus (Mo-MuLV) particles (41), and the extent of Vif incorporation into virions is proportional to cellular Vif expression levels (228). Collectively, these studies suggest that packaging of Vif is neither specific nor necessary for Vif function. Furthermore, when HIV-1 virions are subject to a velocity gradient centrifugation procedure, which promotes better separation of membrane organelles, Vif does not co-sediment with virions (62). A confounding variable in these analyses is the presence of cell-derived microvesicles, which are present in virus preparations and which co-sediment with gradient-fractionated virus particles (22, 84). Thus, many of the components that co-localize to HIV-1 virions in such gradients may be vesicle associated rather than virion associated, and as such, co-sedimentation may not necessarily signify virion packaging. Nevertheless, the possibility that small amounts of Vif functionally associate with virions cannot be ruled out. Answers to this question will require the identification of mutations that concomitantly impair both virion incorporation of Vif and Vif activity.

Of all the accessory gene mutants, SIV variants bearing an inactivated *vif* gene exhibit the greatest defect in terms of replication and pathogenicity in vivo (61). HIV-1 ΔVif variants also exhibit the greatest replication defect in primary T cells and macrophages in vitro (71, 77, 235, 246, 264). Vif is essential for the replication of feline immunodeficiency virus (FIV) in T-cell lines and in primary peripheral blood lymphocytes (257). Similarly, replication of caprine arthritis-encephalitis virus (CAEV) in both synovial membrane cells and monocyte/macrophages is Vif-dependent (102). In contrast to the phenotype observed for primate lentiviral Vif mutants in which the extent of virus production is not affected, CAEV mutants containing an inactivated *vif* gene exhibit lower levels of virus formation under single-cycle conditions (102). Intriguingly, Vif is dispensable for HIV-1 replication in some cell lines (70, 71, 77, 203, 227, 231, 237, 264). As a consequence, cells have been classified as "permissive" and "nonpermissive." Permissive cells such as CEM-SS T cells and C8166 T cells produce ΔVif viruses whose infectivities approximate those of wild-type viruses. In contrast, ΔVif viruses produced from nonpermissive cells, which include primary macrophages, peripheral blood lymphocytes, H9 T cells, and HUT 78 T cells, are noninfectious (Fig. 9.3). It is possible that permissive cells contain a factor that compensates for Vif and that is missing in nonpermissive cells. Alternatively, nonpermissive cells may contain a factor that, in the absence of Vif, inhibits HIV-1 infectivity, and this factor is absent in permissive cells. To address these possibilities, the infectivity phenotype of ΔVif viruses produced from heterokaryons that had been formed between permissive and nonpermissive cells was examined (160, 226). ΔVif viruses produced from these heterokaryons were markedly impaired in infectivity. This result is consistent with the hypothesis that nonpermissive cells express an activity that, in the absence of Vif, negatively influences viral infectivity. Thus, Vif may counteract this negative factor so as to restore viral replication capacity (see Fig. 9.4).

The negative cellular factor that is counteracted by Vif appears to be species restricted. Thus, Vif of SIV from macaques can functionally complement Vif-defective HIV-1; however, Vif proteins from nonprimate lentiviruses, including Visna, bovine immunodeficiency virus (BIV), and FIV, do not complement Vif-defective HIV (231). The species restriction appears to be dictated by species-specific interactions between Vif and the cellular "negative factor" cell rather than between Vif and viral components (229). Thus, HIV-1 Vif modulates the infectivity of HIV-1, HIV-2, and SIV$_{agm}$ in human cells. In contrast, Vif of SIV$_{agm}$ cannot complement HIV-1 infectivity in human cells but can do so in African green monkey cells. The ability of Vif to complement HIV-1 and SIV$_{agm}$ infectivity in human cells suggests that the negative activity that is present in human cells impairs the replication of HIV-1 and SIV$_{agm}$ and argues against species-specific interaction between Vif activity and virus components. The inability of SIV$_{agm}$ Vif to function in human cells argues for species-specific interaction between Vif and the negative activity that is present in human cells (Fig. 9.4). The presence of a species-specific restriction to Vif function has implications for the zoonotic origin of HIV-1. Similarities between HIV-1 and SIV$_{cpz}$ suggest that HIV-1 emerged in humans following transmission of SIV$_{cpz}$ from chimpanzees (79). There is, however, no evidence for transmission of SIV$_{agm}$ to humans, and it has been proposed that the in-

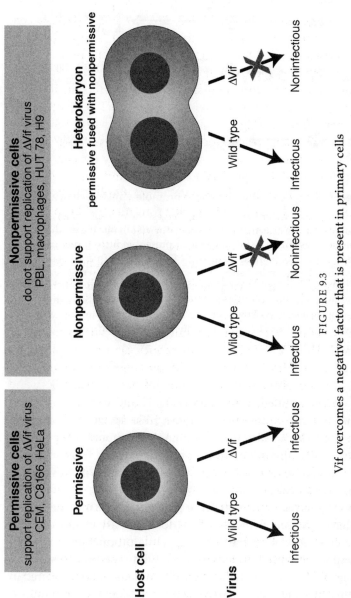

FIGURE 9.3

Vif overcomes a negative factor that is present in primary cells

Permissive cells promote the release of infectious virions regardless of their *vif* genotype. In contrast, ΔVif viruses produced from nonpermissive cells are unable to establish infection in either permissive or nonpermissive cells. When permissive and nonpermissive cells are fused, ΔVif virions produced from such heterokaryons are noninfectious. This is consistent with a model in which nonpermissive cells contain an endogenous activity that renders HIV-1 virions noninfectious in the absence of Vif. Vif blocks this endogenous inhibitory activity, thus allowing the production of infectious virions (160, 226).

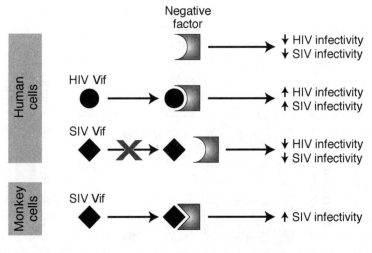

FIGURE 9.4

Vif targets a negative cellular factor to promote viral infectivity

Experiments with heterokaryons (160, 226) suggest the presence of an activity in nonpermissive cells that in the absence of Vif inhibits the production of infectious virions. The negative factor present in human cells can impair the infectivity of both HIV-1 and SIV (226, 229). Vif interacts with the negative cellular factor in a species-specific manner so as to negate its effect on viral infectivity. HIV-1 Vif counteracts the negative activity in human cells to augment both HIV and SIV infectivity. In contrast, SIV Vif does not counteract the negative factor in human cells and is unable to augment the infectivity of HIV-1 or SIV virions produced from human cells. (For a more complete description, see references 226 and 229.)

ability of SIV_{agm} Vif to function in human cells would ultimately restrict the establishment of SIV_{agm} in humans were a cross-species transmission to occur (229). A similar species restriction has been reported for the cell cycle arrest activity of primate lentiviral Vpr proteins (245). Thus, it is quite likely that the action of several accessory proteins restricts virus establishment following zoonotic infection.

A major hurdle in the identification of a function for Vif is the lack of any obvious defect in noninfectious ΔVif virions that are produced from nonpermissive cells. Although the extent of virus production from ΔVif proviruses compares favorably with that from wild-type proviruses (227, 237, 264), virions produced from ΔVif proviruses are markedly impaired in infectivity. While the infectivity defect can be complemented by the expression of Vif in *trans*, ΔVif virus infectivity cannot be rescued when Vif is expressed in the target cell (77, 264). Although the presence of Vif is essential for the production of an infectious virion, there is no clear consensus as to the exact nature of the defect in ΔVif virions. Electron-microscopic examination suggests that ΔVif virions lack a characteristic cone-shaped core morphology. Vif has further been implicated in proteolytic processing of the

Gag p55 precursor (26, 223) in that ΔVif viruses derived from peripheral blood lymphocytes contain a higher proportion of unprocessed Gag precursors (26, 30, 108). However, other investigators have been unable to discern any qualitative or quantitative differences with respect to Gag, Pol, or Env proteins between wild-type and ΔVif virions (74). Nevertheless, an inability to complement the Vif defect in the target cell in *trans* indicates that the Vif defect is determined in the virus-producing cell and that the infectious characteristics of the virion are negatively influenced in the absence of Vif (Fig. 9.5). This defect is most apparent when viral cDNA synthesis in the target cell is compared between ΔVif and wild-type viruses (57, 88, 227, 237). The rate and extent of viral cDNA synthesis are impaired in ΔVif relative to wild-type-virus-infected cells (237). In the absence of Vif, late products of reverse transcription can be detected (88, 227). However, these late reverse transcription products undergo rapid degradation (227). Several explanations can be forwarded for these experimental findings. The stability of the reverse transcription complex may be impaired following infection by ΔVif viruses. Fusion or uncoating may be affected such that viral nucleic acids enter a nonproductive compartment within the target cell and are rapidly degraded. Viral cDNAs within the reverse transcription complex may be more accessible to cellular nucleases. Whatever the defect, the precipitating event occurs in the virus-producing cell and could involve, for example, an effect of Vif on posttranslational modification of a virion protein, an effect of Vif on an essential cellular cofactor that has to be packaged within virions for them to be infectious, and/or an effect of Vif on the appropriate spatial organization of virion components. Given the degree to which viral replication and virulence are impaired by inactivation of Vif, the identification of Vif inhibitors is of the highest priority.

Vpu

vpu, which is found only in HIV-1 and SIV$_{cpz}$ (see Fig. 9.1), encodes an 80-amino-acid protein of 16 kDa (52, 247). Vpu and Env are translated from different translation frames of the same mRNA (219). Vpu is an amphipathic membrane protein that forms oligomeric structures in vitro and in vivo (162, 248). Vpu is phosphorylated on one or more serines by casein kinase 2 (215). The protein localizes predominantly to the Golgi complex (135) but has also been found in association with the plasma membrane (76). Although Vpu associates with the plasma membrane, it does not appear to be incorporated into virus particles (248).

Vpu and Virus Particle Release

Vpu enhances virus particle release (82, 135, 248, 254, 286). HIV-1 variants lacking an intact *vpu* gene are impaired in virion release, and as a result, virions accumulate on intracytoplasmic vesicles (135, 254). Vpu-mediated

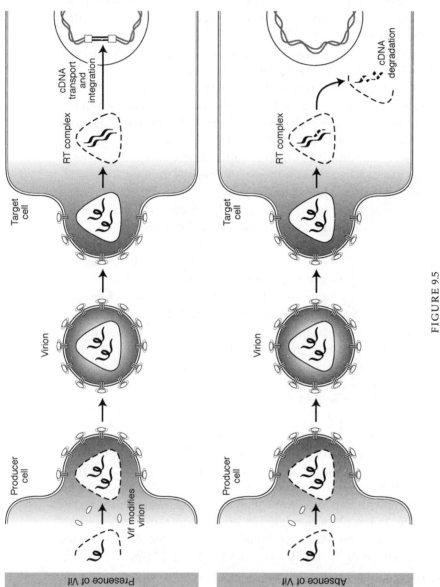

FIGURE 9.5

Vif promotes virus infectivity

In the presence of Vif, a component of the virion or a stage leading up to formation of the virion is modified by Vif through an undefined mechanism. Following infection of the target cell by Vif-modified virions, viral cDNA is synthesized and translocated to the host cell nucleus. Following infection of cells by virions produced in the absence of Vif, viral cDNA appears to be synthesized but subsequently undergoes degradation. Infectivity of ΔVif virions cannot be restored by expression of Vif in the target cell.

CD4 degradation requires the hydrophilic cytoplasmic domain of Vpu and involves the trapping of CD4 in the endoplasmic reticulum (ER) (131) (Fig. 9.6). The effect of Vpu on virus particle release involves a post-ER compartment (215), requires the transmembrane domain of Vpu, and appears to be mediated through the Gag protein. Expression of Gag in mammalian cells is sufficient for immature formation of viral capsids, which can be increased in the presence of Vpu. A Vpu-binding protein (UBP) belonging to the tetratricopeptide repeat family of proteins has been identified in a yeast two-hybrid screen (40). UBP also interacts directly with HIV-1 Gag, and this interaction is diminished in the presence of Vpu. Overexpression of UBP in virus-producing cells greatly impairs HIV-1 particle release (40) (Fig. 9.7). It has been suggested that the interaction between UBP and Gag

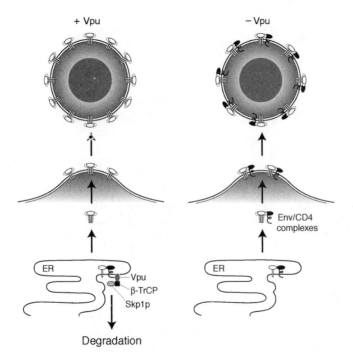

FIGURE 9.6

Vpu effects on stability of intracellular Env/CD4 complexes

The viral envelope glycoprotein binds to CD4 during transport in the ER. Within the ER, Vpu interacts with the cytoplasmic tail of CD4. Upon interaction with β-TrCP and Skp1p, Vpu targets CD4/Env complexes to the ubiquitin-proteosome pathway, where these complexes are degraded. As a consequence, only Env glycoproteins that have not bound CD4 are free to translocate to the plasma membrane for incorporation into assembling virus particles. In the absence of Vpu, Env/CD4 complexes that are formed in the ER ultimately translocate to the plasma membrane rather than being targeted for degradation. During virus assembly, Env/CD4 complexes are incorporated into virions. This ultimately may affect the infectivity of the virion by reducing the number of available receptor occupancy sites for CD4 engagement on the target cell. (Adapted from reference 68a.)

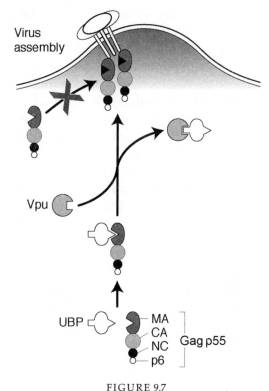

FIGURE 9.7

Vpu effects on virus assembly

A cellular Vpu-binding protein (UBP) first interacts with Gag p55 precursors via the N-terminal matrix domain. Subsequent interaction of Vpu with UBP promotes its dissociation from Gag. Gag molecules that have undergone interaction with UBP and subsequently undergone Vpu-mediated dissociation from UBP may be more efficiently translocated to the site of virus assembly, thereby enhancing virus release. In the absence of Vpu, the interaction of Gag precursors with UBP may impair their translocation and reduce the efficiency of particle release. Thus, UBP may be considered a negative cellular factor that Vpu counteracts. As shown in Fig. 9.4, a similar model has been proposed to account for the role of Vif in particle infectivity. (Adapted from reference 40, which contains a more complete description of the UBP model.)

leads to an irreversible change in Gag that further renders Gag incapable of interaction with UBP (40). As such, UBP represents a factor required for correct particle formation and release (Fig. 9.7). The N-terminal matrix domain of Gag p55 is required for Vpu-mediated enhancement of virus particle release (147). A prediction of this is that UBP also interacts with Gag via the matrix domain. Given analogies with immunophilins that are involved in protein folding (75, 157, 255), it has been proposed that UBP acts by promoting proper folding of Gag (40). *vpu* is contained in the genomes of HIV-1 and the related SIV$_{cpz}$ but is not found in HIV-2 and all other SIV isolates characterized to date (Fig. 9.1). However, the Env glycoprotein of HIV-2 appears to contain a Vpu-like activity (29). Thus, exchanging the Gag-Pol region of HIV-1 with the corresponding region of HIV-2 confers Vpu responsiveness on the chimeric HIV-2. HIV-2 Env glycoprotein enhances HIV-2 particle release to an extent comparable with that of HIV-1 Vpu. Inactivation of HIV-2 Env impairs virus particle release to a similar extent when Vpu is deleted in HIV-1 isolates (29). In some HIV-1 isolates, the enhancement of virus release can be influenced by either Vpu or Env (214). The primary HIV-1 isolate, AD8, does not express Vpu because of a mutation in the Vpu initiation codon. AD8 particle release is, however, enhanced when AD8 Env glycoprotein is provided in *trans*, and the level of Env expression varies depending on whether AD8 contains a functional Vpu initiation codon (214). This suggests that the coordinated expression of Env can compensate for inactivating mutations in Vpu so as to restore virus release to maximal levels. The conservation of a Vpu-like activity across lentiviral lineages provides strong evidence that this activity influences viral fitness. The effect of Vpu on virus particle release likely increases virion "burst size," thereby augmenting the efficiency of virus spread.

Vpu and CD4 Downregulation

Two genetically separable biological activities have been described for Vpu. First, Vpu promotes rapid degradation of the HIV-1 receptor, CD4, both in cell-free systems (46) and in vivo (215, 277). Vpu binds to CD4 in the ER (278) and recruits CD4 to the cytosolic ubiquitin-proteasome pathway, where it is subsequently degraded (212). Vpu-mediated CD4 degradation requires a hydrophilic cytoplasmic domain in Vpu (213). In addition, degradation of CD4 in the presence of Vpu can be abrogated by the removal of lysine residues, the target of ubiquitination, from the cytoplasmic tail of CD4. Recruitment of CD4/Vpu complexes to the proteasome is mediated through a protein termed β-TrCP, which itself binds to the proteasome targeting factor Skp1p. Trimolecular complexes comprising CD4, Vpu, and β-TrCP can be isolated from cells (166). Furthermore, Vpu-induced degradation of CD4 is impaired in the presence of a β-TrCP variant that is unable to bind Skp1p (166).

Presumably, downmodulation of cell surface CD4 expression is necessary for some aspect of virus replication, since the virus has evolved three mechanistically and genetically distinct mechanisms to regulate cell surface CD4. Newly synthesized Env glycoprotein binds directly to CD4 in the ER and impairs its translocation to the cell membrane (110, 113, 241, 243). As discussed later, the accessory protein Nef recruits preexisting CD4 from the cell surface to clathrin-coated pits and eventually to degradative lysosomes (3, 81, 89, 97, 148, 184). There are at least two possible consequences of CD4 downregulation from the cell surface: induction of superinfection resistance and inhibition of CD4 uptake into virus particles. Superinfection resistance is a process by which a virus, upon downregulating its receptor on the host cell, prevents subsequent reinfection of that cell by progeny virions. This interference phenomenon is exhibited by a number of retroviruses including human T-cell leukemia virus types 1 and 2, avian leukosis virus, and bovine leukemia virus (64, 263, 262, 272, 273, 275). Infected cells are rapidly turned over (49, 50, 107, 271) by a combination of viral cytopathic effects and destruction of infected cells by cytotoxic T cells (65, 99, 103, 183, 293). Thus, the induction of superinfection resistance, through downregulation of CD4, may ultimately prevent reinfection of a short-lived cell. The combined effects of Vpu, Nef, and Env on surface CD4 expression may also reduce the incorporation of CD4 molecules into virions. Interaction between Env and CD4 within the ER and cytosol and subsequent incorporation of Env-CD4 complexes into virions would lead to occupancy of receptor binding sites on Env that are available for engaging CD4 on the target cell (Fig. 9.6). Vpu therefore promotes rapid degradation of Env-CD4 complexes, thereby ensuring that free Env (i.e., not bound to CD4) reaches the cell surface for incorporation into virions. Nef rapidly shuttles CD4 from the cell surface, thus minimizing chances for CD4-Env interaction on the surface of the producer cell. Consistent with this is the demonstration that when high levels of CD4 are expressed on the surface of HIV-1-infected cells, there is a dramatic reduction in virion infectivity due primarily to the occupancy of receptor binding sites by producer-cell-derived CD4 (140). Thus, efforts on the part of the virus to downregulate CD4 may be to combat this "envelope interference" (140).

Vpr/Vpx Proteins

Within the genomes of HIV-1, SIV_{cpz}, SIV_{agm}, SIV_{syk}, and SIV_{mnd}, the region overlapping the *vif* and *tat* open-reading frames (the so-called central viral region) contains a single small open-reading frame that is usually termed *vpr* (see Fig. 9.1). In HIV-2 and several other SIV strains (SIV_{sm}, SIV_{mac}) the central viral region encodes two small open-reading frames that are termed *vpr* and *vpx*. Based on their homology and their juxtaposition, it was suggested that *vpr* and *vpx* genes were the result of a gene duplication event (258). Phylogenetic analysis of a more comprehensive sequence database indicates that the ancestor to SIV_{sm} acquired a *vpx* gene through nonhomologous recombination with SIV_{agm} (most likely sabaeus) (221). The acquisition of a *vpx* gene may have conferred a more efficient replication capacity, which promoted the predominance of viruses containing both *vpr* and *vpx* genes. Most of the information regarding properties of Vpr and Vpx proteins has been generated from studies of HIV-1 Vpr. When expressed in mammalian cells, Vpr localizes to the nuclear Env (73, 261) and to the nucleoplasm (63, 116, 220, 250, 287). As discussed later, the association of Vpr with the nucleus may underscore the ability of this protein to promote localization of viral reverse transcription complexes to the nucleus. An α-helical structure at the N-terminus of Vpr has been implicated in the nuclear localization of Vpr (63, 161, 287). This motif does not, however, bear a strong similarity to basic nuclear localization signals (NLS) characteristic of other viral nuclear proteins (44). Both Vpr and Vpx are packaged within virions in amounts stoichiometrically equivalent to Gag primarily through their interaction with the C-terminal p6 domain of the *gag* precursor (51, 137, 143, 156, 182, 282, 289). A conserved LXXLF motif within Gag p6 mediates the interaction of Vpr with Gag and incorporation of Vpr into virions (136). Vpx has further been shown to associate with HIV-2 cores (128). The ability of Vpr and Vpx proteins to promote packaging of functional integrase and reverse transcriptase in *trans* further suggests that these proteins are being directed to virion cores (152, 283).

Three well-characterized properties have been described for primate lentiviral Vpr and Vpx proteins. These include induction of cell cycle arrest (104, 119, 194, 200), association with uracil DNA glycosylase (UDG) (28, 220), and nuclear targeting of viral reverse transcription complexes (42, 72, 105, 173, 192, 193, 261). Insight into the independent contributions of these activities to viral replication and pathogenicity has been promoted by the demonstration that these functions segregate between Vpr and Vpx proteins of primate lentiviruses. Thus, activities of cell cycle arrest and UDG association are governed by HIV-2/SIV$_{sm}$ Vpr (72, 189, 220), while nuclear targeting of viral DNA in nondividing cells is governed by HIV-2/SIV$_{sm}$ Vpx (72). In HIV-1, these functions are all contained within the single Vpr allele. It is not known whether these properties are all exhibited by the single Vpr protein of SIV$_{agm}$.

Interaction of Vpr with UDG

Vpr proteins of HIV-1 (28) and of HIV-2/SIV$_{sm}$ (220) have been shown in the yeast two-hybrid system to interact with the DNA repair enzyme, UDG. UDG specifically removes the RNA-base uracil from DNA. Interaction of Vpr with UDG does not appear to compromise the enzymatic activity of UDG (28). In addition, the binding of Vpr to UDG is not necessary for the effects of Vpr on cell cycle progression (220). The demonstration that UDG-associating activity of Vpr is conserved across primate lentiviral lineages argues that this activity plays an important role in virus replication, although the actual role is undefined. Inactivation of this activity in HIV-2/SIV$_{sm}$ does not appear to compromise viral replication in either primary lymphocytes or primary macrophages (72). However, some clues may be provided by studies on an apparently analogous function encoded by the genomes of nonprimate lentiviruses and onco-retroviruses. The *pol* genes of Visna (21, 68, 168), EIAV (256), FIV, CAEV (150, 256), and ovine lentiviruses (259) contain a deoxyuridine triphosphatase (dUTPase) domain. dUTPase hydrolyzes dUTP to dUMP, which is subsequently used for synthesis of TTP by thymidylate synthase. The action of dUTPase promotes the maintenance of a low dUTP/TTP ratio, thus minimizing misincorporation of uracil into DNA. This becomes particularly acute in noncycling cells, which have a relatively high dUTP/TTP ratio relative to cycling cells (253). As a consequence, retroviruses that replicate in nondividing cells face conditions that increase the likelihood of misincorporation of uracil into cDNA. The dUTPase activity within the *pol* genes of onco-retroviruses and nonprimate lentiviruses may have evolved to combat this hazard. dUTPase-deficient mutants of FIV and EIAV replicate with wild-type kinetics in continuous cell lines but are markedly impaired in macrophages (150, 256, 266). Similarly, dUTPase mutants of caprine and ovine lentiviruses replicate with wild-type kinetics in dividing cells but are attenuated in primary macrophages (259).

UDG is the first enzyme in the base excision repair pathway for removal of uracil from DNA. Although UDG and dUTPase are mechanically distinct enzymes, they ultimately minimize misincorporation of uracil into DNA. A prediction of this is that primate lentiviral variants that are unable to associate with UDG should be impaired in nondividing cells such as primary macrophages. However, variants of SIV_{sm} that, as a result of inactivation of Vpr, no longer associate with UDG replicate with wild-type kinetics in primary macrophages (72). On the other hand, simple replication assays may not reveal the actual replication defect in macrophages infected with ΔVPR viruses. For example, non-UDG-associating mutants may exhibit an increased misincorporation of uracil into cDNA. If allowed to accumulate, such misincorporations could impair replication fitness and, as such, be selected against over multiple rounds of virus replication. Simple replication assays may not reveal these qualitative effects on the virus life cycle.

Additional evidence for an effect of Vpr on the integrity of viral cDNA is the demonstration that Vpr reduces the rate of UV-induced deletions in a plasmid shuttle vector (118). Vpr also reduces the mutation rate of an HIV-1 shuttle vector by approximately fourfold (165). At present, it is unclear whether the influence of Vpr on the fidelity of reverse transcription (165) or on the repair of UV-damaged DNA (118) is related to the ability of Vpr to associate with UDG. These issues notwithstanding, the question still remains as to how HIV-1 reverse transcription proceeds in low-dNTP environments such as that encountered in nondividing macrophages. Primate lentiviruses may have adapted to this environment such that the reverse transcription can proceed in low-dNTP environments. Some viruses

have adapted to the resting cell environment by encoding proteins that regulate nucleic acid metabolism and synthesis. These viral proteins fall into
two categories: proteins that are essential for amplification of viral DNA
and enzymes that influence nucleic acid metabolism of the cell such as
thymidine kinase, ribonucleotide reductase, dUTPase, and UDG. The large
herpes viruses encode their own ribonucleotide reductase as well as other
enzymes required for DNA synthesis (reviewed in reference 201). Since
many of these enzymes required for DNA synthesis are inactive in nondividing cells (reviewed in reference 195), the ability of herpes viruses to
regulate deoxyribonucleotide production positively promotes their ability
to replicate within resting cells that are deficient in these enzymes. Thus, it
would seem appropriate to examine the fidelity of viral cDNA synthesis in
nondividing cells infected with lentiviral mutants that do not associate
with UDG.

Vpr and Cell Cycle Progression

By virtue of the Vpr protein, primate lentiviruses join a long list of other
viruses that influence cell cycle progression (for reviews, see references
120, 158, 171, 265). Continuous passage of viruses containing intact Vpr
alleles leads to the outgrowth of viruses containing mutations that trun-
cate the Vpr open-reading frame. This is a consequence of the accumulation of CD4[+] T cells in the G_2 stage of the cell cycle in the presence of Vpr
(104, 119, 194, 200). Cells harboring wild-type proviruses divide more
slowly than those harboring defective *vpr* genes and are selected against.
Cell cycle arrest activity of Vpr is conserved among primate lentiviruses
(189, 245). In addition, when expressed in fission yeast, Vpr induces G_2
arrest (292, 294), indicating a high degree of conversation in the pathway
through which Vpr mediates cycle arrest. Vpr-mediated cell cycle delay is
manifest in primary and transformed T-cell lines but not in terminally differentiated macrophages (95). The mechanism through which Vpr induces
cell cycle arrest is still undefined. It has been suggested that Vpr inhibits
the activation and phosphorylation state of CDC2 kinase, which controls
the entry of the cell into mitosis (104, 119, 194). Several groups have examined the fate of cells that, through the action of Vpr, accumulate in the G_2
phase of the cell cycle. For example, it has been demonstrated that cell
cycle arrest leads to the induction of apoptosis (244). Paradoxically, it has
been suggested that Vpr suppresses immune activation and apoptosis
through regulation of nuclear factor 5B (11). However, that study examined
the effects of exogenous recombinant Vpr on cell function. It has been suggested that the cell cycle block that is induced by Vpr is qualitatively similar to the DNA damage checkpoint control that is induced by, for example, DNA damaging agents (191). In contrast, it was suggested that the
effects of Vpr are cytostatic rather than cytotoxic and that the mitotic block

is mechanistically distinct from the DNA damage checkpoint control because it is independent of p53 (16).

Studies are beginning to reveal how manipulation of the cell cycle by Vpr would be advantageous to virus replication. The ultimate goal of the cell cycle delay activity of Vpr may be to extend the phase of the cell cycle in which the LTR is most active (86). Vpr increases HIV-1 LTR activity (1, 51, 249, 270). The enhancement of HIV-1 LTR transcription by Vpr may be due to increased levels of transcription factors in the G_2 phase that act on the LTR. The ability of Vpr to upregulate viral transcription is dependent on a functional TATA box and an enhancer (95). As the LTR is more active in the G_2 phase of the cell cycle, the rate of virus production in G_2 is increased accordingly (86). Over a single cycle of cell division, virus production from a wild-type provirus is twofold higher than that from a provirus containing an inactivated *vpr* gene (Fig. 9.8). At face value, this level of augmentation would appear to be modest; however, over multiple rounds of virus replication, the slight increase in replicative fitness conferred by Vpr would maintain selective pressure for those viruses that contain functional Vpr alleles. Consistent with this is the demonstration that coinfection of pigtailed macaques with wild-type and ΔVPR SIV variants results in prevalence of wild-type genomes (106). Although inactivation of Vpr in that study presumably affected both cell cycle arrest and UDG-associating activities of Vpr, the results argue for an important role of Vpr in viral fitness. The amount of Vpr that is packaged into virions is sufficient to induce cell cycle arrest without the requirement for de novo synthesis of Vpr (190). This has prompted the suggestion that cell-free virions, whether infectious or noninfectious, may have the ability to influence the cell cycle state of cells with which they come in contact. This could form the basis for a previously proposed contribution of Vpr to immune dysfunction (244). Since the effect of virion-associated Vpr on host cell function does not require that the virion be infectious, it would be insensitive to antiretroviral agents. Thus, in patients undergoing antiretroviral therapy, residual reservoirs of virus production could still affect immune function (190).

Vpr/Vpx Proteins and Nuclear Transport of Viral DNA

CD4$^+$ T lymphocytes and tissue macrophages are the predominant host cells for primate lentivirus replication. The infection of macrophage lineage cells by primate lentiviruses poses unique obstacles to the replication of the latter. In addition to problems in reverse transcription in low-dNTP environments that were discussed earlier, lentiviruses must overcome the nondividing nucleus as they translocate their viral cDNA from the point of virus entry to the nucleoplasm. In the retrovirus life cycle, viral cDNA synthesis occurs within a high molecular weight nucleoprotein complex

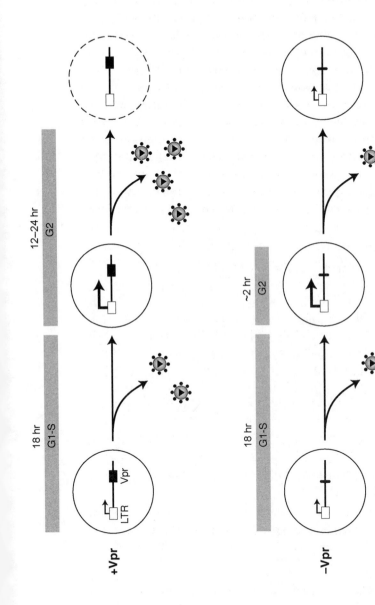

FIGURE 9.8

Consequences of HIV-1 Vpr-mediated cell cycle delay for virion output

In cells harboring a wild-type provirus, the action of Vpr extends the G_2 phase of the cell cycle—in which the LTR is transcriptionally more active and, consequently, in which virus production is more efficient—from approximately 2 hours to 12–20 hours. An extended period of G_2 ultimately results in death of the cell through Vpr-mediated apoptosis. In contrast, in cells harboring a ΔVPR provirus, the period of increased LTR activity and virus production is limited to approximately 2 hours. As a consequence, the average rate of virus production for each round of the cell cycle is increased in the presence of Vpr. (Adapted from reference 86, which contains a more complete discussion.)

(also referred to as a reverse transcription or preintegration complex). These large, ribosome-size (160S) nucleoprotein complexes (31, 38, 122) have a Stokes diameter of 30–50 nM. Since nuclear uptake is limited to proteins of less than around 60 kDa, lentiviruses must go to extraordinary measures in order to access the nucleus of a nondividing cell. In the case of onco-retroviruses, viral reverse transcription complexes are held in the cytoplasm until the host cell goes through mitosis, at which time the nuclear Env breaks down and viral DNA can access the nucleus (149, 199). However, in the case of HIV-1, viral reverse transcription complexes are able to access the nucleus of growth-arrested cells (38, 149). As a consequence, HIV-1-based lentivirus vectors have been used for transduction of various nondividing cells including muscle, macrophages, and neurons (24, 172). The ability of primate lentiviruses to access the nucleus has been attributed to nucleophilic viral proteins that associate with, and promote, nuclear uptake of the complex (37). The Vpr protein of HIV-1 and the Vpx protein of HIV-2/SIV$_{sm}$ have been implicated as such nucleophilic proteins. A number of independent lines of experimental evidence are consistent with this model:

- HIV-1 Vpr and SIV$_{sm}$ Vpx proteins associate with viral reverse transcription complexes in acutely infected cells (72, 101, 105).
- Inactivation of HIV-1 Vpr and SIV$_{sm}$ Vpx impairs virus replication in primary macrophages but not in activated T cells (15, 42, 56, 72, 83, 98, 105, 290). Although some studies have suggested that Vpr and Vpx mutants are impaired in primary lymphocytes (42, 98, 121), these effects appear to be donor dependent and manifest only in peripheral blood mononuclear cell (PBMC) cultures that inefficiently replicate virus.
- The defect in macrophage infection by HIV-1 Vpr and SIV$_{sm}$ Vpx mutants is at the level of nuclear targeting of viral cDNA (72, 105, 173, 192, 193, 250, 261).
- When expressed in cells, HIV-1 Vpr localizes to the nucleus (116, 287), the nuclear Env (261), or the nuclear pore complex (NPC) (73). Vpr contains a transferable NLS-like motif that functions in both somatic cells and xenopus oocytes (73).
- Vpr interacts with components of the cellular nuclear import apparatus. Vpr interacts with the NLS receptor, importin-α, in vitro (192, 193, 261). HIV-1 Vpr has further been shown to interact with POM121, a protein that localizes to the NPC (73).

The interaction of Vpr with the NLS receptor, importin-α, and with the nuclear pore protein, POM121, suggests two possible models for nuclear uptake of reverse transcription complexes by Vpr (Fig. 9.9). Macromolecules that access the nucleus by active transport interact, either directly or indirectly, with some component of the NPC. Thus, macromolecules larger than 50 kDa may cross the NPC either through specific interaction with the

NPC or by interacting with an intermediary carrier (receptor-mediated import). In the first model (Fig. 9.9A), Vpr, as a component of the preintegration complex, may interact directly with the NPC without requiring an intermediary carrier. Localization of Vpr to the nuclear rim and interaction with POM121 would be consistent with such a model. Interaction of Vpr with the NPC would promote docking of the reverse transcription complex at the NPC but may not be sufficient to promote transport of the reverse transcription complex to the nucleoplasm. Thus, the coordinated activity of other components of the reverse transcription complex such as Gag matrix or integrase (39, 78) may mediate subsequent nucleoplasmic localization. In an alternate model (Fig. 9.9B), Vpr interacts with an intermediary receptor that itself interacts with the components of the NPC. The best characterized of this type of receptor-mediated nuclear import involves recognition of an NLS by a component of the karyopherin-β/

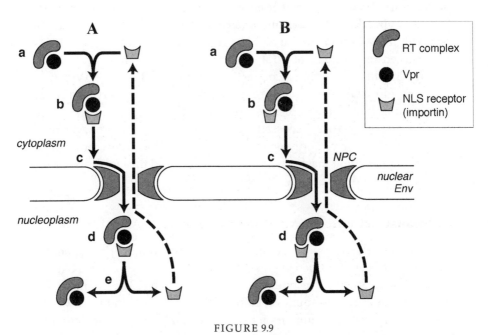

FIGURE 9.9

Models for Vpr-mediated nuclear translocation
of viral reverse transcription complexes

In model A, Vpr, as a component of the viral reverse transcription complex, interacts with the NLS receptor (importin) via the importin-α subunit to form an import-competent complex (b). The NLS receptor then mediates docking of the reverse transcription complex with the NPC (c). The reverse transcription complex is subsequently translocated to the nucleus (d) and dissociates from the NLS receptor (e). In model B, interaction with the NLS receptor is not mediated by Vpr but by other components within the reverse transcription complex such as integrase (78) or matrix (39). Following formation of the import-competent complex (b), Vpr mediates interaction of the complex with the NPC, for example, through the binding of Vpr to POM121 within the membrane of the NPC.

importin-β superfamily (for review, see reference 281). Upon binding the import substrate by importin-α via the NLS, subsequent interaction with importin-β promotes docking at the NPC. Evidence for such a model is the demonstration that Vpr interacts with importin-α and that Vpr localizes to the nucleoplasm (63, 220, 287). The interaction of Vpr with importin-α contributes to the ability of Vpr to support macrophage infection in that a Vpr F34I mutant that does not interact with importin-α does not localize to the nuclear Env and inefficiently infects primary macrophages (261). Vpr does not contain a classical NLS and appears to interact with importin-α at a site distinct from the classical NLS-binding site (192). Recent studies have suggested an NLS-independent mechanism for Vpr import (116). Vpr contains two discrete nuclear targeting signals that use two different import pathways, both of which are distinct from the classical NLS-mediated pathway (116). By directly engaging the NPC at two discrete sites, Vpr may bypass many of the soluble receptors that mediate nuclear import (116).

Vpx-mediated infection of nondividing macrophages appears to be essential for viral dissemination and replication in vivo (106). Inactivation of Vpx within the genome of the highly pathogenic variant SIV$_{sm}$ PBj leads to a marked impairment of viral dissemination, replication, and pathogenicity. In addition, within a coinfection setting, an SIV$_{sm}$ PBj ΔVpx mutant is rapidly overtaken by wild-type virus (106). One interpretation of these results is that macrophages are essential target cells for primate lentiviral replication. As discussed later in the chapter, macrophages may serve as centers for viral dissemination (252), and the ability of primate lentiviruses to exploit macrophages may be regulated through another accessory gene product, namely, the Nef protein.

Additional Activities of Vpr/Vpx Proteins

In addition to UDG, importin-α, and POM121, two other Vpr-interacting proteins have been identified in yeast two-hybrid screens. Lysine-tRNA synthetase, interacts with Vpr both in vitro and in vivo (239). Lysine-tRNA synthetase catalyzes the aminoacylation of tRNA^{Lys}, and binding of Vpr to lysine-tRNA synthetase impairs its ability to catalyze aminoacylation of tRNA^{Lys}. Since tRNA^{Lys} is a primer for initiation of HIV-1 reverse transcription, it has been suggested that this interaction may impair viral reverse transcription (239). Vpr also interacts in vitro and in vivo with the protein HHR23A, which is involved in nucleotide excision repair (280). Vpr and HHR23A co-localize to the nuclear membrane. Mutagenesis of a C-terminal 45-amino-acid domain in HHR23A that mediates interaction with Vpr results in partial alleviation of Vpr-mediated G$_2$ arrest (280). Since HHR23A participates in DNA repair, it has been suggested that the interaction of Vpr with HHR23A impairs the repair of damaged DNA. As a consequence, pathways that signal progression of the cell cycle into mitosis may not be transmitted, thereby arresting cells at the G_2 checkpoint. Extracellular Vpr has been implicated in the formation of ion channels in artificial lipid bilayers (187) and in neurons (186, 188). Although the physiological significance of this activity is unclear, it raises the possibility that the presence of soluble Vpr within, for example, the cerebrospinal fluid may effect some of the neuropathologies that have been observed in AIDS patients.

The Nef Protein

Nef is one of the earliest detectable gene products after transcriptional activation of the provirus (197). Nef exists as a homodimer in infected cells as a result of intermolecular disulfide bonds between highly conserved cysteine residues (130). The protein is myristylated and localized on the plasma membrane of the infected cell (174). Nef is phosphorylated, but no function has been attributed to this modification (97, 288). HIV-1 Nef contains proline residues (PXX) that have similarities to Src-homology 3 (SH3) binding motifs that mediate interaction with the SH3 domain of Src tyrosine kinases (222). These motifs are highly conserved across lentiviral lineages including HIV-1, HIV-2, and SIV. In addition, SIV *nef* genes contain an additional SH2 binding motif that mediates interaction with kinases through phosphotyrosine-containing sequences (236). Nef can be detected in virions, where it is proteolytically processed by the viral protease (36, 180, 210, 274). Proteolytic processing of Nef does not appear to be required for the effects of Nef on CD4 downregulation (179) or for the ability of Nef to enhance virion infectivity (47).

Nef inactivation leads to the impairment of viral replication in vivo to a level that is not readily apparent in in vitro systems. Nef mutants of SIV exhibit marked attenuation in terms of both replication and virulence (61, 127). Point mutations in Nef (e.g., premature stop codon) rapidly revert in vivo to restore viral virulence. Furthermore, infection of macaques with an SIV$_{mac}$ clone containing a deletion in Nef results in repair of the deletion in vivo and resumption of virulence (276). SIV variants lacking a functional *nef* gene induce disease in both infant and adult macaques (12, 14), suggesting that Nef greatly facilitates but is not essential for viral virulence. The characteristics of humans infected with variants containing defective *nef* alleles provide further evidence that Nef profoundly influences virus replication and pathogenicity. Individuals naturally infected with Nef mutant viruses exhibit a long-term nonprogressor phenotype (60, 134). HIV-1 variants containing inactive *nef* alleles are also markedly attenuated in the SCID-Hu thymus model of HIV-1 infection and pathogenicity (5, 6, 115). Indeed, the relative impact on viral pathogenicity in this model parallels the degree to which various accessory gene mutations impair SIV pathogenicity in macaques (6, 61). A comparison of Nef consensus sequences derived from long-term nonprogressors and individuals with progressive HIV-1 infection indicates the presence of amino acid variations in Nef that correlate with CD4+ T-cell count and the level of viremia (133). This further underscores a relationship between Nef function and the immune and virologic status of the infected individual. Intriguingly, HIV-1 Nef is able to substitute for SIV$_{mac}$ Nef in vivo in conferring pathogenic infection (7). The possibility that Nef harbors a determinant for primate lentiviral pathogenicity has been suggested from studies in transgenic animals. Mice transgenic for SIV Nef had an increased mortality rate following challenge with pathogenic herpes simplex virus type I and, in addition, exhibited an immunologic defect such as decreased proliferative responses to phytohemagglutinin (PHA) (142). In addition, mice transgenic for HIV-1 Nef exhibited AIDS-like pathologies including wasting, loss of CD4+ T cells, and premature death. Nef-expressing thymocytes were activated and exhibited hyperresponsiveness to CD3 stimulation (100). Given the role of Nef in virus replication and virulence, a number of research groups have focused their efforts on identification of properties of Nef that may explain how it promotes these activities.

Nef and Downregulation of CD4 and Major Histocompatibility Complex Class I (MHC-I)

The expression of Nef within cells promotes downregulation of two important immunoregulatory molecules, namely, CD4 (3, 9, 20, 32, 45, 80, 81, 93, 97, 112, 167, 184, 196, 205, 216) and MHC-I (55, 90, 148, 153, 163, 218). Genetically distinct subregions of Nef appear to mediate the downregulation of CD4 and MHC-I (Fig. 9.10). A dileucine sequence (LL[164, 165]) in Nef acts as an internalization signal for CD4 downregulation (33, 58, 90) but is dispensable for MHC-I downregulation (90, 148, 163). Conversely, MHC-I but not CD4 downregulation requires a proline-rich domain, the N-terminal α-helical domain, and a cluster of acidic amino acids at the N-terminus of Nef (90, 148, 163). CD4 downregulation involves interaction between the sequence WL[57, 58] in Nef and the tail of the CD4 receptor (94, 111). In addition, the cytoplasmic domain of CD4 is sufficient for its responsiveness to Nef-mediated downregulation (10). A diacidic (EE[155, 156]) motif at positions 155 and 156 of HIV-1 Nef acts as a lysosomal sorting signal during CD4 downregulation (185). SIV Nef appears to utilize both leucine- and tyrosine-based protein sorting pathways for downregulation of CD4 (153).

The downregulation of CD4 and MHC-I is mediated through a combination of accelerated endocytosis and, additionally, in the case of CD4, targeting from the Golgi apparatus to the endocytic pathway (3, 163, 196, 218) (Figs. 9.11, 9.12). Endocytosis of these proteins is mediated through interaction of signals in the cytoplasmic tail of CD4 and MHC-I with clathrin-coated pits. The assembly of these pits at the plasma membrane and on the

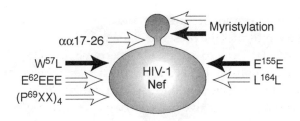

FIGURE 9.10

Domains in Nef that mediate downregulation of CD4 and MHC-I

Regions of Nef that, when mutated, influence cell surface expression of CD4 (solid arrowheads) or MHC-I (open arrowheads) are indicated. (Adapted from reference 185.)

Golgi apparatus involves an interaction between cytosolic clathrin and adapter complexes (see reference 198). Both HIV-1 and SIV Nef are able to form complexes with the clathrin adapters AP-1 and AP-2 (33, 58, 90). These adapters interact with tyrosine-based (Y-X-X-hydrophobic amino acid) and leucine-based (L-X, where X may be L, I, M, V, or F) motifs in the cytoplasmic domain of Nef. Although SIV Nef utilizes two tyrosine-based motifs at the N-terminus (153, 184), HIV-1 Nef lacks these tyrosine-based motifs but uses a highly conserved leucine-based motif near the C-terminus, and mutation in this motif leads to a loss of CD4 downregulation and interaction with clathrin adapters (33, 58, 90). SIV Nef has recently been reported to contain a leucine-based motif that acts in a redundant manner with the previously reported tyrosine-based signal to downregulate CD4 (34).

Two distinct consequences have been hypothesized to occur as a result of CD4 and MHC-I downregulation. As discussed previously for the Vpu protein, downregulation of CD4 may lead to the establishment of superinfection resistance and prevent incorporation of CD4 into virions so as to prevent masking of receptor binding sites on virion Env glycoproteins by virion-associated CD4. MHC-I downregulation likely confers protection from immune surveillance (Fig. 9.13). Surface MHC-I molecules are responsible for presenting peptides after their synthesis in the cell to cytotoxic T lymphocytes (CTLs). This mechanism forms the chief component of the acquired antiviral immune response and allows for the destruction of cells that express foreign antigens. Downregulation of cell surface MHC-I expression by Nef protects infected cells from killing by cytotoxic T cells (55) (for review, see reference 54). Nef appears to downmodulate HLA-A2 antigens selectively and does not modulate, for example, HLA-C or HLA-E antigens. Any delay in lysis of an infected cell by CTL could prolong virion production time, thus enhancing virus replication (Fig. 9.13). The degree of immune escape afforded by Nef in vivo is at present unknown. For example, Borrow and colleagues (27) analyzed a patient who exhibited

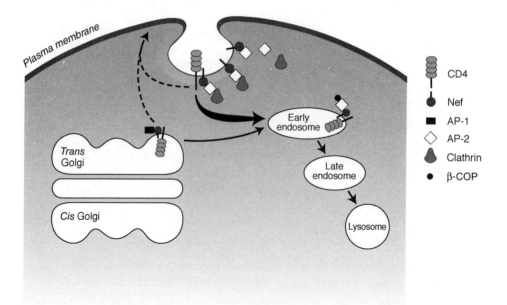

FIGURE 9.11

Mechanism of Nef-mediated CD4 downregulation

The major pathway for downregulation of cell surface CD4 by Nef involves direction of CD4 to the endosomal apparatus by Nef. In this process, Nef mediates the attachment of CD4 to AP-2 and to clathrin. This results in a rapid acceleration of CD4 endocytosis. In early endosomes, Nef interacts with β-COP. As a result, internalized complexes are directed from early endosomes to late endosomes and, ultimately, to the lysosome for degradation. Nef directs a minor population of CD4 molecules from the Golgi to the endosomal apparatus following interaction with AP-1.

a high frequency of precursor CTLs that were directed to a specific HIV-1 Env epitope. Presumably, as a consequence of pressure from CTL killing, there was a rapid and complete replacement of the CTL-sensitive virus population with a CTL-resistant virus pool, and the rate with which the CTL-sensitive virus pool was replaced paralleled that observed when a drug-sensitive virus population is replaced by a drug-resistant virus pool during antiretroviral drug therapy (107, 271). Furthermore, long-term nonprogressors infected with HIV-1 variants lacking a functional *nef* gene maintain low but sustained levels of virus replication (60, 134). The absence of a *nef* gene would predict that this low degree of virus replication would be better controlled by CTLs if indeed HIV-1 Nef is affording some protection from CTL surveillance. The answer to the question as to whether HIV-1 Nef through MHC-I downregulation protects infected cells from immune surveillance will be better appreciated when the phenotype of SIV-1 variants containing *nef* alleles incapable of downregulating MHC-I is examined in vivo. Depletion of CD8+ T cells from SIV-infected macaques

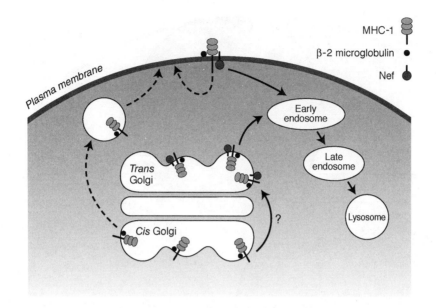

FIGURE 9.12

Mechanism of Nef-mediated MHC downregulation

MHC-I, which covalently associates with β-2 microglobulin, is assembled in the ER/*cis*-Golgi apparatus. Normally, this complex is shuttled to the cell surface. In the presence of Nef, MHC-I is retained within the *trans* Golgi and additionally may be shuttled to the endosomal pathway and degraded. In addition, interaction of Nef with MHC-I on the cell surface may expose a cryptic endocytosis motif in MHC-I, thus increasing the rate of MHC-I internalization and degradation in lysosomes.

using an anti-CD8 monoclonal antibody results in an increase of plasma viremia of 1 to 3 logs (117). It appears, then, that CD8+ T cells effectively suppress SIV replication in vivo. Thus, it will be important to determine whether the replication of SIV variants incapable of downregulating MHC-I is affected to the same degree as wild-type virus following ablation of CD8+ T cells.

Nef and Virion Infectivity Enhancement

Nef has been shown to enhance virus infectivity under two circumstances. Nef increases infectivity of virions for HeLa cells expressing CD4 (4, 217). In the absence of Nef, reverse transcription of viral cDNA in the target cell is impaired, suggesting that Nef may act in producer cells to facilitate the production of fully infectious virions (4, 217). When HIV-1 ΔNef viruses are pseudotyped with Env glycoprotein of vesicular stomatitis virus, full infectivity is restored (2). Thus, the endocytic pathway either circumvents the stage of the HIV-1 life cycle that is affected by Nef or, alternatively, restores

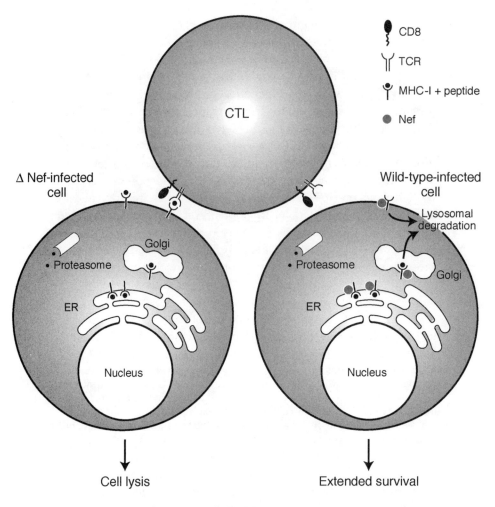

FIGURE 9.13

Consequences of Nef-mediated MHC-I downregulation and CTL recognition

Viral antigens are processed within the proteasome. Trimolecular complexes between MHC-I, β-microglobulin, and viral peptide are formed in the ER/Golgi. Through the TCR and CD8 receptor, CTLs recognize these foreign peptide antigens in the groove of MHC-I. In wild-type-infected cells, Nef interacts with MHC-I/peptide complexes and either retains them in the Golgi or targets them for lysosomal degradation. In addition, MHC-I complexes on the plasma membrane are rapidly internalized after binding the Nef protein. As a consequence, CTL may inefficiently recognize wild-type HIV-1-infected cells, which may influence infected cell turnover. Alternatively, the release of soluble substances from CTLs that inhibit HIV-1 infection may be impaired as a result of Nef-mediated MHC-I downregulation (177, 267, 269, 285).

a function that is otherwise impaired in ΔNef viruses during fusion-mediated entry. Nef also promotes virion infectivity in more physiologically relevant primary CD4+ T cells (48, 169, 202, 232, 238). As in HeLa CD4+ cells, enhancement of viral infectivity for T cells is at the level of virus entry. Whether the infectivity enhancement effect of Nef is dependent on the activation state of the T cell is still unclear. In resting cells, HIV-1 infection results in a nonproductive infection characterized by a labile intracellular replication intermediate (242, 291). Virus replication can be restored upon activation of the cell. When cells are infected in the quiescent state and activated at various intervals after infection, the efficiency of virus recovery from the cell drops precipitously as the interval between infection and subsequent activation is extended. Inactivation of Nef shortens the interval between the time when resting cells are infected and the time when virus can be recovered after cell activation (169, 238). These studies suggest that Nef influences the stability of the replication intermediate that is formed in resting cells. Treatment of resting cells with certain combinations of cytokines can confer permissiveness to productive HIV-1 infection without apparent full-blown activation (260). The manifestation of a replication defect in the absence of Nef appears to depend on the nature of the T-cell activating stimulus. For example, when primary CD4+ T cells are activated with anti-CD3 in the presence of interleukin-2 (IL-2), replication of the ΔNef virus is markedly impaired relative to the wild-type variant (125). The increased growth rate of the wild-type virus reflects increases in the level of viral DNA synthesis in the target cell and depends on an intact acidic amino-acid-rich domain from amino acids 69–75. This region of Nef also forms part of the SH3 binding domain; however, the infectivity enhancement does not appear to require SH3 binding, since proline residues in this acidic region are dispensable for the Nef effect (125). Inactivation of Nef can further impair virus replication in both activated T cells and macrophages when cells are infected at low multiplication of infection (MOI) (48, 202, 232). In contrast, inactivation of Nef does not affect SIV or HIV replication in primary PBMC or in macrophages at high MOI (61, 252).

Nef Association with Cellular Kinases

The presence of highly conserved SH3 recognition motifs in HIV-1 Nef and SH2 and SH3 recognition motifs in SIV Nef has prompted the suggestion that Nef proteins of primate lentiviruses influence signaling pathways in the cell. Nef interacts with and activates protein tyrosine kinases in vitro (17, 23, 35, 53, 124, 145, 146, 164, 170, 204) and in vivo (35, 170). The best characterized of these interactions involves the interaction of HIV-1 Nef with the myeloid-specific tyrosine kinase Hck (35, 94, 145, 170, 204) (for review, see reference 181). The proline repeat motif in HIV-1 Nef is necessary and sufficient for full activation of Hck (35, 170). Hck is one of the earliest kinases expressed after monocyte activation (295). Knockout mice with simultaneous deletions in Hck and Src exhibit developmental defects and impaired immunity (154). The biological significance of Nef-Hck interaction is unclear. Macrophage lineage cells may be important for viral dissemination and replication (106, 252). However, there is no direct evidence that Hck is activated upon HIV-1 infection of primary macrophages. Despite these uncertainties, the extremely high affinity of Nef for Hck (kDa of 0.25 µM) (146, 204) supports the notion that this interaction may be functionally significant. Nef interacts with the protein tyrosine kinase Lck (17, 53, 67, 92). A prediction of the interaction is that Nef may influence the activation state of the T cell by modulating the activity of Lck. When Nef is localized to the cytoplasm, T-cell receptor (TCR)–mediated induction of tyrosine phosphorylation and calcium mobilization is inhibited. However, when Nef is localized to membranes, T cells are in an activated state (17, 18).

Although SH2 and SH3 motifs of primate lentiviral Nefs are well conserved, the degree to which they are required for Nef-mediated pathogenicity is unknown. As discussed earlier, Nef is necessary for viral replication and pathogenicity in the SCID-Hu mouse model (5, 6, 115). In the case of HIV-1 Nef, there is a central proline repeat motif (PXXP4) and a C-terminal proline repeat motif (PXXP2). Inactivation of either of these motifs does not significantly affect virus replication and pathogenicity, but inactivation of both motifs impairs replication and pathogenicity to the same extent as inactivation of the myristylation signal (5). Mutagenesis of the proline repeat motif in SIV Nef (SIV_{mac} 239-$P^{104}A$/$P^{107}A$) impairs association of Nef with a Nef-associated serine/threonine kinase in vitro (207). In macaques infected with such an SIV_{mac} Nef proline mutant, there is rapid reversion to a wild-type genotype and the renewed induction of high virus loads and AIDS (129, 208). In a separate study, infection of macaques with a SIV variant containing a proline repeat mutant of Nef resulted in induction of AIDS without reversions in the Nef mutant sequences (141). Therefore, there is as yet no clear consensus on the impact of the proline repeat motif on Nef-mediated viral replication and pathogenicity. Furthermore, this motif is expected to mediate interaction of Nef with various protein tyrosine kinases and serine/threonine kinases, and, as such, it may be difficult to ascribe inactivation of this motif to loss of a specific activity of Nef. The recent availability of pathogenic SHIV variants together with a demonstration that SIV Nef and HIV Nef are functionally interchangeable (232) will provide a useful system to examine the contribution of SH3 recognition motifs to Nef function in vivo.

A number of studies have demonstrated interaction of primate lentiviral Nef proteins with cellular serine/threonine kinases (17, 25, 69, 92, 155, 159, 164, 175, 206, 208, 234, 279). The best characterized of these interactions involves a binding of HIV-1 Nef to a kinase that is related to p21-activated kinase (PAK) (155, 175, 208). Interaction of Nef with this serine/

threonine kinase (also known as Nef-associated kinase, or NAK) requires the core domain of Nef, which contains the proline repeat motif and a di-arginine motif (RR) (164, 207, 279). Recent studies indicate that interaction of Nef with the guanine nucleotide exchange factor Vav and NAK cooperates to induce cytoskeletal rearrangements that lead to activation of the JNK/SAPK cascade. This, in turn, leads to increased transcription from the HIV-1 LTR and increased HIV production (69) (Fig. 9.14). Thus, the interaction between Nef and Vav may explain how Nef promotes increased levels of viral transcription and replication, both in vitro and in vivo (129, 204). The interaction between Nef and Vav also demonstrates that alteration of signaling cascades by Nef may affect the infected cell in both structural and physiologic terms. Recently, it has been suggested that the process of HIV-1 infection may induce transcription factors such as the nuclear factor of activated T cells (NFAT) and, further, that the expression of NFAT in nonactivated T cells promotes their susceptibility to productive infection (132). However, it is unclear whether the activation of NFAT is influenced by Nef.

Nef and Lymphocyte Activation

Perhaps one of the most intriguing yet poorly understood activities of Nef is its involvement in lymphocyte activation. As discussed earlier, resting (G_0) T lymphocytes do not support productive HIV-1 infection, whereas, at least in vitro, T cells from the G_{1b} cell cycle stage onward appear to support efficient HIV-1 infection (138, 139, 242, 291). Although the interaction of Nef with cellular protein tyrosine kinases and serine/threonine kinases may provide the basis for the modulation of host cell activation pathways, there is little clear evidence that HIV directly influences lymphocyte activation status through the Nef protein. Through its ability to augment lymphocyte activation, Nef would be predicted to promote a productive infection in resting lymphocytes; however, at least in vitro, this is not the case (138, 242, 291). In addition, the possibility that Nef, through its influence on lymphocyte activation, could increase permissiveness of resting T cells to productive infection raises a paradox. Since resting T cells are not capable of supporting a productive HIV-1 infection, they are unable to express Nef de novo unless activated prior to infection. In addition, there is no evidence that virion-associated Nef is functional in this regard. Nef production in suboptimally activated T cells may directly increase the activation state and promote viral gene expression. Consistent with this model is the demonstration that *nef* genes of SIV and HIV stimulate the production of IL-2 in an IL-2-dependent rhesus T-cell line (8). Further evidence that Nef influences the activation state of the T cell comes from the demonstration that mice transgenic for Nef exhibit perturbations in T-cell signaling (233). Nef is important for HIV-1 replication in human tonsillar histocultures ex

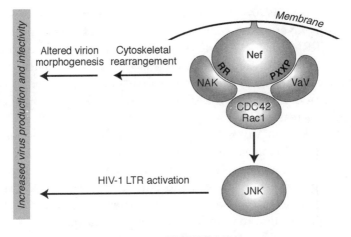

FIGURE 9.14

Possible consequences of Nef interaction with Vav and NAK

Nef, which is localized to the cell membrane by virtue of its N-terminal myristic acid, interacts via its PXXP motif with the SH3 domain of Vav. Subsequent activation of guanine nucleotide exchange factor activity leads to activation of CDC42-GTP and RAC1-GTP proteins. These small GTPases in turn activate the Nef-associated serine/threonine kinase, NAK, which interacts with Nef via the double arginine motif. Activation of NAK activity triggers a series of events that ultimately results in rearrangement of the cytoskeleton and activation of the JNK/SAPK kinase cascade. Cytoskeletal rearrangement may influence the process of HIV-1 assembly and morphogenesis, thereby rendering virions more infectious. Concomitantly, increased HIV-1 LTR transcription following activation of JNK/SAPK may augment production of virion components. (Adapted from reference 69, which contains a fuller description.)

vivo (85). Intriguingly, the replication of wild-type HIV-1 in human tonsillar histocultures is augmented by the addition of exogenous IL-2, whereas the ΔNef variant is only marginally affected by IL-2 addition. These studies suggest that Nef may increase HIV replication by augmenting the responsiveness of T cells to IL-2 stimulation. Expression of Nef within primary T cells increases their activation status, as evidenced by increased IL-2 generation following CD3/CD28 costimulation (211). This is due to an increase in the number of cells that become fully activated rather than augmentation of IL-2 production, suggesting that Nef lowers the threshold of stimulation through the dual-receptor T-cell activation pathway (Fig. 9.15). Collectively, these studies are beginning to shed some light on how the presence of Nef could augment the permissiveness of the host to productive infection.

nef genes of SIV and HIV-2 but not of HIV-1 interact in vitro and in vivo with the zeta chain of the TCR (19, 109). The binding site maps to the central core domain of Nef (amino acids 98–235) (109). Active tyrosine kinase can be co-precipitated with Nef-TCR zeta chain complexes from cells containing but not from cells lacking functional Lck. The interaction of Nef

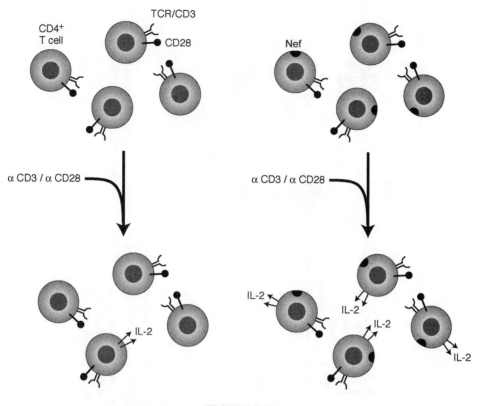

FIGURE 9.15

The effect of Nef on the threshold of dual-receptor-mediated T-cell activation

Stimulation of resting CD4+ T lymphocytes through the TCR/CD3 complex and the CD28 coreceptor (by CD3 and CD28 antibodies) results in full activation in a fraction of these cells as evidenced by IL-2 production. When cells express Nef, CD3/CD28 costimulation leads to an increase in the percentage of cells that reach full activation. This increase in activation, which is dependent on Nef myristylation, does not affect the amount of IL-2 secreted per cell (211). Consistent with this model, HIV-1 infection of human peripheral blood lymphocytes renders them hypersensitive to T-cell receptor and CD28 stimulation (178).

with the zeta chain of the TCR promotes its downmodulation from the surface of the T cell. The TCR zeta chain promotes transport of assembled TCR complexes to the cell surface (251). In addition, the TCR zeta chain contains three immunoreceptor tyrosine-based activation motifs (ITAMs). Following ligation by MHC and antigenic peptide or through CD3 cross-linking, the sequential phosphorylation of tyrosines in these ITAMs is a central step in the initiation of lymphocyte activation (126). Thus, the downmodulation of the TCR zeta chain in the presence of Nef raises the possibility that Nef impairs the response of the cell to activating stimuli received through the TCR/CD3 complex. It is unclear whether the TCR is downmodulated in

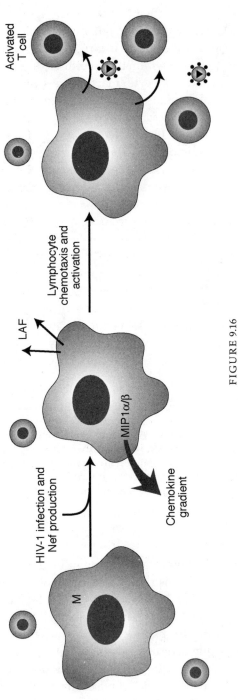

FIGURE 9.16

Nef induces macrophages to release agents that promote lymphocyte migration and activation

In HIV-1-infected macrophages, Nef stimulates the release of the chemokines MIP-1α and MIP-1β. Stimulation of chemokine production leads to the formation of a chemokine gradient for the chemotaxis of both resting and activated T cells. Nef further stimulates the production of an as yet unidentified lymphocyte activating factor (LAF), which promotes the activation of neighboring T cells. As a consequence, virions released from the infected cell encounter permissive (activated) T lymphocytes. This may enhance virus dissemination between cells. (For an expanded discussion, see references 59 and 252.)

SIV-infected cells or whether these cells exhibit impaired responses to activating stimuli.

There is accumulating evidence that Nef influences lymphocyte activation state indirectly. The *nef* gene of the highly cytopathic and acutely pathogenic SIV isolate PBj 14 confers on this virus the ability to grow in resting PBMC cultures. Replication within these cultures, which are a mixture of resting lymphocytes and monocyte/macrophages, requires macrophages because their removal prevents resting cell infection (66). Infection of macrophages by HIV-1 leads to elevated production of the chemokines, macrophage inflammatory protein-1α and -1β (43, 209). Expression of Nef within primary macrophages is sufficient for chemokine induction (252). HIV-1-infected macrophages or macrophages expressing Nef protein are chemotactic for T cells (252). Furthermore, Nef induces the release of an as yet unidentified factor that is able to promote the activation of resting T cells, thus rendering them permissive to productive HIV-1 infection (252). These studies suggest a model in which Nef acts to promote recruitment of lymphocytes to sites of virus replication and activation of T lymphocytes at those sites, thereby augmenting viral replication and dissemination (Fig. 9.16). This activity of Nef appears to be independent of highly conserved SH3 recognition motifs within Nef (252). Validation of this model will require the identification of an effector domain in Nef that controls the release of T-cell activating agents by macrophages and the demonstration that SIV variants lacking such an activity are impaired in a pathogenic model of SIV infection.

REFERENCES

1. Agostini, I., J. M. Navarro, F. Rey, M. Bouhamdan, B. Spire, R. Vigne, and J. Sire. 1996. The human immunodeficiency virus type 1 Vpr transactivator: cooperation with promoter-bound activator domains and binding to TFIIB. J. Mol. Biol. 261:599–606.

2. Aiken, C. 1997. Pseudotyping human immunodeficiency virus type 1 (HIV-1) by the glycoprotein of vesicular stomatitis virus targets HIV-1 entry to an endocytic pathway and suppresses both the requirement for Nef and the sensitivity to cyclosporin A. J. Virol. 71:5871–5877.

3. Aiken, C., J. Konner, N. R. Landau, M. E. Lenburg, and D. Trono. 1994. Nef induces CD4 endocytosis: requirement for a critical dileucine motif in the membrane-proximal CD4 cytoplasmic domain. Cell 76:853–864.

4. Aiken, C., and D. Trono. 1995. Nef stimulates human immunodeficiency virus type 1 proviral DNA synthesis. J. Virol. 69:5048–5056.

5. Aldrovandi, G. M., L. Gao, G. Bristol, and J. A. Zack. 1998. Regions of human immunodeficiency virus type 1 nef required for function in vivo. J. Virol. 72:7032–7039.

6. Aldrovandi, G. M., and J. A. Zack. 1996. Replication and pathogenicity of human immunodeficiency virus type 1 accessory gene mutants in SCID-hu mice. J. Virol. 70:1505–1511.

7. Alexander, L., Z. Du, A. Y. M. Howe, S. Czajak, and R. C. Desrosiers. 1999. Induction of AIDS in rhesus monkeys by a recombinant simian immunodeficiency virus expressing Nef of human immunodeficiency virus type 1. J. Virol. 73:5814–5825.

8. Alexander, L., Z. Du, M. Rosenweig, J. U. Jung, and R. C. Desrosiers. 1997. A role for natural simian immunodeficiency virus and human immunodeficiency virus type 1 nef alleles in lymphocyte activation. J. Virol. 71: 6094–6099.

9. Anderson, S., D. C. Shugars, R. Swanstrom, and J. V. Garcia. 1993. Nef from primary isolates of human immunodeficiency virus type 1 suppresses surface CD4 expression in human and mouse T cells. J. Virol. 67:4923–4931.

10. Anderson, S. J., M. Lenburg, N. R. Landau, and J. V. Garcia. 1994. The cytoplasmic domain of CD4 is sufficient for its down-regulation from the cell surface by human immunodeficiency virus type 1 nef. J. Virol. 68:3092–3101.

11. Ayyavoo, V., A. Mahboubi, S. Mahalingam, R. Ramalingam, S. Kudchodkar, W. V. Williams, D. R. Green, and D. B. Weiner. 1997. HIV-1 Vpr suppresses immune activation and apoptosis through regulation of nuclear factor kappa B. Nature Med. 3:1117–1123.

12. Baba, M., O. Nishimura, N. Kanzaki, M. Okamoto, H. Sawada, Y. Iizawa, M. Shiraishi, Y. Aramaki, K. Okonogi, Y. Ogawa, K. Meguro, and M. Fujino. 1999. A small-molecule, nonpeptide CCR5 antagonist with highly potent and selective anti-HIV-1 activity. Proc. Natl. Acad. Sci. USA 96:5698–5703.

13. Baba, T. W., Y. S. Jeong, D. Penninck, R. Bronson, M. F. Greene, and R. M. Ruprecht. 1995. Pathogenicity of live, attenuated SIV after mucosal infection of neonatal macaques. Science 267:1820–1825.

14. Baba, T. W., V. Liska, A. H. Khimani, N. B. Ray, P. J. Dailey, D. Penninck, R. Bronson, M. F. Greene, H. M. McClure, L. N. Martin, and R. M. Ruprecht. 1999. Live attenuated, multiply deleted simian immunodeficiency virus causes AIDS in infant and adult macaques. Nature Med. 5:194–203.

15. Bailliet, J. W., D. L. Kolson, G. Eiger, F. M. Kim, K. A. McGann, A. Srinivasan, and R. Collman. 1994. Distinct effects in primary macrophages and lymphocytes of the human immunodeficiency virus type I accessory genes *vpr*, *vpu* and *nef*: mutational analysis of a primary HIV-1 isolate. Virology 200: 623–631.

16. Bartz, S. R., M. E. Rogel, and M. Emerman. 1996. Human immunodeficiency virus type 1 cell cycle control: Vpr is cytostatic and mediates G_2 accumulation by a mechanism which differs from DNA damage checkpoint control. J. Virol. 70:2324–2331.

17. Baur, A. S., G. Sass, B. Laffert, D. Willbold, C. Cheng-Mayer, and B. M. Peterlin. 1997. The N-terminus of Nef from HIV-1/SIV associates with a protein complex containing Lck and a serine kinase. Immunity 6:283–291.

18. Baur, A. S., E. T. Sawai, P. Dazin, W. J. Fanti, C. Cheng-Mayer, and B. M. Peterlin. 1994. HIV-1 Nef leads to inhibition or activation of T cells depending on its intracellular localization. Immunity 1:373–384.

19. Bell, I., C. Ashman, J. Maughan, E. Hooker, F. Cook, and T. A. Reinhart. 1998. Association of simian immunodeficiency virus Nef with the T-cell receptor (TCR) zeta chain leads to TCR down-modulation. J. Gen. Virol. 79:2717–2727.

20. Benson, R. E., A. Sanfridson, J. S. Ottinger, C. Doyle, and B. R. Cullen. 1993. Downregulation of cell-surface CD4 expression by simian immunodeficiency virus nef prevents viral super infection. J. Exp. Med. 177:1561–1566.

21. Bergman, A. C., O. Björnberg, J. Nord, P. O. Nyman, and A. M. Rosengren. 1994. The protein p30, encoded at the *gag-pro* junction of mouse mammary tumor virus, is a dUTPase fused with a nucleocapsid protein. Virology 204:420–424.

22. Bess, J. W., R. J. Gorelick, W. J. Bosche, L. E. Henderson, and L. O. Arthur. 1997. Microvesicles are a source of contaminating cellular proteins found in purified HIV-1 preparations. Virology 230:134–144.

23. Biggs, T. E., S. J. Cooke, C. H. Barton, M. P. Harris, K. Saksela, and D. A. Mann. 1999. Induction of activator protein 1 (AP-1) in macrophages by human immunodeficiency virus type-1 NEF is a cell-type-specific response that requires both Hck and MAPK signaling events. J. Mol. Biol. 290:21–35.

24. Blomer, U., L. Naldini, T. Kafri, D. Trono, I. M. Verma, and F. H. Gage. 1997. Highly efficient and sustained gene transfer in adult neurons with a lentivirus vector. J. Virol. 71:6641–6649.

25. Bodéus, M., A. Marie-Cardine, C. Bougeret, F. Ramos-Morales, and R. Benarous. 1995. *In vitro* binding and phosphorylation of human immunodeficiency virus type 1 Nef protein by serine/threonine protein kinase. J. Gen. Virol. 76:1337–1344.

26. Borman, A. M., C. Quillent, P. Charneau, C. Dauguet, and F. Clavel. 1995. Human immunodeficiency virus type 1 Vif⁻ mutant particles from restrictive cells: role of Vif in correct particle assembly and infectivity. J. Virol. 69:2058–2067.

27. Borrow, P., H. Lewicki, X. Wei, M. S. Horwitz, N. Peffer, H. Meyers, J. A. Nelson, J. E. Gairin, B. H. Hahn, M. B. Oldstone, and G. M. Shaw. 1997. Antiviral pressure exerted by HIV-1-specific cytotoxic T lymphocytes (CTLs) during primary infection demonstrated by rapid selection of CTL escape virus. Nature Med. 3:205–211.

28. Bouhamdan, M., S. Benichou, F. Rey, J. M. Navarro, I. Agostini, B. Spire, J. Camonis, G. Slupphaug, R. Vigne, R. Benarous, and J. Sire. 1996. Human immunodeficiency virus type 1 Vpr protein binds to the uracil DNA glycosylase DNA repair enzyme. J. Virol. 70:697–704.

29. Bour, S., U. Schubert, K. Peden, and K. Strebel. 1996. The envelope glycoprotein of human immunodeficiency virus type 2 enhances viral particle release: a Vpu-like factor? J. Virol. 70:820–829.

30. Bouyac, M., M. Courcoul, G. Bertoia, Y. Baudat, D. Gabuzda, D. Blanc, N. Chazal, P. Boulanger, J. Sire, R. Vigne, and B. Spire. 1997. Human immunodeficiency virus type 1 Vif protein binds to the Pr55Gag precursor. J. Virol. 71:9358–9365.

31. Bowerman, B., P. O. Brown, J. M. Bishop, and H. E. Varmus. 1989. A nucleoprotein complex mediates the integration of retroviral DNA. Genes Dev. 3:469–478.

32. Brady, H. J. M., D. J. Pennington, C. G. Miles, and E. A. Dzierzak. 1993. CD4 cell surface downregulation in HIV-1 Nef transgenic mice is a consequence of intracellular sequestration. EMBO J. 12:4923–4932.

33. Bresnahan, P. A., W. Yonemoto, S. Ferrell, D. Williams-Herman, R. Geleziu-nas, and W. C. Greene. 1998. A dileucine motif in HIV-1 Nef acts as an internalization signal for CD4 downregulation and binds the AP-1 clathrin adaptor. Curr. Biol. 8:1235–1238.

34. Bresnahan, P. A., W. Yonemoto, and W. C. Greene. 1999. Cutting edge: SIV nef protein utilizes both leucine- and tyrosine-based protein sorting pathways for down-regulation of CD4. J. Immunol. 163:2977–2981.

35. Briggs, S. D., M. Sharkey, M. Stevenson, and T. E. Smithgall. 1997. SH3-mediated Hck tyrosine kinase activation and fibroblast transformation by the Nef protein of HIV-1. J. Biol. Chem. 272:17899–17902.

36. Bukovsky, A. A., T. Dorfman, A. Weimann, and H. G. Göttlinger. 1997. Nef association with human immunodeficiency virus type 1 virions and cleavage by the viral protease. J. Virol. 71:1013–1018.

37. Bukrinsky, M., S. Haggerty, M. P. Dempsey, N. Sharova, A. Adzhubei, L. Spitz, P. Lewis, D. Goldfarb, M. Emerman, and M. Stevenson. 1993. A nuclear localization signal within HIV-1 matrix protein that governs infection of nondividing cells. Nature 365:666–669.

38. Bukrinsky, M. I., N. Sharova, M. P. Dempsey, T. L. Stanwick, A. G. Bukrin-skaya, S. Haggerty, and M. Stevenson. 1992. Active nuclear import of human immunodeficiency virus type 1 preintegration complexes. Proc. Natl. Acad. Sci. USA 89:6580–6584.

39. Bukrinsky, M. I., N. Sharova, T. L. McDonald, T. Pushkarskaya, W. G. Tarpley, and M. Stevenson. 1993. Association of integrase, matrix, and reverse transcriptase antigens of human immunodeficiency virus type 1 with viral nucleic acids following acute infection. Proc. Natl. Acad. Sci. USA 90: 6125–6129.

40. Callahan, M. A., M. A. Handley, Y. H. Lee, K. J. Talbot, J. W. Harper, and A. T. Panganiban. 1998. Functional interaction of human immunodeficiency virus type 1 Vpu and Gag with a novel member of the tetratricopeptide repeat protein family. J. Virol. 72:5189–5197.

41. Camaur, D., and D. Trono. 1996. Characterization of human immunodeficiency virus type 1 Vif particle incorporation. J. Virol. 70:6106–6111.

42. Campbell, B. J., and V. M. Hirsch. 1997. Vpr of simian immunodeficiency virus of African green monkeys is required for replication in macaque macrophages and lymphocytes. J. Virol. 71:5593–5602.

43. Canque, B., M. Rosenzwajg, A. Gey, E. Tartour, W. H. Fridman, and J. C. Gluckman. 1996. Macrophage inflammatory protein-1alpha is induced by human immunodeficiency virus infection of monocyte-derived macrophages. Blood 87:2011–2019.

44. Chelsky, D., R. Ralph, and G. Jonak. 1989. Sequence requirements for synthetic peptide-mediated translocation to the nucleus. Mol. Cell. Biol. 9:2487–2492.

45. Chen, B. K., R. T. Gandhi, and D. Baltimore. 1996. CD4 down-modulation during infection of human T cells with human immunodeficiency virus type 1 involves independent activities of *vpu, env,* and *nef.* J. Virol. 70:6044–6053.

46. Chen, H.-H., and M. M. Fluck. 1993. Cell cycle control of polymomavirus-induced transformation. J. Virol. 67:1996–2005.

47. Chen, Y. L., D. Trono, and D. Camaur. 1998. The proteolytic cleavage of human immunodeficiency virus type 1 Nef does not correlate with its ability to stimulate virion infectivity. J. Virol. 72:3178–3184.

48. Chowers, M. Y., C. A. Spina, T. J. Kwoh, N. J. S. Fitch, D. D. Richman, and J. C. Guatelli. 1994. Optimal infectivity *in vitro* of human immunodeficiency virus type 1 requires an intact *nef* gene. J. Virol. 68:2906–2914.

49. Coffin, J. M. 1995. HIV population dynamics *in vivo*: implications for genetic variation, pathogenesis, and therapy. Science 267:483–489.

50. Coffin, J. M. 1995. Lines drawn in epitope wars. Nature 375:534–535.

51. Cohen, E. A., G. Dehni, J. G. Sodroski, and W. A. Haseltine. 1990. Human immunodeficiency virus *vpr* product is a virion-associated regulatory protein. J. Virol. 64:3097–3099.

52. Cohen, E. A., E. F. Terwilliger, J. G. Sodroski, and W. A. Haseltine. 1988. Identification of a protein encoded by the *vpu* gene of HIV-1. Nature 334: 532–534.

53. Collette, Y., H. Dutartre, A. Benziane, F. Ramos-Morales, R. Benarous, M. Harris, and D. Olive. 1996. Physical and functional interaction of Nef with Lck. J. Biol. Chem. 271:6333–6341.

54. Collins, K. L., and D. Baltimore. 1999. HIV's evasion of the cellular immune response. Immunol. Rev. 168:65–74.

55. Collins, K. L., B. K. Chen, S. A. Kalams, B. D. Walker, and D. Baltimore. 1998. HIV-1 Nef protein protects infected primary cells against killing by cytotoxic T lymphocytes. Nature 391:397–401.

56. Connor, R. I., B. K. Chen, S. Choe, and N. R. Landau. 1995. Vpr is required for efficient replication of human immunodeficiency virus type-1 in mononuclear phagocytes. Virology 206:935–944.

57. Courcoul, M., C. Patience, F. Rey, D. Blanc, A. Harmache, J. Sire, R. Vigne, and B. Spire. 1995. Peripheral blood mononuclear cells produce normal amounts of defective vif⁻ human immunodeficiency virus type 1 particles which are restricted for the preretrotranscription steps. J. Virol. 69:2068–2074.

58. Craig, H. M., M. W. Pandori, and J. C. Guatelli. 1998. Interaction of HIV-1 Nef with the cellular dileucine-based sorting pathway is required for CD4 down-regulation and optimal viral infectivity. Proc. Natl. Acad. Sci. USA 95:11229–11234.

59. Cullen, B. R. 1999. HIV-1 Nef protein: an invitation to a kill. Nature Med. 5:985–986.

60. Deacon, N. J., A. Tsykin, A. Solomon, K. Smith, M. Ludford-Menting, D. J. Hooker, D. A. McPhee, A. L. Greenway, A. Ellett, C. Chatfield, V. A. Lawson, S. Crowe, A. Maerz, S. Sonza, J. Learmont, J. S. Sullivan, A. Cunningham, D. Dwyer, D. Dowton, and J. Mills. 1995. Genomic structure of an attenuated quasi species of HIV-1 from a blood transfusion donor and recipients. Science 270:988–991.

61. Desrosiers, R. C., J. D. Lifson, J. S. Gibbs, S. C. Czajak, A. Y. Howe, L. O. Arthur, and R. P. Johnson. 1998. Identification of highly attenuated mutants of simian immunodeficiency virus. J. Virol. 72:1431–1437.

62. Dettenhofer, M., and X. F. Yu. 1999. Highly purified human immunodeficiency virus type 1 reveals a virtual absence of Vif in virions. J. Virol. 73:1460–1467.

63. Di Marzio, P., S. Choe, M. Ebright, R. Knoblauch, and N. R. Landau. 1995. Mutational analysis of cell cycle arrest, nuclear localization and virion packaging of human immunodeficiency virus type 1 Vpr. J. Virol. 69:7909–7916.

64. Dorner, A. J., and J. M. Coffin. 1986. Determinants for receptor interaction and cell killing on the Avian retrovirus glycoprotein gp85. Cell 45:365–374.

65. Douek, D. C., R. D. Macfarland, P. H. Keiser, E. A. Gage, J. M. Massey, B. F. Haynes, M. A. Polis, A. T. Haase, M. B. Feinberg, J. L. Sullivan, B. D. Jamieson, J. A. Zack, L. J. Picker, and R. A. Koup. 1998. Changes in thymic function with age and during the treatment of HIV infection. Nature 396:690–695.

66. Du, Z., S. M. Lang, V. G. Sasseville, A. A. Lackner, P. O. Ilynskii, M. D. Daniel, J. U. Jung, and R. C. Desrosiers. 1995. Identification of a *nef* allele that causes lymphocyte activation and acute disease in macaque monkeys. Cell 82: 655–674.

67. Dutartre, H., M. Harris, D. Olive, and Y. Collette. 1998. The human immunodeficiency virus type 1 Nef protein binds the Src-related tyrosine kinase Lck SH2 domain through a novel phosphotyrosine independent mechanism. Virology 247:200–211.

68. Elder, J. H., D. L. Lerner, C. S. Hasselkus-Light, D. J. Fontenot, E. Hunter, P. A. Luciw, R. C. Montelaro, and T. R. Phillips. 1992. Distinct subsets of retroviruses encode dUTPase. J. Virol. 66:1791–1794.

68a. Emerman, M., and M. H. Malim. 1998. HIV-1 regulatory/accessory genes: keys to unraveling viral and host cell biology. Science 280:1880–1884.

69. Fackler, O. T., W. Luo, M. Geyer, A. S. Alberts, and B. M. Peterlin. 1999. Activation of Vav by Nef induces cytoskeletal rearrangements and downstream effector functions. Mol. Cell 3:729–739.

70. Fan, N., J. Gavalchin, B. Paul, K. H. Wells, M. J. Lane, and B. J. Poiesz. 1992. Infection of peripheral blood mononuclear cells and cell lines by cell-free human T-cell lymphoma/leukemia virus type I. J. Clin. Microbiol. 30:905–910.

71. Fisher, A. G., B. Ensoli, L. Ivanoff, M. Chamberlain, S. Pettway, L. Ratner, R. C. Gallo, and F. Wong-Staal. 1987. The *sor* gene of HIV-1 is required for efficient virus transmission in vitro. Science 237:888–893.

72. Fletcher, T. M., B. Brichacek, N. Sharova, M. A. Newman, G. Stivahtis, P. M. Sharp, M. Emerman, B. H. Hahn, and M. Stevenson. 1996. Nuclear import and cell cycle arrest functions of the HIV-1 Vpr protein are encoded by two separate genes in HIV-2/SIV$_{SM}$. EMBO J. 15:6155–6165.

73. Fouchier, R. A., B. E. Meyer, J. H. Simon, U. Fischer, A. V. Albright, F. Gonzalez-Scarano, and M. H. Malim. 1998. Interaction of the human immunodeficiency virus type 1 Vpr protein with the nuclear pore complex. J. Virol. 72:6004–6013.

74. Fouchier, R. A. M., J. H. M. Simon, A. B. Jaffe, and M. H. Malim. 1996. Human immunodeficiency virus type 1 Vif does not influence expression or virion incorporation of *gag*-, *pol*-, and *env*-encoded proteins. J. Virol. 70:8263–8269.

75. Franke, E. K., H. E. H. Yuan, and J. Luban. 1994. Specific incorporation of cyclophilin A into HIV-1 virions. Nature 372:359–362.

76. Friborg, J., A. Ladha, H. G. Gottlinger, W. A. Haseltine, and E. A. Cohen. 1995. Functional analysis of the phosphorylation sites on the human immunodeficiency virus type 1 Vpu protein. AIDS Res. Hum. Retroviruses 8:10–22.

77. Gabuzda, D. H., K. Lawrence, E. Langhoff, E. Terwilliger, T. Dorfman, W. A. Haseltine, and J. Sodroski. 1992. Role of *vif* in replication of human immuno-deficiency virus type 1 in CD4[+] T lymphocytes. J. Virol. 66:6489–6495.

78. Gallay, P., T. Hope, D. Chin, and D. Trono. 1997. HIV-1 infection of nondividing cells through the recognition of integrase by the importin/karyopherin pathway. Proc. Natl. Acad. Sci. USA 94:9825–9830.

79. Gao, F., E. Bailes, D. L. Robertson, Y. Chen, C. M. Rodenburg, S. F. Michael, L. B. Cummins, L. O. Arthur, M. Peeters, G. M. Shaw, P. M. Sharp, and B. H. Hahn. 1999. Origin of HIV-1 in the chimpanzee Pan troglodytes troglodytes. Nature 397:436–441.

80. Garcia, J. V., J. Alfano, and A. D. Miller. 1993. The negative effect of human immunodeficiency virus type 1 nef on cell surface CD4 expression is not species specific and requires the cytoplasmic domain of CD4. J. Virol. 67:1511–1516.

81. Garcia, J. V., and A. D. Miller. 1991. Serine phosphorylation independent downregulation of cell-surface CD4 by Nef. Nature 350:508–511.

82. Geraghty, R. J., and A. T. Panganiban. 1993. Human immunodeficiency virus type 1 Vpu has a CD4- and an envelope glycoprotein-independent function. J. Virol. 67:4190–4194.

83. Gibbs, J. S., D. A. Regier, and R. C. Desrosiers. 1994. Construction and in vitro properties of HIV-1 mutants with deletions in "nonessential" genes. AIDS Res. Hum. Retroviruses 10:343–350.

84. Gluschankoff, P., I. Mondor, H. R. Gelderblom, and Q. J. Sattentau. 1997. Cell membrane vesicles are a major contaminant of gradient-enriched human immunodeficiency virus type-1 preparations. Virology 230:125–133.

85. Glushakova, S., J. C. Grivel, K. Suryanarayana, P. Meylan, J. D. Lifson, D. R. Desrosiers, and L. Margolis. 1999. Nef enhances human immunodeficiency virus replication and responsiveness to Interleukin-2 in human lymphoid tissue ex vivo. J. Virol. 73:3968–3974.

86. Goh, W. C., M. E. Rogel, C. M. Kinsey, S. F. Michael, P. N. Fultz, M. A. Nowak, B. H. Hahn, and M. Emerman. 1998. HIV-1 Vpr increases viral expression by manipulation of the cell cycle: a mechanism for selection of Vpr in vivo. Nature Med. 4:65–71.

87. Goncalves, J., P. Jallepalli, and D. H. Gabuzda. 1994. Subcellular localization of the Vif protein of human immunodeficiency virus type 1. J. Virol. 68:704–712.

88. Goncalves, J., Y. Korin, J. Zack, and D. Gabuzda. 1996. Role of Vif in human immunodeficiency virus type 1 reverse transcription. J. Virol. 70:8701–8709.

89. Greenberg, M. E., S. Bronson, M. Lock, M. Neumann, G. N. Pavlakis, and J. Skowronski. 1997. Co-localization of HIV-1 Nef with the AP-2 adaptor protein complex correlates with Nef-induced CD4 down-regulation. EMBO J. 16:6964–6976.

90. Greenberg, M. E., A. J. Iafrate, and J. Skowronski. 1998. The SH3 domain-binding surface and an acidic motif in HIV-1 Nef regulate trafficking of class I MHC complexes. EMBO J. 17:2777–2789.

91. Greenough, T. C., J. L. Sullivan, and R. C. Desrosiers. 1999. Declining CD4 T-cell counts in a person infected with nef-deleted HIV-1. N. Engl. J. Med. 340:236–237.

92. Greenway, A., A. Azad, and D. McPhee. 1995. Human immunodeficiency virus type 1 nef protein inhibits activation pathways in peripheral blood mononuclear cells and T cell lines. J. Virol. 69:1842–1850.

93. Greenway, A. L., D. A. McPhee, E. Grgacic, D. Hewish, A. Lucantoni, I. Macreadie, and A. Azad. 1994. Nef 27, but not the Nef 25 isoform of human immunodeficiency virus-type 1 pNL4.3 down-regulates surface CD4 and IL-2R expression in peripheral blood mononuclear cells and transformed T cells. Virology 198:245–256.

94. Grzesiek, S., A. Bax, G. M. Clore, A. M. Gronenborn, J. S. Hu, J. Kaufman, I. Palmer, S. J. Stahl, and P. T. Wingfield. 1996. The solution structure of HIV-1 Nef reveals an unexpected fold and permits delineation of the binding surface for the SH3 domain of Hck tyrosine protein kinase. Nat. Struct. Biol. 3:340–345.

95. Gummuluru, S., and M. Emerman. 1999. Cell cycle- and Vpr-mediated regulation of human immunodeficiency virus type 1 expression in primary and transformed T-cell lines. J. Virol. 73:5422–5430.

96. Guy, B., M. Geist, K. Dott, D. Spehner, M.-P. Kieny, and J.-P. Lecocq. 1991. A specific inhibitior of cysteine proteases impairs a vif-dependent modification of human immunodeficiency virus type 1 env protein. J. Virol. 65:1325–1331.

97. Guy, B., M. P. Kieny, Y. Riviere, C. LePeuch, K. Dott, M. Girard, L. Montagnier, and J.-P. Lecocq. 1987. HIV F/3' orf encodes a phosphorylated GTP-binding protein resembling an oncogene product. Nature 330:266–269.

98. Guyader, M., M. Emerman, L. Montagnier, and K. Peden. 1989. VPX mutants of HIV-2 are infectious in established cell lines but display a severe defect in peripheral blood lymphocytes. EMBO J. 8:1169–1175.

99. Haase, A. T. 1986. Pathogenesis of lentivirus infections. Nature 322:130–136.

100. Hanna, Z., D. G. Kay, N. Rebai, A. Guimond, S. Jothy, and P. Jolicoeur. 1998. Nef harbors a major determinant of pathogenicity for an AIDS-like disease induced by HIV-1 in transgenic mice. Cell 95:163–175.

101. Hansen, M. S. T., and F. D. Bushman. 1997. Human immunodeficiency virus type 2 preintegration complexes: activities in vitro and response to inhibitors. J. Virol. 71:3351–3356.

102. Harmache, A., M. Bouyac, G. Audoly, C. Hieblot, P. Peveri, R. Vigne, and M. Suzan. 1995. The vif gene is essential for efficient replication of caprine arthritis encephalitis virus in goat synovial membrane cells and affects the late steps of the virus replication cycle. J. Virol. 69:3247–3257.

103. Harousoe, J. M., A. Gettie, R. C. H. Tan, J. Blanchard, and C. Cheng-Mayer. 1999. Distinct pathogenic sequela in rhesus macaques infected with CCR5 or CXCR4 utilizing SHIVs. Science 284:816–819.

104. He, J., S. Choe, R. Walker, P. DiMarzio, D. O. Morgan, and N. R. Landau. 1995. Human immunodeficiency virus type 1 viral protein R (Vpr) arrests cells in the G_2 phase of the cell cycle by inhibiting p34^{cdc2} activity. J. Virol. 69: 6705–6711.

105. Heinzinger, N., M. Bukrinsky, S. Haggerty, A. Ragland, M.-A. Lee, V. Kewal-Ramani, H. Gendelman, L. Ratner, M. Stevenson, and M. Emerman. 1994. The Vpr protein of human immunodeficiency virus type 1 influences nuclear localization of viral nucleic acids in nondividing host cells. Proc. Natl. Acad. Sci. USA 91:7311–7315.

106. Hirsch, V. M., M. E. Sharkey, C. R. Brown, B. Brichacek, S. Goldstein, J. Wakefield, R. Byrum, W. R. Elkins, B. H. Hahn, J. D. Lifson, and M. Stevenson. 1998. Vpx is required for dissemination and pathogenesis of SIV$_{SM}$ PBj: evidence of macrophage-dependent viral amplification. Nature Med. 4:1401–1408.

107. Ho, D. D., A. U. Neumann, A. S. Perelson, W. Chen, J. M. Leonard, and M. Markowitz. 1995. Rapid turnover of plasma virions and CD4 lymphocytes in HIV-1 infection. Nature 373:123–126.

108. Hoglund, S., A. Ohagen, K. Lawrence, and D. Gabuzda. 1994. Role of vif during packing of the core of HIV-1. Virology 201:349–355.

109. Howe, A. Y., J. U. Jung, and R. C. Desrosiers. 1998. Zeta chain of the T-cell receptor interacts with nef of simian immunodeficiency virus and human immunodeficiency virus type 2. J. Virol. 72:9827–9834.

110. Hoxie, J. A., J. D. Alpers, J. L. Rackowski, K. Huebner, B. S. Haggarty, A. J. Cedarbaum, and J. C. Reed. 1986. Alterations in T4 (CD4) protein and mRNA synthesis in cells infected with HIV. Science 234:1123–1127.

111. Hua, J., W. Blair, R. Truant, and B. R. Cullen. 1997. Identification of regions in HIV-1 Nef required for efficient downregulation of cell surface CD4. Virology 231:231–238.

112. Inoue, M., Y. Koga, D. Djordjijevic, T. Fukuma, E. P. Reddy, M. M. Yokoyama, and K. Sagawa. 1993. Down-regulation of CD4 molecules by the expression of nef: a quantitative analysis of CD4 antigens on the cell surfaces. Int. Immunol. 5:1067–1073.

113. Jabbar, M. A., and D. P. Nayak. 1990. Intracellular interaction of human immunodeficiency virus type 1 (ARV-2) envelope glycoprotein gp160 with CD4 blocks the movement and maturation of CD4 to the plasma membrane. J. Virol. 64:6297–6304.

114. Jacqué, J.-M., A. Mann, H. Enslen, N. Sharova, B. Brichacek, R. J. Davis, and M. Stevenson. 1998. Modulation of HIV-1 infectivity by MAPK, a virion-associated kinase. EMBO J. 17:2607–2618.

115. Jamieson, B. D., G. M. Aldrovandi, V. Planelles, J. B. M. Jowett, L. Gao, L. M. Bloch, I. Chen, and J. A. Zack. 1994. Requirement of human immunodeficiency virus type 1 *nef* for *in vivo* replication and pathogenicity. J. Virol. 68:3478–3485.

116. Jenkins, Y., M. McEntee, K. Weis, and W. C. Greene. 1998. Characterization of HIV-1 vpr nuclear import: analysis of signals and pathways. J. Cell. Biol. 143:875–885.

117. Jin, X., D. E. Bauer, S. E. Tuttleton, S. Lewin, A. Gettie, J. Blanchard, C. E. Irwin, J. R. Safrit, J. Mittler, L. Weinberger, L. E. Kostrikis, L. Zhang, A. S. Perelson, and D. D. Ho. 1999. Dramatic rise in plasma viremia after CD8$^+$ T cell depletion in simian immunodeficiency virus-infected macaques. J. Exp. Med. 189:991–998.

118. Jowett, J. B., Y. Xie, and I. S. Y. Chen. 1999. The presence of human immunodeficiency virus type 1 Vpr correlates with a decrease in the frequency of mutations in a plasmid shuttle vector. J. Virol. 73:7132–7137.

119. Jowett, J. B. M., V. Planelles, B. Poon, N. P. Shah, M.-L. Chen, and I. S. Y. Chen. 1995. The human immunodeficiency virus type 1 vpr gene arrests infected T cells in the G$_2$ + phase of the cell cycle. J. Virol. 69:6304–6313.

120. Jung, J. U., M. Stager, and R. C. Desrosiers. 1994. Virus-encoded cyclin. Mol. Cell. Biol. 14:7235–7244.

121. Kappes, J. C., J. A. Conway, S.-W. Lee, G. M. Shaw, and B. H. Hahn. 1991. Human immunodeficiency virus type 2 vpx protein augments viral infectivity. Virology 184:197–209.

122. Karageorgos, L., P. Li, and C. Burrell. 1993. Characterization of HIV replication complexes early after cell-to-cell infection. AIDS Res. Hum. Retroviruses 9:817–823.

123. Karczewski, M. K., and K. Strebel. 1996. Cytoskeleton association and virion incorporation of the human immunodeficiency virus type 1 Vif protein. J. Virol. 70:494–507.

124. Karn, T., B. Hock, U. Holtrich, M. Adamski, K. Strebhardt, and H. Rubsamen-Waigmann. 1998. Nef proteins of distinct HIV-1 or -2 isolates differ in their binding properties for Hck: isolation of a novel Nef binding factor with characteristics of an adaptor protein. Virology 246:45–52.

125. Kawano, Y., Y. Tanaka, N. Misawa, R. Tanaka, J. I. Kira, T. Kimura, M. Fukushi, K. Sano, T. Goto, M. Nakai, T. Kobayashi, N. Yamamoto, and Y. Koyanagi. 1997. Mutational analysis of human immunodeficiency virus type 1 (HIV-1) accessory genes: requirement of a site in the nef gene for HIV-1 replication in activated CD4+ T cells in vitro and in vivo. J. Virol. 71:8456–8466.

126. Kersh, E. N., A. S. Shaw, and P. M. Allen. 1998. Fidelity of T cell activation through multistep T cell receptor zeta phosphorylation. Science 281: 572–575.

127. Kestler, H. W., D. J. Ringler, K. Mori, D. L. Panicali, P. K. Sehgal, M. D. Daniel, and R. C. Desrosiers. 1991. Importance of the nef gene for maintenance of high virus loads and for development of AIDS. Cell 65:651–662.

128. Kewal-Ramani, V. N., and M. Emerman. 1996. Vpx association with mature core structures of HIV-2. Virology 218:159–168.

129. Khan, I. H., E. T. Sawai, E. Antonio, C. J. Weber, C. P. Mandell, P. Montbriand, and P. A. Luciw. 1998. Role of the SH3-ligand domain of simian immunodeficiency virus Nef in interaction with Nef-associated kinase and simian AIDS in rhesus macaques. J. Virol. 72:5820–5830.

130. Kienzle, N., J. Freund, H. R. Kalbitzer, and N. Mueller-Lantzsch. 1993. Oligomerization of the Nef protein from human immunodeficiency virus (HIV) type 1. Eur. J. Biochem. 214:451–457.

131. Kimura, T., M. Nishikawa, and A. Ohyama. 1994. Intracellular membrane traffic of human immunodeficiency virus type 1 envelope glycoproteins: vpu liberates Golgi-targeted gp160 from CD4-dependent retention in the endoplasmic reticulum. J. Biochem. 115:1010–1020.

132. Kinoshita, S., B. K. Chen, H. Kaneshima, and G. P. Nolan. 1998. Host control of HIV-1 parasitism in T cells by the nuclear factor of activated T cells. Cell 95:595–604.

133. Kirchhoff, F., P. J. Easterbrook, N. Douglas, M. Troop, T. C. Greenough, J. Weber, S. Carl, J. L. Sullivan, and R. S. Daniels. 1999. Sequence variations in human immunodeficiency virus type 1 nef are associated with different stages of disease. J. Virol. 73:5497–5508.

134. Kirchhoff, F., T. C. Greenough, D. B. Brettler, J. L. Sullivan, and R. C. Desrosiers. 1995. Brief report: absence of intact nef sequences in a long-term survivor with nonprogressive HIV-1 infection. N. Engl. J. Med. 332:228–232.

135. Klimkait, T., K. Strebel, M. D. Hoggan, M. A. Martin, and J. M. Orenstein. 1990. The human immunodeficiency virus type 1-specific protein *Vpu* is required for efficient virus maturation and release. J. Virol. 64:621–629.

136. Kondo, E., and H. G. Gottlinger. 1996. A conserved LXXLF sequence is the major determinant in p6^{gag} required for the incorporation of human immunodeficiency virus type 1 vpr. J. Virol. 70:159–164.

137. Kondo, E., F. Mammano, E. A. Cohen, and H. G. Gottlinger. 1995. The p6^{gag} domain of human immunodeficiency virus type 1 is sufficient for the incorporation of vpr into heterologous viral particles. J. Virol. 69:2759–2764.

138. Korin, Y. D., and J. A. Zack. 1998. Progression to the G1b phase of the cell cycle is required for completion of human immunodeficiency virus type 1 reverse transcription in T cells. J. Virol. 72:3161–3168.

139. Korin, Y. D., and J. A. Zack. 1999. Nonproductive human immunodeficiency virus type 1 infection in nucleoside-treated G0 lymphocytes. J. Virol. 73:6526–6532.

140. Lama, J., A. Mangasarian, and D. Trono. 1999. Cell-surface expression of CD4 reduces HIV-1 infectivity by blocking Env incorporation in a Nef- and Vpu-inhibitable manner. Curr. Biol. 9:622–631.

141. Lang, S. M., A. J. Iafrate, C. Stahl-Hennig, E. M. Kuhn, T. Nisslein, F. J. Kaup, M. Haupt, G. Hunsmann, J. Skowronski, and F. Kirchhoff. 1997. Association of simian immunodeficiency virus Nef with cellular serine/threonine kinases is dispensable for the development of AIDS in rhesus macaques. Nature Med. 3:860–865.

142. Larsen, N. B., H. W. Kestler, and J. J. Docherty. 1998. Mice transgenic for simian immunodeficiency virus *nef* are immunologically compromised. J. Biomed. Sci. 5:260–266.

143. Lavallée, C., X. J. Yao, A. Ladha, H. Gottlinger, W. A. Haseltine, and E. A. Cohen. 1994. Requirement of the Pr55^{gag} precursor for incorporation of the Vpr product into human immunodeficiency virus type 1 viral particles. J. Virol. 68:1926–1934.

144. Learmont, J. C., A. F. Geczy, J. Mills, L. J. Ashton, C. H. Raynes-Greenow, R. J. Garsia, W. B. Dyer, L. McIntyre, R. B. Oelrichs, D. I. Rhodes, N. J. Deacon, and J. S. Sullivan. 1999. Immunologic and virologic status after 14 to 18 years of infection with an attenuated strain of HIV-1. A report from the Sydney Blood Bank Cohort. N. Engl. J. Med. 340:1715–1722.

145. Lee, C., B. Leung, M. A. Lemmon, J. Zheng, D. Cowburn, J. Kuriyan, and K. Saksela. 1995. A single amino acid in the SH3 domain of Hck determines its high affinity and specificity in binding to HIV-1 Nef protein. EMBO J. 14:5006–5015.

146. Lee, C. H., K. Saksela, U. A. Mirza, B. T. Chait, and J. Kuriyan. 1996. Crystal structure of the conserved core of HIV-1 nef complexed with a Src family SH3 domain. Cell 85:931–942.

147. Lee, Y. H., M. D. Schwartz, and A. T. Panganiban. 1997. The HIV-1 matrix domain of Gag is required for Vpu responsiveness during particle release. Virology 237:46–55.

148. Le Gall, S., L. Erdtmann, S. Benichou, C. Berlioz-Torrent, L. Liu, R. Benarous, J. M. Heard, and O. Schwartz. 1998. Nef interacts with the mu subunit of

clathrin adaptor complexes and reveals a cryptic sorting signal in MHC I molecules. Immunity 8:483–495.

149. Lewis, P. F., and M. Emerman. 1994. Passage through mitosis is required for oncoretroviruses but not for the human immunodeficiency virus. J. Virol. 68:510–516.

150. Lichtenstein, D. L., K. E. Rushlow, R. F. Cook, M. L. Raabe, C. J. Swardson, G. J. Kociba, C. J. Issel, and R. C. Montelaro. 1995. Replication in vitro and in vivo of an equine infectious anemia virus mutant deficient in dUTPase activity. J. Virol. 69:2881–2888.

151. Liu, H., X. Wu, M. Newman, G. M. Shaw, B. H. Hahn, and J. C. Kappes. 1995. The Vif protein of human and simian immunodeficiency viruses is packaged into virions and associates with viral core structures. J. Virol. 69:7630–7638.

152. Liu, H., X. Wu, H. Xiao, J. A. Conway, and J. C. Kappes. 1997. Incorporation of functional human immunodeficiency virus type 1 integrase into virions independent of the Gag-Pol precursor protein. J. Virol. 71:7704–7710.

153. Lock, M., M. E. Greenberg, A. J. Iafrate, F. Kirchhoff, N. Shohdy, and J. Skowronski. 1999. Two elements target SIV Nef to the AP-2 clathrin adaptor complex, but only one is required for the induction of CD4 endocytosis. EMBO J. 18:2722–2733.

154. Lowell, C. A., M. Niwa, P. Soriano, and H. E. Varmus. 1996. Deficiency of the Hck and Src tyrosine kinases results in extreme levels of extramedullary hematopoiesis. Blood 87:1780–1792.

155. Lu, X., X. Wu, A. Plemenitas, H. Yu, E. T. Sawaii, A. Abo, and B. M. Peterlin. 1996. CDC42 and Rac1 are implicated in the activation of the Nef-associated kinase and replication of HIV-1. Curr. Biol. 6:1677–1684.

156. Lu, Y.-L., P. Spearman, and L. Ratner. 1993. Human immunodeficiency virus type 1 viral protein R localization in infected cells and virions. J. Virol. 67:6542–6550.

157. Luban, J., K. L. Bossolt, E. K. Franke, G. V. Kalpana, and S. P. Goff. 1993. Human immunodeficiency virus type 1 *gag* protein binds to cyclophilins A and B. Cell 73:1067–1078.

158. Ludlow, J. W. 1993. Interactions between SV40 large-tumor antigen and the growth suppressor proteins pRB and p53. FASEB J. 7:866–871.

159. Luo, T., and J. V. Garcia. 1996. The association of Nef with a cellular serine/ threonine kinase and its enhancement of infectivity are viral isolate dependent. J. Virol. 70:6493–6496.

160. Madani, N., and D. Kabat. 1998. An endogenous inhibitor of human immunodeficiency virus in human lymphocytes is overcome by the viral Vif protein. J. Virol. 72:10251–10255.

161. Mahalingam, S., S. A. Khan, R. Murali, M. A. Jabbar, C. E. Monken, R. G. Collman, and A. Srinivasan. 1995. Mutagenesis of the putative a-helical domain of the Vpr protein of human immunodeficiency virus type 1: effect on stability and virion incorporation. Proc. Natl. Acad. Sci. USA 92: 3794–3798.

162. Maldarelli, F., M.-Y. Chen, R. L. Willey, and K. Strebel. 1993. Human immunodeficiency virus type 1 Vpu protein is an oligomeric type I integral membrane protein. J. Virol. 67:5056–5061.

163. Mangasarian, A., V. Piguet, J. K. Wang, Y. L. Chen, and D. Trono. 1999. Nef-induced CD4 and major histocompatibility complex class I (MHC-I) down-regulation are governed by distinct determinants: N-terminal alpha helix and proline repeat of Nef selectively regulate MHC-I trafficking. J. Virol. 73:1964–1973.

164. Manninen, A., M. Hiipakka, M. Vihinen, W. Lu, B. J. Mayer, and K. Saksela. 1998. SH3-domain binding function of HIV-1 Nef is required for association with a PAK-related kinase. Virology 250:273–282.

165. Mansky, L. M. 1996. The mutation rate of human immunodeficiency virus type 1 is influenced by the *vpr* gene. Virology 222:391–400.

166. Margottin, F., S. P. Bour, H. Durand, L. Selig, S. Benichou, V. Richard, D. Thomas, K. Strebel, and R. Benarous. 1998. A novel human WD protein, h-beta TrCp, that interacts with HIV-1 Vpu connects CD4 to the ER degradation pathway through an F-box motif. Mol. Cell 1:565–574.

167. Mariani, R., and J. Skowronski. 1993. CD4 down-regulation by *nef* alleles isolated from human immunodeficiency virus type 1-infected individuals. Proc. Natl. Acad. Sci. USA 90:5549–5553.

168. McGeoch, D. J. 1990. Protein sequence comparisons show that the "pseudo proteases"encoded by poxviruses and certain retroviruses belong to the deoxyuridine triphosphatase family. Nucleic Acids Res. 18:4105–4110.

169. Miller, M. D., M. T. Warmerdam, I. Gaston, W. C. Greene, and M. B. Feinberg. 1994. The human immunodeficiency virus-1 *nef* gene product: a positive factor for viral infection and replication in primary lymphocytes and macrophages. J. Exp. Med. 179:101–113.

170. Moarefi, I., M. LaFevre-Bernt, F. Sicheri, M. Huse, C.-H. Lee, J. Kuriyan, and W. T. Miller. 1997. Activation of the Src-family tyrosine kinase Hck by SH3 domain displacement. Nature 385:650–653.

171. Moran, E. 1993. Interaction of adenoviral proteins with pRB and p53. FASEB J. 7:880–885.

172. Naldini, L., U. Blomer, F. H. Gage, D. Trono, and I. M. Verma. 1996. Efficient transfer, integration, and sustained long-term expression of the transgene in adult rat brains injected with a lentiviral vector. Proc. Natl. Acad. Sci. USA 93:11382–11388.

173. Nie, Z., D. Bergeron, R. A. Subbramanian, X. J. Yao, F. Checroune, N. Rougeau, and E. A. Cohen. 1998. The putative alpha helix 2 of human immunodeficiency virus type 1 Vpr contains a determinant which is responsible for the nuclear translocation of proviral DNA in growth-arrested cells. J. Virol. 72:4104–4115.

174. Niederman, T. M., W. R. Hastings, and L. Ratner. 1993. Myristylation-enhanced binding of the HIV-1 nef protein to T cell skeletal matrix. Virology 197:420–425.

175. Nunn, M. F., and J. W. Marsh. 1996. Human immunodeficiency virus type 1 Nef associates with a member of the p21-activated kinase family. J. Virol. 70:6157–6161.

176. Oberste, M. S., and M. A. Gonda. 1992. Conservation of amino-acid sequence motifs in lentivirus Vif proteins. Virus Genes 6:95–102.

177. Ogg, G. S., X. Jin, S. Bonhoeffer, P. R. Dunbar, M. A. Nowak, S. Monard, J. P.

Segal, Y. Cao, S. L. Rowland-Jones, V. Cerundolo, A. Hurley, M. Markowitz, D. D. Ho, D. F. Nixon, and A. J. McMichael. 1998. Quantitation of HIV-1-specific cytotoxic T lymphocytes and plasma load of viral RNA. Science 279:2103–2106.

178. Ott, M., S. Emiliani, C. Van Lint, G. Herbein, J. Lovett, N. Chirmule, T. Mc-Closkey, S. Pahwa, and E. Verdin. 1997. Immune hyperactivation of HIV-1-infected T cells mediated by Tat and the CD28 pathway. Science 275:1481–1485.

179. Pandori, M., H. Craig, L. Moutouh, J. Corbeil, and J. Guatelli. 1998. Virological importance of the protease-cleavage site in human immunodeficiency virus type 1 Nef is independent of both intravirion processing and CD4 down-regulation. Virology 251:302–316.

180. Pandori, M., N. J. S. Fitch, H. M. Craig, D. D. Richman, C. A. Spina, and J. C. Guatelli. 1996. Producer-cell modification of human immunodeficiency virus type 1: Nef is a virion protein. J. Virol. 70:4283–4290.

181. Pawson, T. 1997. New impressions of Src and Hck. Nature 385:582–585.

182. Paxton, W., R. I. Connor, and N. R. Landau. 1993. Incorporation of Vpr into human immunodeficiency virus type 1 virions: requirement for the p6 region of *gag* and mutational analysis. J. Virol. 67:7229–7237.

183. Perelson, A. S., P. Essunger, Y. Cao, M. Vesanen, A. Hurley, K. Saksela, M. Markowitz, and D. D. Ho. 1997. Decay characteristics of HIV-1-infected compartments during combination therapy. Nature 387:188–191.

184. Piguet, V., Y. L. Chen, A. Mangasarian, M. Foti, J. L. Carpentier, and D. Trono. 1998. Mechanism of Nef-induced CD4 endocytosis: Nef connects CD4 with the mu chain of adaptor complexes. EMBO J. 17:2472–2481.

185. Piguet, V., F. Gu, M. Foti, N. Demaurex, J. Gruenberg, J. L. Carpentier, and D. Trono. 1999. Nef-induced CD4 degradation: a diacidic-based motif in Nef functions as a lysosomal targeting signal through the binding of b-COP in endosomes. Cell 97:63–73.

186. Piller, S. C., G. D. Ewart, D. A. Jans, P. W. Gage, and G. B. Cox. 1999. The amino-terminal region of Vpr from human immunodeficiency virus type 1 forms ion channels and kills neurons. J. Virol. 73:4230–4238.

187. Piller, S. C., G. D. Ewart, A. Premkumar, G. B. Cox, and P. W. Gage. 1996. Vpr protein of human immunodeficiency virus type 1 forms cation-selective channels in planar lipid bilayers. Proc. Natl. Acad. Sci. USA 93:111–115.

188. Piller, S. C., P. Jans, P. W. Gage, and D. A. Jans. 1998. Extracellular HIV-1 virus protein R causes a large inward current and cell death in cultured hippocampal neurons: implications for AIDS pathology. Proc. Natl. Acad. Sci. USA 95:4595–4600.

189. Planelles, V., J. B. M. Jowett, Q. Li, Y. Xie, B. Hahn, and I. S. Y. Chen. 1996. Vpr-induced cell cycle arrest is conserved among primate lentiviruses. J. Virol. 70:2516–2524.

190. Poon, B., K. Grovit-Ferbas, S. A. Stewart, and I. S. Y. Chen. 1998. Cell cycle arrest by Vpr in HIV-1 virions and insensitivity to antiretroviral agents. Science 281:266–269.

191. Poon, B., J. B. M. Jowett, S. A. Stewart, R. W. Armstrong, G. M. Rishton, and I. S. Y. Chen. 1997. Human immunodeficiency virus type 1 *vpr* gene induces phenotypic effects similar to those of the DNA alkylating agent, nitrogen mustard. J. Virol. 71:3961–3971.

192. Popov, S., M. Rexach, L. Ratner, G. Blobel, and M. Bukrinsky. 1998. Viral protein R regulates docking of the HIV-1 preintegration complex to the nuclear pore complex. J. Biol. Chem. 273:13347–13352.

193. Popov, S., M. Rexach, G. Zybarth, N. Reiling, M.-A. Lee, L. Ratner, C. M. Lane, M. S. Moore, G. Blobel, and M. Bukrinsky. 1998. Viral protein R regulates nuclear import of the HIV-1 pre-integration complex. EMBO J. 17:909–917.

194. Re, F., D. Braaten, E. K. Franke, and J. Luban. 1995. Human immunodeficiency virus type 1 Vpr arrests the cell cycle in G_2 by inhibiting the activation of p34^{cdc2}-cyclin B. J. Virol. 69:6859–6864.

195. Reichard, P. 1988. Interactions between deoxyribonucleotide and DNA synthesis. Annu. Rev. Biochem. 57:349–374.

196. Rhee, S. S., and J. W. Marsh. 1994. Human immunodeficiency virus type 1 nef-induced down-modulation of CD4 is due to rapid internalization and degradation of surface CD4. J. Virol. 68:5156–5163.

197. Robert-Guroff, M., M. Popovic, S. Gartner, P. Markham, R. C. Gallo, and M. S. Reitz. 1990. Structure and expression of *tat-*, *rev-*, and *nef*-specific transcripts of human immunodeficiency virus type 1 in infected lymphocytes and macrophages. J. Virol. 64:3391–3398.

198. Robinson, M. S. 1994. The role of clathrin, adaptors and dynamin in endocytosis. Curr. Opin. Cell Biol. 6:538–544.

199. Roe, T., T. C. Reynolds, G. Yu, and P. O. Brown. 1993. Integration of murine leukemia virus DNA depends on mitosis. EMBO J. 12:2099–2108.

200. Rogel, M. E., L. I. Wu, and M. Emerman. 1995. The human immunodeficiency virus type 1 *vpr* gene prevents cell proliferation during chronic infection. J. Virol. 69:882–888.

201. Roizman, B., and A. E. Sears. 1996. Herpes simplex viruses and their replication, p. 2231–2295. *In* B. N. Fields, D. M. Knipe, and P. M. Howley (ed.), Fields virology, 3rd ed., vol. 2. Lippincott-Raven Publishers, Philadelphia.

202. Ryan-Graham, M. A., and K. W. C. Peden. 1995. Both virus and host components are important for the manifestation of a nef-phenotype in HIV-1 and HIV-2. Virology 213:158–168.

203. Sakai, H., M. Kawamura, J.-I. Sakuragi, S. Sakuragi, R. Shibata, A. Ishimoto, N. Ono, S. Ueda, and A. Adachi. 1993. Integration is essential for efficient gene expression of human immunodeficiency virus type 1. J. Virol. 67:1169–1174.

204. Saksela, K., G. Cheng, and D. Baltimore. 1995. Proline-rich (PxxP) motifs in HIV-1 Nef bind to SH3 domains of a subset of Src kinases and are required for the enhanced growth of Nef+ viruses but not for down-regulation of CD4. EMBO J. 14:484–491.

205. Sanfridson, A., B. R. Cullen, and C. Doyle. 1993. The simian immunodeficiency virus nef protein promotes degradation of CD4 in human T cells. J. Biol. Chem. 269:3917–3920.

206. Sawai, E. T., A. Baur, H. Struble, B. M. Peterlin, J. A. Levy, and C. Cheng-Mayer. 1994. Human immunodeficiency virus type 1 Nef associates with a cellular serine kinase in T lymphocytes. Proc. Natl. Acad. Sci. USA 91: 1539–1543.

207. Sawai, E. T., A. S. Baur, B. M. Peterlin, J. A. Levy, and C. Cheng-Mayer. 1995. A conserved domain and membrane targeting of Nef from HIV and SIV are

required for association with a cellular serine kinase activity. J. Biol. Chem. 270:15307–15314.

208. Sawai, E. T., I. H. Khan, P. M. Montbriand, B. M. Peterlin, C. Cheng-Mayer, and P. A. Luciw. 1996. Activation of PAK by HIV and SIV Nef: importance for AIDS in rhesus macaques. Curr. Biol. 6:1519–1527.

209. Schmidtmayerova, H., H. S. L. M. Nottet, G. Nuovo, T. Raabe, C. R. Flanagan, L. Dubrovsky, H. E. Gendelman, A. Cerami, M. Bukrinsky, and B. Sherry. 1996. Human immunodeficiency virus type 1 infection alters chemokine b peptide expression in human monocytes: implications for recruitment of leukocytes into brain and lymph nodes. Proc. Natl. Acad. Sci. USA 93: 700–704.

210. Schorr, J., R. Kellner, O. Fackler, J. Freund, J. Konvalinka, N. Kienzle, H.-G. Kräusslich, N. Mueller-Lantzsch, and H. R. Kalbitzer. 1996. Specific cleavage sites of Nef proteins from human immunodeficiency virus types 1 and 2 for the viral proteases. J. Virol. 70:9051–9054.

211. Schrager, J. A., and J. W. Marsh. 1999. HIV-1 Nef increases T cell activation in a stimulus-dependent manner. Proc. Natl. Acad. Sci. USA 96:8167–8172.

212. Schubert, U., L. C. Anton, I. Bacik, J. H. Cox, S. Bour, J. R. Bennink, M. Orlowski, K. Strebel, and J. W. Yewdell. 1998. CD4 glycoprotein degradation induced by human immunodeficiency virus type 1 Vpu protein requires the function of proteasomes and the ubiquitin-conjugating pathway. J. Virol. 72:2280–2288.

213. Schubert, U., S. Bour, A. V. Ferrer-Montiel, M. Montal, F. Maldarelli, and K. Strebel. 1996. The two biological activities of human immunodeficiency virus type 1 Vpu protein involve two separable structural domains. J. Virol. 70: 809–819.

214. Schubert, U., S. Bour, R. L. Willey, and K. Strebel. 1999. Regulation of virus release by the macrophage-tropic human immunodeficiency virus type 1 AD8 isolate is redundant and can be controlled by either Vpu or Env. J. Virol. 73:887–896.

215. Schubert, U., and K. Strebel. 1994. Differential activities of the human immunodeficiency virus type 1-encoded Vpu protein are regulated by phosphorylation and occur in different cellular compartments. J. Virol. 68: 2260–2271.

216. Schwartz, O., A. Dautry-Varsat, B. Goud, V. Marechal, A. Subtil, J.-M. Heard, and O. Danos. 1995. Human immunodeficiency virus type 1 nef induces accumulation of CD4 in early endosomes. J. Virol. 69:528–533.

217. Schwartz, O., V. Marechal, O. Danos, and J.-M. Heard. 1995. Human immunodeficiency virus type 1 nef increases the efficiency of reverse transcription in the infected cell. J. Virol. 69:4053–4059.

218. Schwartz, O., V. Marechal, S. Le Gall, F. Lemonnier, and J.-M. Heard. 1996. Endocytosis of major histocompatibility complex class I molecules is induced by the HIV-1 Nef protein. Nature Med. 2:338–342.

219. Schwartz, S., B. K. Felber, D. M. Benko, E.-M. Fenyo, and G. N. Pavlakis. 1990. Cloning and functional analysis of multiply spliced mRNA species of human immunodeficiency virus type 1. J. Virol. 64:2519–2529.

220. Selig, L., B. Benichou, M. E. Rogel, L. I. Wu, M. A. Vodicka, J. Sire, R. Benarous, and M. Emerman. 1997. Uracil DNA glycosylase specifically interacts with

Vpr of both human immunodeficiency virus type 1 and simian immunodeficiency virus of sooty mangabeys, but binding does not correlate with cell cycle arrest. J. Virol. 71:4842–4846.

221. Sharp, P. M., E. Bailes, M. Stevenson, M. Emerman, and B. H. Hahn. 1996. Gene acquisition in HIV and SIV. Nature 383:586–587.

222. Shugars, D. C., M. S. Smith, D. H. Glueck, P. V. Nantermet, F. Seillier-Moiseiwitsch, and R. Swanstrom. 1993. Analysis of human immunodeficiency virus type 1 *nef* gene sequences present in vivo. J. Virol. 67:4639–4650.

223. Simm, M., M. Shahabuddin, W. Chao, J. S. Allan, and D. J. Volsky. 1995. Aberrant gag protein composition of a human immunodeficiency virus type 1 *vif* mutant produced in primary lymphocytes. J. Virol. 69:4582–4586.

224. Simon, J. H. M., E. A. Carpenter, R. A. M. Fouchier, and M. H. Malim. 1999. Vif and the p55^{Gag} polyprotein of human immunodeficiency virus type 1 are present in colocalizing membrane-free cytoplasmic complexes. J. Virol. 73:2667–2674.

225. Simon, J. H. M., R. A. M. Fouchier, T. E. Southerling, C. B. Guerra, C. K. Grant, and M. H. Malim. 1997. The Vif and Gag proteins of human immunodeficiency virus type 1 colocalize in infected human T cells. J. Virol. 71:5259–5267.

226. Simon, J. H. M., N. C. Gaddis, R. A. M. Fouchier, and M. H. Malim. 1998. Evidence for a newly discovered cellular anti-HIV-1 phenotype. Nature Med. 4:1397–1400.

227. Simon, J. H. M., and M. H. Malim. 1996. The human immunodeficiency virus type 1 Vif protein modulates the postpenetration stability of viral nucleoprotein complexes. J. Virol. 70:5297–5305.

228. Simon, J. H. M., D. L. Miller, R. A. M. Fouchier, and M. H. Malim. 1998. Virion incorporation of human immunodeficiency virus type-1 Vif is determined by intracellular expression level and may not be necessary for function. Virology 248:182–187.

229. Simon, J. H. M., D. L. Miller, R. A. M. Fouchier, M. A. Soares, K. W. Peden, and M. H. Malim. 1998. The regulation of primate immunodeficiency virus infectivity by Vif is cell species restricted: a role for Vif in determining virus host range and cross-species transmission. EMBO J. 17:1259–1267.

230. Simon, J. H. M., A. M. Sheehy, E. A. Carpenter, R. A. M. Fouchier, and M. H. Malim. 1999. Mutational analysis of the human immunodeficiency virus type 1 Vif protein. J. Virol. 73:2675–2681.

231. Simon, J. H. M., T. E. Southerling, J. C. Peterson, B. E. Meyer, and M. H. Malim. 1995. Complementation of *vif*-defective human immunodeficiency virus type 1 by primate, but not nonprimate, lentivirus *vif* genes. J. Virol. 69:4166–4172.

232. Sinclair, E., P. Barbosa, and M. B. Feinberg. 1997. The *nef* gene products of both simian and human immunodeficiency viruses enhance virus infectivity and are functionally interchangeable. J. Virol. 71:3641–3651.

233. Skowronski, J., D. Parks, and R. Mariani. 1993. Altered T cell activation and development in transgenic mice expressing the HIV-1 *nef* gene. EMBO J. 12:703–713.

234. Smith, B. L., B. W. Krushelnycky, D. Mochly-Rosen, and P. Bergs. 1996. The HIV Nef protein associates with protein kinase C theta. J. Biol. Chem. 271:16753–16757.

235. Sodroski, J., W. C. Goh, C. Rosen, A. Tartar, D. Portelle, A. Burny, and W. Haseltine. 1986. Replicative and cytopathic potential of HTLV-III/LAV with *sor* gene deletions. Science 231:1549–1553.

236. Songyang, Z., S. E. Shoelson, M. Chaudhuri, G. Gish, T. Pawson, W. G. Haser, F. King, T. Roberts, S. Ratnofsky, and R. J. Lechleider. 1993. SH2 domains recognize specific phosphopeptide sequences. Cell 72:767–778.

237. Sova, P., and D. J. Volsky. 1993. Efficiency of viral DNA synthesis during infection of permissive and nonpermissive cells with *vif*-negative human immunodeficiency virus type 1. J. Virol. 67:6322–6326.

238. Spina, C. A., T. J. Kwoh, M. Y. Chowers, J. C. Guatelli, and D. D. Richman. 1994. The importance of *nef* in the induction of human immunodeficiency virus type 1 replication from primary quiescent CD4 lymphocytes. J. Exp. Med. 179:115–123.

239. Stark, L. A., and R. T. Hay. 1998. Human immunodeficiency virus type 1 (HIV-1) viral protein R (Vpr) interacts with Lys-tRNA synthetase: implications for priming of HIV-1 reverse transcription. J. Virol. 72:3037–3044.

240. Steinhauer, D. A., and J. J. Holland. 1987. Rapid evolution of RNA viruses. Annu. Rev. Microbiol. 41:409.

241. Stevenson, M., C. Meier, A. M. Mann, N. Chapman, and A. Wasiak. 1988. Envelope glycoprotein of HIV induces interference and cytolysis resistance in CD4$^+$ cells: mechanism for persistence in AIDS. Cell 53:483–496.

242. Stevenson, M., T. L. Stanwick, M. P. Dempsey, and C. A. Lamonica. 1990. HIV-1 replication is controlled at the level of T cell activation and proviral integration. EMBO J. 9:1551–1560.

243. Stevenson, M., X. H. Zhang, and D. J. Volsky. 1987. Downregulation of cell surface molecules during noncytopathic infection of T cells with human immunodeficiency virus. J. Virol. 61:3741–3748.

244. Stewart, S. A., B. Poon, J. B. M. Jowett, and I. S. Y. Chen. 1997. Human immunodeficiency virus type 1 Vpr induces apoptosis following cell cycle arrest. J. Virol. 71:5579–5592.

245. Stivahtis, G. L., M. A. Soares, M. A. Vodicka, B. H. Hahn, and M. Emerman. 1997. Conservation and host specificity of Vpr-mediated cell cycle arrest suggest a fundamental role in primate lentivirus evolution and biology. J. Virol. 71:4331–4338.

246. Strebel, K., D. Daugherty, K. Clouse, D. Cohen, T. Folks, and M. A. Martin. 1987. The HIV "A" (*sor*) gene product is essential for virus infectivity. Nature 328:728–730.

247. Strebel, K., T. Klimkait, and M. A. Martin. 1988. A novel gene of HIV-1, vpu, and its 16-kilodalton product. Science 241:1221–1223.

248. Strebel, K., T. Klimkait, T. F. Maldarelli, and M. A. Martin. 1989. Molecular and biochemical analyses of human immunodeficiency virus type 1 *vpu* protein. J. Virol. 63:3784–3791.

249. Subbramanian, R. A., A. Kessous-Elbaz, R. Lodge, J. Forget, X. J. Yao, D. Bergeron, and E. A. Cohen. 1998. Human immunodeficiency virus type 1 Vpr is a positive regulator of viral transcription and infectivity in primary human macrophages. J. Exp. Med. 187:1103–1111.

250. Subbramanian, R. A., X. J. Yao, H. Dilhuydy, N. Rougeau, D. Bergeron, Y. Robitaille, and E. A. Cohen. 1998. Human immunodeficiency virus type 1

Vpr localization: nuclear transport of a viral protein modulated by a putative amphipathic helical structure and its relevance to biological activity. J. Mol. Biol. 278:13–30.

251. Sussman, J. J., J. S. Bonifacino, J. Lippincott-Schwartz, A. M. Weissman, T. Saito, R. D. Klausner, and J. D. Ashwell. 1988. Failure to synthesize the T cell CD3-zeta chain: structure and function of a partial T cell receptor complex. Cell 52:85–95.

252. Swingler, S., A. Mann, J.-M. Jacqué, B. Brichacek, V. G. Sasseville, K. Williams, A. A. Lackner, E. N. Janoff, R. Wang, D. Fisher, and M. Stevenson. 1999. HIV-1 Nef mediates lymphocyte chemotaxis and activation by infected macrophages. Nature Med. 5:997–1003.

253. Terai, C., and D. A. Carson. 1991. Pyrimidine nucleotide and nucleic acid synthesis in human monocytes and macrophages. Exp. Cell Res. 193:375–381.

254. Terwilliger, E. F., E. A. Cohen, Y. Lu, J. G. Sodroski, and W. A. Haseltine. 1989. Functional role of human immunodeficiency virus type 1 *vpu*. Proc. Natl. Acad. Sci. USA 86:5163–5167.

255. Thali, M., A. Bukovsky, E. Kondo, B. Rosenwirth, C. T. Walsh, J. Sodroski, and H. G. Gottlinger. 1994. Functional association of cyclophilin A with HIV-1 virions. Nature 372:363–365.

256. Threadgill, D. S., W. K. Steagall, M. T. Flaherty, F. J. Fuller, S. T. Perry, K. E. Rushlow, S. F. J. Le Grice, and S. L. Payne. 1993. Characterization of equine infectious anemia virus dUTPase: growth properties of a dUTPase-deficient mutant. J. Virol. 67:2592–2600.

257. Tomonaga, K., T. Miyazawa, J. Sakuragi, T. Mori, A. Adachi, and T. Mikami. 1993. The feline immunodeficiency virus ORF-A gene facilitates efficient viral replication in established T-cell lines and peripheral blood lymphocytes. J. Virol. 67:5889–5895.

258. Tristem, M., C. Marshall, A. Karpas, J. Petrik, and F. Hill. 1990. Origin of *vpx* in lentiviruses. Nature 347:341–342.

259. Turelli, P., G. Petursson, F. Guiguen, J.-F. Mornex, R. Vigne, and G. Querat. 1996. Replication properties of dUTPase-deficient mutants of caprine and ovine lentiviruses. J. Virol. 70:1213–1217.

260. Unutmaz, D., V. N. Kewal-Ramani, S. Marmon, and D. R. Littman. 1999. Cytokine signals are sufficient for HIV-1 infection of resting human T lymphocytes. J. Exp. Med. 189:1735–1746.

261. Vodicka, M. A., D. M. Koepp, P. A. Silver, and M. Emerman. 1998. HIV-1 Vpr interacts with the nuclear transport pathway to promote macrophage infection. Genes Dev. 12:175–185.

262. Vogt, P. K., and R. Ishizaki. 1965. Reciprocal patterns of genetic resistance to avian tumor viruses in two lines of chickens. Virology 26:664–672.

263. Vogt, P. K., and R. Ishizaki. 1966. Patterns of viral interference in the avian leukosis and sarcoma complex. Virology 30:368–374.

264. von Schwedler, U., J. Song, C. Aiken, and D. Trono. 1993. *vif* is crucial for human immunodeficiency virus type 1 proviral DNA synthesis in infected cells. J. Virol. 67:4945–4955.

265. Vousden, K. 1993. Interactions of human papillomavirus transforming proteins with the products of tumor suppressor genes. FASEB J. 7:872–879.

266. Wagaman, P. C., C. S. Hasselkus-Light, M. Henson, D. L. Lerner, T. R. Phillips, and J. H. Elder. 1993. Molecular cloning and characterization of deoxyuridine triphosphatase from feline immunodeficiency virus (FIV). Virology 196:451–457.

267. Wagner, L., O. O. Yang, E. A. Garcia-Zepeda, Y. Ge, S. A. Kalams, B. D. Walker, M. S. Pasternack, and A. D. Luster. 1998. Beta-chemokines are released from HIV-1-specific cytolytic T-cell granules complexed to proteoglycans. Nature 391:908–911.

268. Wain-Hobson, S. 1992. Human immunodeficiency virus type 1 quasispecies in vivo and ex vivo. Curr. Top. Microbiol. Immunol. 176:181.

269. Walker, C. M., D. J. Moody, D. P. Stites, and J. A. Levy. 1986. CD8+ lymphocytes can control HIV infection in vitro by suppressing virus replication. Science 234:1563–1566.

270. Wang, B., Y. C. Ge, P. Palasanthiran, S.-H. Xiang, J. Ziegler, D. E. Dwyer, C. Randle, D. Dowton, A. Cunningham, and N. K. Saksena. 1996. Gene defects clustered at the C-terminus of the vpr gene of HIV-1 in long-term nonprogressing mother and child pair: *in vivo* evolution of vpr quasispecies in blood and plasma. Virology 223:224–232.

271. Wei, X., S. K. Ghosh, M. E. Taylor, V. A. Johnson, E. A. Emini, P. Deutsch, J. D. Lifson, S. Bonhoeffer, M. A. Nowak, B. H. Hahn, M. S. Saag, and G. M. Shaw. 1995. Viral dynamics in human immunodeficiency virus type 1 infection. Nature 373:117–122.

272. Weiss, R. 1984. Tissue-specific transformation by human T-cell leukemia virus. Nature 310:273–274.

273. Weiss, R. A., P. Clapham, K. Nagy, and H. Hoshino. 1985. Envelope properties of human T-cell leukemia viruses. Curr. Top. Microbiol. Immunol. 115: 235–246.

274. Welker, R., H. Kottler, H. R. Kalbitzer, and H.-G. Kräusslich. 1996. Human immunodeficiency virus type 1 Nef protein is incorporated into virus particles and specifically cleaved by the viral proteinase. Virology 219:228–236.

275. Weller, S. K., A. E. Joy, and H. M. Temin. 1980. Correlation between cell killing and massive second-round superinfection by members of some subgroups of avian leukosis virus. J. Virol. 33:494–506.

276. Whatmore, A. M., N. Cook, G. A. Hall, S. Sharpe, E. W. Rud, and M. P. Cranage. 1995. Repair and evolution of nef in vivo modulates simian immunodeficiency virus virulence. J. Virol. 69:5117–5123.

277. Willey, R. L., F. Maldarelli, M. A. Martin, and K. Strebel. 1992. Human immunodeficiency virus type 1 Vpu protein regulates the formation of intracellular gp160-CD4 complexes. J. Virol. 66:226–234.

278. Willey, R. L., M. A. Martin, and K. W. C. Peden. 1994. Increase in soluble CD4 binding to and CD4-induced dissociation of gp120 from virions correlates with infectivity of human immunodeficiency virus type 1. J. Virol. 68:1029–1039.

279. Wiskerchen, M., and C. Cheng-Mayer. 1996. HIV-1 Nef association with cellular serine kinase correlates with enhanced virion infectivity and efficient proviral DNA synthesis. Virology 224:292–301.

280. Withers-Ward, E. S., J. B. Jowett, S. A. Stewart, Y. M. Xie, A. Garfinkel, Y. Shibagaki, S. A. Chow, N. Shah, F. Hanaoka, D. G. Sawitz, R. W. Armstrong,

L. M. Souza, and I. S. Chen. 1997. Human immunodeficiency virus type 1 Vpr interacts with HHR23A, a cellular protein implicated in nucleotide excision DNA repair. J. Virol. 71:9732–9742.

281. Wozniak, R. W., M. P. Rout, and J. D. Aitchison. 1998. Karyopherins and kissing cousins. Trends Cell Biol. 8:184–188.

282. Wu, X., J. A. Conway, J. Kim, and J. C. Kappes. 1994. Localization of the Vpx packaging signal within the C terminus of the human immunodeficiency virus type 2 gag precursor protein. J. Virol. 68:6161–6169.

283. Wu, X., H. Liu, H. Xiao, J. A. Conway, E. Hunter, and J. C. Kappes. 1997. Functional RT and IN incorporated into HIV-1 particles independently of the Gag/Pol precursor protein. EMBO J. 16:5113–5122.

284. Yang, X., and D. Gabuzda. 1998. Mitogen-activated protein kinase phosphorylates and regulates the HIV-1 Vif protein. J. Biol. Chem. 273:29879–29887.

285. Yang, X., J. Goncalves, and D. Gabuzda. 1996. Phosphorylation of Vif and its role in HIV-1 replication. J. Biol. Chem. 271:10121–10129.

286. Yao, X. J., H. Gottlinger, W. A. Haseltine, and E. A. Cohen. 1992. Envelope glycoprotein and CD4 independence of *vpu*-facilitated human immunodeficiency virus type 1 capsid export. J. Virol. 66:5119–5126.

287. Yao, X. J., R. A. Subbramanian, N. Rougeau, F. Boisvert, D. Bergeron, and E. A. Cohen. 1995. Mutagenic analysis of human immunodeficiency virus type 1 Vpr: role of a predicted N-terminal alpha-helical structure in Vpr nuclear localization and virion incorporation. J. Virol. 69:7032–7044.

288. Yu, G., and R. L. Felsted. 1992. Effect of myristylation on p27*nef* subcellular distribution and suppression of HIV-LTR transcription. Virology 187:46–55.

289. Yu, X.-F., S. Ito, M. Essex, and T.-H. Lee. 1988. A naturally immunogenic virion-associated protein specific for HIV-2 and SIV. Nature 335:262–265.

290. Yu, X.-F., Q.-C. Yu, M. Essex, and T.-H. Lee. 1991. The *vpx* gene of simian immunodeficiency virus facilitates efficient viral replication in fresh lymphocytes and macrophages. J. Virol. 65:5088–5091.

291. Zack, J. A., S. J. Arrigo, S. R. Weitsman, A. S. Go, A. Haislip, and I. S. Y. Chen. 1990. HIV-1 entry into quiescent primary lymphocytes: molecular analysis reveals a labile, latent viral structure. Cell 61:213–222.

292. Zhang, C., C. Rasmussen, and L. J. Chang. 1997. Cell cycle inhibitory effects of HIV and SIV Vpr and Vpx in the yeast *Schizosaccharomyces pombe*. Virology 230:103–112.

293. Zhang, L., P. J. Dailey, T. He, A. Gettie, S. Bonhoaffar, A. S. Perelson, and D. D. Ho. 1998. Rate of SIV particle clearance in rhesus macaques. Presented at the Fifth Conference on Retroviruses and Opportunistic Infections, Chicago.

294. Zhao, Y., J. Cao, M. R. G. O'Gorman, M. Yu, and R. Yogev. 1996. Effect of human immunodeficiency virus type 1 protein R (*vpr*) gene expression on basic cellular function of fission yeast *Schizosaccharomyces pombe*. J. Virol. 70:5821–5826.

295. Ziegler, S. F., C. B. Wilson, and R. M. Perlmutter. 1988. Augmented expression of a myeloid-specific protein tyrosine kinase gene (Hck) after macrophage activation. J. Exp. Med. 168:1801–1810.

10

The Interface
between the
Pathogenesis
and Treatment
of HIV Infection

MARK B. FEINBERG

Twenty Years of Progress

In the 20 years since the first description of the acquired immunodeficiency syndrome (AIDS), substantial progress has been made in the identification of the etiologic agent of the disease, the discovery of key aspects of the natural history and pathogenesis of HIV infection, and the derivation of an array of effective antiretroviral drugs and treatment strategies. With the introduction of new, more effective antiviral drugs, therapeutic strategies can be designed to accomplish lengthy and near complete suppression of virus replication in many HIV-infected persons. The inherent tendency of HIV to generate drug-resistant variants, due to the poor fidelity of its mechanisms of genome replication and the multiple rounds of virus replication occurring each day in HIV-infected individuals, remains the main obstacle limiting the ability of antiviral drugs to inhibit virus replication and delay disease progression. However, recent insights into the biology of HIV replication and the molecular basis of antiviral drug resistance suggest approaches for the use of antiviral agents in ways that delay or even prevent the emergence of drug-resistant viruses. Although substantial uncertainties remain about key aspects of the pathogenesis of AIDS, it is likely that more is now known about the virology and immunology of HIV infection than any other viral disease affecting humans. In addition, the interface between the emerging understanding of disease pathogenesis and efforts to develop increasingly successful strategies to treat the infection has been exploited more productively in the case of HIV infection than for the treatment of any other infectious disease. Indeed, insights into the in vivo biology of HIV infection have enabled the development of effective strategies to treat an infection that seemed, for a time, to present numerous insurmountable challenges. Likewise, the development of potent antiretroviral drugs provided invaluable tools with which to probe fundamental aspects of AIDS pathogenesis in HIV-infected persons in ways that had never before been attempted or accomplished for any other virus infection. As a result of this mutually informative and beneficial flow of information, it has been possible to derive principles for the treatment of HIV infection that are predicated on key insights into the biology of HIV infection (26, 33, 110). Given the rapidly evolving nature of the field of HIV therapeutics, this chapter focuses on discussion of basic aspects of AIDS pathogenesis that are relevant to the treatment of infected persons and of fundamental biological principles underlying the optimal use of antiretroviral drugs. It is highly likely that these insights into pathogenic mechanisms of HIV infection and the therapeutic approaches derived from them will continue to be refined and extended in the future. However, their pace of change is not expected to be as substantial as in the area of optimal use of specific available (or newly available) antiretroviral drugs and monitoring strategies used to gauge therapeutic success.

There are currently 15 antiretroviral drugs approved by the U.S. Food and Drug Administration (FDA), as well as three coformulated preparations. In addition, active ongoing basic and clinical research efforts to develop newer agents are expected to lead to the availability of a steady flow of new drugs in the future. Given the large and growing number of antiretroviral drugs and continuing discovery of important new aspects of HIV pathogenesis, implementation of clinical treatment practices for the care of HIV-infected persons has commonly outpaced the conduct of clinical trials to define optimal available treatment strategies. As such, contemporary treatment recommendations often reflect a complex balance struck between basic insights into the in vivo biology of HIV infection, data obtained from well-controlled clinical trials, and the practical challenges facing patients using complex and sometimes toxic combination antiretroviral therapy regimens. Consequently, clinicians must struggle to balance those approaches they think are the best for the treatment of HIV-infected patients with those that have been formally demonstrated, through rigorous clinical trials, actually to be the best. Moreover, as our understanding of HIV disease has advanced and the availability of beneficial therapies has increased in both number and intricacy, the complexity of caring for HIV-infected patients has increased substantially. Recent evidence indicates that practitioners familiar with HIV disease treatment provide more effective care for HIV-infected patients than do those with less experience or understanding of the disease process. This disparity will likely continue to widen in the future as therapeutic success increasingly depends on a thorough understanding of HIV disease pathogenesis and on familiarity with when and how to use increasingly effective drugs and monitoring tools to treat HIV infection and its complications. Expert panels convened by the International AIDS Society–USA (http://www.iasusa.org) and the

Department of Health and Human Services (DHHS)/Kaiser Family Foundation (http://hivatis.org) strive to accommodate the rapidly evolving field of clinical treatment of HIV-infected individuals through the issuance of updated treatment guidelines that include guidance concerning the use of current FDA-approved drugs, their specific indications and associated toxicities, and application of monitoring tools to guide initiation and modification of antiretroviral therapy. Readers are referred to these sources for information concerning current treatment recommendations.

Paradigm Shifts and Treatment Advances

The first antiretroviral agents to be developed belonged to the class of drugs referred to as nucleoside analog reverse transcriptase inhibitors (NRTIs; see Chapter 3 in this volume). The earliest available drugs of the NRTI class (e.g., zidovudine, zalcitabine, and didanosine) are now known to possess only modest and transient antiviral activity in vivo. However, the initial availability of these drugs predated the development of sensitive and reliable laboratory measures of plasma HIV RNA levels (so-called virus load assays) that enable accurate assessments of the levels of HIV replication taking place in HIV-infected individuals. Thus, it was not possible at the time for clinicians to gauge the true antiviral effect of therapy in treated patients, and they had to rely on indirect surrogate markers such as CD4$^+$ T-cell counts to discern any evidence of drug efficacy. Furthermore, the NRTIs then available were initially used as single agents in a strategy that is now referred to, since the advent of combination antiretroviral therapy regimens, as "monotherapy." Typically, when an HIV-infected patient would show signs of clinical progression while being treated with a single NRTI, he or she would then be switched to monotherapy with an alternative NRTI. Given that such surrogate markers are an imperfect tool to monitor HIV therapy and that the therapies themselves when used as monotherapies are now appreciated to exert limited, at best, antiretroviral activity, it is not surprising in retrospect that therapeutic benefits of antiviral treatment were so limited and so fleeting at the time (39, 67). Although combinations of two NRTIs (e.g., zidovudine and didanosine or lamivudine) were subsequently shown to afford greater clinical benefits, they too failed to confer substantial and durable improvements in surrogate markers or clinical outcomes (6, 26, 35, 56).

The derivation of more effective treatment strategies would await the development of more potent drugs and the availability of more accurate and sensitive measures of HIV replication in vivo. Furthermore, in the absence of sensitive measures of HIV replication, the natural history of HIV disease and the dynamics and pathogenic consequences of HIV replication remained obscure. Unfortunately, once more effective drugs and treatment strategies emerged, those patients who had followed the recommended course of sequential monotherapy or combination therapy with two NRTIs were often compromised in their ability to benefit from more potent combination antiretroviral therapies as a result of their harboring HIV variants that had accumulated mutations conferring resistance to multiple NRTIs.

The development of substantially more potent antiretroviral drugs, particularly the effective and bioavailable protease inhibitors (PIs; ritonavir and indinavir were the first drugs of this type available), provided the foundation for derivation of far more successful treatment strategies (40). The advent of these drugs alone was not sufficient to alter the long-term clinical outcomes, but key insights about how to do so emerged from thoughtful analyses of the virologic and immunologic data obtained in the course of early-phase clinical trials of these agents (see below). Initial clinical trials of PIs, as well as of the potent non-nucleoside reverse transcriptase inhibitors (NNRTIs; e.g., nevirapine; see Chapter 4 in this volume), that utilized newly developed plasma HIV RNA assays to measure directly antiviral drug activity helped reveal the impressive magnitude of virus replication that takes place each day in HIV-infected persons (58, 87, 111, 137). These studies also helped establish the fundamental relationship regarding how continuing HIV replication in the presence of drug therapy leads to the inevitable selection of drug-resistant viral variants (33, 81, 87, 114, 131, 137).

In addition, analyses of the magnitude and duration of suppression of HIV replication accomplished by different agents led to the recognition that important distinctions exist between the potency of a given antiviral drug and the durability of viral suppression that are based on the number of mutations needed for an HIV variant to display substantially reduced susceptibility to the agent used. Initial studies in which the more potent antiviral agents in the PI and NNRTI classes were used as single agents in "monotherapy" trial designs demonstrated substantially greater, but also frequently transient, antiviral activity in vivo. Study of the viral variants that emerged coincident with the eventual waning antiviral suppression seen in patients treated with PIs or NNRTIs helped define the pattern of genetic alterations in the target genes for the antiviral drugs that are responsible for the observed decreased susceptibility to the drugs employed. These studies yielded the important insight that while certain antiretroviral agents require only a single nucleotide change in the viral genome to confer high-level drug resistance (e.g., the NNRTIs and lamivudine), other agents require the simultaneous presence of multiple mutations in the HIV genome to enable high-level drug resistance (e.g., the PIs) (17, 18, 114). These observations led to the formulation of the very useful concept of the relative "genetic barrier" to resistance development characteristic of a given antiretroviral drug (15). According to this theoretically and practically important concept, agents that require that only single or few mutations be present in the HIV genome to enable high-level resistance are recognized to present "low genetic barriers" to the outgrowth of drug-resistant HIV variants, while those drugs that require multiple mutations for high-level resistance present a "high genetic barrier." Given appreciation of this relationship and the recognition that even the newly available potent agents were by themselves typically unable to suppress HIV replication sufficiently to the extent that emergence of drug-resistant viral variants could be prevented, it was realized that the development of drug-resistant variants and consequent loss of clinical benefit could be avoided only if HIV replication could be maximally suppressed, to below the detection limits of the most sensitive plasma HIV RNA tests available (currently with detection limits of 50 copies of HIV RNA/ml), through the use of logical combinations of multiple antiretroviral drugs that both possess substantial antiviral potency and exert a high genetic barrier to the development of antiviral drug resistance (33, 50). In this way, the likelihood that HIV variants that possess multiple mutations associated with resistance to the sum of the drugs used in the combination are already present in infected individuals *before* initiation of therapy is greatly reduced. Further, once profound suppression of HIV replication is achieved by combination antiretroviral therapy, the ability of the resident virus population to generate new, multiply resistant variants through continuing replication and attendant genetic diversification is greatly limited. Achievement of this goal is now commonly pursued in HIV-infected patients by using the simultaneous initiation and maintenance of anti-HIV therapy with combinations of antiretroviral drugs that inhibit essential HIV-specific enzymes acting at specific phases of the virus life cycle, such as the viral reverse transcriptase (RT) and protease (7, 100).

Given the availability of more potent drugs and a far more complete understanding of HIV replication dynamics and the processes that underlie the emergence of drug-resistant HIV variants, the concept of "highly active antiretroviral therapy" (HAART) emerged. The development of HAART regimens resulted in a veritable revolution in the extent to which antiviral treatment could benefit HIV-infected individuals. Although it was once imagined that the inherent predisposition of HIV to generate drug-resistant variants represented an insurmountable obstacle for the long-term utility of any anti-HIV therapies, it became clear that this tendency could be circumvented by the profound degree of suppression of HIV replication that could be achieved in many infected individuals able to adhere to the demanding treatment regimens. A growing number of antiretroviral drugs have been demonstrated to be effective when used as constituents in a variety of combination antiretroviral therapy regimens to treat HIV-infected individuals. Therapies are now available that effectively and durably suppress HIV replication to below the limits of detection of sensitive plasma HIV RNA assays and that have been clearly shown to be efficacious in increasing CD4 counts, slowing progression to AIDS, and substantially reducing AIDS-associated morbidity and mortality (67, 74, 99).

Along with a rapidly evolving appreciation of the dynamics of virus replication in vivo and the understandable enthusiasm that greeted the advent of HAART therapy, mathematical models predicting the declination of infected cell populations following initiation of combination antiviral therapies led to optimistic predictions about the potential for ultimate eradication of the infection in drug-treated individuals (103). Such optimism soon faded with the recognition that virus replication continues at low levels even in individuals with undetectable levels of plasma HIV RNA and that latently infected cell populations appear to be present in infected persons and are estimated to decay so slowly as to make eradication of the infection by HAART alone exceedingly unlikely (reviewed in reference 106). Further, the practical complexities of adhering to often complicated HAART regimens and dealing with the not infrequent side effects and toxicities associated with their use have made it difficult for many HIV-infected individuals to realize the impressive benefits of HAART observed in some treated patients.

Current Therapeutic Challenges

When used appropriately, combination antiretroviral therapy can result in durable suppression of HIV replication without the development of antiviral drug resistance. However, the emergence within treated individuals of HIV variants that are resistant to multiple antiretroviral drugs is inevitable when adherence to the complicated antiretroviral treatment regimens is insufficient. Successful response to HAART (defined as achievement of durably undetectable levels of plasma HIV RNA) is reported to require that a patient take 90–95% of the recommended drug doses, with lesser degrees of adherence associated with increased risk of virologic failure (101). In addition, individuals who have been treated previously or who have been unsuccessfully treated with incompletely suppressive antiretroviral regimens (such as prior NRTI monotherapy or insufficiently potent combinations of NRTIs) harbor HIV variants that are resistant to important constituent drugs in the available HAART regimens and are at increased risk of virologic failure.

The failure to achieve durable suppression of HIV replication, and consequent development of drug-resistant viral variants (so-called virologic failure), are reported to occur during initial combination therapy of 50% or more of HIV-infected individuals studied in clinic-based cohorts (75, 80). As a result of the widespread use of combination antiretroviral therapies, the relatively high frequency with which virologic failure occurs in routine clinical practice, and the persistent engagement of some treated individuals in behaviors that transmit HIV infection to others, increasing evidence of transmission of drug-resistant HIV variants to newly infected individuals has been observed (62, 69, 77, 119, 139). Widespread dissemination of HIV variants that are resistant to multiple potent antiretroviral drugs will represent a major public health setback, and there is currently no reason to expect that recent trends in this direction will not continue. Furthermore, as indicated previously, although available HAART regimens can accomplish durable suppression of HIV replication, they are unable to eradicate the infection. As such, long-term, likely lifelong, therapy will likely be essential to achieve durable preservation of health. However, in addition to the inconvenience of long-term therapy, available antiretroviral drugs are each associated with known toxicities, and they may also lead to potential yet-to-be-discovered long-term toxicities (100). Last, from a global perspective, the most important limitation of available therapies is the fact that the high cost of effective combination antiretroviral treatment regimens and the requisite intensity of clinical and laboratory monitoring needed to ensure their successful and safe use limit the availability and use of effective HAART regimens in resource-poor countries where more than 95% of all HIV-infected people live (108).

HIV: The Etiologic Agent of AIDS

Taxonomy and Origin of HIV

The etiologic agents of AIDS, HIV-1 and HIV-2, are retroviruses belonging to the subfamily known as Lentivirinae (also known as lentiviruses) (55). Lentiviruses cause a number of naturally occurring, slowly progressive disorders in animals, including various neurologic, musculoskeletal, hematologic, respiratory, and wasting diseases of ungulate (hoofed) mammals. Like HIV-induced AIDS, these lentiviruses establish persistent infections that are not cleared by host immune responses and lead to diseases that are characterized by long incubation periods and protracted symptomatic phases. Prior to the emergence of the AIDS epidemic in 1981 and the discovery of the etiologic agents of the disease, HIV-1 in 1983 and HIV-2 in 1986, lentiviruses had not been known to cause infections in primates or to lead to the development of immunodeficiency diseases. However, the appearance of AIDS and the isolation of HIVs led to analyses of other animal species, particularly nonhuman primates, in a quest to identify the origins of these novel human pathogens, as well as to define model systems that would enable experimental study of the pathogenesis of AIDS and the evaluation of candidate antiviral drugs and vaccines. These studies led to the recognition that HIV-1 and HIV-2 entered human populations via multiple episodes of cross-species (zoonotic) transmission of $CD4^+$ T-cell tropic lentiviruses that originated in chimpanzees (*Pan troglodytes*) and sooty mangabey monkeys (*Cercocebus atys*), respectively (55). Further study of nonhuman primates in Africa has revealed that a startlingly diverse array of species harbor viruses related to HIV in both their genome structures and their tropism for CD4$^+$ cells of the immune system. Genetic analyses of these viruses suggest that they have been present in these natural hosts for tens of thousands of years or longer. Importantly, in all known instances of natural host infection, the virus infection does not lead to immunodeficiency diseases or other AIDS-associated complications. Interestingly, SIV$_{cpz}$-infected chimpanzees and SIV$_{sm}$-infected sooty mangabeys have been shown to exhibit substantial levels of ongoing virus replication and yet do not suffer progressive CD4$^+$ T-cell depletion. Thus, the natural host species that have harbored these viruses for tens of thousands of years or more have evolved host-virus equilibria wherein preservation of health is not dependent on effective immunologic containment of virus replication. Although the mechanisms by which natural hosts for the viral progenitors of HIV-1 and HIV-2 remain healthy have yet to be determined, it appears that the viruses themselves are not inherently pathogenic. Rather, the fact that AIDS arises following zoonotic transfer of these infections to other species (such as humans) suggests that the development of progressive immunodeficiency seen in "non-natural" species is the result of the specific nature of the interaction between both viral *and* host factors. Certainly, AIDS would not be the disease that it is were it not for the evolutionary choice of CD4 as the primary virus receptor made over the millennia in natural nonhuman primate host species. However, the targeting of CD4$^+$ T cells and their death as the direct result of virus infection alone does not appear to be causally sufficient for the development of AIDS. Indeed, accumulating insights into the pathogenesis of AIDS indicate that the disease arises as a result of both the direct cytopathic effects of HIV infection of CD4$^+$ T-cell populations and the deleterious indirect effects that arise following infection as an apparent inadvertent result of the active but ultimately ineffective pro-inflammatory antiviral immune response mounted by the human host.

Both HIV-1 and HIV-2 infections can lead to AIDS, although HIV-1 does so more rapidly and more reproducibly and now represents the most prevalent cause of AIDS worldwide (108, 137). These viruses possess related but distinct genome structures, as HIV-2 lacks the *vpu* gene present in HIV-1 but includes a gene termed *vpx*, which is absent in HIV-1 (55). HIV-1 is responsible for the majority of cases of human immunodeficiency infection and AIDS worldwide, and far more is known about the pathogenesis and treatment of HIV-1 than HIV-2 infection. For this reason, the generic term "HIV" is used to refer to HIV-1 in this chapter. Although the pathogenic mechanisms of HIV-1 and HIV-2 infections are likely to be similar, given described differences in genome structures and in the rates and frequency of disease progression seen in the two infections, it is also likely that important biological differences may exist between them. Most of the antiretroviral agents developed to treat HIV-1 infection (e.g., NRTIs and

PIs) are also active against HIV-2 in vitro, but less is known about how effective they are in treating HIV-2-infected individuals. Furthermore, available NNRTIs that provide very useful drugs for the treatment of HIV-1 infection do not inhibit the replication of HIV-2.

The HIV Life Cycle and Predisposition for Genetic Variation

Replication of HIV depends on a virally encoded enzyme, RT, which is an RNA-dependent DNA polymerase that copies the single-stranded viral RNA genome into a double-stranded DNA in an early and essential step in the virus life cycle (33, 44). Retroviral RTs have an inherently greater rate of nucleotide misincorporation than do the host cell DNA polymerases used to copy host cell chromosomal DNA during the course of cellular replication. Further, unlike cellular DNA polymerases, retroviral RTs lack a 3′–5′ exonuclease activity that serves a "proofreading" function to repair errors made during transcription of the viral genome. As a result, the HIV RT is an "error-prone" enzyme, making frequent errors while copying the RNA into DNA and giving rise to numerous mutations in the progeny virus genomes produced from infected cells. Estimates of the mutation rate of HIV RT predict that an average of one mutation is introduced in every one to three HIV genomes copied (13, 82). Additional variation is introduced into the replicating population of HIV variants as a result of genetic recombination that occurs during the process of reverse transcription via template switching between the two HIV RNA molecules that are included in each virus particle (13, 92). The generation of recombinant HIV variants depends on a host target cell being simultaneously infected with at least two genetically distinct HIV variants and the resultant incorporation of two distinct RNA genomes within single virus particles. The actual process of recombination occurs within a newly infected target cell following infection with such heterozygous virions. Recombination enables favorable mutations to be "mixed and matched" such that the favorable mutations initially present on different viral genomes can be included within the same genome. In this way, detrimental mutations can be repaired, and beneficial mutations can accumulate rapidly within the population of actively replicating HIV variants. Importantly, both pathways for genetic diversification of HIV populations, either through introduction of mutations in the course of reverse transcription or as a result of genetic recombination, are dependent on ongoing virus replication. As such, antiretroviral therapies that effectively block new rounds of virus infection can prevent continued diversification of resident HIV populations that would otherwise inevitably lead to the outgrowth of viral variants with progressively increasing levels of resistance to the antiviral drugs used.

Because of the error-prone nature of HIV replication and the magnitude of HIV replication seen in infected persons, the population of viral variants present in infected persons is highly diverse (13). The rate of appearance of genetic variants of HIV within infected persons is a function of the number of cycles of virus replication that occur during a person's infection. As a result of the substantial magnitude of HIV replication in vivo (see below), it is estimated that a mutation is probably introduced into every position of the HIV genome many times each day within an infected person (13). Indeed, the populations of HIV present within infected persons are best described as "quasi species" of viral variants of distinct genotypes and potentially biological functions. Many mutations introduced into the HIV genome during the process of reverse transcription will compromise or abolish the infectivity of the virus as a result of disruption of the function of essential gene products. However, many other mutations are compatible with virus infectivity. Indeed, the ability of HIV to accommodate a wide array of mutations introduced in the course of virus replication is remarkable and represents a great challenge to the development and application of effective antiretroviral therapies. In HIV-infected persons, the actual frequency with which different genetic variants of HIV are seen is a function of their replicative vigor (or "fitness") and the nature of the selective pressures that may be acting on the existing swarm of genetic variants present (13). Important selective pressures present in HIV-infected persons include the magnitude and specificity of their anti-HIV immune responses, the availability of host cells that are susceptible to virus infection in different tissues, and the use of antiretroviral drug treatments. HIV variants that are well adapted to prevailing selective pressures will come to predominate within the resident virus population during successive cycles of virus replication. However, even less fit viral variants can persist at low levels in infected persons, either through persistent low-level replication or as a result of being "archived" within the population of proviral sequences present in latently infected cells (106). In vivid and clinically significant ways, the processes of natural selection for the most "fit" genetic variants postulated long ago by Darwin are demonstrated each day in the application of antiretroviral therapy for the treatment of HIV infection.

The Identity and Consequences of HIV's Target Cell Preference

Infection with HIV typically leads to the progressive depletion of CD4$^+$ T lymphocytes from peripheral blood and lymphoid organs, ultimately resulting in a state of profound immunodeficiency characterized by susceptibility to a wide variety, but interestingly not all types, of opportunistic infections and neoplasms (8, 54, 132). The same CD4 cell surface molecule that plays an essential role in helper/inducer T-cell antigen recognition though interaction with major histocompatibility (MHC) class II molecules on antigen-presenting cells also serves as the initial cell surface protein that interacts with the HIV surface envelope (Env) glycoprotein, gp120 (44, 54,

137). As such, HIV infection is targeted to cell populations that express CD4 on their cell surfaces, including the helper/inducer T lymphocytes and macrophages (and their counterparts within the central nervous system, the microglial cells). In addition to their expression of the CD4 cell surface protein, HIV infection is focused to CD4$^+$ T cells and macrophages by virtue of their expression of specific chemokine receptors that serve as essential coreceptors for HIV entry into target cells (54). Genetic polymorphisms within the HIV gp120 Env protein determine the preference of a given viral variant for chemokine receptor that is utilized as a coreceptor for virus entry into host cells. The chemokine receptor CCR5 is expressed on activated CD4$^+$ T cells and on macrophages and represents the predominant coreceptor used by most HIV variants, particularly those that are transmitted between individuals and that predominate in the earlier stages of the infection (see Chapter 7 in this volume). The ability to utilize the chemokine receptor CXCR4 as a coreceptor (in addition to CCR5) for entry into target cells is manifest by HIV variants that arise in some (but not all) HIV-infected persons. CXCR4-using HIV variants possess an expanded host range for infection that includes naive CD4$^+$ T-cell populations, and their appearance in infected persons is associated with an accelerated rate of CD4$^+$ T-cell depletion (see below). It is not known why CXCR4-using HIV variants are detectable only in some infected persons and typically only in the later stages of the infection, as given the tremendous ongoing genetic diversification of resident HIV populations, CXCR4-using viral variants are likely to be generated multiple times each day in infected persons. Although both CD4$^+$ T cells and macrophages are readily susceptible to HIV infection in culture, CD4$^+$ T cells represent the substantial majority of all HIV-infected cells in vivo (at least of those present outside the central nervous system) (54). The fact that HIV employs CD4 and the coreceptor molecules CCR5 and CXCR4 as essential host cell surface proteins to gain entry into target cells thus focuses virus-induced pathology on essential cellular components of the immune system.

In addition to CD4 and chemokine receptor molecules used by HIV as primary receptors and coreceptors for entry into target cells, HIV gp120 Env has been recently shown to interact with an additional molecule referred to as DC-SIGN, which is expressed on the surface host dendritic cells that serve as central antigen-presenting cells essential for activation of antigen-specific host immune responses (48). Dendritic cells themselves do not appear to be commonly infected with HIV, but they traffic widely to key lymphoid organs throughout the body and are able to potentiate greatly the susceptibility to HIV infection of adjacent CD4$^+$ T cells within the lymphoid tissues. As such, the interaction of HIV and dendritic cells via gp120 Env–DC-SIGN interactions likely facilitates the dissemination and propagation of HIV infection in vivo. Further, within the peripheral lymphoid organs, such as lymph nodes and spleen, HIV is effectively trapped by and accumulates on the surface of follicular dendritic cells (FDCs) within lymphoid follicles (54). The binding of HIV to FDCs within lymphoid follicles is thought to be primarily mediated by antibody and complement included in immune complexes with HIV and that interact with Fc and complement receptors expressed on the surface of FDCs. Although HIV-coated FDCs are not infected with HIV, they act to place the virus at the precise location where $CD4^+$ T cells become activated in the generation of antigen-specific immune responses.

The fact that most infection events appear to occur in vivo at close proximity and in the setting of immune activation has important implications for our understanding of the pathogenesis of AIDS, as it provides yet another mechanism by which important host immune responses may be compromised. In addition, evidence that many $CD4^+$ T cells become infected in the setting of local episodes of immune activation may also limit the effectiveness of antiviral therapies, as short-range virus transmission may be less effectively inhibited by antiretroviral therapies given the high local concentrations of virus and the proximate availability of highly susceptible target cells (49).

HIV infection exerts direct cytopathic effects on infected $CD4^+$ T cells, and studies of virus replication dynamics suggest that many HIV-infected $CD4^+$ T cells may die shortly after they begin to produce virus particles (see below). Although the precise nature of these cytopathic effects is incompletely understood, specific interactions occurring between the HIV gp120/gp41 Env proteins and the target cell CD4 and CCR5 or CXCR4 coreceptors are believed to play important roles. HIV variants that preferentially utilize the CXCR4 coreceptor for entry are more efficient at mediating fusion of $CD4^+$ T cells (so-called syncytia formation) in tissue culture, and, as mentioned above, their emergence in the course of HIV infection in vivo is associated with an accelerated rate of $CD4^+$ T-cell decline (54). Macrophages are more resistant to the cytopathic consequences of HIV infection than $CD4^+$ T cells and are widely distributed throughout the body. As a result, they may play critical roles in the persistence of HIV infection by providing a reservoir of chronically infected cells, even if they do not represent the predominant target cell for virus infection in vivo. In addition, the microglial cells present in the central nervous system are known to be susceptible to HIV infection and may provide a sanctuary for virus persistence in the setting of antiretroviral therapy, as many of the available antiviral drugs do not cross the blood-brain barrier efficiently. For as yet unclear reasons, early concerns that HIV-infected cells within the central nervous system might also serve as important sites for generation of drug-resistant viral variants, given that ongoing virus replication within this anatomic compartment may occur in the setting of subtherapeutic drugs concentrations, do not appear to have been borne out in the clinical use of HAART therapies.

Susceptibility of target cells to HIV infection, and the amount of virus they produce following infection, are enhanced by the induction of immune activation of CD4$^+$ T cells (44, 54). HIV can enter resting T cells, but efficient progression through the virus replication cycle does not occur unless the target cells are activated by exposure to their cognate antigens or to stimulatory cytokines and proliferating. Once the cells are infected, production of HIV-1 RNA, protein, and virions is augmented by activation of the target T cells. The link between target cell activation and the facility of HIV replication is the cumulative result of processes operative at multiple levels in the virus life cycle. Activation of CD4$^+$ T cells results in increased CCR5 coreceptor expression, enhanced efficiency of the reverse transcription process as a result of increased intracellular nucleotide concentrations, facilitation of the nuclear transport of newly reverse-transcribed HIV genomes, and augmented NF-kB-mediated transcriptional activity of integrated HIV proviruses (44, 54, 106). As a result, HIV infection in vivo is focused on those CD4 T lymphocytes that are activated and actively proliferating. In addition, exposure of HIV-infected individuals to exogenous antigens as a result of infections or immunizations can result in transient increases in the levels of virus replication measured by plasma HIV RNA assays as the likely result of an increased pool of susceptible target cells (127, 128).

CD4$^+$ T-cell activation in HIV-infected individuals can result from a variety of influences, including the generation of immune responses to contemporary antigenic exposures, host compensatory responses to ongoing attrition of overall CD4$^+$ T-cell populations, and the overall heightened state of generalized immune activation seen in the setting of HIV infection (see below). In addition, because HIV itself represents a major antigenic stimulus in HIV-infected persons, it is believed that HIV-specific CD4$^+$ T cells represent important targets for HIV infection and depletion. Depletion of HIV-specific CD4$^+$ T-cell responses is thought to occur early in the course of the initial infection period in most infected persons (116, 117). As CD4$^+$ T cells play critical roles in the induction and maintenance of CD8$^+$ cytotoxic T-lymphocyte (CTL) responses, loss of HIV-specific CD4$^+$ T-cell responses may limit the magnitude and duration of effective HIV-specific CTL responses (116, 135). As a result, the ultimate failure of long-term host containment of HIV replication by the CD8$^+$ CTLs in most infected individuals may be predetermined by substantial damage to the HIV-specific CD4$^+$ T-cell response that appears to occur during the primary infection period. Importantly, recent evidence indicates that the initiation of antiretroviral therapy during primary HIV infection may enable preservation of HIV-specific CD4$^+$ T-cell responses and, potentially, improvement in the treated individual's subsequent ability to contain HIV replication immunologically (see below) (116).

Memory CD4$^+$ T cells are preferential targets for HIV infection in vivo, as evidenced by the preferential localization of HIV proviral load and magnitude of HIV RNA expression within this population (54, 121). As a likely consequence of the preferential infection of immunologically activated cells, early loss of CD4 memory T-cell responses to recall antigens is observed in HIV-infected individuals, even before there are significant decreases in total T-cell numbers. While memory CD4$^+$ T cells may harbor the bulk of the actively replicating pool of HIV, depletion of naive CD4$^+$ and CD8$^+$ T-cell populations is also characteristic of HIV infection (54, 61, 115). Depletion of naive T-cell populations is believed to be the cumulative result of the suppressed bone marrow and thymic function observed in HIV-infected persons, the drain on the naive T-cell populations as a result of a host compensatory response to destruction of mature CD4$^+$ T cells, and the aberrant lymphocyte proliferation associated with the generalized immune system activation seen in HIV-infected persons (30, 54, 61, 85). This generalized state of immune activation evident in HIV-infected individuals leads not only to increased rates of proliferation of CD4$^+$ T cells but to increases in proliferation of CD8$^+$ T cells, B cells, and natural killer (NK) cells as well (61). Although the primary process driving host immune activation is not clear, it likely derives from the ongoing active but incompletely effective attempt made by the host immune system to contain persistent HIV replication.

Although most of the immunologic and virologic assessments of HIV-infected persons have focused on studies of peripheral blood lymphocytes, these cells present in this compartment are estimated to represent only about 2% of the total lymphocyte population of the body (54). The importance of lymphoid organs, which contain the majority of the body's CD4$^+$ T cells, has been highlighted by the finding that the concentrations of virus and percentages of HIV-infected CD4$^+$ T cells are substantially higher in peripheral lymphoid tissues than in peripheral blood (such as lymph nodes and gut-associated lymphoid tissues [GALT], where immune responses are generated and where activated and proliferating CD4$^+$ T cells that are highly susceptible to HIV infection are prevalent). For as yet unidentified reasons, normal lymphoid tissue architecture is gradually damaged over time, which compromises the ability of an HIV-infected person to generate effective immune responses and to replace CD4$^+$ T cells lost through the direct and indirect consequences of HIV infection through the expansion of mature T-cell populations in the peripheral lymphoid compartments (54). In addition to the damage exacted on peripheral T-cell compartments that leads to compromised generation of immune responses and impaired capacity for compensatory expansion of mature CD4$^+$ T cells, HIV infection also affects key tissue compartments essential for lymphocyte production and differentiation (63, 85). The productive capacity of the bone marrow is compromised in the setting of HIV infection, which likely constrains the number of lymphoid progenitor cells available for trafficking to the thymus. The thymus itself is believed to be an early target of HIV infection and damage, thereby limiting T-cell production even in younger persons in whom thymic capacity for production of T lymphocytes remains active. In all, while the depletion of CD4$^+$ T cells following HIV infection is most readily revealed by sampling peripheral blood, damage to the host immune system is exacted in key lymphoid organs throughout the body. Thus, HIV infection compromises multiple anatomic and functional sources of T-cell production, so that the rate of T-cell replenishment cannot match the rate of cell loss. Consequently, total CD4$^+$ T-cell counts decline inexorably in most HIV-infected persons (54).

After initial infection, the pace at which immunodeficiency develops is associated with the rate of decline of CD4$^+$ T-cell counts (34, 54, 129). The rate at which CD4$^+$ T-cell counts decline differs considerably between individuals and is not constant throughout all stages of HIV infection. In the earlier stages of HIV infection, a relative increase of total CD8$^+$ T-cell levels is observed that likely reflects the generalized state of immune activation manifest in individuals experiencing untreated HIV infection (61). In addition, homeostatic regulatory mechanisms that serve to regulate the size of T-cell populations are believed to mount a compensatory response acting to maintain normal levels of total CD3$^+$ T cells through relative increases in the size of the CD8$^+$ T-cell population in the setting of progressive CD4$^+$ T-cell depletion (83). Acceleration in the rate of decline of CD4$^+$ T cells heralds the progression of HIV disease, as does the breakdown of lymphocyte homeostasis manifest by declining CD8$^+$ T cells (and thus total CD3$^+$ T cells). The point of onset of a more rapid fall in CD4 T-cell counts is referred to as the "inflection point" (83). The virologic and immunologic events that occur around this time are incompletely understood at present. However, increasing levels of HIV replication, an even more pronounced state of generalized immune activation, the emergence of HIV variants that exhibit increased cytopathic effects of CD4$^+$ T cells (so-called syncytium-including variants that utilize the CXCR4 coreceptor in addition to CCR5), and declining cell-mediated anti-HIV immune responses are often seen.

Susceptibility to specific opportunistic infections is characteristically manifest at specific ranges of CD4$^+$ T-cell deficiency (132). Although clinical evidence of immunodeficiency can be found even at higher CD4$^+$ T-cell levels (e.g., greater susceptibility to bacterial infections and increased risk of reactivation of latent infections such as those caused by herpes viruses and *Mycobacterium tuberculosis*), susceptibility to disabling or life-threatening opportunistic infections is typically seen once CD4$^+$ T-cell counts fall below 200 cells/mm^3 (e.g., *Pneumocystis carinii* pneumonia). At even lower levels of CD4$^+$ T-cell counts (<50 cells/mm^3), opportunistic infections characteristic of more pronounced immune deficiency are seen (e.g., cytomegalovirus retinitis, and *Mycobacterium avium* complex and serious fungal infections).

Although the progression of HIV disease is most readily gauged by tracking diminishing CD4[+] T-cell counts, numerical defects in specific CD4[+] T-cell subpopulations as well as functional defects in the ability to generate specific types of immune responses have also been described (43, 54, 61). Furthermore, with advancing immunodeficiency, increasing evidence of constriction and skewing of the normally highly diverse CD4[+] T-cell repertoire for antigen recognition is seen (19, 47).

Mechanisms of CD4[+] T-Cell Depletion

The direct cytopathic effect of HIV is well established, but earlier models of AIDS pathogenesis that were predicated solely on the direct HIV-induced killing of CD4[+] T cells (66) have been challenged by a large body of evidence indicating that HIV infection is also associated with major losses of *uninfected* T lymphocytes of both CD4[+] and CD8[+] T-cell lineages (54, 61, 63, 85). Losses of uninfected CD4[+] and CD8[+] T cells are thought to result primarily from abnormally high levels of activation-induced programmed cell death or apoptosis, which in turn appear to be associated with chronic high levels of host immune activation (54, 61). According to recent estimates, more uninfected CD4[+] T cells die as a result of inappropriate apoptosis in HIV-infected persons than as a result of the direct cytopathic effects of virus infection (54). Perhaps not surprisingly, elevated levels of immune activation and lymphocyte apoptosis have been shown to be associated with increased risk of disease progression (78). Indeed, the level of CD8[+] T cell activation in HIV-infected individuals (as assessed by levels of CD38 expression on CD8[+] T cells) has been found to be as strong a predictor of disease progression as plasma virus load, and in the later stages of the disease is even more predictive of subsequent immune deterioration than plasma virus load (78). Upon initiation of HAART, levels of ongoing virus replication fall precipitously, but so do levels of HIV-specific cellular immune responses, and the generalized state of host immune activation similarly resolves (54). Thus, it seems that both the antigen specific immune responses and the attendant generalized immune activation are driven by ongoing virus replication. Thus, HIV disease is not simply the result of viral factors alone, but rather results from a complex balance between the direct impact of the virus infection and the indirect consequences of the host response to infection.

The observation that HIV viremia is maintained by continuous rounds of viral infection and destruction of virus-infected cells led to the formulation of a model in which active HIV replication induces CD4[+] T-cell destruction at a very high rate ($>10^9$ cells/day), resulting in the exhaustion of host capacity for lymphocyte regeneration and ultimately in the collapse of the immune system (66). However, others have suggested that CD4$^+$ T-cell depletion primarily results from the inability of the infected host to replace CD4$^+$ T cells lost to virus infection, rather than from excess CD4$^+$ T-cell destruction alone (63, 85). In this latter model, a key factor would be the extent of direct or indirect HIV-induced interference with proper generative function of bone marrow, thymus, and peripheral sites of lymphocyte proliferation and differentiation. Destruction of proper lymph node structures that accrues during the course of HIV infection, as well as the prevailing increased propensity for lymphocyte apoptosis, may lead to progressive compromise of peripheral T-cell expansion (54). Progressively severe suppression of bone marrow function may contribute to the exhaustion of the CD4$^+$ T-cell regenerative capacity by limiting the production of pre-thymic T-lymphocyte progenitors (85). Observed decreases in recent thymic emigrants in HIV-infected humans assessed by quantitative assessment of T-cell receptor excision circles (TRECs) within CD4 and CD8 T-cell populations suggest that HIV infection results either in the decreased thymic production of naive T cells or in an increased proliferative drain on the pool of naive cells (due to pressure to maintain total T-cell homeostasis and/or due to the prevailing generalized state of immune activation), or both (30, 61). In addition to the compromised production of naive T cells, the regenerative capacity of the mature peripheral T-cell pool, as well as the ability of peripheral T cells to generate effective immune responses, is believed to be impaired as a result of progressive damage to lymph node architecture that accrues with advancing HIV disease (54, 60). Overall, there is compelling evidence that HIV infection results in a significant compromise of the regenerative capacity of the lymphoid compartment.

Coincident with declining levels of both viremia and immune activation induced by HAART, CD4 T-cell counts rise in many treated individuals, but rarely to normal levels and sometimes hardly at all (54, 85). Increased CD4 T-cell counts reflect the cumulative result of a number of beneficial processes including the sparing of uninfected CD4$^+$ T cells from direct destruction by HIV infection, the amelioration of the impairment of lymphocyte regeneration due to lower levels of chronic immune activation, and the decreased levels of lymphocyte apoptosis seen after initiation of HAART (86). The extent to which restoration of CD4$^+$ T-cell populations is achieved in HAART-treated patients varies substantially between individuals and likely depends on a number of important variables, including the degree of virus suppression, the residual structural and functional integrity of essential immune regenerative compartments, and the extent to which the damage inflicted on key immunologic regulatory mechanisms during the preceding period of unopposed HIV infection can be reversed (see below).

Establishment and Maintenance of Persistent Infection

HIV causes a persistent infection that, once established, cannot be cleared by host immune responses and that also appears to be refractory to clearance by seemingly potent antiviral therapies. Multiple mechanisms by which HIV may evade host immune responses have been described. These include escape from cellular and humoral immune responses resulting from the constantly evolving genetic diversity of HIV populations present in infected persons; the fact that the conformation of the gp120 surface Env protein shields key structural domains involved in critical interactions with the chemokine coreceptors for virus entry (e.g., CCR5), making HIV infection refractory to neutralization by the host antibody response; the ability of the HIV *nef* gene product to downmodulate the expression of class I human leukocyte antigen (HLA) molecules on infected cells, making them less readily recognized by HIV-specific CD8$^+$ T cells; and the ability of HIV to establish an immunologically "invisible" latent state of infection in target cells (see Chapter 12 in this volume and reference 87). Furthermore, as HIV infection is known to be facilitated by immune activation of CD4$^+$ T-cell targets, HIV-specific CD4$^+$ T cells may be preferentially infected and lost (54). Indeed, HIV-specific CD4$^+$ T-cell responses appear to be lost early in the course of HIV infection (117). Given that maintenance of antigen-specific CD8$^+$ T-cell responses is known to depend on provision of "help" from antigen-specific CD4$^+$ T cells, the early loss of HIV-specific CD4$^+$ T-cell responses may compromise the magnitude and subsequent durability of the antiviral CD8$^+$ T-cell response (71, 87). Importantly, while initiation of HAART during the first weeks of primary HIV infection appears able to protect HIV-specific CD4$^+$ T-cell responses from being acutely deleted or anergized, these responses do not return once HAART is initiated during the chronic phase of the infection (1, 116). Although it might be hoped that cellular immune responses would provide an effective adjunct to HAART in facilitating clearance of the persistent reservoir of HIV infection, the association between falling viremia and decreasing magnitude of host immune responses likely limits any beneficial role that immune responses might play toward accomplishing this goal (87).

Natural History of HIV Infection

AIDS as a Disease of Progressive CD4$^+$ T-Cell Loss

As detailed above, HIV infection ultimately leads to the development of profound immunodeficiency disease through the attrition of the host's capacity to maintain normal T-lymphocyte populations and to mount protective antigen-specific immune responses (Fig. 10.1). In the absence of effective therapy, the length of time between initial HIV infection and AIDS

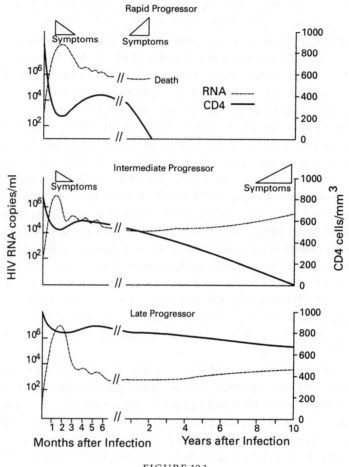

FIGURE 10.1

Generalized time course of HIV infection
and disease progression

Schematic representations of three different patterns of HIV disease
progression: rapid, intermediate, and late progression. A strong direct
relationship is seen between plasma RNA levels and rates of CD4+
T-cell loss and risk of disease progression. However, a number of additional factors have also been identified that influence rates of progression to AIDS, including host genetic background, age, and levels
of cellular immune activation. (Adapted from reference 36.)

averages between 7 and 10 years (34). However, some individuals (~20%)
manifest full-blown AIDS within 5 years of infection, whereas others (<5%)
have sustained long-term (>10 years) asymptomatic HIV-1 infection without significant decline in CD4 counts. Overall, HIV-1 infection results in
progressive immune deficiency, AIDS, and death in 98% or more of all infected but untreated individuals (60). As such, it is likely one of the most

virulent virus infections affecting human populations even if there is a relatively long time interval between initial infection and death.

Only 2% or fewer of HIV-infected persons seem to be able to contain viral replication to extremely low levels and maintain stable CD4 counts within the normal range for lengthy periods (>12–15 years) (5, 60). Within this group commonly referred to as "long-term nonprogressors" (LTNPs), very rare individuals have been found to be infected with HIV-1 variants harboring genetic defects (e.g., *nef* gene deletions) (5). However, most instances of slowly progressive or apparently nonprogressive HIV infection are believed to result from more effective host antiviral immune responses. These individuals tend to have preserved CD4$^+$ T-cell responses to HIV antigens and active and broadly reactive CTL responses against HIV-1-infected cells. An additional important feature of the host virus equilibrium in LTNPs is their ability to control HIV replication effectively without the substantially increased levels of generalized immune activation and lymphocyte apoptosis that accompany progressive HIV disease (19, 87, 117). Whether the maintenance of active and seemingly effective HIV-specific CD4 and CD8 immune responses is directly responsible for preservation of the integrity of host immune system function seen in LTNPs or merely the reflection of it remains unclear (see below and Chapter 12 in this volume).

Certain combinations of MHC genes (referred to as HLAs in humans) that are essential for presentation of antigenic peptides to antigen-specific CD8$^+$ cytotoxic T cells are associated with either relatively rapid or delayed progression to AIDS in infected persons (reviewed in reference 95). Possession of HLA-B27 and HLA-B57 types is associated with slow progression of HIV disease, whereas HLA-B35 is associated with increased rates of progression to AIDS. Individuals who are homozygous at HLA class I loci tend to progress to AIDS more rapidly than those who are heterozygous, presumably as the result of limitations imposed on generation of a diverse antiviral CD8$^+$ T-cell response. These observations indicate that specific aspects of the host immune response to HIV infection may be important determinants of the rate of disease progression (87). However, the precise nature and mechanisms of action of these genetically determined factors have yet to be defined precisely. Inheritance of specific genes other than HLA genes has also been shown to affect the rate of progression of HIV-1 disease, including chemokine coreceptor mutations (both in structural [e.g., CCR5Δ32, CCR5-64I, or CX3CR1] and presumed regulatory regions of certain chemokine receptor genes [e.g., SDF1-3'A]) as well as certain cytokine gene promoter polymorphisms (e.g., IL-10-5'A) (reviewed in reference 95). It is likely that additional important genetic polymorphisms that determine HIV progression rates will be identified as a result of the recent availability of the human genome sequence, the development of high-resolution genetic mapping methods (e.g., analyses of single nucleotide polymorphisms [SNPs]), and the advent of high-throughput technologies to assess patterns of gene expression.

Measuring HIV Replication in Vivo

Levels of ongoing virus replication are most readily and most accurately assessed by quantitative determination of levels of HIV genomic RNA present within virus particles (with each virion containing two copies of HIV genomic RNA) in the plasma fraction of a peripheral blood specimen (36, 44, 105, 118, 132). Plasma HIV RNA concentrations can be quantified by either target amplification methods (e.g., quantitative RT polymerase chain reaction [RT-PCR]) or nucleic acid sequence-based amplification [NASBA]) or signal amplification methods (e.g., branched DNA [bDNA]) (93, 98, 133). Versions of both types of assays are now commercially available, and suggested guidelines for the use of plasma HIV RNA assays in clinical practice have been published (1, 23, 118).

The level of viremia, as measured by the amount of HIV RNA in the plasma, accurately reflects the extent of virus replication in an infected person (66, 103, 136). Although the lymphoid tissues (e.g., lymph nodes and other compartments of the reticuloendothelial system) provide the major sites of active virus production in HIV-infected persons, virus produced in these tissues is released into the peripheral circulation, where it can be readily sampled (54). Immune system activation (by immunizations or intercurrent infections) can lead to increased numbers of activated CD4+ T cells and thereby result in increased levels of HIV replication (reflected by significant elevations of plasma HIV RNA levels) that may persist for as long as the inciting stimulus remains (118, 127, 128, 132). Similarly, initiation of potent antiretroviral therapy leads to rapid decreases in the level of plasma RNA. Thus, measurement of plasma HIV RNA concentrations provides a meaningful and near contemporaneous measure of the level of ongoing virus replication throughout the body, although it is not known whether specific compartments (e.g., the central nervous system) represent sites of infection that are not in direct communication with the peripheral pool of virus.

Predictors of Rates of Progression to AIDS

Plasma HIV RNA can be detected in virtually all HIV-infected persons, although its concentration can vary widely depending on the stage of the infection (Fig. 10.1) and on incompletely understood aspects of the host-virus interactions. During primary infection in adults, when there are numerous target cells susceptible to HIV infection without a countervailing host immune response, plasma HIV RNA levels can exceed 10^7 copies/ml (71, 120). During this period, HIV disseminates widely throughout the body, and many newly infected persons display symptoms of an acute viral illness, including fever, fatigue, pharyngitis, rash, myalgias, and headache (71, 120). Coincident with the emergence of antiviral immune responses, of which the antiviral CTL response is believed to be the most important, plasma HIV RNA levels decline substantially (by 2–3 $\log_{10}$ copies).

After a period of fluctuation, often lasting six months or more, plasma HIV RNA levels usually stabilize around a steady-state "set point" (Fig. 10.1) (88, 89, 90, 96, 97, 120, 130, 131). Although terms such as "steady-state set point" imply a rather static process of HIV infection, important studies that estimated the turnover rates of virus in circulation and the longevity of HIV-infected cells based on the rates of decline of plasma viremia following initiation of HAART indicate that, to the contrary, HIV infection in vivo is a remarkably dynamic process (see Fig. 10.4 and below) (66, 103, 136).

Different infected persons display different steady-state levels of HIV replication. In established HIV infection, concentrations of plasma HIV RNA can range from less than 200 copies/ml in extraordinary persons who have apparently nonprogressive HIV infection to greater than 10^6 copies/ml in persons who are in the advanced stages of immunodeficiency or are at risk for very rapid disease progression. In most HIV-infected and untreated adults, set-point plasma HIV RNA levels range between 10^3 and 10^5 copies/ml. Individuals who have higher steady-state set-point levels of plasma HIV RNA generally lose CD4[+] T cells more quickly, progress to AIDS more rapidly, and die sooner than those with lower HIV RNA set-point levels (70, 88, 89, 90, 96, 97) (Figs. 10.1 and 10.2). Plasma HIV RNA levels provide more powerful predictors of risk for progression to AIDS and death than do CD4[+] T-cell counts; however, the combined measurement of the two values provides an even more accurate method to assess the prognosis of HIV-infected persons (Fig. 10.2) (89). Progressive loss of CD4[+] T cells is observed in all strata of baseline plasma HIV RNA concentrations, but substantially more rapid rates of decline are seen in persons who have higher baseline levels of plasma HIV RNA (89). Likewise, a clear gradient in risk for disease progression and death is seen with increasing baseline plasma HIV RNA levels (Fig. 10.2).

Once established, set-point HIV RNA levels can remain fairly constant for months to years. However, studies of populations of HIV-infected persons suggest a gradual trend toward increasing HIV RNA concentrations with time after infection (97). Within individual HIV-infected persons, rates of increase of plasma HIV RNA levels can change gradually, abruptly, or hardly at all. Progressively increasing HIV RNA concentrations can signal the development of advancing immunodeficiency, regardless of the initial set-point value (97).

That plasma HIV-1 RNA concentrations measured within six months of initial infection are predictive of the rate of CD4 decline and of time to AIDS and death indicates that fundamental aspects of the host-virus rela-

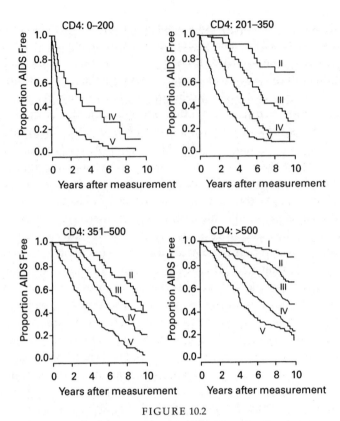

FIGURE 10.2

**AIDS-free survival by baseline plasma
HIV RNA and CD4⁺ T-cell levels**

Kaplan-Meier curves showing AIDS-free survival by baseline measures of plasma HIV RNA and CD4⁺ T-cell counts among groups of persons followed in the Multicenter AIDS Cohort Study demonstrate the strong direct relationship between "set-point" viral load measures and risk of progression to AIDS (89). The five categories of baseline plasma HIV RNA levels (in copies/ml) were (I) <500, (II) 501–3,000, (III) 3,001–10,000, (IV) 10,001–30,000, and (V) >30,000. Within each CD4⁺ T-cell category, baseline plasma HIV RNA concentrations provided significant discrimination of AIDS-free survival times. In the lowest CD4⁺ T-cell category (<200 cells/mm³), there were too few participants with HIV RNA levels of <10,000 copies/ml to provide reliable estimates for RNA categories I to III. In the next lowest CD4⁺ T-cell categories (201–350 and 351–500 cells/mm³), there were too few participants with HIV RNA levels of <500 copies/ml (category I) to provide reliable estimates.

tion for each infected person are established early in the course of the infection. This observation is in accord with additional clinical and laboratory evidence indicating that an individual's initial encounter with HIV-1 in the course of his or her primary infection may herald his or her subsequent rate of disease progression (71). Individuals with severe symptoms of primary HIV-1 infection seem more likely to progress rapidly to AIDS than those with asymptomatic primary infections. Rapid progression may be more likely in persons with a high level of CD8 T lymphocytosis, those who have an impaired or clonally restricted cellular antiviral immune response, or those who mount a limited serological response to the virus. Delineation of the events that occur early in infection and the underlying host-specific factors are essential topics for future research. Likewise, the ability with which antiviral therapy initiated during primary HIV-1 infection, or during the stabilization period that follows, might alter the set point of virus replication and ameliorate the progression of HIV-1 disease is also a critically important issue (see below) (116).

The determinants of viral load set points are incompletely understood but probably include the number of susceptible $CD4^+$ target cells available for infection, the degree of immune activation extant, and the tropism and replicative vigor (fitness) of the prevailing population of HIV variants at various times after the initial infection, as well as the effectiveness of the host anti-HIV immune response (see below). Interestingly, the host-virus relationship responsible for determination of set-point levels of viremia does appear to be relatively characteristic for each individual's HIV infection, as even individuals treated with antiretroviral therapy will return to levels close to or the same as their original pretherapy viremia baselines when they temporarily stop treatment or when treatment fails as a result of development of drug resistance (see below).

Levels of HIV-specific CD4 and CD8 T-cell responses have been reported to be inversely correlated with levels of virus replication, suggesting that the efficacy of the host immune response is an important variable in modulating set-point levels of HIV replication in different infected persons (71, 87, 116). However, precise definition of the role that cellular immune responses play in the determination of ongoing set-point levels of HIV replication has been complicated by both technical and biological issues. For example, it is not known to what extent the reported inverse association between specific cellular immune responses and relative containment of viremia is the cause or consequence of the extent of observed immune system preservation. Furthermore, the use of different assay methods to quantitate HIV-specific $CD4^+$ and $CD8^+$ T-cell responses has led to the generation of apparently conflicting results concerning the relationship between specific cellular responses and in vivo control of HIV replication. Traditional assays for both antigen-specific $CD4^+$ (e.g., proliferative responses) and $CD8^+$ T cell (e.g., limiting dilution chromium-release assays) require that the antigen-specific cells be able to proliferate for a period of time in tissue culture. However, given that lymphocytes obtained from HIV-infected individuals display, to varying degrees, an increased propensity to undergo apoptosis ex vivo, they can be impaired in their ability to proliferate in tissue culture, thereby leading to potential inaccuracies in the estimation (the magnitude of which may differ in different individuals) of the number of HIV-specific lymphocytes actually present in vivo. While assessment of HIV-specific CD4+ T-cell responses by standard antigen-specific proliferative responses in culture clearly finds an inverse association between the magnitude of HIV-specific proliferation and levels of plasma HIV RNA (117), measurement of HIV-specific CD4+ T-cell responses by flow cytometric determination of HIV-antigen-induced intracellular cytokine (e.g., interferon-gamma production by CD4+ T cells) fails to demonstrate a clear association between cellular responses and viremia in many HIV-infected individuals (109). Similarly, when traditional chromium-release assays are used for assessment of HIV-specific CD8+ cytotoxic T cells, an inverse correlation between cellular responses and plasma viremia has been reported (87). However, more recent measurements of HIV-specific CD8+ T-cell responses by intracellular cytokine production assays have disclosed high-level HIV-specific CD8+ T-cell responses in patients with chronic low, as well as high, levels of viremia (46). Such evidence indicating that different individuals with similar levels of HIV-specific CD8+ T cells assessed by available immune function assays can have substantially different levels of plasma viremia suggests that HIV-specific immune responses may differ in important qualitative as well as quantitative ways (46). Furthermore, although host cellular immune responses may help modulate the levels of ongoing virus replication and thus potentially slow the rate of disease progression, they most often fail in the long run, as the vast majority of HIV-infected individuals will ultimately progress to AIDS in the absence of effective antiretroviral therapy.

HIV Replication Dynamics

The steady-state concentration of HIV-1 RNA present in the plasma is a function of the rates of production and clearance (collectively referred to as "turnover") of the virus in circulation. Assessment of kinetic rates of virus turnover requires that some disturbance of the steady-state system—for example, that provided by the initiation of effective antiviral therapy—be used to allow measurement of viral clearance, the magnitude of virus production, and the longevity of virus-producing cells. Influential studies estimating virus turnover rates in this way have revealed a very dynamic process of virus production and clearance that underlies the seemingly static steady-state level of HIV-1 virions in the plasma (66, 136). Measurement of the slope of the initial fall in viremia after initiation of potent antiviral therapy was utilized to formulate mathematical models that enabled estimation of the rates of clearance and half-lives of HIV-1 virions (66, 102, 103, 136). The actual turnover and identity of various compartments of viruses and infected cells were inferred for the time course of decline of plasma viremia, as these cannot be measured directly in vivo because of methodological limitations. Thus, the primary utility of such models is to help clarify concepts of HIV replication dynamics and guide future experimental study, and they do not necessarily describe the actual in vivo circumstances of HIV infection. In this regard, the initial modeling studies of HIV replication dynamics resulted in substantial advances in our appreciation of the nature and magnitude of HIV replication that occurs daily within infected individuals, and the predictions of these models have had profound effects on the formulation of more effective treatment strategies for HIV infection. More recently, however, a number of these fundamental assumptions that underlie the initial models of HIV dynamics, and some of the predictions derived from them, have been questioned on both experimental and theoretical grounds (10, 11, 29, 37, 38, 45, 49, 52, 106, 112, 126, 138, 140). In particular, these models assumed that the antiretroviral treatment regimens employed in the studies completely blocked new cycles of infection of target cells in HIV-infected individuals and that the rate of decline of viremia observed reflected the progressive diminution of distinct populations of cells that were infected *before* the initiation of treatment (66, 103). Yet recent data indicate that the rates of decline of viremia (and thus the rates of turnover of different compartments of cells and virus calculated using original dynamic models) are influenced by the potency of the antiviral regimen used and that HIV replication continues at a low level even in treated patients with plasma HIV RNA levels below the limit of detection of sensitive quantitative assays (29, 49, 106, 112, 126, 140). Further, these models were predicated on the assumption that the decline, or "decay," of infected cells could be ascribed a "half-life" analogous to the decay of radioactive elements, wherein an infected cell would have an equal chance of dying at any moment after infection (66, 136). Application of such terminology to describe the longevity of HIV-infected cells has been questioned, as the timing of cell death following HIV infection is likely better described as an aging process in which cells that have been infected for longer periods of time have a higher chance of dying (49). Nevertheless, the approaches and predictions of these initial modeling efforts are still worth considering in detail, especially in light of how vividly they highlight the challenges confronted in the treatment of HIV infection and how accessibly they clarify the contemporary principles of HIV therapy that enable a number of these important obstacles to be overcome (see Fig. 10.4).

Within two weeks of initiation of potent antiretroviral therapy, plasma HIV RNA levels usually decrease to approximately 1% of their initial values (Fig. 10.3). The slope of this initial decline has been proposed to reflect

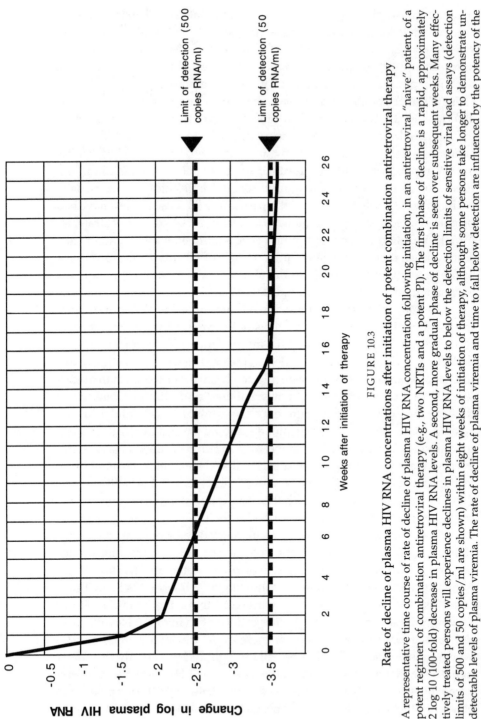

FIGURE 10.3

Rate of decline of plasma HIV RNA concentrations after initiation of potent combination antiretroviral therapy

A representative time course of rate of decline of plasma HIV RNA concentration following initiation, in an antiretroviral "naive" patient, of a potent regimen of combination antiretroviral therapy (e.g., two NRTIs and a potent PI). The first phase of decline is a rapid, approximately 2 log 10 (100-fold) decrease in plasma HIV RNA levels. A second, more gradual phase of decline is seen over subsequent weeks. Many effectively treated persons will experience declines in plasma HIV RNA levels to below the detection limits of sensitive viral load assays (detection limits of 500 and 50 copies/ml are shown) within eight weeks of initiation of therapy, although some persons take longer to demonstrate undetectable levels of plasma viremia. The rate of decline of plasma viremia and time to fall below detection are influenced by the potency of the antiretroviral combination used and the initial plasma HIV RNA values. Even when plasma RNA levels are below the limits of quantitation of sensitive assays, recent evidence indicates that HIV replication may continue at very low levels in patients who are treated successfully from a clinical perspective.

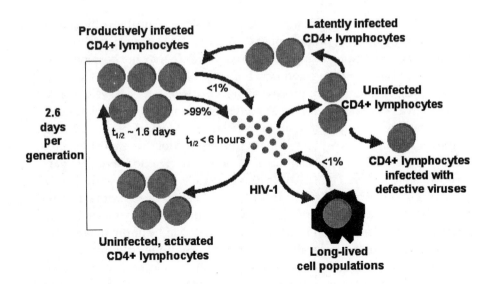

FIGURE 10.4

HIV and CD4+ T-cell population dynamics in vivo

The steady-state level of HIV RNA in the plasma is a function of the rates of production and clearance (i.e., the turnover) of the virus in circulation. Effective antiretroviral therapy perturbs this steady state and allows an assessment of the kinetic events that underlie it. Using data describing rates of decline of plasma HIV RNA levels following potent antiretroviral therapy, mathematical modeling approaches have been employed to estimate the rates of virus clearance, the magnitude of virus production, and the longevity of virus-producing cells (103). These studies indicate that HIV replication in vivo is a very dynamic process involving rapid turnover of virus in the plasma and multiple cycles of virus infection of previously uninfected cells that survived for only a short period following production of new virions. Additional minor sources of virus found in plasma, including production from long-lived macrophages or recently activated latently infected cells, are also envisioned by these models. Such formulations are conceptually very important, but it is important to note that they remain "models" of HIV infection and that the precise identity and fate of virus-infected cells in HIV infected persons, and how these are affected by antiretroviral therapy, are still being elucidated. (Adapted from reference 103.)

the clearance of virus from the circulation and the longevity of recently infected CD4+ T cells (66, 102, 103). The half-life of virions in circulation is calculated to be exceedingly short—in the range of less than 6 hours. Thus, on average, half of the population of plasma virions turns over every 6 hours or less. With the definition of such a short and rather constant half-life of HIV virions in circulation, it appears that the main determinant of steady-state concentrations of HIV in an infected person is the amount of virus production taking place in his or her body at any point in time. Given such a rapid rate of virus clearance, it has been estimated that up to 10^{10} (or more) virions are produced each day to maintain the steady-state plasma HIV RNA levels typically found in persons who have moderate to advanced HIV disease. Clearance rates do not vary substantially among persons with different pretreatment CD4 counts or plasma HIV RNA concentrations, suggesting that plasma virus clearance may not be dependent on specific host immune responses. Rather, virion clearance may be via a high-capacity, nonimmune process of the reticuloendothelial system or result from a potential inherent thermodynamic instability of the virus.

When new rounds of virus replication are blocked by potent antiretroviral drugs, it is estimated that virus production from most infected cells (approximately 99%) continues for only a short period, averaging approximately 2 days (102, 103). In these models, the slope of decline of viremia is thought to reflect the loss of CD4[+] T cells infected with HIV, presumably resulting from the direct cytopathic effects of virus infection, with the average half-life of an infected cell estimated to be approximately 1.6 days. The estimated generation time of HIV (the time from release of a virion until it infects another cell and results in the release of a new generation of virions) is approximately 2.5 days, which implies that the virus is replicating at a rate of approximately 140 or more cycles per year in an infected person (13, 102, 103). Thus, at the median period between initial infection and the diagnosis of AIDS, it is estimated that each virus genome present in an HIV-infected person is removed by more than 1,000 generations from the virus that initiated the infection (13).

After the initial rapid decline in plasma HIV RNA levels following initiation of potent antiretroviral therapy, a slower decay of the remaining 1% of initial plasma HIV RNA levels is observed (Fig. 10.3). The length of this second phase of virus decay differs among different persons, lasting approximately 8 to 28 days. According to initial models, most of the residual viremia measured during this second phase of decay was proposed to have been produced by infected macrophages (102, 103). It was estimated that these infected macrophages are lost with an average half-life of about 2 weeks, whereas the remainder of the residual viremia has been suggested to be produced after activation of latently infected CD4[+] T cells that decay with an average half-life of about 8 days. Alternatively, it has been suggested by others that virus released from FDCs in the lymph nodes may also contribute to this second phase of decay of viremia (54, 106). Depending on the potency of the antiretroviral regimen used and the initial baseline level of plasma HIV RNA, plasma HIV RNA levels commonly decrease below the levels of detection of even the most sensitive plasma HIV RNA assays available (sensitivity of 50 copies of HIV RNA/ml of plasma) within 8–14 weeks of initiation of potent antiretroviral therapy (in previously untreated patients), indicating that new rounds of HIV infection are profoundly suppressed (Fig. 10.3) (7, 132). Fortunately, this level of suppression of HIV replication appears to be maintained in most previously untreated patients who are able to adhere to effective combination antiretroviral drug regimens (51).

The slope of the initial rate of decline in levels of plasma HIV RNA observed following initiation of therapy is influenced by the potency of the drugs used in combination in the HAART regimen employed (49). More potent antiretroviral regimens have been shown to lead to faster rates of decline of plasma viremia following initiation of therapy and more rapid attainment of undetectable levels of plasma HIV RNA. In addition, individuals with higher baseline levels of plasma HIV RNA (e.g., >100,000 copies/ml) or lower $CD4^+$ T-cell counts, or both, may take longer to reach undetectable levels of viremia and are less likely to maintain them durably if achieved (9, 23, 110). Patients who have been treated previously with other antiviral regimens (and who may harbor HIV variants with reduced overall susceptibility to the HAART regimen employed) may experience more gradual rates of decline and may also be less likely to reach and maintain undetectable levels of plasma viremia. From a practical perspective, individuals with higher baseline levels of plasma HIV RNA and those with histories of prior antiretroviral drug use should be treated with HAART regimens of greater-than-usual potency, such as those that include more drugs (than the "standard" three-drug regimens of two NRTIs plus one PI or NNRTI) and agents from additional classes (e.g., NNRTIs in addition to NRTIs and PIs).

Although HAART can achieve suppression of HIV replication to below the limits of detection of sensitive plasma HIV RNA assays in many treated patients, this marked pharmacological interference with HIV replication does not lead to eradication of the infection and does not necessarily even mean that virus replication has been blocked entirely. Individuals who discontinue effective combination antiretroviral therapy after even prolonged periods with undetectable levels of plasma HIV RNA typically show rapid rebounds in HIV replication, clearly indicating that the infection persists despite the most effective antiretroviral therapies available. Futhermore, infectious HIV can still be isolated from $CD4^+$ T cells obtained from antiretroviral-treated persons whose plasma HIV RNA levels have been suppressed to undetectable levels (<50 copies/ml) for prolonged periods (10, 11, 37, 38, 138). Viruses recovered from such individuals most often exhibit preserved susceptibility to the antiretroviral drugs used, suggesting that a reservoir of latently infected resting $CD4^+$ T cells exists in infected persons and can maintain HIV infection for prolonged periods even when new cycles of virus replication are blocked (see below) (106). It is not known whether infected persons have additional reservoirs of residual HIV infection that can permit persistence of HIV infection despite profound inhibition of virus replication by effective combination antiretroviral therapies. Infection with HIV within the central nervous system represents an additional potential sanctuary for virus persistence because many of the antiretroviral drugs now available do not efficiently cross the blood-brain barrier. However, the actual contribution of this reservoir to the persistence of HIV infection has been difficult to determine directly owing to its inaccessibility to sampling in living persons (106).

Latently infected cells cannot be visualized directly but rather are defined experimentally as purified resting CD4+ T cells from which replication-competent HIV can be isolated following activation of these cells in tissue culture (reviewed in reference 106). It is imagined that latently infected cells defined by this method harbor HIV proviruses that are maintained in a transcriptionally inactive state. As viral RNA, and thus HIV proteins, would not be expressed in this setting, latently infected CD4+ T cells would not be recognized and cleared by host HIV-specific immune responses (87, 106). Furthermore, because all available antiretroviral drugs act through inhibition of stages of the HIV replication cycle, they have no activity against latently infected cells. The majority of CD4+ T cells detected in HIV-infected individuals that are found to harbor HIV proviruses have integrated genomes that are replication defective and are likely to have been produced as a result of the acquisition of lethal mutations due to error-prone RT-dependent replication (13, 54). In contrast, the numerically less common population of latently infected cells is thought to harbor genetically intact proviruses whose transcription is induced following immunologic activation of the cell and can subsequently be transmitted to new target cells (54, 106). Most of the latently infected pool of infected CD4+ T cells is contained within the memory T-cell population, as is expected given that the cells would have had to have been activated previously in order to have become infected initially (54, 106). Measurement of the rate of decline of the latently infected reservoir of CD4+ T cells determined by this method suggests that it has a very long half-life, estimated to be approximately 44 months (106). If these estimates are accurate, eradication of this reservoir of latently infected CD4+ T cells by available HAART regimens would require more than 60 years of treatment, thus rendering prospects for clearance of the infection by antiretroviral therapy alone unrealistic.

In addition to the revelation of an apparent long-lived pool of latently infected CD4+ T cells, application of highly sensitive molecular amplification methods indicates that plasma HIV RNA can still be persistently detected in a proportion of treated individuals whose plasma RNA levels are (and remain) below the limits of *quantitation* of the sensitive commercially available viral load assays currently available (<50 copies RNA/ml) (45). Persistently very low levels of HIV RNA are detected in the plasma of some patients, "blips" of detectable virus are observed in others, and still other HAART-treated individuals do not have any plasma HIV RNA detected at any time. Additionally, recent studies indicate that persistent evidence of HIV RNA transcription, as well as unintegrated DNA intermediates in the HIV replication cycle that provide molecular markers of recent de novo infection events, can be detected within peripheral blood and lymph node cells in individuals with "undetectable" plasma HIV RNA (29, 45, 112, 126, 140). Nucleotide sequence analysis of HIV genomes detected under these circumstances displays evidence of continuing (but relatively slow) genetic evolution, and this evidence is also consistent with the notion that ongoing low-level HIV replication takes place in individuals who are being effectively treated, from a clinical perspective, with HAART (52, 60, 74, 129). Interestingly, individuals with persistently detectable HIV RNA and those with periodic "blips" of virus replication display reservoirs of "latently" infected cells that are estimated to decline more slowly in the setting of HAART therapy (112). This observation calls into question the true meaning of HIV "latency," as it is currently impossible to distinguish between a long-lived reservoir of latently infected cells and a pool of shorter-lived infected cells that is continuously replenished by ongoing low-level HIV replication. Should persistence of HIV infection be maintained by the inability of current antiretroviral therapies to inhibit HIV replication completely and thus enable cessation of constant low-level propagation of the infection, it is conceivable that the development of even more potent anti-retroviral regimens (or perhaps immunologic interventions) may ultimately enable eventual eradication of the infection (49). However, should HIV latency within infected cells in vivo be experimentally proven to be a reality, in addition to theoretical construct, then this optimistic suggestion will be invalidated.

It is not yet known whether ongoing replication during HAART is the result of anatomic sanctuaries where antiviral drugs do not adequately penetrate, the result of activation of HIV production from latently infected cells, or the difficulty of inhibiting the transmission of HIV between cells that are in close proximity, which is postulated to be a major mode of HIV transmission in vivo (49, 106). More recently developed models of HIV replication dynamics that accommodate the notion that HAART does not completely block new rounds of HIV infection of target cells (a foundation of initial models described above) and their predications are also consistent with the observed rates of decline of plasma viremia following initiation of therapy (49). These newer models imagine that HAART therapy decreases the amplitude of HIV infection cycles but does not completely block new rounds of infection. As such, it suggests that rates of decline of viremia actually track the virus produced by cells that were infected *after,* rather than before, the initiation of therapy (as had been proposed in initial dynamic models). In this model, multiple and difficult-to-inhibit bursts of HIV replication are proposed to occur in infected persons in association with localized immune activation events. In this setting, the ability of HAART to decrease the amplitude of ongoing HIV infection cycles can progressively attenuate with time and may cease altogether at a lower steady-state level of virus load. This model predicts that more potent drug combinations would lead to more rapid reductions in levels of plasma viremia following initiation of therapy and is consistent with recent data obtained in clinical studies. However, like the initially described mathematical models of HIV replication dynamics, these newer models will be useful primarily if their predictions can be evaluated experimentally and help lead to new insights into AIDS pathogenesis and improvements in the therapy of HIV infection.

Importantly, the levels of virus replication observed in individuals with evidence of ongoing virus replication (detected by exceptionally sensitive methods but below the quantitation limits of the most sensitive commercially available plasma HIV RNA assays [<50 copies HIV RNA/ml]) do not seem to be sufficient to enable the development and eventual outgrowth of drug-resistant HIV variants. Thus, if HIV replication is suppressed to below the limit of detection of sensitive viral load assays, potent HAART regimens now available appear to be able to prevent the development of resistance durably, even in instances in which they do not completely block new rounds of HIV infection (51, 60, 74, 107, 111, 129). It will be important to evaluate in future studies whether the ultimate long-term risk of outgrowth of drug-resistant HIV variants in treatments is made even less likely if more potent HAART regimens are employed.

Therapeutic Implications of HIV Replication and Population Dynamics

Emerging insights into the dynamics of HIV replication in vivo raise a number of issues of great practical importance to optimal therapeutic application of antiretroviral therapy in clinical practice (7, 36, 132). Because of the error-prone nature of the HIV RT used to replicate the viral RNA genome into a DNA copy with each cycle of virus infection, the rate of appearance of genetic variants of HIV-1 within infected persons is a function of the number of cycles of virus replication that take place during the course of an individual's infection. That numerous rounds of replication are taking place every day in infected persons thus provides the opportunity to generate large numbers of variant viruses, including those that may display diminished sensitivity to antiviral drugs. Indeed, it is believed that a mutation is probably introduced at every position in the HIV genome many times each day within an infected person (13). Further, as the process of retroviral recombination is also inherently linked to ongoing cycles of virus replication, it is likely that frequent recombination events occur each day among the diverse constituency of viral quasi species that represent the replicating pool of HIV within infected individuals (92). Importantly, as a result of the great genetic diversity and dynamic nature of the resident virus population, viruses harboring mutations that confer resistance to individual antiretroviral drugs (and possibly combinations of drugs) are often present in infected individuals *before* therapy is initiated. Indeed, mutations that confer resistance to NRTIs, NNRTIs, and PIs have been identified in HIV-infected persons who have never been treated with antiretroviral drugs (58, 73). For drugs such as lamivudine and nevirapine (and other NNRTIs), single nucleotide changes in the HIV RT gene (and that give rise to single amino acid changes in the protein) can confer 100- to 1,000-fold reductions in drug susceptibility (114, 123). Thus, although these agents may be potent inhibitors of HIV replication, their antiretroviral activity when they are used alone (or in incompletely suppressive regimens) is largely reversed within four weeks of initiation of therapy owing to the rapid outgrowth of drug-resistant variants (58, 123, 136). The rapidity with which drug-resistant variants emerge in this setting is consistent with the predictions of the existence of drug-resistant subpopulations of the HIV within infected patients *before* the initiation of treatment (13, 58). The likelihood that drug-resistant variants are present in an infected person decreases as the number of non-cross-resistant antiviral drugs used in combination is increased (13, 36).

Should therapy effectively inhibit HIV replication in an infected person, a fall in plasma HIV RNA should be observed within the first days of treatment (see Fig. 10.3) (7, 132). Likewise, if drug-resistant variants are present and possess sufficient replicative ability, decreases in plasma HIV RNA will not be seen or will be of limited magnitude and of very short duration. With potent combinations of antiviral drugs now available, plasma HIV RNA concentrations become undetectable after initiation of HAART in most previously untreated patients within two to three months of initiation of therapy (see Fig. 10.3) (7, 132). Should drug-resistant viruses not appear and HIV RNA levels remain below detectable levels for months, drug-resistant viruses are unlikely to emerge as long as therapy is continued at effective doses. Incomplete suppression of HIV-1 replication (as indicated by the continued presence of detectable plasma HIV-1 RNA while on therapy) will afford the opportunity for continued accumulation of mutations that may confer high-level drug resistance and thereby facilitate the eventual outgrowth of the resistant virus population during continued therapy.

The most effective and only reliable method to accomplish durable suppression of HIV replication to undetectable levels is to use logical combinations of antiretroviral drugs that possess sufficient potency and present a sufficiently high genetic barrier to the outgrowth of HIV variants that harbor multiple mutations responsible for conferring diminished susceptibility to the agents included in the HAART regimen (Fig. 10.5) (7, 15, 36, 132). Thus, the clear goal of antiretroviral therapy is to suppress HIV replication to below the levels of detection of the most sensitive plasma HIV RNA assays available. While this does not necessarily mean that HIV replication has been completely abrogated, it does appear to represent a sufficiently severe restriction on virus growth to be able to prevent the emergence of viral variants that are simultaneously resistant to multiple

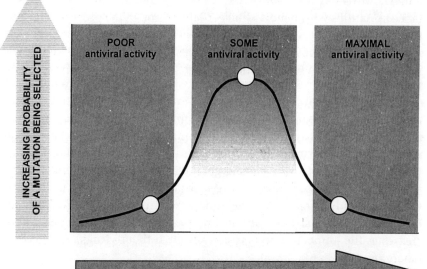

FIGURE 10.5

Relationship between antiviral drug potency
and selection of drug-resistant viral variants

Potent suppression of HIV replication is necessary to prevent the emergence of drug-resistant HIV variants. The selective pressure exerted on resident HIV quasi species by HIV therapy depends on both the potency of the regimen used and the number of mutations required for a given viral variant to exhibit high-level drug resistance. The relationship between antiviral activity and probability of resistant virus selection is shown. At low levels of antiviral potency, selection pressures for drug resistance are relatively low, but inhibition of virus replication is ineffective, and no durable clinical benefit is seen. Increasing levels of antiviral activity increase the probability that drug-resistant variants will be selected, but only up to a point. At high levels of antiviral activity, virus replication is inhibited to the extent that the chances of resistant virus generation through accumulation of new mutations generated by RT errors and recombination (which both depend on ongoing replication) are reduced. To achieve durable suppression of HIV replication and prevent the emergence of drug-resistant variants effectively, it is essential that potent drugs be used in combination so as to block new rounds of virus replication effectively. It is also essential that the drugs used exert a high "genetic barrier," requiring that variant viruses harbor multiple mutations in order to be simultaneously resistant to all the antiretroviral agents used in combination. The higher the genetic barrier, the less likely it is that variant viruses will preexist in infected persons that will already be resistant to combination therapy. If new rounds of replication are blocked, new resistant viruses cannot be generated. (Adapted from reference 15.)

antiviral drugs. If HIV cannot replicate, it cannot accumulate new resistance mutations within individual genomes through the process of reverse transcription, and it cannot create hybrid genomes that manifest high-level multidrug resistance by assembling diverse mutations that were initially present on distinct viral genomes through the process of genetic recombination.

The initiation and maintenance of antiretroviral therapy with optimum doses of combinations of potent antiviral drugs provide the only reliable strategy to forestall (or prevent) the emergence of drug-resistant viruses and achieve maximum protection from HIV-induced immune system damage. From a practical perspective, combination therapy should be initiated with all drugs started simultaneously. Once therapy is initiated, it must be continued at recommended effective doses. At any time after initiation of therapy, underdosing with any one agent in a combination or administering fewer than all drugs of a combination at any one time should be avoided. Antiretroviral drug resistance is less likely to occur if all antiretroviral therapy is temporarily stopped than if the dosage of one or more of the components is reduced or if one component of an effective suppressive regimen is withheld. Importantly, adherence to therapy must be actively encouraged through extensive patient education about the goals of and rationale for therapy, as inadequate adherence greatly increases the risk of development of drug-resistant HIV variants (7, 132). Efforts to increase the simplicity and tolerability of combination antiretroviral therapy regimens will likely facilitate patient adherence.

Because many of the available antiretroviral drugs select for HIV variants that harbor the same or related mutations, specific treatments can select for the outgrowth of HIV variants that are resistant to drugs of the same class of antiretroviral agents (e.g., NRTIs, NNRTIs, and PIs) with which the patient has not been treated (referred to as "cross-resistance") (7, 65, 132). Cross-resistance is a major limitation of the NNRTIs (see Chapter 4 in this volume). Although drugs such as nevirapine and efavirenz are potent, they are quite "fragile" in the sense that they present only a low genetic barrier to the selection of (preexisting) highly resistant viruses. Further, once the outgrowth of NNRTI-resistant viruses occurs, the degree of cross-resistance seen between available agents precludes the subsequent ability of any available members of this drug class to inhibit replication (7, 65, 132). Cross-resistance to PIs is also a critical concern; however, it is a genetically more complex phenomenon (see Chapter 5 in this volume) (17, 18, 31, 81, 91, 94). The initial mutations in the protease gene that are present in HIV variants with reduced susceptibility to PIs that emerge in patients whose levels of HIV replication are inadequately suppressed on PI-containing regimens are typically those that affect the binding of the drug to the active site of the enzyme (so-called primary mutations). While replication of these variants is less susceptible to inhibition by PIs, they are typically also impaired in their ability to replicate and are therefore less fit. However, when they are provided with the opportunity to continue to replicate as a result of inadequate drug inhibition of new cycles of HIV infection, additional mutations will accumulate in the protease genes of the replicating pool of HIV variants that enable the virus to become increasingly fit and to replicate to progressively higher levels. These secondary, so-called compensatory mutations do not affect drug action per se but do enable substantial increases in the activity of the protease function in variants that harbor primary resistance mutations and thereby facilitate the ability of the resistant viruses to replicate in the presence of the drug (17, 81, 84). As such, high-level resistance to PIs requires the acquisition of *multiple* mutations in the resident population of HIV, thus explaining the high genetic barrier exerted by drugs of this class (15). Because multiple mutations are required to achieve high-level resistance to PIs, some of which notably impair the fitness of the virus, variants that simultaneously harbor all the requisite mutations associated with reduced susceptibility to PIs, along with the mutations required for compensated fitness, likely do not preexist in PI-naive individuals.

Viral variants that harbor mutations associated with reduced fitness will, by definition, grow less efficiently and will be less well represented among the resident HIV quasi species (13). However, once drug treatment is initiated, preexisting populations of drug-resistant viruses can rapidly predominate, and individual mutations associated with drug resistance or that enable greater viral fitness in the presence of other mutations conferring drug resistance can be rapidly exchanged within the replicating pool of HIV variants to generate viruses that are best adapted to grow in the presence of incompletely suppressive antiretroviral drug pressure. Antiretroviral drugs that select for partially disabled (less fit) viruses may benefit the host by decreasing the amount of virus replication (and consequent damage) that occurs even after drug-resistant mutants have overgrown drug-sensitive viruses. In this regard, recent evidence suggests that such less fit, drug-resistant viruses may be temporarily less able to suppress $CD4^+$ T-cell levels in persons who continue on therapy (24).

Evidence for decreased fitness of drug-resistant viruses has been gleaned from studies of PI-treated or lamivudine-treated patients (81, 84, 123). However, this effect has not been as apparent in patients who were treated with NNRTIs as single agents in the early clinical development of these drugs (e.g., nevirapine or efavirenz), before the "fragility" of these agents was appreciated. In this setting, levels of plasma viremia quickly returned to baseline levels following the outgrowth of preexisting NNRTI-resistant variants after initiation of NNRTI monotherapy, suggesting that the resistant variants were not particularly fitness impaired (or that somehow the fitness of the NNRTI-resistant variants is paradoxically greater in the presence of the drug than in its absence) (136). However, NNRTI-resistant viruses must possess some degree of fitness impairment compared with the predominant drug-sensitive "wild-type" variants, or they would be present at readily detectable levels in untreated patients and would not decline in frequency (which they do) once NNRTI therapy is stopped.

Once HIV variants with reduced susceptibility to a given antiretroviral drug are selected for, their relative representation among the resident HIV quasi species present in an infected person will increase from their initial levels (13). The actual steady-state level of replication of such drug-resistant variants will be determined by their overall frequency, their relative levels of fitness, and whether continued therapy is still able to inhibit their replication partially. Depending on its relative fitness, the drug-resistant variant can persist at appreciable levels even after the antiretroviral therapy that selected for its outgrowth is withdrawn (13, 113). Variants of HIV resistant to NNRTIs have been found to persist at lower but detectable levels for more than a year after withdrawal of treatment (58). Because HIV variants that are resistant to PIs often appear to be less fit than drug-sensitive viruses, their prevalence in patients who develop PI resistance may decline after withdrawal of the drug. However, although such variants may decline after drug withdrawal, they also may persist in patients at higher levels than their original levels and can be rapidly selected for should the same antiretroviral agent (or a PI demonstrating cross-resistance to the original drug employed) be used again (17, 25). In addition, HIV resistance to individual antiretroviral drugs, as well as multiple drugs, has been shown to persist in infected persons and to replicate well enough to be transmitted from one person to another (3, 14, 20, 62, 69, 139). In addition, the genetic sequences associated with drug resistance are soon "archived" after their emergence within the pool of CD4+ T cells that are latently infected with replication-competent proviruses as well as in those cells that harbor defective proviruses but that are able to be subsequently "superinfected" (and thus rescued) by a replication-competent HIV variant (106). For all these reasons, it is clear that because of the genetics of HIV variants generated and maintained in vivo, the process of HIV drug resistance has a "memory." Once drug-resistant variants emerge, they can persist even if they are below the limit of detection of sensitive resistance assays. Further, the resistant variants will rapidly reemerge if therapy with the same drug, or an agent with which the initially employed drug shares a genetic pattern of cross-resistance, is employed subsequently. For these reasons, every therapeutic decision made in the treatment of HIV infection must be viewed within the context of how it will influence future treatment options (36, 132).

Different PIs tend to select for somewhat different primary and compensatory mutations (17, 18, 65, 81, 84, 91, 132; see Chapter 5 in this volume). However, there is a great degree of overlap between the mutations associated with decreased susceptibility to the available PIs, and additional common mutations are selected for along the evolutionary path to increased levels of resistance and fitness (4, 17, 18, 31, 91). For this reason, patients who develop resistant variants while being treated with a given PI are predisposed to develop resistance rapidly to a second PI and thus substantially compromised in their ability to respond clinically to a "second-line" HAART regimen that includes another PI as an essential component. Thus, there remains an essential need to develop new PIs that select for very distinct genetic patterns of resistance (see Chapter 5 in this volume). Importantly, recent advances in the pharmacological manipulation of the effective potency of PIs in treated patients have been achieved through combination PI therapy that acts to increase blood levels of the drugs substantially (see below and Figs. 10.6 and 10.7) (42). Given that antiviral drug resistance is a relative rather than absolute phenomenon and that PI-resistant viruses typically need to accumulate multiple mutations before high-level resistance is manifest, it is now often possible to increase the concentrations of PIs in treated patients (the so-called drug exposure) to levels at which even partially resistant viruses can be suppressed effectively (16, 42).

All available PIs (ritonavir, indinavir, saquinavir, amprenavir, lopinavir, and nelfinavir) are, to varying degrees, inhibitors of cytochrome P450 (CYP3A4), which provides the primary pathway responsible for their metabolism (40, 42, 126). Of the available PIs, ritonavir is the most potent inhibitor of CYP3A4. In addition to their effects on CYP3A4, all available PIs have been reported to be substrates for the multidrug resistance-1 transporter system that mediates the efflux of these drugs from within cells (42, 76). The activity of this efflux system is also inhibited by ritonavir. Thus, when even low doses of ritonavir are used in combination with certain other PIs, substantial increases in drug levels, including peak (C_{max}), trough (C_{min}), and cumulative plasma concentration over time (or "area under the curve" [AUC]), can be achieved (see Figs. 10.6 and 10.7). (Effects on nelfinavir concentrations are less substantial because of its primary metabolism by P450 systems other than CYP3A4 [16, 42, 68].) As a result of improved pharmacokinetic (PK) properties achieved by combinations of other PIs with ritonavir, combination therapy with PIs can permit more efficient suppression of the wild-type viruses than is achieved by individual PIs. More important, however, the improvements in PK afforded by appropriate PI combinations enable improvements in in vivo drug exposures in treated patients to the point where even relatively drug-resistant HIV variants may be inhibited (16, 42).

The definition of mutations associated with resistance to specific antiretroviral drugs and the advent of genetic methods to detect drug-resistant variants in treated patients have raised the possibility of screening HIV-infected patients for the presence of HIV variants as a tool to guide therapeutic decisions (reviewed in references 25, 65, 79). This type of

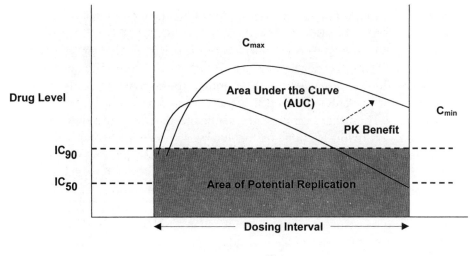

FIGURE 10.6

Utilizing PI interactions to improve drug PKs

Available PIs are substrates for metabolism by the cytochrome P450 drug-metabolizing enzymes in the liver and the gut wall. To varying extents, these drugs also inhibit the cytochrome P450 system. Of available PIs, ritonavir is the most potent inhibitor of cytochrome P450 enzymes and when used in combination with other PIs can alter their metabolism in substantial and beneficial ways (16, 42). Combination of ritonavir with other PIs (e.g., lopinavir, indinavir, amprenavir, or saquinavir) can result in significant improvements in PK properties, including increased maximum concentration (C_{max}), trough concentrations (C_{min}), and the overall level of drug exposure (depicted as "area under the curve" [AUC] of the plasma concentration versus time curve). As a result, high levels of drug concentrations can be achieved that can exceed levels needed to inhibit HIV replication (depicted as inhibitory concentration 50 [IC_{50}] or 90 [IC_{90}]). In addition, such PK improvement permits suppression of partially resistant viral strains and less frequent or simpler drug administration or both. The consequent simplification of treatment regimens may also improve medication adherence. (Adapted from reference 41.)

"genotypic" assay for drug resistance examines the nucleotide sequences of the pool of replicating HIV variants present in the plasma of a treated patient at a given time (53, 122). A substantial body of genetic information concerning mutations in the HIV genome associated with reduced susceptibility of HIV to specific antiretroviral drugs has been generated and continues to accumulate with further study and the development of new antiviral agents. An extensive, up-to-date database of these data can be found at www.hiv-web.kanl.gov. While these data provide high-resolution analyses of precise mutations found in HIV variants resistant to specific drugs, it is often challenging to translate such information effectively into routine clinical practice (65). Important reasons for this difficulty are that, as previously described, drug resistance is a relative rather than absolute

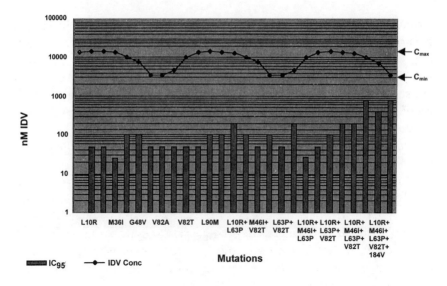

FIGURE 10.7

Improving drug exposure to inhibit replication of PI-resistant HIV variants

PK enhancement strategies employing logical combinations of PIs can substantially increase peak and trough drug concentrations achieved, as well as the overall drug exposure, in treated patients. In many instances, the C_{min} and C_{max} will be sufficient to exceed the concentrations needed to suppress replication of HIV variants that are highly resistant to PIs. For example, the addition of low doses of ritonavir to indinavir can alter the metabolism of indinavir so that substantially higher drug concentrations are achieved throughout the dosing interval. Indinavir levels reached in treated patients are sufficient to inhibit the replication of HIV variants that harbor various mutations associated with indinavir resistance and manifest diminished sensitivity to the drug (shown as IC_{95} levels) (data courtesy of Merck & Co.) (16).

phenomenon. As such, the use of the alternative description of "reduced susceptibility" to an antiviral drug is, in a number of ways, of greater practical utility than "resistance"(see below) (16). However, the determinants of reduced susceptibility are complex and determined by genetic variations in multiple, often interacting, regions of the HIV genome. While high-level resistance to certain drugs (e.g., NNRTIs or lamivudine) is accomplished through characteristic single nucleotide changes within the RT gene, other agents (such as PIs) select for viral variants with multiple mutations that can progressively accumulate in the viral genome in course of acquisition of increased fitness through ongoing replication in the presence of the drug (17, 18, 81, 91, 94, 114, 123). As the evolution of HIV variants toward increasing levels of resistance (and in vivo fitness) does not always follow the same pattern or sequence in different patients, and because the actual functional relationship between mutational patterns and resistance to a number of important drugs is incompletely understood, viral resistance patterns predictive of clinical responses often cannot be reliably inferred from genotypic data alone (65). As a likely result of these challenges, data from some clinical trials have indicated that genotypic resistance testing can improve short-term clinical outcomes in patients changing their HAART for reasons of virologic failure, while other studies have provided less sanguine endorsements of this technology (2, 12, 32). More recent studies of genotypic resistance testing highlight the value of expert advice in interpreting the data, a feature that will need to be accommodated as use of this method extends to physicians with less familiarity with the genetic basis of antiretroviral drug resistance (65).

In addition to genotypic assays, so-called phenotypic assays have also been developed to assess drug susceptibility of patient-derived HIV isolates (16, 65, 104). Phenotypic assays are based on a strategy in which specific HIV sequences (from key target genes for antiviral drugs such as RT or protease) present in the population of HIV found in the plasma of a treated patient are molecularly cloned and inserted into recombinant indicator viruses, and the relative susceptibility of these recombinant viruses to infect target cells in the presence of various concentrations of antiviral drugs is then determined in the laboratory (65, 104). Results of phenotypic assays are reported as the concentration (known as the "inhibitory concentration" [IC]) of drug required to inhibit spread of virus in cell culture. Reduced susceptibility to a given drug manifest by a given patient-derived HIV isolate (or more accurately by the target gene sequences cloned from the predominant replicating pool of HIV present in the patient's plasma) is reflected by an increase in the inhibitory concentration to a level substantially higher than that of a reference "wild-type," drug-sensitive HIV isolate. Results of phenotypic assays are commonly reported as the IC_{50} or IC_{90}, or the concentration of the drug needed to inhibit virus infection in cell culture by 50% or 90%, respectively. Although phenotypic assays for reduced susceptibility provide a useful working definition for resistance, it is not yet known to what extent (and in which ways) the parameters measured in tissue culture settings will accurately predict the response to therapy within the far more complicated in vivo environment of the treated patient. Within patients, important additional variables that will determine the outcome of therapy—including issues of pharmacology (drug potency, absorption, clearance, metabolism, protein binding, and tissue distribution), virology (interactions with coadministered antiviral drugs, prevailing replication dynamics, and potential sanctuaries and reservoirs), and the patient's level of adherence to therapy—can all vary in ways that are not modeled in the tissue culture settings employed in available resistance tests.

Application of both methods for so-called resistance testing can potentially be useful in two important clinical situations (65). In the clinical scenario that is most often of interest, analysis of the genotype of the replicating population of virus may enable determination of the nature of the observed treatment failure in HAART-treated patients who display persistent evidence of ongoing HIV replication while on therapy (as determined by plasma RNA assay repeatedly above the assay detection limits) and may help guide the selection of more effective, alternative HAART regimens. In many instances treatment failure will likely be due to the outgrowth of HIV variants with reduced susceptibility to all the drugs included in the combination HAART regimen used. However, in other instances, determination of the genotypes of the persistently detectable HIV population will identify characteristic mutations associated with resistance to only some of the components of the treatment regimen (27, 59). Such a result can emerge because of the differential ease with which certain drug resistance mutations can come to predominate in the setting of incompletely suppressive HAART regimens (due to differences in relative fitness of resistant viruses or the magnitude of the genetic barriers imposed by a specific drug, or both), differences in the PK properties of the different drugs, or when treated patients are adherent to some but not all of the components of the treatment regimen (as resistant viruses will be the predominant virus population only in the presence of the drug). In this setting, information about the susceptibility can potentially help guide the clinician in tailoring an alternative HAART combination that makes important changes in certain key drugs included in the regimen, but not necessarily changing all of them (7, 132). Alternatively, if some degree of reduced susceptibility is detected, it may be possible to overcome that level of resistance through increasing the relevant concentrations of drug (e.g., the level of "drug exposure"; see Figs. 10.6 and 10.7) to the point where even the replication of relatively resistant viruses can be inhibited (16).

Importantly, the appropriate application of resistance testing also needs to be conducted within the context of what is known about the population dynamics of HIV quasi species present within infected individuals. As previously discussed, the most fit viral variants will predominate at any given time, but less fit variants can persist even if they cannot be detected by the most sensitive available molecular methods. An essential corollary of these lessons is that the antiviral susceptibility of the prevailing virus population needs to be assessed while the patient continues treatment with the drugs of interest. Once a specific regimen of therapy is stopped or changed, viral variants with reduced susceptibility to antiretroviral drugs (whose relative fitness is much reduced in the absence of the drug pressure) will rapidly decrease in number and often fall below the detection limits of available resistance assays (13, 28). However, these variants may continue to replicate at low levels and are likely to have already been archived in latently infected cells, only to reemerge rapidly once therapy is instituted with the original drugs or ones to which the drug-resistant viral variants possess cross-resistance (13, 17, 135).

Although newly developed technologies for resistance testing provide very useful adjuncts for the performance of clinical trials, their application to routine clinical practice is complicated by a number of issues. First, all available assays lack the sensitivity to detect genetic variants that are relatively rare (~<20% of the replicating quasi species) and as such cannot detect resistant variants that are below this level but that can rapidly come to predominate following changes in therapy (65). Second, the assays are expensive, and their accurate interpretation requires substantial expertise that is not commonly available to the average practitioner. Third, the practical utility of genotypic assays is limited by uncertainties in the in vivo correlates of the genetic mutations associated with resistance, while the utility of phenotypic assays is limited by uncertainties concerning how the tissue culture environment in which they are performed mirrors the virologically, pharmacologically, and immunologically far more complex environment present within a treated patient. Fourth, given that HIV is constantly evolving in infected persons, delays between when the samples are obtained and the results reported (particularly for the slower-to-perform phenotypic assays [typically two weeks or more]) may not predict the precise composition of the relevant virus populations at the time therapy is altered. Delays in data reporting for resistance tests may be particularly important with respect to their use in the setting of primary infection, in which, for immunologic reasons, it appears to be essential to initiate therapy as early as possible to obtain desired immunologic effects. Nevertheless, resistance testing is gaining widespread use in clinical care of HIV-infected persons, and a number of clinical trials have demonstrated that it can confer therapeutic benefit in some clinical circumstances over that obtained by a careful review of treatment history alone. In reality, the true value of resistance testing in improving clinical outcomes will become clear only when new antiretroviral drugs are developed that select for distinct patterns of drug resistance mutations. Until this time, limitations of the beneficial impact of resistance testing may reflect current limitations in the available repertoire of antiviral drugs, rather than an inherent limitation in the concept of defining the antiviral susceptibility of HIV quasi species present in treated individuals at a given time. Recommendations concerning the clinical interpretation and use of antiretroviral drug resistance testing have recently been published (65).

Future Research Challenges

A remarkable degree of progress has been realized in the development of effective antiretroviral therapies for HIV infection, but a number of important challenges remain. The inherent tendency of HIV to generate drug-resistant viral variants continues to be an essential issue limiting therapeutic success. Individuals who fail to respond to their initial HAART regimens, owing to virologic or immunologic factors or to nonadherence, often fail to respond to subsequent "salvage" regimens. Further, those individuals who acquire drug-resistant HIV variants in their initial infection are predisposed to a greater risk of virologic failure once they initiate HAART. Continuing drug development efforts are focusing on derivation of new agents that are active against HIV variants resistant to available drugs, and given the extensive accumulated data concerning the genetic basis of HIV drug resistance and the demonstrated power of structure-based drug design strategies, these efforts are likely to be successful. Further, the derivation of new drugs active against novel essential targets in the HIV life cycle is being actively pursued (such as entry inhibitors [see Chapter 7 in this volume] and integrase inhibitors [see Chapter 6 in this volume], as well as inhibitors of HIV regulatory [see Chapter 8 in this volume] and accessory gene functions [see Chapter 9 in this volume]). The fact that HIV has been able to develop resistance to all the antiretroviral drugs developed to date is quite remarkable. However, it may still be possible to develop new agents for which the virus cannot tolerate the mutations that would be required for manifestation of resistance or for which resistance mutations would confer a loss of fitness on the resistant virus that could not be compensated by accumulation of additional mutations.

Important additional challenges in HIV therapeutics include the development of newer agents or combinations of existing agents that exhibit increased antiviral potency and that exert even more stringent genetic as well as pharmacological barriers to the outgrowth of drug-resistant HIV variants. Efforts along these lines, such as recently developed strategies for PK enhancement of the level and effective duration of antiretroviral activity exerted by combinations of PIs in vivo, have already validated the utility of an approach that can now be further developed and refined in the future (see Figs. 10.6 and 10.7) (16, 42). Similarly, the development of newer agents or combinations of existing agents that enable simpler, more convenient dosing schedules should promote greater adherence on the part of treated patients and allow increased rates of long-term therapeutic success. Continued efforts are needed to define and ameliorate the long-term toxicities of HAART regimens, and efforts to develop new anti-HIV drugs with substantially improved side effects profiles will be essential to ensure that improvements in both the quality and quantity of life achieved as a result of HAART continue to increase in the future.

When simpler, more convenient, and less toxic antiviral therapies for HIV infection are developed, it is likely that treatment recommendations will evolve to include more individuals at earlier stages of HIV infection and those with lower short-term risk of disease progression (7, 132). Such a trend will be important if it proves, with long-term follow-up of treated patients, that immune reconstitution achieved after initiation of HAART in the later stages of the infection is incomplete (because of restrictions in the T-cell repertoire) or transient (because of accelerated senescence of the immune system) as sequelae of the prolonged period of unopposed HIV replication experiences prior to initiation of therapy.

In addition to the numerous practical and virologic limitations of current HAART regimens, important uncertainties remain concerning the degree to which beneficial immunologic responses follow use of virologically successful antiretroviral therapies (85). While treatment advances achieved to date have arisen from a focus on the virologic aspects of HIV infection, there remains a need to define strategies to increase the number, to improve the function, and to enable increased diversification of the host CD4+ T-cell populations above and beyond the results achieved by HAART alone. Further, efforts to augment the magnitude and effectiveness of the host immune response to HIV itself as an adjunct to or substitute for antiretroviral drug therapy represent an essential but challenging topic for future research (125).

Perhaps the most vexing future research challenge relates to the fact that the vast majority of HIV-infected individuals live in countries where complex and costly HAART regimens are unlikely to be made generally available or able to be implemented within existing infrastructures for health care delivery (108). As a result, efforts to define the simplest, most effective, and most affordable antiretroviral therapy regimens are essential if recent treatment advances are ever to benefit all those in need. Based on the substantial advances that have been achieved in our understanding of the pathogenic mechanisms of HIV infection that underlie disease progression and response to antiretroviral therapy, substantial efforts should now be mounted to define highly effective and safe treatment strategies that can be practically implemented in resource-poor countries to benefit the tens of millions of individuals currently living with HIV infection worldwide (108).

REFERENCES

1. Altfeld, M., and B. D. Walker. 2001. Less is more? STI in acute and chronic HIV-1 infection. Nature Med. 7:881–884.
2. Baxter, J. D., D. L. Mayers, D. N. Wentworth, J. D. Neaton, M. L. Hoover, M. A. Winters, S. B. Mannheimer, M. A. Thompson, D. I. Abrams, B. J. Brizz, J. P. Ioannidis, and T. C. Merigan. 2000. A randomized study of antiretroviral management based on plasma genotypic antiretroviral resistance testing in patients failing therapy. CPCRA 046 Study Team for the Terry Beirn Community Programs for Clinical Research on AIDS. AIDS 14:F83–93.
3. Boden, D., A. Hurley, L. Zhang, Y. Cao, Y. Guo, E. Jones, J. Tsay, J. Ip, C. Farthing, K. Limoli, N. Parkin, and M. Markowitz. 1999. HIV-1 drug resistance in newly infected individuals [see comments]. JAMA 282:1135–1141.
4. Brown, A. J., B. T. Korber, and J. H. Condra. 1999. Associations between amino acids in the evolution of HIV type 1 protease sequences under indinavir therapy. AIDS Res. Hum. Retroviruses 15:247–253.

5. Buchbinder, S., and E. Vittinghoff. 1999. HIV-infected long-term non-progressors: epidemiology, mechanisms of delayed progression, and clinical and research implications. Microbes and Infection 1(13):1113–1120.

6. CAESAR Coordinating Committee. 1997. Randomised trial of addition of lamivudine or lamivudine plus lovirride to zidovudine-containing regimens for patients with HIV-1 infection: the CAESAR trial. Lancet 349:1413–1421.

7. Carpenter, C. C., et al. 2000. Antiretroviral therapy in adults: updated recommendations of the International AIDS Society-USA Panel [see comments]. JAMA 283:381–390.

8. Centers for Disease Control and Prevention. 1993. 1993 revised classification system for HIV infection and expanded surveillance case definition for AIDS among adolescents and adults. Morbid. Mortal. Weekly Rep. 41:1–19.

9. Chaisson, R., J. Keruly, and R. Moore. 2000. Association of initial CD4 cell count and viral load with response to highly active antiretroviral therapy. JAMA 284:3128–3129.

10. Chun, T. W., et al. 1997. Quantification of latent tissue reservoirs and total body viral load in HIV-1 infection [see comments]. Nature 387:183–188.

11. Chun, T. W., L. Stuyver, S. B. Mizell, L. A. Ehler, J. A. Mican, M. Baseler, A. L. Lloyd, M. A. Nowak, and A. S. Fauci. 1997. Presence of an inducible HIV-1 latent reservoir during highly active antiretroviral therapy. Proc. Natl. Acad. Sci. USA 94:13193–13197.

12. Clevenbergh, P., J. Durant, P. Halfon, P. del Giudice, V. Mondain, N. Montagne, J. M. Schapiro, C. A. Boucher, and P. Dellamonica. 2000. Persisting long-term benefit of genotype-guided treatment for HIV-infected patients failing HAART. The Viradapt Study: week 48 follow-up. Antiviral Therapy 5:65–70.

13. Coffin, J. M. 1995. HIV population dynamics in vivo: implications for genetic variation, pathogenesis, and therapy [see comments]. Science 267:483–489.

14. Cohen, O. J., and A. S. Fauci. 1998. Transmission of multidrug-resistant human immunodeficiency virus—the wake-up call [editorial; comment]. N. Engl. J. Med. 339:341–343.

15. Condra, J., and E. Emini. 1997. Preventing HIV-1 drug resistance. Science and Medicine (January/February):14–23.

16. Condra, J., C. Petropoulos, R. Ziermann, W. Schleif, M. Shivaprakash, and E. Emini. 2000. Drug resistance and predicted virologic responses to human immunodeficiency virus type 1 protease inhibitor therapy. J. Infect. Dis. 182:758–765.

17. Condra, J. H., et al. 1996. Genetic correlates of in vivo viral resistance to indinavir, a human immunodeficiency virus type 1 protease inhibitor. J. Virol. 70:8270–8276.

18. Condra, J. H., W. A. Schleif, O. M. Blahy, L. J. Gabryelski, D. J. Graham, J. C. Quintero, A. Rhodes, H. L. Robbins, E. Roth, and M. Shivaprakash. 1995. In vivo emergence of HIV-1 variants resistant to multiple protease inhibitors [see comments]. Nature 374:569–571.

19. Connors, M., J. A. Kovacs, S. Krevat, J. C. Gea-Banacloche, M. C. Sneller, M. Flanigan, J. A. Metcalf, R. E. Walker, J. Falloon, M. Baseler, I. Feuerstein, H. Masur, and H. C. Lane. 1997. HIV infection induces changes in CD4+ T-cell phenotype and depletions within the CD4+ T-cell repertoire that are not im-

mediately restored by antiviral or immune-based therapies [see comments]. Nature Med. 3:533–540.

20. Conway, B., V. Montessori, D. Rouleau, J. S. Montaner, M. V. O'Shaughnessy, S. Fransen, A. Shillington, O. Weislow, and D. L. Mayers. 1999. Primary lamivudine resistance in acute/early human immunodeficiency virus infection. Clin. Infect. Dis. 28:910–911.

21. Cooper, D. A., J. M. Gatell, S. Kroon, N. Clumeck, J. Millard, F. D. Goebel, J. N. Bruun, G. Stingl, R. L. Melville, and J. Gonzalez-Lahoz. 1993. Zidovudine in persons with asymptomatic HIV infection and CD4+ cell counts greater than 400 per cubic millimeter. The European-Australian Collaborative Group [see comments]. N. Engl. J. Med. 329(5):297–303.

22. Deeks, S. G. 2001. Durable HIV treatment benefit despite low-level viremia. Reassessing definitions of success or failure. JAMA 286:224–226.

23. Deeks, S. G., N. S. Hellmann, R. M. Grant, N. T. Parkin, C. J. Petropoulos, M. Becker, W. Symonds, M. Chesney, and P. A. Volberding. 1999. Novel four-drug salvage treatment regimens after failure of a human immunodeficiency virus type 1 protease inhibitor-containing regimen: antiviral activity and correlation of baseline phenotypic drug susceptibility with virologic outcome. J. Infect. Dis. 179:1375–1381.

24. Deeks, S. G., T. Wrin, T. Liegler, R. Hoh, M. Hayden, J. D. Barbour, N. S. Hellmann, C. J. Petropoulos, J. M. McCune, M. K. Hellerstein, and R. M. Grant. 2001. Virologic and immunologic consequences of discontinuing combination antiretroviral-drug therapy in HIV-infected patients with detectable viremia [see comments]. N. Engl. J. Med. 344:472–480.

25. DeGruttola, V., et al. 2000. The relation between baseline HIV drug resistance and response to antiretroviral therapy: re-analysis of retrospective and prospective studies using a standardized data analysis plan. Antiviral Therapy 5:41–48.

26. Delta Coordinating Committee. 1996. Delta: a randomized double-blind controlled trial comparing combinations of zidovudine plus didanosine or zalcitabine with zidovudine alone in HIV-infected individuals. Lancet 348: 283–291.

27. Descamps, D., P. Flandre, V. Calvez, G. Peytavin, V. Meiffredy, G. Collin, C. Delaugerre, S. Robert-Delmas, B. Bazin, J. P. Aboulker, G. Pialoux, F. Raffi, and F. Brun-Vezinet. 2000. Mechanisms of virologic failure in previously untreated HIV-infected patients from a trial of induction-maintenance therapy. Trilege (Agence Nationale de Recherches sur le SIDA 072) Study Team [see comments]. JAMA 283:205–211.

28. Devereux, H. L., M. Youle, M. A. Johnson, and C. Loveday. 1999. Rapid decline in detectability of HIV-1 drug resistance mutations after stopping therapy. AIDS 13:F123–127.

29. Dornadula, G., H. Zhang, B. Van Uitert, J. Stern, L. Livornese, Jr., M. J. Ingerman, J. Witek, R. J. Kedanis, J. Natkin, J. DeSimone, and R. J. Pomerantz. 1999. Residual HIV-1 RNA in blood plasma of patients taking suppressive highly active antiretroviral therapy [see comments]. JAMA 282:1627–1632.

30. Douek, D. C., R. D. McFarland, P. H. Keiser, E. A. Gage, J. M. Massey, B. F. Haynes, M. A. Polis, A. T. Haase, M. B. Feinberg, J. L. Sullivan, B. D. Jamieson,

J. A. Zack, L. J. Picker, and R. A. Koup. 1998. Changes in thymic function with age and during the treatment of HIV infection [see comments]. Nature 396:690–695.

31. Dulioust, A., S. Paulous, L. Guillemot, A. M. Delavalle, F. Boue, and F. Clavel. 1999. Constrained evolution of human immunodeficiency virus type 1 protease during sequential therapy with two distinct protease inhibitors. J. Virol. 73:850–854.

32. Durant, J., P. Clevenbergh, P. Halfon, P. Delgiudice, S. Porsin, P. Simonet, N. Montagne, C. A. Boucher, J. M. Schapiro, and P. Dellamonica. 1999. Drug-resistance genotyping in HIV-1 therapy: the VIRADAPT randomised controlled trial [see comments]. Lancet 353:2195–2199. (Erratum, 354:1128.)

33. Emerman, M., and M. H. Malim. 1998. HIV-1 regulatory/accessory genes: keys to unraveling viral and host cell biology. Science 280:1880–1884.

34. Enger, C., N. Graham, Y. Peng, J. S. Chmiel, L. A. Kingsley, R. Detels, and A. Munoz. 1996. Survival from early, intermediate, and late stages of HIV infection. JAMA 275:1329–1334.

35. Eron, J. J., S. L. Benoit, J. Jemsek, R. D. MacArthur, J. Santana, J. B. Quinn, D. R. Kuritzkes, M. A. Fallon, and M. Rubin 1995. Treatment with lamivudine, zidovudine, or both in HIV-positive patients with 200 to 500 CD4+ cells per cubic millimeter. North American HIV Working Party [see comments]. N. Engl. J. Med. 333(25):1662–1669.

36. Feinberg, M., C. Carpenter, A. Fauci, S. Stanley, O. Cohen, J. Bartlett, J. Kaplan, and E. Abrutyn. 1998. Report of the NIH Panel to Define Principles of Therapy of HIV Infection. Ann. Intern. Med. 128(12):1056–1078.

37. Finzi, D., et al. 1997. Identification of a reservoir for HIV-1 in patients on highly active antiretroviral therapy [see comments]. Science 278:1295–1300.

38. Finzi, D., et al. 1999. Latent infection of CD4+ T cells provides a mechanism for lifelong persistence of HIV-1, even in patients on effective combination therapy [see comments]. Nature Med. 5:512–517.

39. Fischl, M. A., D. D. Richman, M. H. Grieco, M. S. Gottlieb, P. A. Volberding, O. L. Laskin, J. M. Leedom, J. E. Groopman, D. Mildvan, and R. T. Schooley. 1987. The efficacy of azidothymidine (AZT) in the treatment of patients with AIDS and AIDS-related complex. A double-blind, placebo-controlled trial. N. Engl. J. Med. 317(4):185–191.

40. Flexner, C. 1998. HIV-protease inhibitors [see comments]. N. Engl. J. Med. 338(18):1281–1292.

41. Flexner, C. 2000. Drug interactions: Better living through pharmacology?, p. 75–85. In Medscape HIV/AIDS Annual Update 2000, J. P. Phair and E. King (ed.), Medscape, Inc., New York.

42. Flexner, C. 2000. Dual protease inhibitor therapy in HIV-infected patients: pharmacologic rationale and clinical benefits. Annu. Rev. Pharmacol. Toxicol. 40:649–674.

43. Fogelman, I., V. Davey, H. D. Ochs, M. Elashoff, M. B. Feinberg, J. Mican, J. P. Siegel, M. Sneller, and H. C. Lane. 2000. Evaluation of CD4+ T cell function in vivo in HIV-infected patients as measured by bacteriophage phiX174 immunization. J. Infect. Dis. 182:435–441.

44. Frankel, A. D., and J. A. Young. 1998. HIV-1: fifteen proteins and an RNA. Annu. Rev. Biochem. 67:1–25.

45. Furtado, M. R., D. S. Callaway, J. P. Phair, K. J. Kunstman, J. L. Stanton, C. A. Macken, A. S. Perelson, and S. M. Wolinsky. 1999. Persistence of HIV-1 transcription in peripheral-blood mononuclear cells in patients receiving potent antiretroviral therapy [see comments]. N. Engl. J. Med. 340:1614–1622.

46. Gea-Banacloche, J. C., S. A. Migueles, L. Martino, W. L. Shupert, A. C. Mc-Neil, M. S. Sabbaghian, L. Ehler, C. Prussin, R. Stevens, L. Lambert, J. Altman, C. W. Hallahan, J. C. de Quiros, and M. Connors. 2000. Maintenance of large numbers of virus-specific CD8+ T cells in HIV-infected progressors and long-term nonprogressors. J. Immunol. 165:1082–1092.

47. Gea-Banacloche, J. C., E. E. Weiskopf, C. Hallahan, J. C. Lopez Bernaldo de Quiros, M. Flanigan, J. M. Mican, J. Falloon, M. Baseler, R. Stevens, H. C. Lane, and M. Connors. 1998. Progression of human immunodeficiency virus disease is associated with increasing disruptions within the CD4+ T cell receptor repertoire. J. Infect. Dis. 177:579–585.

48. Geijtenbeek, T. B., D. S. Kwon, R. Torensma, S. J. van Vliet, G. C. van Duijnhoven, J. Middel, I. L. Cornelissen, H. S. Nottet, V. N. Kewal-Ramani, D. R. Littman, C. G. Figdor, and Y. van Kooyk. 2000. DC-SIGN, a dendritic cell-specific HIV-1-binding protein that enhances trans-infection of T cells [see comments]. Cell 100:587–597.

49. Grossman, Z., M. Polis, M. B. Feinberg, I. Levi, S. Jankelevich, R. Yarchoan, J. Boon, F. de Wolf, J. M. Lange, J. Goudsmit, D. S. Dimitrov, and W. E. Paul. 1999. Ongoing HIV dissemination during HAART. Nature Med. 5:1099–1104.

50. Gulick, R. M., J. W. Mellors, D. Havlir, J. J. Eron, C. Gonzalez, D. McMahon, D. D. Richman, F. T. Valentine, L. Jonas, A. Meibohm, E. A. Emini, and J. A. Chodakewitz. 1997. Treatment with indinavir, zidovudine, and lamivudine in adults with human immunodeficiency virus infection and prior antiretroviral therapy [see comments]. N. Engl. J. Med. 337:734–739.

51. Gulick, R. M., J. W. Mellors, D. Havlir, J. J. Eron, A. Meibohm, J. H. Condra, F. T. Valentine, D. McMahon, C. Gonzalez, L. Jonas, E. A. Emini, J. A. Chodakewitz, R. Isaacs, and D. D. Richman. 2000. 3-year suppression of HIV viremia with indinavir, zidovudine, and lamivudine. Ann. Intern. Med. 133:35–39.

52. Gunthard, H. F., S. D. Frost, A. J. Leigh-Brown, C. C. Ignacio, K. Kee, A. S. Perelson, C. A. Spina, D. V. Havlir, M. Hezareh, D. J. Looney, D. D. Richman, and J. K. Wong. 1999. Evolution of envelope sequences of human immunodeficiency virus type 1 in cellular reservoirs in the setting of potent antiviral therapy. J. Virol. 73:9404–9412.

53. Gunthard, H. F., J. K. Wong, C. C. Ignacio, D. V. Havlir, and D. D. Richman. 1998. Comparative performance of high-density oligonucleotide sequencing and dideoxynucleotide sequencing of HIV type 1 pol from clinical samples. AIDS Res. Hum. Retroviruses 14:869–876.

54. Haase, A. T. 1999. Population biology of HIV-1 infection: viral and CD4+ T cell demographics and dynamics in lymphatic tissues. Annu. Rev. Immunol. 17:625–656.

55. Hahn, B. H., G. M. Shaw, K. M. De Cock, and P. M. Sharp. 2000. AIDS as a zoonosis: scientific and public health implications. Science 287:607–614.

56. Hammer, S. M., D. A. Katzenstein, M. D. Hughes, H. Gundacker, R. T. Schooley, R. H. Haubrich, W. K. Henry, M. M. Lederman, J. P. Phair, M. Niu, M. S.

Hirsch, and T. C. Merigan. 1996. A trial comparing nucleoside monotherapy with combination therapy in HIV-infected adults with CD4 cell counts from 200 to 500 per cubic millimeter. AIDS Clinical Trials Group Study 175 Study Team [see comments]. N. Engl. J. Med. 335(15):1081–1090.

57. Havlir, D. V., R. Bassett, D. Levitan, P. Gilbert, P. Tebas, A. C. Collier, M. S. Hirsch, C. Ignacio, J. Condra, H. F. Gunthard, D. D. Richman, and J. K. Wong. 2001. Prevalence and predictive value of intermittent viremia with combination HIV therapy. JAMA. 286:171–179.

58. Havlir, D. V., S. Eastman, A. Gamst, and D. D. Richman. 1996. Nevirapine-resistant human immunodeficiency virus: kinetics of replication and estimated prevalence in untreated patients. J. Virol. 70:7894–7899.

59. Havlir, D. V., N. S. Hellmann, C. J. Petropoulos, J. M. Whitcomb, A. C. Collier, M. S. Hirsch, P. Tebas, J. P. Sommadossi, and D. D. Richman. 2000. Drug susceptibility in HIV infection after viral rebound in patients receiving indinavir-containing regimens [see comments]. JAMA 283:229–234.

60. Haynes, B. F., G. Pantaleo, and A. S. Fauci. 1996. Toward an understanding of the correlates of protective immunity to HIV infection [see comments]. Science 271:324–328.

61. Hazenberg, M. D., D. Hamann, H. Schuitemaker, and F. Miedema. 2000. T cell depletion in HIV-1 infection: how CD4+ T cells go out of stock. Nat. Immunol. 1(4):285–289.

62. Hecht, F. M., R. M. Grant, C. J. Petropoulos, B. Dillon, M. A. Chesney, H. Tian, N. S. Hellmann, N. I. Bandrapalli, L. Digilio, B. Branson, and J. O. Kahn. 1998. Sexual transmission of an HIV-1 variant resistant to multiple reverse-transcriptase and protease inhibitors [see comments]. N. Engl. J. Med. 339: 307–311.

63. Hellerstein, M. K., and J. M. McCune. 1997. T cell turnover in HIV-1 disease. Immunity 7(5):583–589.

64. Hermankova, M., S. C. Ray, C. Ruff, M. Powell-Davis, R. Ingersoll, R. T. D'Aquila, T. C. Quinn, J. D. Siliciano, R. F. Siliciano, and D. Persaud. 2001. HIV-1 drug resistance profiles in children and adults with viral load of <50 copies/ml receiving combination therapy. JAMA 286:196–207.

65. Hirsch, M. S., F. Brun-Vezinet, R. T. D'Aquila, S. M. Hammer, V. A. Johnson, D. R. Kuritzkes, C. Loveday, J. W. Mellors, B. Clotet, B. Conway, L. M. Demeter, S. Vella, D. M. Jacobsen, and D. D. Richman. 2000. Antiretroviral drug resistance testing in adult HIV-1 infection: recommendations of an International AIDS Society-USA Panel [see comments]. JAMA 283: 2417–2426.

66. Ho, D. D., A. U. Neumann, A. S. Perelson, W. Chen, J. M. Leonard, and M. Markowitz. 1995. Rapid turnover of plasma virions and CD4 lymphocytes in HIV-1 infection [see comments]. Nature 373:123–126.

67. Hogg, R. S., K. V. Heath, B. Yip, K. J. Craib, M. V. O'Shaughnessy, M. T. Schechter, and J. S. Montaner. 1998. Improved survival among HIV-infected individuals following initiation of antiretroviral therapy [see comments]. JAMA 279:450–454.

68. Hsu, A., G. R. Granneman, G. Cao, L. Carothers, T. el-Shourbagy, P. Baroldi, K. Erdman, F. Brown, E. Sun, and J. M. Leonard. 1998. Pharmacokinetic inter-

actions between two human immunodeficiency virus protease inhibitors, ritonavir and saquinavir. Clinical Pharmacology and Therapeutics 63(4): 453–464.

69. Imrie, A., A. Beveridge, W. Genn, J. Vizzard, and D. A. Cooper. 1997. Transmission of human immunodeficiency virus type 1 resistant to nevirapine and zidovudine. Sydney Primary HIV Infection Study Group. J. Infect. Dis. 175:1502–1506.

70. Jurriaans, S., B. Van Gemen, G. J. Weverling, D. Van Strijp, P. Nara, R. Coutinho, M. Koot, H. Schuitemaker, and J. Goudsmit. 1994. The natural history of HIV-1 infection: virus load and virus phenotype independent determinants of clinical course? Virology 204:223–233.

71. Kahn, J. O., and B. D. Walker. 1998. Acute human immunodeficiency virus type 1 infection. N. Engl. J. Med. 339:33–39.

72. Kalams, S. A., S. P. Buchbinder, E. S. Rosenberg, J. M. Billingsley, D. S. Colbert, N. G. Jones, A. K. Shea, A. K. Trocha, and B. D. Walker. 1999. Association between virus-specific cytotoxic T-lymphocyte and helper responses in human immunodeficiency virus type 1 infection. J. Virol. 73:6715–6720.

73. Kozal, M. J., N. Shah, N. Shen, R. Yang, R. Fucini, T. C. Merigan, D. D. Richman, D. Morris, E. Hubbell, M. Chee, and T. R. Gingeras. 1996. Extensive polymorphisms observed in HIV-1 clade B protease gene using high-density oligonucleotide arrays. Nature Med. 2:753–759.

74. Ledergerber, B., M. Egger, V. Erard, R. Weber, B. Hirschel, H. Furrer, M. Battegay, P. Vernazza, E. Bernasconi, M. Opravil, D. Kaufmann, P. Sudre, P. Francioli, and A. Telenti. 1999. AIDS-related opportunistic illnesses occurring after initiation of potent antiretroviral therapy: the Swiss HIV Cohort Study [see comments]. JAMA 282:2220–2226.

75. Ledergerber, B., M. Egger, M. Opravil, A. Telenti, B. Hirschel, M. Battegay, P. Vernazza, P. Sudre, M. Flepp, H. Furrer, P. Francioli, and R. Weber. 1999. Clinical progression and virological failure on highly active antiretroviral therapy in HIV-1 patients: a prospective cohort study. Swiss HIV Cohort Study. Lancet 353:863–868.

76. Lee, C. G., M. M. Gottesman, C. O. Cardarelli, M. Ramachandra, K. T. Jeang, S. V. Ambudkar, I. Pastan, and S. Dey. 1998. HIV-1 protease inhibitors are substrates for the MDR1 multidrug transporter. Biochemistry 37:3594–3601.

77. Little, S. J., E. S. Daar, R. T. D'Aquila, P. H. Keiser, E. Connick, J. M. Whitcomb, N. S. Hellmann, C. J. Petropoulos, L. Sutton, J. A. Pitt, E. S. Rosenberg, R. A. Koup, B. D. Walker, and D. D. Richman. 1999. Reduced antiretroviral drug susceptibility among patients with primary HIV infection [see comments]. JAMA 282:1142–1149.

78. Liu, Z., W. G. Cumberland, L. E. Hultin, A. H. Kaplan, R. Detels, and J. V. Giorgi. 1998. CD8+ T-lymphocyte activation in HIV-1 disease reflects an aspect of pathogenesis distinct from viral burden and immunodeficiency. J. Acquired Immune Defic. Syndr. 18:332–340.

79. Lorenzi, P., M. Opravil, B. Hirschel, J. P. Chave, H. J. Furrer, H. Sax, T. V. Perneger, L. Perrin, L. Kaiser, and S. Yerly. 1999. Impact of drug resistance mutations on virologic response to salvage therapy. Swiss HIV Cohort Study. AIDS 13:F17–21.

80. Lucas, G. M., R. E. Chaisson, and R. D. Moore. 1999. Highly active antiretroviral therapy in a large urban clinic: risk factors for virologic failure and adverse drug reactions. Ann. Intern. Med. 131:81–87.

81. Mammano, F., V. Trouplin, V. Zennou, and F. Clavel. 2000. Retracing the evolutionary pathways of human immunodeficiency virus type 1 resistance to protease inhibitors: virus fitness in the absence and in the presence of drug. J. Virol. 74:8524–8531.

82. Mansky, L. M., and H. M. Temin. 1995. Lower in vivo mutation rate of human immunodeficiency virus type 1 than that predicted from the fidelity of purified reverse transcriptase. J. Virol. 69:5087–5094.

83. Margolick, J. B., A. Munoz, A. D. Donnenberg, L. P. Park, N. Galai, J. V. Giorgi, M. R. O'Gorman, and J. Ferbas. 1995. Failure of T-cell homeostasis preceding AIDS in HIV-1 infection. The Multicenter AIDS Cohort Study [see comments]. Nature Med. 1:674–680.

84. Martinez-Picado, J., A. V. Savara, L. Sutton, and R. T. D'Aquila. 1999. Replicative fitness of protease inhibitor-resistant mutants of human immunodeficiency virus type 1. J. Virol. 73:3744–3752.

85. McCune, J. 2001. The dynamics of CD4+ T-cell depletion in HIV disease. Nature 410:974–979.

86. McCune, J. M., M. B. Hanley, D. Cesar, R. Halvorsen, R. Hoh, D. Schmidt, E. Wieder, S. Deeks, S. Siler, R. Neese, and M. Hellerstein. 2000. Factors influencing T-cell turnover in HIV-1-seropositive patients [see comments]. J. Clin. Invest. 105:R1–8.

87. McMichael, A., and S. Rowland-Jones. 2001. Cellular immune responses to HIV. Nature 410:980–987.

88. Mellors, J. W., L. A. Kingsley, C. R. Rinaldo, Jr., J. A. Todd, B. S. Hoo, R. P. Kokka, and P. Gupta. 1995. Quantitation of HIV-1 RNA in plasma predicts outcome after seroconversion. Ann. Intern. Med. 122:573–579.

89. Mellors, J. W., A. Munoz, J. V. Giorgi, J. B. Margolick, C. J. Tassoni, P. Gupta, L. A. Kingsley, J. A. Todd, A. J. Saah, R. Detels, J. P. Phair, and C. R. Rinaldo, Jr. 1997. Plasma viral load and CD4+ lymphocytes as prognostic markers of HIV-1 infection [see comments]. Ann. Intern. Med. 126:946–954.

90. Mellors, J. W., C. R. Rinaldo, Jr., P. Gupta, R. M. White, J. A. Todd, and L. A. Kingsley. 1996. Prognosis in HIV-1 infection predicted by the quantity of virus in plasma [see comments]. Science 272:1167–1170. (Erratum, 275:14, 1997.)

91. Molla, A., et al. 1996. Ordered accumulation of mutations in HIV protease confers resistance to ritonavir. Nature Med. 2:760–766.

92. Moutouh, L., J. Corbeil, and D. D. Richman. 1996. Recombination leads to the rapid emergence of HIV-1 dually resistant mutants under selective drug pressure. Proc. Natl. Acad. Sci. USA 93:6106–6111.

93. Mulder, J., N. McKinney, C. Christopherson, J. Sninsky, L. Greenfield, and S. Kwok. 1994. Rapid and simple PCR assay for quantitation of human immunodeficiency virus type 1 RNA in plasma: application to acute retroviral infection. J. Clin. Microbiol. 32(2):292–300.

94. Nijhuis, M., R. Schuurman, D. de Jong, J. Erickson, E. Gustchina, J. Albert, P. Schipper, S. Gulnik, and C. A. Boucher. 1999. Increased fitness of drug re-

sistant HIV-1 protease as a result of acquisition of compensatory mutations during suboptimal therapy. AIDS 13:2349–2359.

95. O'Brien, S., G. Nelson, C. Winkler, and M. Smith. 2000. Polygenic and multifactorial disease gene association in man: lessons from AIDS. Annu. Rev. Genet. 34:563–591.

96. O'Brien, T. R., W. A. Blattner, D. Waters, E. Eyster, M. W. Hilgartner, A. R. Cohen, N. Luban, A. Hatzakis, L. M. Aledort, P. S. Rosenberg, W. J. Miley, B. L. Kroner, and J. J. Goedert. 1996. Serum HIV-1 RNA levels and time to development of AIDS in the Multicenter Hemophilia Cohort Study [see comments]. JAMA 276:105–110.

97. O'Brien, T. R., P. S. Rosenberg, F. Yellin, and J. J. Goedert. 1998. Longitudinal HIV-1 RNA levels in a cohort of homosexual men. J. Acquired Immune Defic. Syndr. 18:155–161.

98. Pachl, C., J. A. Todd, D. G. Kern, P. J. Sheridan, S. J. Fong, M. Stempien, B. Hoo, D. Besemer, T. Yeghiazarian, and B. Irvine. 1995. Rapid and precise quantification of HIV-1 RNA in plasma using a branched DNA signal amplification assay. J. Acquired Immune Defic. Syndr. 8:446–454.

99. Palella, F. J., Jr., K. M. Delaney, A. C. Moorman, M. O. Loveless, J. Fuhrer, G. A. Satten, D. J. Aschman, and S. D. Holmberg. 1998. Declining morbidity and mortality among patients with advanced human immunodeficiency virus infection. HIV Outpatient Study Investigators [see comments]. N. Engl. J. Med. 338:853–860.

100. The Panel on Clinical Practices for Treatment of HIV Infection convened by the Department of Health and Human Services (DHHS) and the Henry J. Kaiser Family Foundation. 2001. Guidelines for the use of antiretroviral agents in HIV-infected adults and adolescents. http://hivatis.org.

101. Paterson, D. L., S. Swindells, J. Mohr, M. Brester, E. N. Vergis, C. Squier, M. M. Wagener, and N. Singh. 2000. Adherence to protease inhibitor therapy and outcomes in patients with HIV infection. Ann. Intern. Med. 133:21–30.

102. Perelson, A. S., P. Essunger, Y. Cao, M. Vesanen, A. Hurley, K. Saksela, M. Markowitz, and D. D. Ho. 1997. Decay characteristics of HIV-1-infected compartments during combination therapy [see comments]. Nature 387:188–191.

103. Perelson, A. S., A. U. Neumann, M. Markowitz, J. M. Leonard, and D. D. Ho. 1996. HIV-1 dynamics in vivo: virion clearance rate, infected cell life-span, and viral generation time. Science 271:1582–1586.

104. Petropoulos, C. J., N. T. Parkin, K. L. Limoli, Y. S. Lie, T. Wrin, W. Huang, H. Tian, D. Smith, G. A. Winslow, D. J. Capon, and J. M. Whitcomb. 2000. A novel phenotypic drug susceptibility assay for human immunodeficiency virus type 1. Antimicrob. Agents Chemother. 44:920–928.

105. Piatak, M., Jr., M. S. Saag, L. C. Yang, S. J. Clark, J. C. Kappes, K. C. Luk, B. H. Hahn, G. M. Shaw, and J. D. Lifson. 1993. High levels of HIV-1 in plasma during all stages of infection determined by competitive PCR [see comments]. Science 259:1749–1754.

106. Pierson, T., J. McArthur, and R. F. Siliciano. 2000. Reservoirs for HIV-1: mechanisms for viral persistence in the presence of antiviral immune responses and antiretroviral therapy. Annu. Rev. Immunol. 18:665–708.

107. Pilcher, C. D., W. C. Miller, Z. A. Beatty, and J. J. Eron 1999. Detectable HIV-

1 RNA at levels below quantifiable limits by amplicor HIV-1 monitor is associated with virologic relapse on antiretroviral therapy. AIDS 13:1337–1342.

108. Piot, P., M. Bartos, P. Ghys, N. Walker, and B. Schwartlander. 2001. The global impact of HIV/AIDS. Nature 410:968–973.

109. Pitcher, C. J., C. Quittner, D. M. Peterson, M. Connors, R. A. Koup, V. C. Maino, and L. J. Picker. 1999. HIV-1-specific CD4+ T cells are detectable in most individuals with active HIV-1 infection, but decline with prolonged viral suppression [see comments]. Nature Med. 5:518–525.

110. Powderly, W. G., M. S. Saag, S. Chapman, G. Yu, B. Quart, and N. J. Clendeninn. 1999. Predictors of optimal virological response to potent antiretroviral therapy. AIDS 13:1873–1880.

111. Raboud, J. M., J. S. Montaner, B. Conway, S. Rae, P. Reiss, S. Vella, D. Cooper, J. Lange, M. Harris, M. A. Wainberg, P. Robinson, M. Myers, and D. Hall. 1998. Suppression of plasma viral load below 20 copies/ml is required to achieve a long-term response to therapy. AIDS 12:1619–1624.

112. Ramratnam, B., J. E. Mittler, L. Zhang, D. Boden, A. Hurley, F. Fang, C. A. Macken, A. S. Perelson, M. Markowitz, and D. D. Ho. 2000. The decay of the latent reservoir of replication-competent HIV-1 is inversely correlated with the extent of residual viral replication during prolonged anti-retroviral therapy. Nature Med. 6:82–85.

113. Richman, D. 2001. HIV chemotherapy. Nature 410:995–1001.

114. Richman, D. D., D. Havlir, J. Corbeil, D. Looney, C. Ignacio, S. A. Spector, J. Sullivan, S. Cheeseman, K. Barringer, and D. Pauletti. 1994. Nevirapine resistance mutations of human immunodeficiency virus type 1 selected during therapy. J. Virol. 68:1660–1666.

115. Roederer, M. 1995. T-cell dynamics of immunodeficiency [letter; comment]. Nature Med. 1:621–622.

116. Rosenberg, E. S., M. Altfeld, S. H. Poon, M. N. Phillips, B. M. Wilkes, R. L. Eldridge, G. K. Robbins, R. T. D'Aquila, P. J. Goulder, and B. D. Walker. 2000. Immune control of HIV-1 after early treatment of acute infection. Nature 407:523–526.

117. Rosenberg, E. S., J. M. Billingsley, A. M. Caliendo, S. L. Boswell, P. E. Sax, S. A. Kalams, and B. D. Walker. 1997. Vigorous HIV-1-specific CD4+ T cell responses associated with control of viremia [see comments]. Science 278:1447–1450.

118. Saag, M. S., M. Holodniy, D. R. Kuritzkes, W. A. O'Brien, R. Coombs, M. E. Poscher, D. M. Jacobsen, G. M. Shaw, D. D. Richman, and P. A. Volberding. 1996. HIV viral load markers in clinical practice. Nature Med. 2:625–629.

119. Salomon, H., M. A. Wainberg, B. Brenner, Y. Quan, D. Rouleau, P. Cote, R. LeBlanc, E. Lefebvre, B. Spira, C. Tsoukas, R. P. Sekaly, B. Conway, D. Mayers, and J. P. Routy. 2000. Prevalence of HIV-1 resistant to antiretroviral drugs in 81 individuals newly infected by sexual contact or injecting drug use. Investigators of the Quebec Primary Infection Study. AIDS 14:F17–23.

120. Schacker, T. W., J. P. Hughes, T. Shea, R. W. Coombs, and L. Corey. 1998. Biological and virologic characteristics of primary HIV infection [see comments]. Ann. Intern. Med. 128:613–620.

121. Schnittman, S. M., H. C. Lane, J. Greenhouse, J. S. Justement, M. Baseler, and A. S. Fauci. 1990. Preferential infection of CD4+ memory T cells by human im-

munodeficiency virus type 1: evidence for a role in the selective T-cell functional defects observed in infected individuals. Proc. Natl. Acad. Sci. USA 87:6058–6062.

122. Schuurman, R., L. Demeter, P. Reichelderfer, J. Tijnagel, T. de Groot, and C. Boucher. 1999. Worldwide evaluation of DNA sequencing approaches for identification of drug resistance mutations in the human immunodeficiency virus type 1 reverse transcriptase. J. Clin. Microbiol. 37(7):2291–2296.

123. Schuurman, R., M. Nijhuis, R. van Leeuwen, P. Schipper, D. de Jong, P. Collis, S. A. Danner, J. Mulder, C. Loveday, and C. Christopherson. 1995. Rapid changes in human immunodeficiency virus type 1 RNA load and appearance of drug-resistant virus populations in persons treated with lamivudine (3TC). J. Infect. Dis. 171:1411–1419.

124. Sharkey, M. E., et al. 2000. Persistence of episomal HIV-1 infection intermediates in patients on highly active anti-retroviral therapy. Nature Med. 6:76–81.

125. Silvestri, G., and M. B. Feinberg. 2001. Immune intervention in AIDS. *In* S. H. E. Kaufmann, A. Sher, and R. A. Ahmed (ed.), Anti-infective immune responses. ASM Press, Washington, D.C.

126. Sommadossi, J. P. 1999. HIV protease inhibitors: pharmacologic and metabolic distinctions. AIDS 13(Suppl. 1):S29–40.

127. Stanley, S., M. A. Ostrowski, J. S. Justement, K. Gantt, S. Hedayati, M. Mannix, K. Roche, D. J. Schwartzentruber, C. H. Fox, and A. S. Fauci. 1996. Effect of immunization with a common recall antigen on viral expression in patients infected with human immunodeficiency virus type 1 [see comments]. N. Engl. J. Med. 334:1222–1230.

128. Staprans, S. I., B. L. Hamilton, S. E. Follansbee, T. Elbeik, P. Barbosa, R. M. Grant, and M. B. Feinberg. 1995. Activation of virus replication after vaccination of HIV-1-infected individuals. J. Exp. Med. 182:1727–1737.

129. Stein, D. S., J. A. Korvick, and S. H. Vermund. 1992. CD4+ lymphocyte cell enumeration for prediction of clinical course of human immunodeficiency virus disease: a review [see comments]. J. Infect. Dis. 165:352–363.

130. Sterling, T. R., C. M. Lyles, D. Vlahov, J. Astemborski, J. B. Margolick, and T. C. Quinn. 1999. Sex differences in longitudinal human immunodeficiency virus type 1 RNA levels among seroconverters. J. Infect. Dis. 180:666–672.

131. Sterling, T. R., D. Vlahov, J. Astemborski, D. R. Hoover, J. B. Margolick, and T. C. Quinn. 2001. Initial HIV-1 RNA level and progression to AIDS in women and men. N. Engl. J. Med. 344:720–725.

132. USPHS/IDSA Prevention of Opportunistic Infections Working Group. 1997. USPHS/IDSA guidelines for the prevention of opportunistic infections in persons infected with human immunodeficiency virus. Morbid. Mortal. Weekly Rep. 46:RR-12.

133. Vandamme, A. M., S. Van Dooren, W. Kok, P. Goubau, K. Fransen, T. Kievits, J. C. Schmit, E. De Clercq, and J. Desmyter. 1995. Detection of HIV-1 RNA in plasma and serum samples using the NASBA amplification system compared to RNA-PCR. J. Virological Methods 52(1–2):121–132.

134. Verhofstede, C., F. V. Wanzeele, B. Van Der Gucht, N. De Cabooter, and J. Plum. 1999. Interruption of reverse transcriptase inhibitors or a switch from reverse transcriptase to protease inhibitors resulted in a fast reappearance of

virus strains with a reverse transcriptase inhibitor-sensitive genotype. AIDS 13:2541–2546.

135. Walker, B. D., and E. S. Rosenberg. 2000. Containing HIV after infection [letter; comment]. Nature Med. 6:1094–1095.

136. Wei, X., S. K. Ghosh, M. E. Taylor, V. A. Johnson, E. A. Emini, P. Deutsch, J. D. Lifson, S. Bonhoeffer, M. A. Nowak, and B. H. Hahn. 1995. Viral dynamics in human immunodeficiency virus type 1 infection [see comments]. Nature 373:117–122.

137. Weiss, R. 2001. Gulliver's travels in HIVland. Nature 410:963–967.

138. Wong, J. K., M. Hezareh, H. F. Gunthard, D. V. Havlir, C. C. Ignacio, C. A. Spina, and D. D. Richman. 1997. Recovery of replication-competent HIV despite prolonged suppression of plasma viremia [see comments]. Science 278:1291–1295.

139. Yerly, S., L. Kaiser, E. Race, J. P. Bru, F. Clavel, and L. Perrin. 1999. Transmission of antiretroviral-drug-resistant HIV-1 variants [see comments]. Lancet 354:729–733.

140. Zhang, L., B. Ramratnam, K. Tenner-Racz, Y. He, M. Vesanen, S. Lewin, A. Talal, P. Racz, A. S. Perelson, B. T. Korber, M. Markowitz, and D. D. Ho. 1999. Quantifying residual HIV-1 replication in patients receiving combination antiretroviral therapy [see comments]. N. Engl. J. Med. 340:1605–1613.

11

CHRIS COLLINS
TODD SUMMERS
TOM COATES

HIV Prevention: Implementing Proven Prevention Interventions to Control the Global Epidemic

In 1999, AIDS achieved the distinction of becoming the number one infectious disease killer in the world. Sadly, this human, public health, and economic catastrophe was largely preventable. In industrialized and lower-income countries alike, reluctance to overturn political constraints, confront social stigmas, and provide adequate funding for prevention interventions have all impeded the full-scale, global HIV prevention effort that was and is needed.

Yet the opportunity still exists to reduce the number of new HIV infections drastically and stem the spread of AIDS in countries across the world. More than two decades of HIV prevention programming and behavioral research provide a substantial armamentarium of effective and cost-effective interventions to reduce risk behaviors. New HIV treatment and testing technologies and growing public awareness offer additional opportunities to slow the onslaught of this deadly virus while biomedical scientists search for a vaccine and a cure. What is needed is political leadership, evidenced-based prevention planning, community mobilization, and increased funding. It is no longer a shortage of knowledge or skills that fuels this pandemic but one of will.

The Human and Social Costs of AIDS

Devastating as the AIDS epidemic has already been, the toll in human suffering has only begun. By the end of 1999, HIV/AIDS had taken the lives of 18.8 million people, 3.8 million of them children under 15 years of age. Many more people face debilitating illness and death over the coming decade. The Joint United Nations Programme on HIV/AIDS (UNAIDS) estimates that 34.3 million people, including 15.7 million women and 1.3 million children, were living with HIV at the beginning of 2000. The number

441

of people living with the disease continues to grow each year. In 1999, 2.8 million people died of AIDS, but there were 5.4 million new infections.

The vast majority (95%) of people with HIV live in developing countries, where access to life-prolonging treatments is almost nonexistent. Sub-Saharan Africa, where 24.5 million people are infected, has been most profoundly affected. In this region more than any other, AIDS is an economic and security crisis as well as a human tragedy. According to the World Bank, the epidemic is responsible for erasing half a century's worth of development in many affected countries. Hard-won reductions in adult and child mortality have been reversed; in Botswana and Zimbabwe, for example, AIDS has shortened life expectancy by 17 years.

Prevalence rates are dramatic. In South Africa, the African continent's most populous nation, one in five people is already infected with HIV. In Botswana, more than a third (35.8%) of the population is HIV-positive. Young people will be the most acutely affected in sub-Saharan Africa. In South Africa and several other African countries, more than one-third of the children who are 15 years old today will die from AIDS by the time they are 50. Each week, 290 infants in the country die from the disease. The epidemic also exacerbates other, already serious health problems in African countries. For example, AIDS has greatly increased the number of people in Africa who are living with, and capable of transmitting, tuberculosis. The World Bank has estimated that one-quarter of tuberculosis deaths among HIV-negative persons in the coming years would not have occurred without the AIDS epidemic. People with HIV in poorer countries are twice as likely to become infected with, and carriers of, the parasite that causes malaria (50). Other regions of the world are also experiencing serious HIV/AIDS epidemics. For example, in the Caribbean 2.3% of the adult population is infected (19), and in Haiti 8% of adults in urban areas are now HIV-positive (23). Infection rates are escalating in the states of the former Soviet Union, where the estimated number of people living with HIV/AIDS increased from 170,000 in 1997 to 700,000 in 2000 (20).

AIDS is undermining the ability of societies to care for their sick, educate future generations, and maintain recent gains in economic development. Increasing numbers of health care workers are falling ill and dying from AIDS even as government spending takes a huge portion of the total health care budget (21). In the Central African Republic, more than half of all the schools have had to be closed because of staff shortages resulting primarily from AIDS-related deaths (21). Largely because of AIDS, Zimbabwe has seen the output of communal agriculture fall by 50% during the five years preceding 2000 (21).

Asia is the next most severely affected region, with more than 6.1 million people living with HIV. Latin America has 1.3 million HIV-positive individuals. In recent years, the epidemic has grown rapidly in countries of the former Soviet Union. In just two years, between 1998 and 2000, the estimated total number of people living with HIV in Ukraine increased from 110,000 to 240,000. In Eastern Europe and Central Asia as a whole, 420,000 people are now living with HIV.

The primary routes of HIV transmission differ around the world. In sub-Saharan Africa the vast majority of HIV transmission is attributed to heterosexual sex. Infection rates are substantially higher for young African women than for men, largely because young women are more likely to have older sexual partners and are more biologically vulnerable to infection during sexual intercourse. The epidemic in Eastern Europe and Central Asia tends to be centered among injection drug users (IDUs). Asia, Latin America, and North America have more diverse epidemics, with injection drug use and homosexual and heterosexual sex all playing important roles in the spread of HIV.

Poverty, racism, homophobia, sexism, disenfranchisement, and lack of access to prevention and health care are important risk factors in each of these regions. These social factors make populations vulnerable to HIV/AIDS in a variety of ways. Examples include people dependent on sex work for income who may not be able to demand that condoms be used; women feeling relatively powerless in relationships and afraid to ask that their husbands or primary sexual partners use condoms; homophobic policies and social attitudes that make it more difficult for gay and bisexual men to receive prevention services or openly discuss safer sex; and young women subjected to sexual abuse and rape. Scarce public health resources can make it extremely difficult for nearly everyone in resource-poor regions to access basic health care and prevention education. In 1995, the late Dr. Jonathan Mann observed that maturing AIDS epidemics around the world shared a common theme: "the increasing concentration of HIV/AIDS among those who before the arrival of AIDS were already marginalized, stigmatized, and discriminated against within society" (32).

The AIDS epidemic will also likely affect the welfare of whole nations and is having an important impact on global political dynamics. As UNAIDS has noted, AIDS will "widen the gulf between rich and poor nations and push already-stigmatized groups closer to the margins of society" (21). Because AIDS is destabilizing political, economic, and health care infrastructures in so many fragile regions, in early 2000 U.S. government leaders identified the pandemic as a threat to national and global security.

The Epidemic in the United States

In the United States more than 430,000 have died of AIDS, and it is estimated that as many as 900,000 people are living with HIV or AIDS. Although HIV surveillance has been only partially implemented, experts estimate that 40,000 Americans are newly infected each year. As in other parts of the world, poverty and lack of access to health care and prevention services are important risk factors for HIV infection in the United States. Although still a significant threat to gay and bisexual men, the domestic epidemic has expanded to IDUs, racial and ethnic minorities, women, and youth. Injection drug abuse accounts for approximately one-third to one-half of the epidemic either directly (through actual injection drug use) or indirectly (through sex partners of IDUs or children of these sex partners). Injection drug use plays a particularly important role in the epidemic among African Americans and Latinos. In 1998, 36% of AIDS cases in these two populations were the result of injection drug use.

Although there has been increasing attention to HIV and AIDS among African Americans, Latinos, and other minorities, these groups have been disproportionately affected since the beginning of the epidemic and today represent a steadily growing share of AIDS cases and new infections. Approximately 1 in 50 African American men, and 1 in 160 African American women, are HIV-positive. The rate of AIDS diagnoses is two times greater among African Americans than among Latinos and eight times greater than for whites. In 1998, nearly half (45%) of all newly reported AIDS cases were among African Americans, and two-thirds of cases in women and in children were African American.

IDUs and heterosexuals account for an increasing share of the domestic epidemic, but men who have sex with men (MSMs) remain the largest single exposure group, with 15,464 newly reported AIDS cases in 1999. Recent studies indicate ongoing and perhaps increasing rates of sexual risk taking and infection among MSMs. Young gay and bisexual men continue to be at high risk. A survey conducted in 1999 found that in six urban counties between 5% and 8% of MSMs ages 15 to 22 were HIV-positive. Among African American MSMs, seroprevalence was 8% to 14%.

One of the most dramatic successes in HIV prevention has been among newborns at risk for perinatal transmission (30, 35). Thanks to a campaign of voluntary counseling and testing (VCT) and the widespread use of zidovudine (azidothymidine, AZT) (and increasing cesarean deliveries) (16) to reduce transmission risk, the number of reported cases of perinatally acquired AIDS declined from 800 in 1995 to 263 in 1999 (4).

Powerful treatments for HIV may also have affected prevention efforts, both positively and negatively. Antiretroviral therapy (ART) allows many persons with HIV to reduce viral load substantially, which also appears to reduce sexual and mother-to-child transmissibility risk. Yet there is also growing evidence that the success of combination therapies is leading to a sense of complacency and increased risky behavior among both HIV-positive and HIV-negative individuals. One study sampled gay men, IDUs, and heterosexuals visiting sexually transmitted disease (STD) clinics. Of those surveyed, 31% were "less concerned" about contracting HIV because of what they had heard about new treatments for HIV (29). One-quarter of gay and bisexual men and 30% of heterosexuals reported being less concerned about AIDS.

Awareness of combination therapy has also affected the sexual-risk-taking behavior of some serodiscordant couples (one HIV-positive, one HIV-negative). A study released in April 2000 reported that more than two-thirds of HIV serodiscordant heterosexual couples surveyed in California said they had engaged in unprotected intercourse during the six months proceeding the survey. Up to 33% of seropositive and 40% of seronegative respondents said they had decreased concerns about transmission because of awareness of new treatments for HIV disease (48).

As biomedical treatments for HIV are changing treatment and prevention, the difficulties of communication between human partners remain a constant issue. The awkwardness of direct communication and the difficulties of negotiation around safer sex are enormous challenges to prevention providers. Interviews with HIV-positive and -negative gay and bisexual men found that many were making assumptions about the serostatus of their partners—and acting on those assumptions—based on nonverbal clues. "In many instances," researchers found, "study participants deferred the responsibility for choosing condom use or discussing HIV serostatus to their sexual partner based on how the partner behaved and what he said or did not say within the context of the sexual episode" (42).

Other recent research has confirmed general increases in sexual risk taking among gay men in several urban areas. The AIDS epidemic peaked relatively early in the city of San Francisco; transmission rates then fell precipitously after concerted prevention campaigns were launched. Yet over the past several years, San Francisco public health officials have documented significant increases in recent HIV seroconversions along with higher rates of unprotected anal intercourse (UAI) (10). Other jurisdictions have reported increases in risk behavior (Vancouver [44]) and STDs among MSMs (Los Angeles [33], Seattle [27]). Nationally, researchers have reported a dramatic rise in STD rates among gay men. For example, the incidence of gonorrhea among gay men nearly tripled between 1992 and 1998. Among HIV-positive gay men, the impact has been even more startling: a 250% increase in gonorrhea diagnoses between 1994 and 1998 (11).

Lessons Learned in Prevention Programming

In the United States and around the world, prevention providers have often struggled with inadequate funding and political and social limitations placed on prevention programming. Still, HIV prevention campaigns have proven widely successful at reducing unsafe behavior and lowering infection rates—even among those at highest risk (7). In many communities, the AIDS epidemic has led to profound changes in risk behavior. In both 1982 and 1983 approximately 8,000 gay men became infected with HIV in San Francisco. Ten years later, there were approximately 1,000 infections per year, and that number continued to fall through the mid-1990s; only recently has the trend changed (as noted earlier). Prevention education programs in schools and through the media have reduced risk taking and increased condom use among high-school-aged young people. Among high school students, self-reported condom use at last intercourse rose from 46% in 1991 to 58% in 1999; high school students reporting any sexual intercourse decreased from 54% in 1991 to 50% in 1999 (2).

More than a decade of behavioral research has identified important lessons about what works and what does not work in HIV prevention. These are discussed in the following sections.

Peer Influence and Community Organizing Are Powerful HIV Prevention Tools

Working on the premise that peer leaders could be effective prevention educators, researchers based in Wisconsin (26) identified popular opinion leaders among gay men in several small cities. The researchers then provided these individuals with specific training on encouraging safer sex practices among others in the community. Impressive changes in the intervention communities were documented: UAI fell by 25% in two months; 18% fewer men reported having more than one sex partner; and condom use increased by 16%.

Another study, in Eugene, Oregon (24, 25), sought to mobilize the community of young gay men to plan and produce their own community-level prevention interventions. Interventions included peer-based outreach at settings frequented by young gay and bisexual men; social events and group meetings; informal outreach through casual conversation; and publicity campaigns. From pre- to postintervention, there were significant reductions in the proportion of young gay men reporting UAI in the past two months with both primary and nonprimary partners. Overall rates of UAI decreased from 38% to 31%. Among nonprimary partners, UAI fell from 19% to 14%, and from 58% to 42% with boyfriends.

Clean Needle Availability Reduces Risks for IDUs, Their Partners, and Their Children without Encouraging Illegal Drug Use

Syringe exchange programs are frequently the subject of fervent political debate, both in the United States and in other countries struggling with IDU-related HIV infections. Although the U.S. Congress has prohibited use of federal funds for such programs, many local communities have chosen to implement needle exchange programs: today more than 100 needle exchange programs are in operation in more than 80 U.S. cities in 30 states. The congressional funding restriction is often cited as an example of how politics and public health can collide. Even though six U.S. government–funded studies have concluded that syringe exchange programs can help to prevent HIV infection and do not promote drug use (12, 31, 36, 38, 39, 47) and the nation's top scientists and public health officials have declared them effective at reducing HIV infections without encouraging illegal drug use, opponents continue to cite those concerns to justify funding restrictions. Syringe exchange programs in other countries have faced similar barriers. A community-based syringe exchange program in St. Petersburg, Russia, had its mobile facility destroyed by arson, despite the fact that it was playing an important role in combating a huge increase in IDU-related HIV and hepatitis infections.

Comprehensive Sex Education for Young People at Risk Is Critical and Should Include, but Not Be Limited to, Abstinence Encouragement

Prevention experts at the U.S. Centers for Disease Control and Prevention (CDC) estimate that as many as half of all new HIV infections in the United States occur among those 25 years of age and younger. Yet school-based HIV and sex education remains a hotbed of political debate. Some, including leaders in the U.S. Congress, push for "abstinence-only" programs, while others insist that young people need "comprehensive sexuality education." Abstinence-only programs typically promote abstinence from sex before marriage or a committed relationship and generally avoid specific discussions of contraception, STDs, abortion, or homosexuality. Comprehensive sexuality education often encourages abstinence but also includes discussion of contraceptives, condom use, abortion, and homosexuality.

A substantial body of current behavioral research indicates that some comprehensive sexuality programs have been effective at delaying the onset of sexual intercourse, decreasing the number of sexual partners, and increasing condom and contraceptive use among young people (28). Abstinence-based programs have been shown effective in reducing self-reported risk taking but have also shown to have less impact over time than comprehensive programs. In the United States, a substantial percentage of youth-specific HIV prevention funding is given directly to school districts (5) in which only a small percentage of programming is tailored specifically to the needs of young people at particularly high risk, including homeless youth, young MSMs, and young women who have older partners.

Drug Treatment Is an Important HIV Prevention Tool

As noted earlier, substance abuse plays an increasingly important role in the HIV epidemic in the United States. A 1997 Consensus Development Conference on HIV prevention sponsored by the National Institutes of Health concluded that drug treatment should be one of the most important weapons in HIV prevention. The consensus statement noted, "Research data are clear that the programs reduce risky drug and alcohol abuse behavior and often eliminate drug abuse itself. Drug and alcohol abuse treatment is a central bulwark in the Nation's defense against HIV/AIDS" (37). Yet it has been estimated that in the United States 48% of the need for drug treatment slots is currently unmet (51).

VCT

Approximately one-quarter to one-third of all people living with HIV in the United States (or about 200,000 people) do not yet know they are infected. VCT programs can be an effective tool for reaching those at risk and helping them determine if they are positive (45). When done correctly, VCT can help reduce unsafe behaviors, particularly when client-centered counseling rather than brief didactic counseling is used. Even when brief client-centered counseling is provided, unsafe behaviors may continue for some recipients. VCT programs can also be used to refer those testing positive or found to be at high risk to more intensive health care and prevention supports (9).

Preventing Mother-to-Child Transmission

Several studies have confirmed that ART given to pregnant women can dramatically reduce the chances that they will pass HIV infection on to their newborns. Ideally, the mother is treated in the third trimester of pregnancy and during labor, and the infant is also treated in the first few days after birth. Early studies of perinatal transmission established that AZT is effective at preventing transmissions between mother and child. More recent research has shown that the less expensive drug nevirapine is also highly effective, raising hopes that this therapy can be used widely in the developing world. Biomedical intervention in the perinatal period is, however, an incomplete approach to the prevention of mother-to-child HIV infection because infants face infection risk from breast-feeding. The risk of HIV transmission during breast-feeding has been shown to decrease when women are receiving ART and achieve reduced HIV viral loads. The most effective approach is therefore to provide perinatal treatment to pregnant women and continue to provide HIV prevention therapies to both the newborn and the mother.

HIV Prevention Is Most Effective When Targeted to Those at Risk

To be effective, HIV prevention interventions should be tailored to reach specific audiences. "One size fits all" models of prevention often fail to reach groups most at risk of infection, including young people of color and gay men. In 1999, the CDC released a "Compendium" of tested and proven effective HIV prevention interventions, most of them targeted to specific groups (3). An intervention studied by John Jemmott III involved African American adolescent boys in one five-hour session that included presentations by African American educators and others, educational videos, and small-group discussions. The intervention was successful in helping these young men increase the use of condoms during sex and reduce their total number of sex partners (17).

Advertising and Marketing Campaigns

Mass-media and targeted media campaigns can change community norms in favor of safer sex and safer needle use. A marketing campaign in Switzerland was credited with increasing condom use with casual sex partners from 8% to 50% between 1987 and 1991 (49). A mass-media campaign in Zaire lead to enormous increases in condoms sales, from 936,000 in 1988 (before the campaign) to more than 4.1 million in 1989 (after the campaign) (13). A project using youth-oriented condom social marketing with young people in Botswana demonstrated positive impacts on several health beliefs, including an increased awareness of the benefits of condom use and a reduction in important barriers to condom use (34).

Access to Condoms

Easy access to condoms, along with programs that help people demand them and use them, can reduce HIV infections. Research has demonstrated that the availability of condoms in high schools does not hasten the initiation of sexual activity or the number of sex partners among adolescents and can increase condom use (15). One published review of five successful pregnancy prevention programs found that the two programs that significantly reduced the proportion of adolescents who became pregnant were the two that put the greatest emphasis on providing access to contraceptive services (14).

Dialogue with Doctors and Other Health Care Providers

Health care workers are a trusted source of information about protective health practices, yet doctors, nurses, and other health professionals are a largely untapped prevention resource. One study found that the majority of adolescents surveyed would find it "very helpful" to talk with a physician about how to avoid getting HIV or other STDs from sex, yet only 39% reported such discussions with doctors. Only 15% reported discussing their sex life with a physician (43).

Interventions at Multiple Levels

HIV prevention interventions are most effective when they reach people on multiple levels (8). For example, the impact of an intensive safer sex workshop is greatly reduced if people leaving the workshop reenter communities where there is little social support for maintaining safer sex or discussing HIV prevention. HIV prevention planners should consider multiple levels of interventions, including

- individual-based interventions offering intensive safer sex and needle use education, skill building in condom use and sexual refusal and negotiation skills, and personal counseling;
- dyadic-familial interventions, including communication skills building, couples counseling, and family skills training;
- institutional-community interventions, providing access to condoms and clean needles, launching media campaigns designed to affect community norms that promote safer sex, needle use, and drug treatment;
- policy-legal interventions that change laws and policies, such as paraphernalia laws, protection from discrimination, regulations on blood donations, and confidentiality protections;
- superstructural changes, including antipoverty, jobs, and educational programs or social movements to combat homophobia, racism, and AIDS phobia and thus change the context of people's lives; and
- medical-technological interventions, including drug and STD treatment, voluntary testing and treatment of pregnant mothers to prevent perinatal transmission, and research to develop microbicides and vaccines.

Prevention Successes in Low- and Middle-Income Countries

Political and health leaders in some developing countries have been slow to recognize the devastation AIDS will bring to their societies or to implement tested prevention interventions widely. Yet many of the most impressive successes in HIV prevention have occurred in low- and middle-income countries. Countries such as Thailand, Uganda, and others have led the way in implementing HIV programs that are credited with preventing millions of infections and demonstrating the power of well-designed prevention interventions.

In 1989 Thailand launched a pilot program to encourage 100% condom use in brothels and other commercial sex establishments. The program seeks to gain the agreement of owners of these establishments to enforce condom use as a condition of commercial sex. Health workers, political leaders, and police work together to develop and enforce the program. Brothel owners who do not cooperate face potential sanctions, including permanent closure of their businesses. Implemented nationwide in Thailand in 1991, the program has been credited with preventing more than 2 million HIV infections (22).

Political leaders in Uganda have long been applauded for their focus on HIV prevention programming. For example, the Family AIDS Education and Prevention through Imams Project is a community mobilization intervention that has increased knowledge about HIV and led to increases in safer sex practices. The project holds workshops with religious leaders in the Muslim community (Imams), bicycle taxi drivers, and market vendors. These individuals are trained to pass on information in the community concerning facts about HIV, personal risk perception, and safer sex practices. Two years after the project was initiated, a follow-up survey found increased knowledge about HIV in the community, lower reported numbers of sexual partners, and increased condom use (18).

Researchers at the National AIDS Research Institute in Pune, India, demonstrated that a VCT intervention was successful in reducing sexual risk behaviors. More than 1,600 heterosexual men agreed to visit a health clinic every three months for HIV counseling and testing. Counselors sought to reinforce messages supporting monogamy and condom use with sexual partners, and participants were given free condoms. After two years of counseling, researchers found that the number of men visiting sex workers declined from 63% to 23%. Those men who continued to see sex workers were more than four times more likely to use a condom with sex workers (1).

Emerging Prevention Issues

Primary Prevention for HIV-Positive Persons

HIV prevention providers have often shied away from designing prevention interventions tailored specifically to help people living with HIV practice safer sex and avoid spreading the virus to others. To a large degree, this avoidance can be attributed to justifiable concern about stigmatizing people living with HIV.

Today, there are important reasons for increased concentration on primary prevention for people living with HIV. Growing numbers of people with the disease are living more healthy, sexual lives, increasing the chances that they will pass on infection. Recent evidence suggests that risk taking among both HIV-positive and -negative people is increasing, with the success of ARTs making some people worry less about becoming infected. Lessons learned from earlier prevention work should inform the design of prevention interventions for people living with HIV. But a number of issues are particularly important for this population, and they must be considered in the design of interventions. The challenges include

- communicating the responsibility to not infect others without promoting shame or stigma against people living with HIV;

- acknowledging the need for intimacy through sex and avoiding simplistic messages (such as "safer sex is hotter sex") that do not acknowledge the psychological challenges of consistent condom use;
- improving communication between partners and discouraging people from using nonverbal cues to make assumptions about the HIV status of their partners;
- considering the diverse opinions on utilizing disclosure of HIV status as a prevention approach (a third or more people living with HIV do not know their status, and many who do know they are positive may have legitimate legal, employment, or safety concerns about revealing that status to all potential partners); and
- communicating clear messages to HIV-positive individuals about biomedical issues in the face of unanswered scientific questions, such as the relative infectivity of sperm of people in ART and the dangers to people with HIV of reinfection with drug-resistant strains of the virus.

New Technology to Advance Prevention

New technologies will play an important role in HIV surveillance and prevention efforts. The recently developed "detuned assay" has been used in combination with the standard HIV ELISA test to determine whether a person was recently infected with the virus. The blood of individuals who test positive on the standard ELISA is retested using the less sensitive detuned assay. Because the body has a progressive antibody response to HIV, the less sensitive assay will show a negative result in people who have been infected within approximately the past four months (129 days). When used at anonymous test sites and other testing venues and coupled with information about the race, sex, risk activities, and area of residence, the detuned assay can point to emerging trends in the epidemic. This information can then be used to target HIV prevention efforts more efficiently.

Technology is also being developed that will allow for "rapid testing" for HIV, providing testing results within a matter of minutes or hours. The substantial percentage of people who fail to return to testing sites for their HIV test results is one of the major challenges in prevention. It is hoped that, when licensed, rapid testing will provide virtual "on the spot" results, increasing opportunities to deliver early treatment intervention and prevention counseling to those who are positive (45).

Securing widespread access to ART may also be an important prevention intervention. Emerging research indicates that HIV-positive individuals with lower viral loads are less likely to transmit HIV to their sexual partners. A study involving 415 heterosexual, serodiscordant couples in

Uganda found that the higher the HIV viral load in the infected partner, the higher the risk of HIV transmission (40). Treatment of STDs can also reduce susceptibility to transmission of HIV and should be part of HIV control programs (41).

Integrating Vaccines into Prevention

A vaccine for AIDS is ultimately the best hope to bring the global epidemic under control. Vaccines have several potential advantages over other HIV prevention interventions: they do not rely on consistent and sustained behavior change, and they can reach populations that have limited access to health care. Yet AIDS vaccines present daunting scientific obstacles to researchers. Traditional approaches to vaccine design are considered too dangerous with HIV; the virus is highly variable and mutates rapidly; recovery from HIV has not been documented; the mechanism for human immunity to HIV has not been identified; and there is no perfect animal model for use in AIDS vaccine research. Still, more than 30 candidate vaccines have entered early-phase human trials, and at this writing a large-scale efficacy trial of one vaccine is under way in the United States and Thailand.

Although vaccines hold great promise, communities battling HIV/AIDS epidemics must appreciate the long timeline for vaccine development, testing, and delivery. In 1997, U.S. President Bill Clinton set a goal of discovering an AIDS vaccine within 10 years, yet many researchers believe a vaccine will not be ready for delivery by that time. In the interim, proven behavioral interventions and VCT remain crucial. It is highly unlikely that the first AIDS vaccines will be 100% efficacious, meaning that behavioral interventions will remain important even when AIDS vaccines are widely available.

With AIDS vaccine science now steadily advancing, the coming years are likely to see a significant growth in the number of human clinical trials in communities throughout the world. With these trials come important opportunities, such as engaging communities in HIV education and prevention and encouraging community dialogue in the ethics of clinical trials. One danger is that the far-off promise of an AIDS vaccine will be offered as a panacea, shifting public and private resources away from behavioral prevention interventions and leading some people to believe that complete protection from HIV is at hand. Instead of undermining traditional HIV prevention, vaccine trials should be integrated into existing prevention efforts. Safer sex counseling is an important component of AIDS vaccine trials, and these interventions can be used as a model for prevention education needed by all those at risk of infection in the community.

The Challenge for Prevention Research: Developing and Transferring Useful Prevention Technology

Prevention research is of limited use unless it answers the specific questions asked by prevention providers and policy makers: what programs work, what is most cost effective, how can interventions be effectively tailored to specific populations? Prevention researchers and practitioners should work collaboratively to design and implement studies, and funders must ensure that research results are translated in a way that enables them to be put to use. Without specific technology transfer programs in place, prevention research and delivery can exist as separate worlds. HIV Community Prevention Planning, funded through the CDC, is intended to bring together prevention researchers and practitioners in order to develop evidence-based prevention plans for states and cities. Technology transfer programs require increased emphasis on both domestic and international HIV prevention.

The Need for Increased Resources

One reason vaccines are often called the "only hope" for the developing world is that existing prevention programs have not yet been fully implemented. Particularly in developing countries, prevention services have been consistently underfunded by international health organizations and home governments. In fiscal year 2000, the U.S. Agency for International Development budget for all HIV/AIDS prevention and care activities in developing countries was $200 million (46). This represents a significant increase over recent years but fails to match the several-billion-dollar effort needed to mount a substantial and sustained prevention effort in the developing world. U.S. spending for domestic HIV prevention efforts at the CDC has remained relatively flat over the past several years (6).

The AIDS epidemic has become one of the greatest public health disasters of our time, killing millions of people, exacerbating other health and social problems, and threatening the fate of whole societies. The disease has challenged governments' willingness to engage marginalized communities, including gays, sex workers, and drug users. Richer countries are only now recognizing the international proportions of the human, economic, and security disaster of AIDS.

Growing political will to fight the AIDS pandemic is the essential ingredient needed to improve the response to AIDS. A wealth of proven-effective prevention interventions are available to help individuals, couples, and societies protect themselves from HIV infection. Properly funded and implemented, these interventions could greatly reduce the number of new HIV infections in countries rich and poor and save literally millions of lives.

REFERENCES

1. Bentley, M. E. 1998. HIV testing and counseling among men attending sexually transmitted disease clinics in Pune, India: Changes in condom use and sexual behavior over time. AIDS 12:1869–1877.
2. Centers for Disease Control and Prevention. 1991 and 1999. Youth risk behavioral survey, 1991 and 1999. CDC, Atlanta.
3. Centers for Disease Control and Prevention. 1999. Compendium of HIV prevention interventions with evidence of effectiveness. Atlanta, November. Available on the Web at http://www.cdc.gov/hiv/pubs/HIV compendium.pdf.
4. Centers for Disease Control and Prevention. 2000. HIV/AIDS surveillance report: 11 (2).
5. Centers for Disease Control and Prevention. Division of Adolescent and School of Health. For information, see http://www.cdc.gov/nccdphp/dash/what.htm. Updated June 2001.
6. Centers for Disease Control and Prevention. Funding for the HIV/AIDS prevention at CDC reached $871 million in fiscal year 2001. "Appropriations: HIV/AIDS Programs," AIDS Action. www.aidsaction.org.
7. Coates, T., and C. Collins. 1998. Preventing HIV infection. Scientific American 279:96–97.
8. Coates, T., and C. Collins. 1999. HIV prevention: we don't need to wait for a vaccine. *In* M. D. Glantz and C. R. Hartel (ed.), Drug abuse: origins and interventions. American Psychological Association, Washington, D.C.
9. Coates, T., O. Grinstead, S. Gregorich, et al. 2000. Efficacy of voluntary HIV-1 counseling and testing in individuals and couples in Kenya, Tanzania, and Trinidad: a randomized trial. Lancet 356:103–112.
10. Coates, T., M. Katz, et al. 2000. The San Francisco Department of Public Health and AIDS Research Institute/UCSF response to the updated estimates of HIV infection in San Francisco. July.
11. Denning, P. 2000. Is the stage being set for a resurgence in the HIV epidemic among men who have sex with men? Abstr. S30. Seventh Conference on Retroviruses and Opportunistic Infections, January 30–February 2, 2000, San Francisco, cited by Mark Schoofs in the Village Voice, February 10.
12. Drug Policy Foundation, comp. 1993. The Clinton administration's internal reviews of research on needle exchange programs: previously unreleased documents plus background material. Drug Policy Foundation, Washington, D.C.
13. Ferreros, C., N. Mivumbi, K. Kakera, and J. Price. 1990. Social marketing of condoms for AIDS prevention in developing countries: the Zaire experience. Abstr. S.C.697. Sixth International Conference on AIDS, San Francisco.
14. Frost, J., and J. Forrest. 1995. Understanding the impact of effective teenage pregnancy prevention programs. Family Planning Perspectives 27(5): 188–195.
15. Guttmacher, S., L. Lieberman, D. Ward, et al. 1997. Condom availability in New York City public schools: relationships to condom use and sexual behavior. Am. J. Public Health 87(9):1427–1433.

16. The International Perinatal HIV Group. 1999. The mode of delivery and the risk of vertical transmission of human immunodeficiency virus type 1—a meta-analysis of 15 prospective cohort studies. N. Engl. J. Med. 340:977–987.

17. Jemmott, J. B., L. S. Jemmott, and G. T. Fong. 1992. Reductions in HIV risk-associated sexual behaviors among black male adolescents: effects of an AIDS prevention intervention. Am. J. Public Health 82(3):372–377.

18. Joint United Nations Programme on HIV/AIDS (UNAIDS). 1998. Family AIDS education and prevention through Imams Project. Available on the Web at http://www.unaids.org/bestpractice/collection/subject/sector/familyaids.html.

19. Joint United Nations Programme on HIV/AIDS (UNAIDS). 2000. Aids epidemic update. December.

20. Joint United Nations Programme on HIV/AIDS (UNAIDS). 2000. Fact sheet: HIV/AIDS in the newly independent states.

21. Joint United Nations Programme on HIV/AIDS (UNAIDS). 2000. Report on the global HIV/AIDS epidemic, Geneva, June.

22. Joint United Nations Programme on HIV/AIDS (UNAIDS). 2000. STI/HIV: 100% condom use programme for sex workers. WHO Regional Office for the Western Pacific. Available on the Web at http://www.unaids.org/bestpractice/digest/files/condoms.html.

23. Joint United Nations Programme on HIV/AIDS (UNAIDS). 2001. Fact sheet: HIV/AIDS in the Caribbean.

24. Kegeles, S. M., and G. J. Hart. 1998. Recent HIV prevention interventions for gay men: individual, small-group and community-level interventions. AIDS 12(Suppl.):S209–215.

25. Kegeles, S. M., R. B. Hays, L. Pollack, and T. J. Coates. 1999. Mobilizing young gay men for HIV prevention: a two community study. AIDS 13:1753–1762.

26. Kelly, J. A., J. S. St. Lawrence, Y. Stevenson, et al. 1992. Community AIDS/HIV risk reduction: the effects of endorsements by popular people in three cities. Am. J. Public Health 82(11):1483–1489.

27. King, W. 2000. No end in sight to syphilis outbreak. Seattle Times, May 10.

28. Kirby, D. 1997. No easy answers, The National Campaign to Prevent Teen Pregnancy, Washington, D.C., March. On the Web at www.teenpregnancy.org.

29. Lehman, S., R. Hecht, et al. 2000. Are at-risk populations less concerned about HIV infection in the HAART era? Abstr. 198. Seventh Conference on Retroviruses and Opportunistic Infections, January 30–February 2, 2000, San Francisco, cited in Kaiser Daily Summary, February 1.

30. Lindergren, M. L., R. H. Byers, P. Thomas, et al. 1999. Trends in perinatal transmission of HIV/AIDS in the United States. JAMA 282:1142–1149.

31. Lurie, P., and A. Reingold. 1993. The public health impact of needle exchange programs in the United States and abroad (prepared for the Centers for Disease Control and Prevention). University of California, School of Public Health, Berkeley, and University of California, Institute for Health Policy Studies, San Francisco.

32. Mann, J., and D. Tarantola (ed.). 1996. AIDS in the world II. Oxford University Press, New York.

33. Marquis, J. 2000. Syphilis outbreak grows in LA, and syphilis cases double among gays. Los Angeles Times, April 8.

34. Meekers, D., G. Stallworthy, and J. Harris. 1997. Changing adolescents' beliefs about protective sexual behavior: the Botswana Tsa Banana Program. Population Services International Research Division Working Paper No. 3; presented at the International Conference on STD/AIDS in Africa, Abidjan, 1997, and at the Eighth International Congress of the World Federation of Public Health Association (WFPHA), Arusha, Tanzania, 1997.

35. Melvin, G., K. Corson, H. Malamud, et al. 1998. Success in implementing public health service guidelines to reduce perinatal transmission of HIV—Louisiana, Michigan, New Jersey, and South Carolina. Morbid. Mortal. Weekly Rep. 47:688–691.

36. National Commission on Acquired Immune Deficiency Syndrome. 1991. The twin epidemics of substance use and HIV. National Commission on Acquired Immune Deficiency Syndrome, Washington, D.C.

37. National Institutes of Health. 1997. Interventions to prevent HIV risk behaviors. National Institutes of Health Consensus Development Conference Statement , Bethesda, Md., February 11–13.

38. National Research Council and Institute of Medicine. 1994. Proceedings, Workshop on Needle Exchange and Bleach Distribution Programs. National Academy Press, Washington, D.C.

39. Office of Technology Assessment. 1995. The effectiveness of AIDS prevention efforts. Office of Technology Assessment, Washington, D.C.

40. Quinn, T. C., M. J. Wawer, N. Sewankambo, et al. 2000. Viral load and heterosexual transmission of human immunodeficiency virus type 1. N. Engl. J. Med. 342(13):921.

41. Rothenberg, R., et al. 2000. The effect of treating sexually transmitted diseases on the transmission of HIV in dually infected persons. Sex. Transm. Dis. 27:411–416.

42. San Francisco AIDS Foundation. 1997. Executive summary: a qualitative interview study of 92 gay and bisexual males regarding HIV risk and sexual behavior. Research sponsored by the San Francisco AIDS Foundation in partnership with the Center for AIDS Prevention Studies, University of California, San Francisco, December.

43. Schuster, M., R. Bell, L. Peterson, et al. 1996. Communication between adolescents and physicians about sexual behavior and risk perception. Arch. Pediatrics and Adolescent Med. 150(9):906–913.

44. Strathdee, S. A., S. L. Martindale, et al. 2000. HIV infection and risk behaviors among young gay and bisexual men. Canadian Medical Assoc. J. 162(1):21–25.

45. Summers, T., F. Spielberg, C. Collins, and T. Coates. Voluntary counseling, testing and referral for HIV: new technologies, research findings create dynamic opportunities, in press.

46. United States Agency for International Development. 2000. Budget justification, FY 2001. USAID, Washington, D.C., http://www.usaid.gov/pubs/bj2001/.

47. U.S. General Accounting Office. 1993. Needle exchange programs: research

suggests promise as an AIDS prevention strategy. U.S. General Accounting Office, Washington, D.C.

48. Van der Straten, A., C. Gomez, et al. 2000. Sexual risk behaviors among heterosexual HIV serodiscordant couples in the era of post-exposure prevention and viral suppressive therapy. AIDS 14:F47–54.

49. Wasserfallen, F., S. T. Stutz, D. Summermatter, M. Hausermann, and F. Dubois-Arber. 1993. Six years of promotion of condom use in the framework of the National Stop AIDS Campaign: experiences and results in Switzerland. Abstr. WS-D27-3. Ninth International Conference on AIDS, Berlin.

50. Whitworth, J., D. Morgan, M. Quigley, et al. 2000. Effect of HIV-1 and increasing immunosuppression on malaria parasitaemia and clinical episodes in adults in rural Uganda: a cohort study. Lancet 356:1051–1056.

51. Woodward, A., J. Epstein, J. Gfroerer, D. Melnick, R. Thoreson, D. Wilson. 1997. The drug abuse treatment gap: recent estimates. Health Care Financing Rev. 18:5–17.

The
12 Immunobiology
NORMAN L. LETVIN | ## of HIV-1 Infection

The immunopathogenesis of AIDS is unique among human viral diseases. Humans mount a vigorous immune response against HIV-1, but containment of the replicating virus is incomplete. The incomplete nature of this immune control of the virus can be explained, at least in part, by the ability of the virus to persist in nonreplicating forms, by its propensity to mutate, and by its eventual destruction of the cellular elements of the immune system. The immunobiology of the virus-host interactions of HIV-1 in humans must be understood if we are to succeed in harnessing the immune response in infected individuals to help contain viral replication. We must also understand these immunopathogenic processes if we are to create a vaccine that will control the worldwide spread of the virus. In this chapter, our current understanding of the immunopathogenesis of HIV-1 is described. This description includes a characterization of the biology of its spread from one infected individual to another, the ramifications of its use of specific cellular receptors, and the immune response that it elicits. Finally, the immunologic consequences of persistent infection are detailed.

Nonhuman Primate Models of HIV-1 Infection

Much of our current understanding of AIDS immunobiology has come from studies of macaques infected with simian immunodeficiency or simian human immunodeficiency viruses. Many African nonhuman primate species are infected with lentivirus isolates that are closely related to HIV-1. These viruses are referred to as simian immunodeficiency viruses (SIVs). Interestingly, these viruses do not induce disease in their natural host African monkey species. However, selected isolates of these viruses induce an AIDS-like illness when inoculated under experimental conditions into certain Asian macaque species. Moreover, it has recently been

459

shown that chimeric viruses that express the HIV-1 envelope can be constructed in the laboratory with an SIV backbone. These viruses are known as simian human immunodeficiency viruses (SHIVs). Selected SHIV isolates induce profound CD4$^+$ T-lymphocyte loss, immunodeficiency, and an AIDS-like illness in macaques. Both the SIV and SHIV/macaque models have proven to be enormously powerful models in which to explore mechanisms of AIDS immunopathogenesis. They have proven particularly useful in characterizing events that occur during the initial days following infection, a period of time during which HIV-1-infected humans are rarely seen by clinical investigators.

HIV and Its Spread

An understanding of the immunobiology of AIDS must be built upon an appreciation that HIV represents an extraordinarily diverse population of antigenically distinct viruses. First, these viruses belong to two quite disparate lineages: the HIV-1 group, introduced into the human population from chimpanzees (22); and the HIV-2 group, introduced into humans from the sootey mangaby, a West African nonhuman primate species (30). These two lineages of viruses are so distinct antigenically that their envelope glycoproteins are usually not immunologically cross-reactive. Second, all HIV isolates undergo a continuous process of mutation. One of every 10,000 nucleotides of the replicating virus mutates because the HIV reverse transcriptase lacks a 3'–exonuclease proofreading activity (78). The virus therefore rapidly becomes an antigenically heterogeneous swarm of viral quasi species even in a single infected individual. To contain HIV, the immune system must deal with this ever-changing population of viruses.

Although we understand the epidemiology of HIV transmission in human populations, its transmission at the cellular level is less well defined. It is well established that HIV is transmitted in sexual secretions and blood products, with most transmission occurring across an intact mucosal surface during sexual contact (11). However, the extent to which HIV associates with cells during the process of transmission remains poorly understood. In infected individuals, viable virus exists both in a cell-free state and in cells. While viral transmission can presumably occur through exposure to either cell-free or cell-associated virus, the form in which the virus is usually transmitted during sexual contact remains unknown.

Whether the transmitted virus is cell free or cell associated, an initial population of cells becomes infected following exposure. Studies in the SIV/macaque model of AIDS initially suggested that the first infected cell is of the dendritic or monocyte/macrophage lineage (73). That observation led to the hypothesis that virus in a dendritic cell or macrophage travels from the mucosal site of initial infection to local draining lymph nodes and that virus then replicates in those lymph nodes. This scenario would explain why there appears to be a selectivity for macrophage-tropic viruses at the time of viral transmission. Although that paradigm is certainly intuitively attractive, two recent studies in the SIV/macaque model have raised questions concerning its validity. In experiments in which SIV was applied to the tonsils or vaginal mucosa and local mucosal tissue was then evaluated, viral RNA was found only in T lymphocytes and not in dendritic cells or macrophages (74, 85). These studies suggest that viral infection might occur in T lymphocytes as well as dendritic cells/macrophages early after viral exposure.

CD4 and Chemokine Receptors

Viral entry into cells usually requires an interaction of the envelope glycoprotein of the virus with the CD4 molecule (17, 37, 47). Since CD4 is a cell-signaling molecule and CD4$^+$ T-lymphocyte dysfunction is a clinical hallmark of HIV-1 infection, considerable experimental work has been invested in determining whether an interaction between CD4 and gp120 is responsible for immune abnormalities in AIDS. While recombinant gp120 added to CD4$^+$ T lymphocytes in vitro has been shown to induce T-lymphocyte abnormalities, there has never been conclusive evidence to suggest that viral gp120, either virion associated or shed, can trigger T-cell abnormalities in vivo.

It was recently demonstrated that HIV-1 makes use of receptors for cell entry in addition to CD4 (1, 21, 42). Those molecules are members of the family of receptors that are referred to as seven-transmembrane G-protein-coupled receptors or chemokine receptors. The chemokine receptor used by a particular HIV-1 isolate has important ramifications for the cellular tropism of that isolate. It has been shown that infection of a transformed T-cell line in vitro can occur only with viral isolates that employ the CXCR4 molecule as their second receptor. Infection of primary macrophage populations occurs with isolates that employ the CCR5 molecule as a second receptor. Entry of viruses into primary human T cells can occur through either the CXCR4 or the CCR5 receptor.

The demonstration that these seven-transmembrane G-protein-coupled receptors are important for HIV-1 entry into cells provided an explanation for some previously puzzling biological properties of HIV-1 isolates. This finding provided a rationale for how CD4$^-$ cells such as endothelial cells can be infected in vivo (19). It explained why HIV-1 replication in lymphocytes can be inhibited in vitro by a number of beta chemokines, including MIP-1α, MIP-1β, and RANTES, since these molecules are ligands for some of the seven-transmembrane G-protein-coupled receptors (15). This understanding of the viral requirement for second receptors also explained some of the well-described idiosyncratic biological events in the process of viral transmission and in clinical progression to

AIDS in those who are infected. It has been known for some time that only a subpopulation of HIV-1 isolates appear to be transmitted by sexual contact. Those viral isolates are almost universally macrophage-tropic (16). It is now clear that the isolates of HIV-1 that are most likely to be transmitted are macrophage-tropic because they are CCR5-tropic. It has also been known for some time that clinical conversion from an asymptomatic infection to AIDS in chronically infected individuals is associated with a phenotypic change in the infecting viral isolates (44). It is now appreciated that this phenotypic change is associated with a change of second-receptor use by the virus from CCR5 to CXCR4. HIV-1 replication increases substantially in the infected individual as that individual progresses clinically to symptomatic AIDS. It is unclear whether the associated conversion from CCR5-tropic to CXCR4-tropic virus in these individuals results in a virus with particularly high replication potential or rather that high levels of replicating virus select for CXCR4-tropic viruses.

Antibody Response to HIV-1

It was assumed at the outset of the AIDS epidemic that an antibody response to HIV-1 would play a crucial role in containing the replication of this virus. However, a number of observations have been made raising doubts about that assumption. It has been clear for some time that the HIV-1 neutralizing antibody response in patient sera against primary patient isolates of HIV-1 is quite weak (50, 51). Moreover, the burst of HIV-1 replication that occurs during the period of primary infection is contained well before the emergence of a neutralizing antibody response in infected individuals (38, 58, 60). These observations suggest that the antibody response may not be of central importance in controlling HIV-1 replication in the setting of infection. Nevertheless, considerable attention has been focused on characterizing virus-specific antibody responses that can neutralize HIV-1, since vaccine elicitation of such antibodies may be of central importance in creating an HIV-1 vaccine. Antibodies against three different neutralizing determinants of HIV-1 envelope have been studied in some depth: the third hypervariable loop of the envelope glycoproteins, the CD4-binding sites of envelope, and the transmembrane gp41 protein.

As a result of the formation of a disulfide bond, the third hypervariable domain of the HIV-1 envelope glycoproteins creates a loop structure (41). This so-called V3 loop has been implicated in the interactions of HIV-1 envelope glycoproteins with chemokine receptors (12). It is therefore reasonable that an antibody that can bind to this loop may interfere with the ability of the virus to bind to and enter a cell. In fact, the earliest antibodies that arise after an infection that are capable of neutralizing HIV-1 appear to recognize this V3 loop sequence (24, 35). Experimental work was done in an attempt to develop the V3 loop as an immunogen for eliciting

protective immune responses against HIV-1. However, a number of observations dampened enthusiasm for this approach. Extreme sequence variability exists among diverse HIV-1 isolates (40). Therefore, V3 loop–
specific antibodies can mediate only type-specific neutralization. Moreover, it has become clear that exposure of the V3 loop to neutralizing antibodies on the intact virion does not occur in primary HIV-1 isolates (6).
Thus, the V3 loop can be quite inaccessible to V3 loop–specific antibodies.
These observations convinced investigators interested in vaccine development to shift their attention to the evaluation of more highly conserved
sequences of the virus that might serve as targets for neutralization.

Because the CD4 molecule is nonpolymorphic, the domains of HIV-1
that bind to CD4 must be relatively conserved among diverse isolates to
maintain the viability of the virus. In fact, antibodies specific for those
CD4-binding domains of gp120 are broadly neutralizing, recognizing and
blocking a diversity of HIV-1 isolates from infecting cell populations in
vitro (36, 65). However, the CD4-binding-site-specific antibodies that have
been assessed in vivo for their ability to protect chimpanzees from HIV-1
challenge have not been protective. Thus, it is assumed that the CD4-
binding-site-specific antibodies are not particularly effective as neutralizing antibodies.

The extraordinary degree of sequence conservation in the transmembrane gp41 protein of the envelope among various HIV-1 isolates makes
that component of the envelope an attractive target for eliciting broadly
neutralizing antibodies through vaccination. In fact, monoclonal antibodies have been developed that bind to the gp41 of a diversity of HIV-1 isolates and neutralize the virus in vitro (75). The recently described model of
Kim and colleagues proposing a series of molecular events leading to HIV-
1 entry suggests that highly conserved amino acid sequences of both the
C- and N-terminal regions of gp41 should prove useful targets for vaccine-
induced neutralizing antibody responses (8, 9).

Evidence in mouse models and humans suggests that neutralizing
antibodies in individuals with established HIV-1 infections have little effect on ongoing viral replication. Immunodeficient mice reconstituted with
human lymphoid tissue have been infected with HIV-1 and then infused
with neutralizing anti-HIV-1 antibodies. These antibody treatments have
little effect on HIV-1 replication (62). Intravenous administration of hyper-
immune globulin with high titers of anti-HIV-1 antibodies in HIV-1-
infected humans, similarly, has little effect on viral load or disease progression. Importantly, however, preexisting circulating antibodies specific
for HIV-1 envelope will likely be able to alter the clinical consequences of
new lentiviral infections. This is most convincingly demonstrated in a number of recent nonhuman primate studies. The infusion into a naive rhesus
monkey of IgG derived from serum of an SIV-infected monkey caused a
damping of viral replication and an attenuation of the pathogenicity of a

subsequent SIV infection (45). Moreover, the infusion of HIV-1 neutralizing monoclonal antibodies in macaques prior to their exposure to a highly
pathogenic SHIV dramatically altered the consequences of both intravenous and mucosally initiated infections (45, 46). In monkeys in which
very high serum concentrations of neutralizing monoclonal antibodies are
achieved, SHIV infections can be blocked, or the pathogenic consequences
of the infections can be significantly attenuated. These observations suggest that neutralizing antibodies specific for HIV-1 may have utility in the
setting of vaccination to prevent HIV-1 infection.

CD8⁺ T-Lymphocyte Response to HIV-1

Although few data have been generated to suggest that anti-HIV-1 antibodies play a role in containing replication of the virus in infected individuals, a number of studies have implicated HIV-1-specific CD8⁺ cytotoxic T lymphocytes (CTLs) in controlling HIV-1 replication. HIV-1-specific
CTLs have been found in large numbers in a variety of anatomic compartments in both HIV-1-infected humans and SIV-infected macaques: in peripheral blood lymphocytes, bronchoalveolar lavage lymphocytes, lymph
nodes, spleen, skin, cerebrospinal fluid, and vaginal mucosal tissue (26, 34,
43, 61, 71, 83). Walker and colleagues first reported that CD8⁺ T lymphocytes inhibit HIV-1 replication in vitro (79). Subsequent studies have implicated a number of mechanisms as being responsible for this inhibition.
The CTL itself has been shown to play an important role in this viral inhibitory activity (76). CTL can lyse HIV-1-infected cells in vitro and block
propagation of the in vitro infection. Soluble factors have also been implicated in this CD8⁺ T-lymphocyte-mediated inhibition (79). The beta
chemokines MIP-1α, MIP-1β, and RANTES have been shown to inhibit
HIV-1 replication in vitro (15). Moreover, other soluble factors probably
also play a role in this CD8⁺ T-lymphocyte-mediated inhibition of HIV-1
replication.

It has also been shown that the clearance of the intense viral replication that occurs during early days following infection correlates with the
emergence of the HIV-1-specific CD8⁺ CTL response (38). A correlation also
has been described between this early viral clearance and the appearance
of an in vivo expansion of clonal or oligoclonal populations of CD8⁺ T lymphocytes. The alpha and beta chains of the T-cell receptors expressed by T
lymphocytes determine the recognition specificity of those cells, and the
particular family of T-cell receptor genes employed by those cells contributes to that antigen specificity. The clonal relatedness of members of a
population of lymphocytes can be assessed by determining the representation of the same T-cell receptor Vβ or Vα gene family in that cell population. Oligoclonal populations of T lymphocytes expressing T-cell receptor genes of the same family have been shown to emerge coincident with

HIV-1 clearance during primary infection (56). Temporal correlations between the emergence of oligoclonal populations of CD8+ CTL and viral clearance are particularly well delineated in the SIV/macaque model of AIDS. Using chromium release–type assays, Vβ repertoire analyses, and the newly developed tetramer assays, a tight correlation has been demonstrated between early viral clearance and the emergence of SIV-specific CTL responses (Fig. 12.1) (10, 39, 84). The clinical status of HIV-1-infected individuals has also been shown to correlate with the strength of their virus-specific CTL responses. In chronically infected individuals, the HIV-1-specific CTL response, as measured with both precursor frequency CTL assays and tetramer-binding assays, has been shown to be associated with clinical status and clinical prognosis (54, 55).

Perhaps the most compelling evidence for the importance of CD8+ T cells in containing lentiviral replication comes from recent studies in the SIV-infected rhesus monkeys. In these studies, in vivo depletion of CD8+ cells in the monkeys, achieved by infusion of monoclonal anti-CD8 antibody, had profound effects on the replication of SIV (Fig. 12.2) (70). When that depletion lasted less than 21 days, the clearance of virus during primary infection was delayed by a full week as compared with control antibody-treated monkeys. When the duration of depletion was greater than 28 days, primary viremia was never cleared following infection. These monkeys died with a rapidly progressive AIDS-like syndrome.

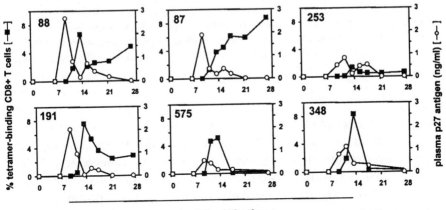

day after infection

FIGURE 12.1

A tight correlation exists between SIV clearance during primary infection and the emergence of SIV-specific CTL responses in rhesus monkeys

CTL are expressed as tetramer-binding CD8+ T lymphocytes and SIV replication as plasma Gag p27 antigen. The percent tetramer binding CD8+ T cells and the p27 antigen in the plasma of six monkeys (88, 87, 253, 191, 575, 348) were analyzed prospectively following SIV infection. CD8+ T lymphocytes were cells gated on CD8αβ+ CD3+ T cells. (From reference 39.)

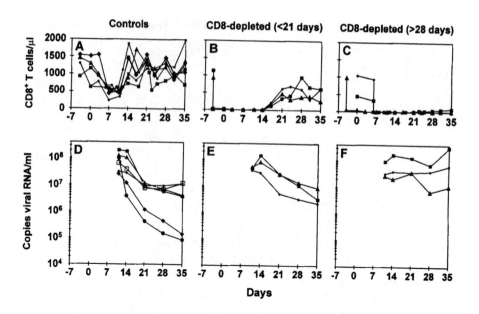

FIGURE 12.2

In vivo depletion of CD8+T lymphocytes in rhesus monkeys
abrogates the monkeys' ability to clear a primary SIV infection

Monkeys were administered an anti-CD8 monoclonal antibody or a control antibody to deplete CD8+ lymphocytes during primary SIV infection. (A) CD8+ T-lymphocyte counts in control antibody-treated monkeys. (B) In three monkeys, treatment with antibody specific for CD8 resulted in near-complete depletion of CD8+ T cells from peripheral blood for 17–21 days. (C) In three monkeys, depletion of CD8+ T cells persisted for 28–60 days. SIV replication was assessed by plasma viral RNA measurement in (D) control antibody-treated monkeys, (E) monkeys depleted of CD8+ lymphocytes for ≤21 days, and (F) monkeys depleted of CD8+ lymphocytes for ≥28 days. (From reference 70.)

Moreover, the transient CD8+ T-lymphocyte depletion of chronically SIV-infected rhesus monkeys was associated with a substantial rise in viral replication that returned to baseline levels with the reemergence of the CD8+ T cell population. These observations illustrate the central role played by CD8+ T lymphocytes in the control of HIV-1 replication.

In view of the ongoing mutation of HIV-1 in infected individuals, it was reasonable to postulate that amino acid substitutions in epitopes of the virus recognized by CD8+ CTL may allow HIV-1 to escape from immune recognition. In fact, studies in HIV-1-infected humans as well as SIV-infected rhesus monkeys have suggested that such escape can sometimes occur (48). However, immune escape of this nature is certainly not inevitable, since some viral epitopes have been shown to be invariable during the course of infection.

CD4⁺ T-Lymphocyte Loss Following HIV-1 Infection

Although HIV-1 replication is controlled in the early weeks following infection by the CD8⁺ T-cell response, the containment of the virus is not complete. The incomplete nature of this containment of viral replication eventually results in the destruction of the immune system by the virus (20). The immunologic hallmark of the persistent replication of HIV-1 infection in humans is a gradual loss of CD4⁺ T lymphocytes. This occurs during the period of clinical latency that follows the primary infection. The duration of the period of clinical latency can extend beyond a decade. No disease is apparent in most infected individuals until the CD4⁺ T-lymphocyte count decreases from a normal of greater than 1,000 to less than 150 cells per microliter of blood. At that time, constitutional symptoms, opportunistic infections, tumors, and eventually death ensue (Fig. 12.3).

The mechanism by which CD4⁺ T cells are lost in the HIV-1-infected individual has remained an issue of considerable controversy. Early in the AIDS epidemic, at a time when the assays for measuring cell-associated virus were quite insensitive, it was assumed that only approximately 1 in 10⁷ peripheral blood CD4⁺ T cells were infected with HIV-1. Explanations

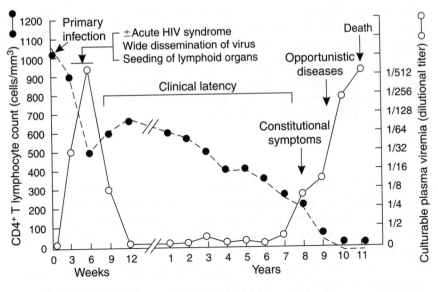

FIGURE 12.3

Disease occurs in HIV-1-infected individuals when peripheral blood
CD4⁺ T-lymphocyte counts decrease to less than approximately 150/μl

The CD4⁺ T-lymphocyte count falls gradually in the years following infection. After an early burst of viral replication during primary infection, as measured by culturable plasma HIV-1, a lower level of replication occurs until late in the clinical course of infection, when it begins to rise precipitously. (From reference 20.)

were therefore sought to account for the occurrence of profound CD4+ T-cell loss in the absence of viral infection of CD4+ T cells. The presumption that insufficient numbers of cells were infected to account for CD4+ T-cell killing led to the suggestion that CD4+ T cells were dying through a secondary, apoptotic process (7). However, as assays for cell-associated virus grew in sensitivity, it became clear that large numbers of CD4+ T cells harbored replicating virus in the infected individual. These observations led some to conclude that the CD4+ T-cell loss in HIV-1-infected individuals occurs solely as a result of virus replicating in and killing individual cells (31). A number of studies have been done in recent years to characterize the mechanism and dynamics of CD4+ T-lymphocyte loss in AIDS. The interpretations of these studies have generated conflicting explanations for this CD4+ T-cell decline.

With the advent of highly active antiretroviral therapy (HAART), it became clear that an early and rapid reconstitution of a percentage of the lost peripheral blood CD4+ T-cell population occurred in HIV-1-infected individuals upon initiation of treatment (32, 59, 81). In fact, carefully observed clinical responses to HAART in HIV-1-infected subjects have been used to draw conclusions concerning AIDS immunopathogenesis. Thus, the observation concerning CD4+ T-lymphocyte repopulation following the institution of HAART lead to the proposal that there is a continuous, high rate of CD4+ T-cell turnover in HIV-1-infected individuals, and the decline in CD4+ T cells in infected individuals occurs as a result of an exhaustion of the capacity to replenish this rapidly turning-over CD4+ T-cell population. The data generated in these studies allowed a calculation of the life span of a CD4+ T cell following infection with HIV-1: a half-life of 1.6 days. Although this explanation for CD4+ T-cell loss in HIV-1-infected individuals was attractive, further studies have not substantiated this model.

The first of the studies to raise doubts about the validity of the model was an experiment done to assess telomere length in CD4+ and CD8+ T cells in HIV-1-infected subjects (82). Telomeres shorten in length as cells age. Therefore, one can approximate the relative age of a lymphocyte by measuring the length of its telomere. When peripheral blood T cells from HIV-1-infected individuals were assessed for their rate of turnover on the basis of telomere length, it was demonstrated that CD4+ T lymphocytes turn over in these individuals at a rate no different from those in uninfected individuals. Interestingly, these studies showed that CD8+ T-cell populations in infected individuals have an increased rate of turnover. Studies were also done to assess the dynamics of CD4+ T-cell loss and repopulation in AIDS in the SIV/macaque model (49, 69). BrdU was employed to measure lymphocyte turnover in both infected and uninfected animals. These studies showed some increase in the rate of CD4+ T-cell turnover in infected as compared with uninfected monkeys. Interestingly, however, the rate of CD8+ T-cell turnover in these infected animals was greater than that of CD4⁺ T cells. Finally, in studies performed using deuterium-labeled lymphocytes in humans, no evidence of an increased rate of CD4⁺ T-cell turnover could be documented in HIV-1-infected subjects (29). In fact, in those studies decreased numbers of circulating CD4⁺ T cells in HIV-1-infected individuals appeared to be attributable to a decrease in the production of those lymphocytes. The ultimate explanation for CD4⁺ T-lymphocyte loss in HIV-1-infected individuals remains unresolved. However, it is likely that this CD4⁺ T-lymphocyte loss is multifactorial in its etiology.

Other facets of the biology of CD4⁺ T lymphocytes in HIV-1-infected individuals are also active areas of investigation. Attempts have been made to characterize the CD4⁺ T lymphocytes that repopulate infected individuals after the initiation of HAART (Fig. 12.4) (2). Early after the institution of therapy, a rise in the memory (CD45RO⁺) CD4⁺ T-cell pool is seen. Later, a reduction in the activation status of all T cells can be demonstrated. Finally, there is a rise in CD4⁺ T lymphocytes with a naive phenotype (CD45RA⁺62L⁺). The early rise in circulating memory CD4⁺ T cells probably reflects the peripheral expansion of preexisting, mature T lymphocytes. The reduction of T-cell activation likely occurs as a consequence of the sustained decrease in production of infecting virus in those individuals. Immune reactivity and the associated T-cell activation are no longer being driven. Finally, the late increase in circulating naive CD4⁺ T cells probably

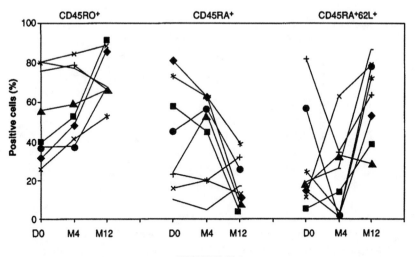

FIGURE 12.4

Successful containment of HIV-1 replication with HAART leads to an early rise in memory and a late rise in naive peripheral blood CD4⁺ T lymphocytes

The proportions of CD4 memory (CD45RO⁺) or naive (CD45RA⁺ and CD45RA⁺CD62L⁺) subsets of T lymphocytes were assessed on peripheral blood lymphocytes. Results are presented as individual percentages of positive cells at day 0 (D0), month 4 (M4), and month 12 (M12) after initiating treatment. (From reference 2.)

reflects repopulation of the periphery with immature, uncommitted lymphocytes from bone marrow and thymus.

Attention has also been focused on characterizing the functional capacity of CD4$^+$ T cells in HIV-1-infected subjects. Early in the AIDS epidemic it was shown that T lymphocytes are functionally abnormal in those infected with the virus. In studies of peripheral blood lymphocytes of subjects with variable degrees of CD4$^+$ T-lymphocyte loss, it was demonstrated that T-lymphocyte responsiveness to soluble protein antigen is lost remarkably early after infection, earlier than responsiveness to alloantigen or mitogen (14). It has recently been shown that an inverse correlation exists in chronically infected individuals between virus load and HIV-1-specific CD4$^+$ T-cell function as measured by viral-protein-driven proliferative responses (Fig. 12.5) (68). Moreover, early institution of HAART during the period of primary infection can result in the preservation of considerable HIV-1-specific CD4$^+$ T-cell function. These observations have led to the suggestion that the preservation of memory HIV-1-specific CD4$^+$ T cells in those infected with this virus will be crucial for the eventual containment of this viral infection.

Other Immunologic Dysfunction in AIDS

While CD4$^+$ T-lymphocyte loss is the best-studied immunologic abnormality seen in those infected with HIV-1, other immunologic dysfunction

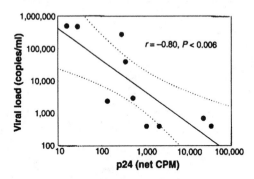

FIGURE 12.5

An inverse correlation exists between plasma viral load and peripheral blood HIV-1-specific CD4$^+$ T-lymphocyte proliferative responses in chronically HIV-1-infected individuals

Proliferative assays and simultaneous plasma HIV-1 viral load measurements (solid circles) were performed on 10 individuals with documented HIV-1 infection with no prior history of antiretroviral therapy. The relation between viral load and proliferative response to p24 antigen was examined by linear regression. The solid line represents the linear regression, and the dotted line represents the 95% confidence interval. (From reference 68.)

clearly occurs in these individuals. Perhaps the most striking of these abnormalities is the destruction of the lymphoid microenvironment (57). As
HIV-1-induced disease progresses clinically, there is an inexorable destruction of lymph node germinal centers. Although the etiology of this germinal center destruction has not been fully explained, the loss of follicular
dendritic cells (FDCs) is prominently seen (6). FDCs are CD4⁻ cells, and, consistent with this, there is no evidence that these cells themselves become infected with HIV-1. FDCs trap viral particles in germinal centers during the
course of infection. This contact with the virus, or local cytokine production
that occurs as a consequence of infection, may contribute to the degenera-
tion of these cells. CD8⁺ T-lymphocyte populations also migrate into the germinal centers of lymph nodes during the course of HIV-1 infection. These
cell populations may secrete cytokines or lytic granules that mediate destruction of FDCs. Whatever the etiology of FDC loss proves to be, the
destruction of the infrastructure upon which the germinal center is built
contributes to germinal center dysfunction and eventual disintegration.

Chronic HIV-1 infection also destroys the thymus (28). Thymic tissue
loss is so marked, it can be demonstrated radiographically (72). The loss of
thymic function in AIDS is also apparent, even at a molecular level. Genetic rearrangements of the antigen recognition domains of the T-cell-
receptor alpha and beta chains of maturing T lymphocytes occur in the thymus as T lymphocytes become committed to a single antigen recognition
specificity. These rearrangements include a splicing out of T-cell-receptor
genetic material, resulting in the generation of so-called T-cell excision circles that can be detected in developing T-lymphocyte populations. High
levels of circulating T lymphocytes containing these excision circles is an
indication of ongoing thymic maturation of T lymphocytes. As AIDS progresses clinically, the proportion of circulating T lymphocytes that contain
these T-cell excision circles decreases (18). This suggests a waning of
thymic function. The etiology of thymic loss and dysfunction in AIDS remains unclear. Importantly, however, both the radiographic evidence of
thymus loss and molecular evidence of thymic dysfunction have been
shown to reverse in HIV-1-infected individuals receiving antiretroviral
therapy (18, 72). These observations suggest that thymic dysfunction is indeed reversible in individuals who respond to antiviral therapy.

Evidence continues to accrue indicating that the bone marrow is also
abnormal in HIV-1-infected individuals. It has been clear since the earliest
clinical descriptions of AIDS that all bone-marrow-derived cell populations are abnormal in infected individuals (27). These abnormalities are
apparent in their number, morphology, and function (52). Anemia, throm-
bocytopenia, and neutropenia are quite commonly seen as clinical manifestations of AIDS. Assays of bone marrow progenitors that assess their
potential to generate mature, functional cells invariably show diminished
activity in infected subjects. Since the major constituent cell populations

that make up the immune system are generated in the bone marrow, there is reason to presume that these cell populations are not produced normally in HIV-1-infected individuals. In fact, recent studies suggest that CD4$^+$ T-cell loss in AIDS may be attributable, at least in part, to decreased production of these cells, presumably in the bone marrow (29). The etiology of this bone marrow dysfunction remains poorly understood. However, studies have shown that bone marrow macrophage populations infected with a lentivirus may contribute to an abnormal microenvironment that is responsible for at least some of this dysfunction (80).

HIV-1 infection also leads to profound cytokine dysregulation. Endogenous cytokines, including TNFα, GM-CSF, IL-6, and IFNγ, have been shown to increase HIV-1 replication in various cell populations in vitro (4, 63, 77). The mechanisms by which this cytokine-induced upregulation of viral replication occurs can differ and sometimes be complementary. For example, TNFα is a transcriptional activator of HIV-1 via NF-κB, while IL-6 induces HIV-1 replication by a posttranscriptional mechanism. It is assumed that immune cells in the infected individual produce increased quantities of many of these cytokines, which in turn increase viral replication in vivo. It has, however, also been shown that other immunologically active cytokines, such as IFNα and IFNβ, can suppress HIV-1 replication in vitro. Therefore, the sum effect of cytokine dysregulation on HIV-1 replication in vivo is difficult to gauge.

Determining the effects of cytokine production on disease progression has been an active and sometimes controversial area of investigation. A number of years ago it was proposed that a bias of immune cells toward the production of specific constellations of cytokines might improve or impede immune control of the virus (13). Work in murine models of the immune control of parasitic infections indicated that a bias toward production of TH2 cytokines interfered with containment of parasites, while a bias toward the production of TH1 cytokines improved containment of those pathogens. Since CTLs have been shown to be of central importance in containing HIV-1 spread and TH1 cytokines are known to support effector T-lymphocyte responses in vivo, it was suggested that a bias toward production of TH1 cytokines may be beneficial for controlling HIV-1 replication. Moreover, it was proposed that a bias toward production of TH2 cytokines may interfere with immune containment of HIV-1 replication. Some even suggested that a vaccine-elicited immune response that was TH2 biased may accelerate disease progression in vaccinated individuals who subsequently become infected with HIV-1. Although this hypothesis generated a substantial amount of investigative work, the consensus of those working in the field has been that there is no evidence to support this paradigm of AIDS pathogenesis (25).

Although B lymphocytes have never been shown to harbor replicating HIV-1 in vivo in infected individuals, B lymphocyte abnormalities have been described in those infected with HIV-1. An increase in circulating B lymphocytes has been described during primary HIV-1 infection as well as during primary infection of macaques with primate lentiviruses (66). Cytokine production by B lymphocytes of infected individuals has also been shown to be abnormal, with increased levels of TNFα and IL-6 spontaneously produced by these cells (5, 67). In fact, it has been suggested that these B-lymphocyte-produced cytokines may actually upregulate HIV-1 replication in CD4$^+$ T lymphocytes and macrophages. It is likely that the B-lymphocyte activation that occurs in HIV-1-infected individuals contributes to the striking incidence of AIDS-related B-cell malignancies (33).

Finally, HIV-1 infects CD4-expressing antigen-presenting cell populations, including monocytes, macrophages, and dendritic cells. Very few circulating cells of these lineages are actually infected by the virus, and this infection does not appear to mediate the obligatory death of these cells. Rather, these infected cells are felt to represent an important reservoir of virus that will probably prove difficult to eradicate by antiviral therapies. Relevant to this postulated role as a reservoir, the infected dendritic cell has been shown to mediate an extremely efficient transfer of virus to normal T-lymphocyte populations, at least under in vitro culture conditions (64). Although very few infected monocyte/macrophages have been documented in the circulation, large numbers of resident macrophages have been shown to be infected in various organs, including lungs and brains.

In light of the infectability of cells of the monocyte/macrophage lineage, it is not surprising that these cells do not function normally in infected individuals. The abnormalities of these cells include problems with oxidative burst response, C3 receptor-mediated clearance, Fc receptor function, and chemotaxis (53). These cells in HIV-1-infected individuals also have been shown to have a decreased ability to mediate antibody-dependent cell-mediated cytotoxicity and antimicrobicidal activity (3). Infection of resident brain macrophages probably initiates a cascade of cytokine abnormalities that change the milieu of the central nervous system, leading to neuronal damage and AIDS dementia (23).

Conclusion

Thus, an extraordinary confluence of immunopathologic events have conspired to create AIDS. HIV-1 continuously accrues mutations in the infected individual that sometimes allow it to escape control by CTLs. The virus is insensitive to neutralization by anti-HIV-1 antibody in the chronically infected individual, leading to persistent, high levels of replication. HIV-1 is selectively tropic for cells of the immune system through its dependence for cell entry on CD4 or chemokine receptors or both. The virus's selective tropism, coupled with its ability to cripple or kill these cells, leads to an immune deficiency syndrome. Finally, the slow pace of the progression of the virus-induced immunodeficiency leads to a prolonged period of clinical latency in the infected individual. It is this long period of asymptomatic infection that facilitates the spread of the virus from an infected to an uninfected person.

REFERENCES

1. Alkhatib, G., C. Combadiere, C. C. Broder, Y. Feng, P. E. Kennedy, P. M. Murphy, and E. A. Berger. 1996. CC CKR5: a RANTES, MIP-1alpha, MIP-1beta receptor as a fusion cofactor for macrophage-tropic HIV-1. Science 272:1955–1958.

2. Autran, B., G. Carcelain, T. S. Li, C. Blanc, D. Mathez, R. Tubiana, C. Katlama, P. Debre, and J. Leibowitch. 1997. Positive effects of combined antiretroviral therapy on CD4+ T cell homeostasis and function in advanced HIV disease [see comments]. Science 277:112–116.

3. Baldwin, G. C., J. Fleischmann, Y. Chung, Y. Koyanagi, I. S. Chen, and D. W. Golde. 1990. Human immunodeficiency virus causes mononuclear phagocyte dysfunction. Proc. Natl. Acad. Sci. USA 87:3933–3937.

4. Biswas, P., G. Poli, A. L. Kinter, J. S. Justement, S. K. Stanley, W. J. Maury, P. Bressler, J. M. Orenstein, and A. S. Fauci. 1992. Interferon gamma induces the expression of human immunodeficiency virus in persistently infected promonocytic cells (U1) and redirects the production of virions to intracytoplasmic vacuoles in phorbol myristate acetate-differentiated U1 cells. J. Exp. Med. 176:739–750.

5. Boue, F., C. Wallon, C. Goujard, F. Barre-Sinoussi, P. Galanaud, and J. F. Delfraissy. 1992. HIV induces IL-6 production by human B lymphocytes. Role of IL-4. J. Immunol. 148:3761–3767.

6. Burton, D. R., and D. C. Montefiori. 1997. The antibody response in HIV-1 infection [see comments]. AIDS 11(Suppl. A):S87–98.

7. Casella, C. R., and T. H. Finkel. 1997. Mechanisms of lymphocyte killing by HIV. Curr. Opin. Hematol. 4 (1):24–31.

8. Chan, D. C., D. Fass, J. M. Berger, and P. S. Kim. 1997. Core structure of gp41 from the HIV envelope glycoprotein. Cell 89:263–273.

9. Chan, D. C., and P. S. Kim. 1998. HIV entry and its inhibition. Cell 93:681–684.

10. Chen, Z. W., Z. C. Kou, C. Lekutis, L. Shen, D. Zhou, M. Halloran, J. Li, J. Sodroski, D. Lee-Parritz, and N. L. Letvin. 1995. T cell receptor V beta repertoire in an acute infection of rhesus monkeys with simian immunodeficiency viruses and a chimeric simian-human immunodeficiency virus. J. Exp. Med. 182:21–31.

11. Chiasson, M. A., R. L. Stoneburner, A. R. Lifson, D. S. Hildebrandt, W. E. Ewing, S. Schultz, and H. W. Jaffe. 1990. Risk factors for human immunodeficiency virus type 1 (HIV-1) infection in patients at a sexually transmitted disease clinic in New York City. Am. J. Epidemiol. 131(2):208–220.

12. Choe, H., M. Farzan, Y. Sun, N. Sullivan, B. Rollins, P. D. Ponath, L. Wu, C. R. Mackay, G. LaRosa, W. Newman, N. Gerard, C. Gerard, and J. Sodroski. 1996. The beta-chemokine receptors CCR3 and CCR5 facilitate infection by primary HIV-1 isolates. Cell 85:1135–1148.

13. Clerici, M., and G. M. Shearer. 1993. A TH1→TH2 switch is a critical step in the etiology of HIV infection [see comments]. Immunol. Today 14:107–111.

14. Clerici, M., N. I. Stocks, R. A. Zajac, R. N. Boswell, D. R. Lucey, C. S. Via, and G. M. Shearer. 1989. Detection of three distinct patterns of T helper cell dysfunction in asymptomatic, human immunodeficiency virus-seropositive patients. Independence of CD4+ cell numbers and clinical staging. J. Clin. Invest. 84:1892–1899.

15. Cocchi, F., A. L. DeVico, A. Garzino-Demo, S. K. Arya, R. C. Gallo, and P. Lusso. 1995. Identification of RANTES, MIP-1 alpha, and MIP-1 beta as the major HIV-suppressive factors produced by CD8+ T cells [see comments]. Science 270:1811–1815.

16. Connor, R. I., and D. D. Ho. 1994. Transmission and pathogenesis of human immunodeficiency virus type 1. AIDS Res. Hum. Retroviruses 10:321–323.

17. Dalgleish, A. G., P. C. Beverley, P. R. Clapham, D. H. Crawford, M. F. Greaves, and R. A. Weiss. 1984. The CD4 (T4) antigen is an essential component of the receptor for the AIDS retrovirus. Nature 312:763–767.

18. Douek, D. C., R. D. McFarland, P. H. Keiser, E. A. Gage, J. M. Massey, B. F. Haynes, M. A. Polis, A. T. Haase, M. B. Feinberg, J. L. Sullivan, B. D. Jamieson, J. A. Zack, L. J. Picker, and R. A. Koup. 1998. Changes in thymic function with age and during the treatment of HIV infection [see comments]. Nature 396:690–695.

19. Edinger, A. L., J. L. Mankowski, B. J. Doranz, B. J. Margulies, B. Lee, J. Rucker, M. Sharron, T. L. Hoffman, J. F. Berson, M. C. Zink, V. M. Hirsch, J. E. Clements, and R. W. Doms. 1997. CD4-independent, CCR5-dependent infection of brain capillary endothelial cells by a neurovirulent simian immunodeficiency virus strain. Proc. Natl. Acad. Sci. USA 94:14742–14747.

20. Fauci, A. S. 1993. Multifactorial nature of human immunodeficiency virus disease: implications for therapy. Science 262:1011–1018.

21. Feng, Y., C. C. Broder, P. E. Kennedy, and E. A. Berger. 1996. HIV-1 entry cofactor: functional cDNA cloning of a seven-transmembrane, G protein-coupled receptor [see comments]. Science 272:872–877.

22. Gao, F., E. Bailes, D. L. Robertson, Y. Chen, C. M. Rodenburg, S. F. Michael, L. B. Cummins, L. O. Arthur, M. Peeters, G. M. Shaw, P. M. Sharp, and B. H. Hahn. 1999. Origin of HIV-1 in the chimpanzee Pan troglodytes troglodytes [see comments]. Nature 397:436–441.

23. Gendelman, H. E., Y. Persidsky, A. Ghorpade, J. Limoges, M. Stins, M. Fiala, and R. Morrisett. 1997. The neuropathogenesis of the AIDS dementia complex. AIDS 11(Suppl. A):S35–45.

24. Goudsmit, J., C. Debouck, R. H. Meloen, L. Smit, M. Bakker, D. M. Asher, A. V. Wolff, C. J. Gibbs, Jr., and D. C. Gajdusek. 1988. Human immunodeficiency virus type 1 neutralization epitope with conserved architecture elicits early type-specific antibodies in experimentally infected chimpanzees. Proc. Natl. Acad. Sci. USA 85:4478–4482.

25. Graziosi, C., G. Pantaleo, K. R. Gantt, J. P. Fortin, J. F. Demarest, O. J. Cohen, R. P. Sekaly, and A. S. Fauci. 1994. Lack of evidence for the dichotomy of TH1 and TH2 predominance in HIV-infected individuals [see comments]. Science 265:248–252.

26. Hadida, F., A. Parrot, M. P. Kieny, B. Sadat-Sowti, C. Mayaud, P. Debre, and B. Autran. 1992. Carboxyl-terminal and central regions of human immunodeficiency virus-1 NEF recognized by cytotoxic T lymphocytes from lymphoid organs. An in vitro limiting dilution analysis. J. Clin. Invest. 89:53–60.

27. Harbol, A. W., J. L. Liesveld, P. J. Simpson-Haidaris, and C. N. Abboud. 1994. Mechanisms of cytopenia in human immunodeficiency virus infection. Blood Rev. 8(4):241–251.

28. Haynes, B. F., L. P. Hale, K. J. Weinhold, D. D. Patel, H. X. Liao, P. B. Bressler, D. M. Jones, J. F. Demarest, K. Gebhard-Mitchell, A. T. Haase, and J. A. Bartlett. 1999. Analysis of the adult thymus in reconstitution of T lymphocytes in HIV-1 infection. J. Clin. Invest. 103:921.

29. Hellerstein, M., M. B. Hanley, D. Cesar, S. Siler, C. Papageorgopoulos, E. Wieder, D. Schmidt, R. Hoh, R. Neese, D. Macallan, S. Deeks, and J. M. Mc-Cune. 1999. Directly measured kinetics of circulating T lymphocytes in normal and HIV-1-infected humans [see comments]. Nature Med. 5:83–89.

30. Hirsch, V. M., R. A. Olmsted, M. Murphey-Corb, R. H. Purcell, and P. R. Johnson. 1989. An African primate lentivirus (SIVsm) closely related to HIV-2. Nature 339:389–392.

31. Ho, D. D. 1997. Perspectives series: host/pathogen interactions. Dynamics of HIV-1 replication in vivo. J. Clin. Invest. 99:2565–2567.

32. Ho, D. D., A. U. Neumann, A. S. Perelson, W. Chen, J. M. Leonard, and M. Markowitz. 1995. Rapid turnover of plasma virions and CD4 lymphocytes in HIV-1 infection [see comments]. Nature 373:123–126.

33. Jacobson, D. L., J. A. McCutchan, P. L. Spechko, I. Abramson, R. S. Smith, A. Bartok, G. R. Boss, D. Durand, S. A. Bozzette, S. A. Spector, et al. 1991. The evolution of lymphadenopathy and hypergammaglobulinemia are evidence for early and sustained polyclonal B lymphocyte activation during human immunodeficiency virus infection. J. Infect. Dis. 163:240–246.

34. Jassoy, C., R. P. Johnson, B. A. Navia, J. Worth, and B. D. Walker. 1992. Detection of a vigorous HIV-1-specific cytotoxic T lymphocyte response in cerebrospinal fluid from infected persons with AIDS dementia complex. J. Immunol. 149:3113–3119.

35. Javaherian, K., A. J. Langlois, C. McDanal, K. L. Ross, L. I. Eckler, C. L. Jellis, A. T. Profy, J. R. Rusche, D. P. Bolognesi, S. D. Putney, et al. 1989. Principal neutralizing domain of the human immunodeficiency virus type 1 envelope protein. Proc. Natl. Acad. Sci. USA 86:6768–6772.

36. Kang, C. Y., P. Nara, S. Chamat, V. Caralli, T. Ryskamp, N. Haigwood, R. Newman, and H. Kohler. 1991. Evidence for non-V3-specific neutralizing antibodies that interfere with gp120/CD4 binding in human immunodeficiency virus 1-infected humans. Proc. Natl. Acad. Sci. USA 88:6171–6175.

37. Klatzmann, D., E. Champagne, S. Chamaret, J. Gruest, D. Guetard, T. Hercend, J. C. Gluckman, and L. Montagnier. 1984. T-lymphocyte T4 molecule behaves as the receptor for human retrovirus LAV. Nature 312:767–768.

38. Koup, R. A., J. T. Safrit, Y. Cao, C. A. Andrews, G. McLeod, W. Borkowsky, C. Farthing, and D. D. Ho. 1994. Temporal association of cellular immune responses with the initial control of viremia in primary human immunodeficiency virus type 1 syndrome. J. Virol. 68:4650–4655.

39. Kuroda, M. J., J. E. Schmitz, W. A. Charini, C. E. Nickerson, M. A. Lifton, C. I. Lord, M. A. Forman, and N. L. Letvin. 1999. Emergence of CTL coincides with clearance of virus during primary simian immunodeficiency virus infection in rhesus monkeys. J. Immunol. 162:5127–5133.

40. LaRosa, G. J., J. P. Davide, K. Weinhold, J. A. Waterbury, A. T. Profy, J. A. Lewis, A. J. Langlois, G. R. Dreesman, R. N. Boswell, P. Shadduck, et al. 1990. Conserved sequence and structural elements in the HIV-1 principal neutralizing determinant. Science 249:932–935. (Erratum, 251:811, 1991.)

41. Leonard, C. K., M. W. Spellman, L. Riddle, R. J. Harris, J. N. Thomas, and T. J. Gregory. 1990. Assignment of intrachain disulfide bonds and characterization of potential glycosylation sites of the type 1 recombinant human immunodeficiency virus envelope glycoprotein (gp120) expressed in Chinese hamster ovary cells. J. Biol. Chem. 265:10373–10382.

42. Littman, D. R. 1998. Chemokine receptors: keys to AIDS pathogenesis? Cell 93:677–680.

43. Lohman, B. L., C. J. Miller, and M. B. McChesney. 1995. Antiviral cytotoxic T lymphocytes in vaginal mucosa of simian immunodeficiency virus-infected rhesus macaques. J. Immunol. 155:5855–5860.

44. Lukashov, V. V., and J. Goudsmit. 1998. HIV heterogeneity and disease progression in AIDS: a model of continuous virus adaptation. AIDS 12(Suppl. A):S43–52.

45. Mascola, J. R., M. G. Lewis, G. Stiegler, D. Harris, T. C. VanCott, D. Hayes, M. K. Louder, C. R. Brown, C. V. Sapan, S. S. Frankel, Y. Lu, M. L. Robb, H. Katinger, and D. L. Birx. 1999. Protection of macaques against pathogenic simian/human immunodeficiency virus 89.6PD by passive transfer of neutralizing antibodies. J. Virol. 73:4009–4018.

46. Mascola, J. R., G. Stiegler, T. C. VanCott, H. Katinger, C. B. Carpenter, C. E. Hanson, H. Beary, D. Hayes, S. S. Frankel, D. L. Birx, and M. G. Lewis. 2000. Protection of macaques against vaginal transmission of a pathogenic HIV-1/SIV chimeric virus by passive infusion of neutralizing antibodies. Nature Med. 6:207–210.

47. McDougal, J. S., M. S. Kennedy, J. M. Sligh, S. P. Cort, A. Mawle, and J. K. Nicholson. 1986. Binding of HTLV-III/LAV to T4+ T cells by a complex of the 110K viral protein and the T4 molecule. Science 231:382–385.

48. McMichael, A. J., and R. E. Phillips. 1997. Escape of human immunodeficiency virus from immune control. Annu. Rev. Immunol. 15:271–296.

49. Mohri, H., S. Bonhoeffer, S. Monard, A. S. Perelson, and D. D. Ho. 1998. Rapid turnover of T lymphocytes in SIV-infected rhesus macaques. Science 279:1223–1227.

50. Montefiori, D. C., G. Pantaleo, L. M. Fink, J. T. Zhou, J. Y. Zhou, M. Bilska, G. D. Miralles, and A. S. Fauci. 1996. Neutralizing and infection-enhancing antibody responses to human immunodeficiency virus type 1 in long-term nonprogressors. J. Infect. Dis. 173:60–67.

51. Moog, C., H. J. Fleury, I. Pellegrin, A. Kirn, and A. M. Aubertin. 1997. Autologous and heterologous neutralizing antibody responses following initial seroconversion in human immunodeficiency virus type 1-infected individuals. J. Virol. 71:3734–3741.

52. Moses, A., J. Nelson, and G. C. Bagby, Jr. 1998. The influence of human immunodeficiency virus-1 on hematopoiesis. Blood 91:1479–1495.

53. Muller, F., H. Rollag, and S. S. Froland. 1990. Reduced oxidative burst responses in monocytes and monocyte-derived macrophages from HIV-infected subjects. Clin. Exp. Immunol. 82(1):10–15.

54. Musey, L., J. Hughes, T. Schacker, T. Shea, L. Corey, and M. J. McElrath. 1997. Cytotoxic-T-cell responses, viral load, and disease progression in early human immunodeficiency virus type 1 infection [see comments]. N. Engl. J. Med. 337:1267–1274.

55. Ogg, G. S., X. Jin, S. Bonhoeffer, P. R. Dunbar, M. A. Nowak, S. Monard, J. P. Segal, Y. Cao, S. L. Rowland-Jones, V. Cerundolo, A. Hurley, M. Markowitz, D. D. Ho, D. F. Nixon, and A. J. McMichael. 1998. Quantitation of HIV-1-specific cytotoxic T lymphocytes and plasma load of viral RNA. Science 279:2103–2106.

56. Pantaleo, G., J. F. Demarest, H. Soudeyns, C. Graziosi, F. Denis, J. W. Adelsberger, P. Borrow, M. S. Saag, G. M. Shaw, R. P. Sekaly, et al. 1994. Major expansion of CD8+ T cells with a predominant V beta usage during the primary immune response to HIV [see comments]. Nature 370:463–467.

57. Pantaleo, G., C. Graziosi, J. F. Demarest, O. J. Cohen, M. Vaccarezza, K. Gantt, C. Muro-Cacho, and A. S. Fauci. 1994. Role of lymphoid organs in the pathogenesis of human immunodeficiency virus (HIV) infection. Immunol. Rev. 140:105–130.

58. Pellegrin, I., E. Legrand, D. Neau, P. Bonot, B. Masquelier, J. L. Pellegrin, J. M. Ragnaud, N. Bernard, and H. J. Fleury. 1996. Kinetics of appearance of neutralizing antibodies in 12 patients with primary or recent HIV-1 infection and relationship with plasma and cellular viral loads. J. Acquired Immune Defic. Syndr. Hum. Retrovirol. 11:438–447.

59. Perelson, A. S., A. U. Neumann, M. Markowitz, J. M. Leonard, and D. D. Ho. 1996. HIV-1 dynamics in vivo: virion clearance rate, infected cell life-span, and viral generation time. Science 271:1582–1586.

60. Pilgrim, A. K., G. Pantaleo, O. J. Cohen, L. M. Fink, J. Y. Zhou, J. T. Zhou, D. P. Bolognesi, A. S. Fauci, and D. C. Montefiori. 1997. Neutralizing antibody responses to human immunodeficiency virus type 1 in primary infection and long-term-nonprogressive infection. J. Infect. Dis. 176:924–932.

61. Plata, F., B. Autran, L. P. Martins, S. Wain-Hobson, M. Raphael, C. Mayaud, M. Denis, J. M. Guillon, and P. Debre. 1987. AIDS virus-specific cytotoxic T lymphocytes in lung disorders. Nature 328:348–351.

62. Poignard, P., R. Sabbe, G. R. Picchio, M. Wang, R. J. Gulizia, H. Katinger, P. W. Parren, D. E. Mosier, and D. R. Burton. 1999. Neutralizing antibodies have limited effects on the control of established HIV-1 infection in vivo. Immunity 10:431–438.

63. Poli, G., and A. S. Fauci. 1992. The effect of cytokines and pharmacologic agents on chronic HIV infection. AIDS Res. Hum. Retroviruses 8:191–197.

64. Pope, M. 1999. Mucosal dendritic cells and immunodeficiency viruses. J. Infect. Dis. 179(Suppl. 3):S427–430.

65. Posner, M. R., T. Hideshima, T. Cannon, M. Mukherjee, K. H. Mayer, and R. A. Byrn. 1991. An IgG human monoclonal antibody that reacts with HIV-

1/GP120, inhibits virus binding to cells, and neutralizes infection. J. Immunol. 146:4325–4332.

66. Reimann, K. A., J. T. Li, G. Voss, C. Lekutis, K. Tenner-Racz, P. Racz, W. Lin, D. C. Montefiori, D. E. Lee-Parritz, Y. Lu, R. G. Collman, J. Sodroski, and N. L. Letvin. 1996. An env gene derived from a primary human immunodeficiency virus type 1 isolate confers high in vivo replicative capacity to a chimeric simian/human immunodeficiency virus in rhesus monkeys. J. Virol. 70:3198–3206.

67. Rieckmann, P., G. Poli, J. H. Kehrl, and A. S. Fauci. 1991. Activated B lymphocytes from human immunodeficiency virus-infected individuals induce virus expression in infected T cells and a promonocytic cell line, U1. J. Exp. Med. 173:1–5.

68. Rosenberg, E. S., J. M. Billingsley, A. M. Caliendo, S. L. Boswell, P. E. Sax, S. A. Kalams, and B. D. Walker. 1997. Vigorous HIV-1-specific CD4+ T cell responses associated with control of viremia [see comments]. Science 278:1447–1450.

69. Rosenzweig, M., M. A. DeMaria, D. M. Harper, S. Friedrich, R. K. Jain, and R. P. Johnson. 1998. Increased rates of CD4(+) and CD8(+) T lymphocyte turnover in simian immunodeficiency virus-infected macaques. Proc. Natl. Acad. Sci. USA 95:6388–6393.

70. Schmitz, J. E., M. J. Kuroda, S. Santra, V. G. Sasseville, M. A. Simon, M. A. Lifton, P. Racz, K. Tenner-Racz, M. Dalesandro, B. J. Scallon, J. Ghrayeb, M. A. Forman, D. C. Montefiori, E. P. Rieber, N. L. Letvin, and K. A. Reimann. 1999. Control of viremia in simian immunodeficiency virus infection by CD8+ lymphocytes. Science 283:857–860.

71. Sethi, K. K., H. Naher, and I. Stroehmann. 1988. Phenotypic heterogeneity of cerebrospinal fluid-derived HIV-specific and HLA-restricted cytotoxic T-cell clones. Nature 335:178–181.

72. Smith, K. Y., H. Valdez, A. Landay, J. Spritzler, H. A. Kessler, E. Connick, D. Kuritzkes, B. Gross, I. Francis, J. M. McCune, and M. M. Lederman. 2000. Thymic size and lymphocyte restoration in patients with human immunodeficiency virus infection after 48 weeks of zidovudine, lamivudine, and ritonavir therapy. J. Infect. Dis. 181:141–147.

73. Spira, A. I., P. A. Marx, B. K. Patterson, J. Mahoney, R. A. Koup, S. M. Wolinsky, and D. D. Ho. 1996. Cellular targets of infection and route of viral dissemination after an intravaginal inoculation of simian immunodeficiency virus into rhesus macaques. J. Exp. Med. 183:215–225.

74. Stahl-Hennig, C., R. M. Steinman, K. Tenner-Racz, M. Pope, N. Stolte, K. Matz-Rensing, G. Grobschupff, B. Raschdorff, G. Hunsmann, and P. Racz. 1999. Rapid infection of oral mucosal-associated lymphoid tissue with simian immunodeficiency virus. Science 285:1261–1265.

75. Trkola, A., A. B. Pomales, H. Yuan, B. Korber, P. J. Maddon, G. P. Allaway, H. Katinger, C. F. Barbas III, D. R. Burton, D. D. Ho, et al. 1995. Cross-clade neutralization of primary isolates of human immunodeficiency virus type 1 by human monoclonal antibodies and tetrameric CD4-IgG. J. Virol. 69:6609–6617.

76. Tsubota, H., C. I. Lord, D. I. Watkins, C. Morimoto, and N. L. Letvin. 1989. A cytotoxic T lymphocyte inhibits acquired immunodeficiency syndrome virus replication in peripheral blood lymphocytes. J. Exp. Med. 169:1421–1434.

77. Tsunetsugu-Yokota, Y., and M. Honda. 1990. Effect of cytokines on HIV release and IL-2 receptor alpha expression in monocytic cell lines. J. Acquired Immune Defic. Syndr. 3:511–516.

78. Wain-Hobson, S. 1996. Running the gamut of retroviral variation [see comments]. Trends Microbiol. 4:135–141.

79. Walker, C. M., D. J. Moody, D. P. Stites, and J. A. Levy. 1986. CD8+ lymphocytes can control HIV infection in vitro by suppressing virus replication. Science 234:1563–1566.

80. Watanabe, M., D. J. Ringler, M. Nakamura, P. A. DeLong, and N. L. Letvin. 1990. Simian immunodeficiency virus inhibits bone marrow hematopoietic progenitor cell growth. J. Virol. 64:656–663.

81. Wei, X., S. K. Ghosh, M. E. Taylor, V. A. Johnson, E. A. Emini, P. Deutsch, J. D. Lifson, S. Bonhoeffer, M. A. Nowak, B. H. Hahn, et al. 1995. Viral dynamics in human immunodeficiency virus type 1 infection [see comments]. Nature 373:117–122.

82. Wolthers, K. C., G. Bea, A. Wisman, S. A. Otto, A. M. de Roda Husman, N. Schaft, F. de Wolf, J. Goudsmit, R. A. Coutinho, A. G. van der Zee, L. Meyaard, and F. Miedema. 1996. T cell telomere length in HIV-1 infection: no evidence for increased CD4+ T cell turnover. Science 274:1543–1547.

83. Yamamoto, H., D. J. Ringler, M. D. Miller, Y. Yasutomi, T. Hasunuma, and N. L. Letvin. 1992. Simian immunodeficiency virus-specific cytotoxic T lymphocytes are present in the AIDS-associated skin rash in rhesus monkeys. J. Immunol. 149:728–734.

84. Yasutomi, Y., K. A. Reimann, C. I. Lord, M. D. Miller, and N. L. Letvin. 1993. Simian immunodeficiency virus-specific CD8+ lymphocyte response in acutely infected rhesus monkeys. J. Virol. 67:1707–1711.

85. Zhang, Z., T. Schuler, M. Zupancic, S. Wietgrefe, K. A. Staskus, K. A. Reimann, T. A. Reinhart, M. Rogan, W. Cavert, C. J. Miller, R. S. Veazey, D. Notermans, S. Little, S. A. Danner, D. D. Richman, D. Havlir, J. Wong, H. L. Jordan, T. W. Schacker, P. Racz, K. Tenner-Racz, N. L. Letvin, S. Wolinsky, and A. T. Haase. 1999. Sexual transmission and propagation of SIV and HIV in resting and activated CD4+ T cells. Science 286:1353–1357.

| 13 | # HIV Vaccines 2000: Prospects and |
SPYROS A. KALAMS
BRUCE D. WALKER

HIV Vaccines 2000: Prospects and Challenges

Efforts to develop an effective AIDS vaccine are being increasingly driven by a better understanding of the immune responses that are associated with control of viremia in infected persons. Important advances have come from both human studies and animal models in the past few years, resulting in an emerging consensus that HIV can be controlled by the immune system. However, the immune responses induced fail to eradicate the virus. Thus, the goal of a vaccine that prevents persistent infection is likely to be difficult to achieve, but a vaccine that attenuates disease may be more realistic. This review addresses recent advances in the understanding of the immune responses likely to be required by an effective vaccine and the advances that have occurred in pursuit of this goal. In addition, it provides a perspective on the potential for therapeutic vaccination in persons who are already infected. The major emphasis is on those advances made in 1999 and 2000.

Rationale for Even Partially Effective AIDS Vaccines

There are a number of ways to measure the effectiveness of a vaccine, ranging from complete prevention of infection to attenuation of disease. In addition, efficacy can be measured by the ability of an incompletely protective vaccine to decrease infectivity and thereby limit spread of infection. Although the ultimate goal of an AIDS vaccine is to prevent infection altogether, increasing data suggest that even partial containment of the initial phase of viremia may have a profound impact on disease progression (116). In humans and animals, viral load early after infection is highly predictive of subsequent disease progression (74). Recent data from the Multicenter AIDS Cohort Study (MACS cohort) indicate that the viral load at six months is similar to that at three years and that disease progression is associated with the early viral load (74). Although some of those with low-level viremia may ultimately progress, cohort studies show a leveling-off of the death rate after eight years of infection, indicating that the effect may be long lived (61).

It remains unclear how some persons achieve lower viral loads at the initial set point after infection and why others end up with high viral loads. It is possible that the level and duration of the initial peak in viremia influence these parameters (117), and this raises the question as to whether interventions aimed at lowering viral load in acute infection will influence disease progression. The earliest such studies involved animal models in which transient treatment with antiviral therapy at the time of acute infection led to improved clinical outcome. Watson et al. infected macaques with a pathogenic strain of HIV-2, treating half of the animals for just 16 weeks with D4T, a nucleoside reverse transcriptase inhibitor (116). The untreated animals had all died within six months of infection, as is typical in this model. In contrast, five of the six animals that had been transiently treated with antiviral therapy are alive and well three years later. All remain viremic, but with persistently low viral set points (N. Haigwood, personal communication, 2000). Although the precise immune responses present in these animals remain to be fully characterized, this experiment suggests that early lowering of viral load can have a dramatic effect on disease progression. Although the lowering of viral load was achieved by antiviral therapy, it is reasonable to hypothesize that even a partially effective vaccine may have a similar effect. Thus, efforts to move forward with a vaccine even in the absence of fully sterilizing immunity appear reasonable.

There are also other examples in which early lowering of viral load led to a chronic steady state in which viremia appeared to be better contained. These include anecdotal cases of persons who were treated with highly active antiviral therapy in the acute stage of HIV-1 infection, have subsequently discontinued therapy, and yet have maintained low viral loads (17, 87, 88). They also include recent studies of transient antiviral therapy in the simian immunodeficiency virus (SIV)–macaque model, in which transient treatment has not only resulted in low viral loads but also protected from superinfection with homologous strains (70). Together these data provide strong rationale for moving forward with vaccines that do not induce complete sterilizing immunity.

What Immune Responses Are Likely to Be Required for an Effective Vaccine?

Since HIV-1 is probably never successfully cleared by the immune system, there is no way to study a truly protective immune response. One might argue that persons who are highly exposed but never become infected might represent cleared infections (56, 76, 98), but it remains unclear as to whether these persons have actually ever been productively infected. Moreover, recent follow-up studies suggest that some of these persons who were apparently protected have gone on to become infected, raising the possibility that even in these persons the protection is not absolute. However, there are persons who have now been infected for more than 20 years and have never developed symptomatic disease (49, 55). A subset of these persons have maintained viral loads below the limits of detection by the most sensitive assays currently available, and emerging data indicate that the immune system is highly activated in these persons (49, 55). Although other factors such as genetic polymorphisms in chemokine receptors (23) and attenuated viruses (33) may account for some of these non-progressing cases, it is becoming clear that the large majority of such cases are associated with strong and persistent virus-specific immune responses.

The immune response to HIV-1 consists of both humoral and cellular arms of the adaptive immune response, which evolve in the setting of rapidly replicating and extremely high titers of virus (72). The most direct way to prevent infection might be through the development of strong and persistent neutralizing antibodies, which would be expected to impair the initial explosive replication. However, generation of effective neutralizing antibodies has proven difficult to achieve with natural infection and is likely to be even harder with a vaccine. Although strong neutralizing antibodies have been identified in some infected persons (22, 89), in general these responses are weak, even in persons with long-term non-progressing infection (50). The majority of responses are actually non-neutralizing and are directed at virion debris (17). The lack of strong responses may in part relate to the heavy glycosylation of the envelope (Env) protein (64). A number of studies have attempted to correlate viral load with the strength of the neutralizing antibody response, but no firm association has been established, suggesting that these responses have little effect on viral set point in chronic infection. Studies in a macaque model of AIDS virus infection have shown that combinations of neutralizing antibodies can protect against maternal-fetal transmission of virus, underscoring the potential for neutralizing antibodies to play a protective role (5). Thus, neutralizing antibodies are an important immune response to be induced with an effective vaccine, but generation of effective neutralizing antibodies remains an unmet challenge.

Another arm of the immune response is virus-specific cytotoxic T lymphocytes (CTLs). These CD8-bearing cells are generated in response to infection and lyse-infected cells by recognition of processed viral antigens presented at the cell surface in association with class I molecules. The best data to date indicating a central role for these cells come from animal experiments in which CD8 cells are removed in vivo through the use of monoclonal antibodies (53, 103). This results in a dramatic increase in steady-state viral load, which subsequently declines again as CD8 cells (and therefore CTLs) recover. If CD8 cells are depleted prior to infection, then viral load stays high and finally drops when CTLs recover (103). Other data indicating the role of CTLs in determining the viral set point come from studies using newly developed techniques to quantitate CTLs precisely (3). The identification of a negative association between viral load and set point again suggests that these cells place immune pressure on the virus during the chronic phase of infection (86). Moreover, the identification of strong and persistent CTL responses in persons who do not progress despite 20 or more years of infection suggests that these cells may be able to exert long-term antiviral control (55). Thus CTLs are likely to be an important component of an effective vaccine, particularly if sterilizing immunity is not achieved.

CTLs not only kill infected cells but also produce antiviral factors that are likely to contribute a direct antiviral effect in the local microenvironment (reviewed in reference 124). These include beta chemokines as well as other CTL-derived proteins that are released when the T-cell receptor on the CTL is triggered by recognition of cognate antigen (115). The potent role of soluble factors in other infections such as hepatitis B virus infection is likely to be mirrored in HIV infection (47). Thus, even though the antiviral effect of CD8-derived soluble factors is far less than that of antiviral therapies in vitro (124), these factors may be particularly important in inhibiting progeny viruses released within the local microenvironment.

In the past few years, a number of studies have shed light on the critical role of T helper cells in immune control of HIV. The potential importance of such cells was noted early in the epidemic, when Clerici, Shearer, and others noted that progressive infection was associated with a striking lack of these responses (26, 27). It was initially thought that HIV simply failed to induce such responses, but then a striking finding by Schwartz et al. indicated that at least one person with nonprogressing infection was able to mount a strong T-helper-cell response against the Env protein of HIV (105). As viral load testing became available and it was possible to identify persons who were successfully controlling viremia, an association between strong Gag-specific T-helper-cell responses and control of viremia was noted (96). Subsequently an association was shown to exist between strong T-helper-cell responses and strong CTL responses (55). In the past two years animal and human studies of chronic viral infections have provided conclusive evidence that virus-specific T helper cells are critical for the maintenance of effective CTL responses in natural viral infections (55a, 96, 125). In the absence of T help, CTLs are not maintained, and a recent study of hepatitis C virus (HCV) infection shows that loss of T helper cells to HCV is associated with recurrence of viremia (42). At least one murine study shows that CTLs may be present but unable to mediate lysis or interferon gamma production in the absence of adequate T-cell help (125), and a recent study of acute HCV infection suggests that such cells lacking full effector function may be present in human viral infections as well (65). Thus, induction of virus-specific T helper cells is likely to be critical for long-term maintenance of CTLs and for effective vaccine protection. The lack of virus-specific T helper cells in chronic HIV infection has been hypothesized to be due to selective loss of these cells when they become stimulated at the time of peak viral load in acute infection, and this notion is supported by preliminary data in an animal model (111).

The potential contribution of other immune responses is less clear. Antibody-dependent cell-mediated cytotoxicity (ADCC) does not appear to correlate with protection against AIDS in at least some HIV-infected cohorts, but the precise role in maintaining viral set point or in potentially protecting against infection remains to be determined (30). It is also important to note that CTL and T-helper-cell responses are associated with control of viremia but are not necessarily causative.

What Should an Effective Vaccine Target?

Most experts would agree that the induction of neutralizing antibodies, CTLs, and T helper cells will be important for an effective vaccine, but significant questions remain as to what viral antigens should serve as targets. There are very few comprehensive studies of the viral epitopes targeted in natural infection, and those that have been performed show narrow focusing of the immune response within areas of targeted proteins such as Gag that differ depending on the ethnic background of the individual (45). There is as yet no firm consensus as to what viral proteins should be targeted by an effective vaccine, although some data are worth noting. Early efforts were all directed at the Env protein, concentrating on the development of neutralizing antibodies. Other antigens are unlikely to be significant targets for this arm of the immune response, and thus neutralizing antibody induction is likely to remain focused on this antigen. Moreover, new attempts to present the Env in different forms may enhance immune responses. Examples include the deglycosylated forms (64) and the fusion intermediates (63), but these approaches await demonstration of efficacy in challenge experiments.

In terms of CTLs, logic would indicate that the broader the response the better, since all viral proteins should be considered to have the potential to be presented for CTL recognition. Gag may be a highly desirable target, in part because it is targeted in a majority of infected persons (18, 55) and thus clearly immunogenic and in part because it is highly conserved. Gag is also the one target antigen for which there has been shown a negative correlation between CTL magnitude and viral load (86), again emphasizing the potential importance of this antigen as a target. One of the largest cohort studies of infected persons to date, the Imunoco Cohort in France, has recently determined that Gag and reverse transcriptase (RT) are the major antigens targeted in a large cohort of infected persons (B. Autran, personal communication). Animals immunized with HIV Gag antigens fail to generate neutralizing antibodies and are infected upon challenge, but their postchallenge viral titers are 50- to 100-fold less than controls, suggesting that Gag may be an important immune target (18). However, if one looks at responses in the early stages of infection, there is some suggestion that CTLs directed against Env are associated with a lower viral set point at steady state (82), and conflicting data from another study suggest that CTLs against Nef may dominate (34, 84). A recent report (67) suggests that increased CD8 antiviral factor may be important in control of subsequent viremia in animals that are vaccinated and then challenged and go on to control viremia partially. Thus, CD8 antiviral activity, which is produced by CTLs following recognition of the cognate epitope, may contribute to protective efficacy of vaccines.

In assessing these data regarding CTL targets in chronic infection, one cannot necessarily draw conclusions regarding the best target antigens for a protective or sterilizing vaccine. Scientific rationale can be stated for attempting to generate responses against early viral proteins such as Nef (34), but there remains no in vitro or in vivo evidence that these would be better able to contain virus. Most studies of chronic infection have focused on responses to Gag, RT, Env, and Nef, and large cohort studies focused on viral regulatory proteins such as Tat, Rev, Vif, and Vpr are needed. Interest in proteins such as Tat has been bolstered by recent experimental animal studies indicating that immunization with Tat can lead to reduced viremia following challenge (19, 25). Immunization of cynomolgus macaques with HIV Tat protein elicited broad humoral and cellular immunity and reduces viremia following challenge with 89.6 P simian human immunodeficiency virus (SHIV) to undetectable levels, and prevents CD4 cell decline. These regulatory proteins are able to serve as CTL targets (1a), and comprehensive studies in persons with chronic infection need to be performed to determine their role, particularly in persons who are able to control viral replication without the need for antiviral therapy.

T helper cells are undoubtedly also important for an effective vaccine, since they are required for maintenance of optimal T- and B-cell function and are associated with control of viremia in persons with chronic HIV infection. Of reported studies thus far, the viral Gag protein appears to be the major target for this response in persons with chronic infection (88, 96). Env-specific responses are rarely detected and never immunodominant (88, 96). The reasons for lack of strong responses to Env remain unclear but could possibly relate to the functional interactions between Env and CD4. More comprehensive studies using a panel of all viral proteins are needed to determine the relative immunogenicity of each. In the meantime, focusing on generation of the broadest possible T-helper-cell responses seems reasonable.

Why Does the Immune System Fail in Infected Persons, and What Are the Implications for an Effective Vaccine?

A number of factors likely contribute to the inability of the immune response to eradicate HIV-1. The virus becomes integrated into the host chromosome and thus can be immunologically silent (37). Sequence variation leads to immune escape from both cellular and humoral immune responses (reviewed in reference 46). The heavy glycosylation of the Env protein makes it a poor target for neutralizing antibodies, and some epitopes are induced only transiently after virion binding to cells (63). HIV infection leads to downmodulation of HLA class I A and B alleles (66), and thus infected cells may become relatively resistant to lysis by CTLs (28). HIV may affect antigen-presenting cells, impairing the ability to maintain effective immunity over time. The infection of CD4 T helper cells (or activation-induced cell death [1]) may diminish these below critical levels required for sustaining CTL responses and for generating new responses. Sequestration of virus at immunologically privileged sites has also been postulated to impair immunologic control, as have host genetic factors such as the particular HLA alleles expressed in an infected person (23). Other studies, the most compelling of which were performed in children, indicate that stimulated CD8 cells are induced to express CD4 and that there is a sufficient level of expression to allow for infection of these cells by virus (123). The extent to which this may contribute to CD8-cell depletion in vivo is not clear, but it represents another potential hit against the immune system.

The likely reasons for failure of the immune system to control or eradicate HIV infection have implications for how we proceed with an HIV vaccine. To the extent that effective neutralizing antibodies might be generated, it might be possible to prevent infection altogether. If this is not possible, then we are likely dealing with the prospect of a vaccine that protects against disease progression rather than providing sterilizing immunity. Thus, components of a vaccine may need to mimic the immune responses observed in long-term nonprogressors (Fig. 13.1). Genetic diversity will have to be dealt with by a vaccine that generates broadly directed immunity able to target diverse quasi species, and CTLs will need to be present in sufficient numbers to encounter cells before class I downregulation occurs. T helper cells will need to be present to sustain effective CTLs. Host genetic factors may be difficult to overcome, although the overall contribution to the ability to control HIV does not appear to be large.

What Are the Most Potent Immune Responses That Have Been Induced by Candidate Vaccine Approaches?

When one compares vaccine-induced immune responses with those induced in natural infection, it is clear that the immunogens tested thus far

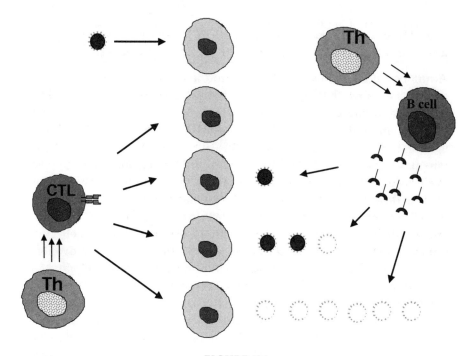

FIGURE 13.1

Immune responses in HIV infection

have been very weak. By far the strongest CTL, T-helper-cell, and neutralizing antibody responses are seen in natural infection. However, achieving these same levels may not be needed with a vaccine. The strong immune responses seen in natural infection may in part reflect the attempts by the immune system to contain the divergent quasi species that develop soon after infection. If virus-specific immune responses are present at the time the virus first enters the host, such diversification may be limited, and less immunity might be able to contain a more homogeneous virus.

Most investigators now agree that HIV vaccine development should be directed at inducing neutralizing antibodies and CTL and T-helper-cell responses; CD8 antiviral factors as well as ADCC also need to be considered. Numerous vaccine trials in which these immune responses have been measured have now been performed in animals and humans. Although all these immune responses have been generated, there is no one vaccine that has been shown to induce strong responses in all categories. However, specific vaccines have shown promise for inducing particular responses.

As noted above, neutralizing antibodies have been difficult to induce with vaccines, and this in part may reflect the lack of strong induction of neutralizing antibodies by natural infection. Neutralization potency seems to be determined largely by antibody affinity for the trimeric Env spike on the virion. Antibody interference with virion attachment seems to be a major mechanism of neutralization by gp120-specific antibodies (102). Studies using viral Env in which specific glycosylation sites have been removed have shown the induction of enhanced neutralizing antibodies, not only against the immunizing strain but also against fully glycosylated native Env (64). At least one other approach has also generated promising preliminary data regarding enhanced induction of broadly cross-reactive neutralizing antibodies (63). This involves the use of fusion intermediates as immunogens. After binding and during virus-cell fusion, new epitopes appear to be induced, and antibodies raised to these intermediates in mice are able to neutralize a broad panel of divergent isolates. Monoclonal antibodies derived from these animals should eventually shed light on the precise mechanism but have not yet been generated. Neutralization has been dramatically enhanced by combining multiple neutralizing antibodies, demonstrating that highly potent combinations of antibodies provide enhanced benefit. In a pathogenic SHIV model, a combination of three passively transferred neutralizing monoclonal antibodies was fully protective in three of six challenged animals (78). This would argue that combination vaccines may provide enhanced benefit.

In terms of vaccine-induced CTLs, many candidates either are likely to induce these or have been shown to induce them, but strong and broadly directed responses such as those likely to be required in an effective vaccine have not been generated. The most immunogenic vaccine for CTLs has been live attenuated virus (54), but the feasibility of using the first- and second-generation attenuated vaccines is doubtful. The most developed vaccines that would be anticipated to induce CTLs are the poxviruses. However, induction of CTLs by these has been strikingly weak (35). Whether coadministration of cytokines or other adjuvants would enhance their immunogenicity needs to be tested. Other important prospects for enhanced induction of CTLs include the use of peptide-pulsed dendritic cells, which have been shown to induce strong and long-lasting CTLs in an influenza model in humans (32). Adenovirus, DNA vaccines, polyepitope vaccines, and combinations of these may also be promising but await further data.

T helper cells will be an important component of an effective vaccine. Early studies showed that proliferative responses to gp120 and gp160 could be induced, but the extent to which these are able to provide help to CTLs and B cells and provide an antiviral effect remains unclear. Newer assay techniques that assess some of the functional characteristics of these cells may be helpful (92) and may also provide a better quantitation of these responses. Data from infected persons would suggest that induction of T-helper-cell responses against Gag may be most important (77, 88, 96). Of the vaccine candidates tested thus far, only whole inactivated virus has been shown to induce strong Gag-specific responses, but the functional activity of these cells has not been assessed.

What Are the Current Vaccine Approaches?

Despite a desperate need for an AIDS vaccine and the testing of numerous candidate immunogens in clinical trials, there is still no clear front-runner. Anecdotal cases of HIV infection occurring in persons after receiving full immunization schedules indicate that some of the present candidates are not fully protective (29), but one cannot yet determine if some degree of disease attenuation may have been achieved. The advent of highly active antiretroviral therapy (HAART) provides an opportunity to test many of the vaccine candidates as therapeutic vaccines as well, and this is supported by increasing data showing that HAART leads to increases in naive cells that might be educated to participate in the antiviral immune response (69). This notion is further supported by the finding that infected persons can generate responses to vaccines such as influenza and that these immunizations do not have an adverse effect on viral load or CD4 counts (38, 113). Numerous vaccine candidates are in various stages of clinical trials, and recent results are reviewed here.

Recombinant Protein

The first vaccines to make it to clinical trials were recombinant proteins, and more persons have now received these than any other HIV vaccine. A large efficacy trial is now under way, using recombinant gp120. Although unlikely to provide sterilizing immunity, this approach may at least decrease infectivity and alter the subsequent course of disease in recipients. Efficacy may be limited because is not likely to induce CTLs, and T help would be directed only at Env. In seronegative persons who have received this vaccine, the pattern of antibody responses is different than in natural infection. Vaccinees display more potent recognition of linear epitopes in V1/V2 and V3 and have strong CD4BS antibodies, but the levels of neutralizing antibodies induced are still weaker than those seen in HIV-positive persons (9). Bivalent vaccines consisting of more than one clade may be able to induce more cross-reactive neutralizing antibodies, but this remains to be proven. At least two studies have shown breakthrough cases of new HIV infection in persons who have received this vaccine, with poor development of autologous neutralizing antibodies in recipients (29, 73).

There is some hope that new technical approaches may enhance immunogenicity of recombinant proteins. Most candidates tested thus far · have been monomeric, whereas the natural protein is an oligomeric structure (122). Deglycosylation may allow for the unmasking of important epitopes and enhanced neutralization of native virus (64). In addition, cautious optimism has been expressed based on results with "fusion competent" vaccines. This approach involves the use of fixation techniques to capture transient Env-CD4-coreceptor structures that are thought to arise during HIV-1 binding and fusion. Immunization of mice with these structures resulted in induction of potent neutralizing antibodies (63). Antibodies to such intermediates that were generated in a transgenic mouse model have been shown to possess potent neutralizing antibody responses that neutralize diverse clades. The generation of monoclonal antibodies from these animals has not yet been successful, which has led to more guarded optimism about this approach. Better definition of the precise targets of these antibody responses remains a high priority.

A similar approach to recombinant proteins is the use of synthetic peptides. HGP-30 is a p17-derived peptide vaccine that, when given in two immunizations to 11 seronegative subjects, resulted in induction of antibody and proliferative responses in about half of the recipients. SCID mice reconstituted with peripheral blood mononuclear cells (PBMCs) from the responders were less likely to become infected upon challenge, suggesting some degree of functional immunity, but the components of this protection remain undefined (101).

Recombinant proteins have also been tried as therapeutic vaccines. Although vaccine recipients may have broader and more robust T-helper-cell responses than placebo recipients (109), a recently reported trial of 800-plus volunteers showed no additional benefit when recombinant Env protein was administered in conjunction with standard of care in infected persons (100). Lack of effect on natural history of disease despite the induction of new lymphoproliferative responses was seen in another trial of 40 asymptomatic persons immunized over a five-year period, but these studies antedated the use of HAART (15). Even in the presence of one- or two-drug therapy, gp160 has not had an effect on natural history, even though lymphoproliferative responses were induced (44). Synthetic Env peptides have also been tested in persons who are seropositive. Increased T-helper-cell responses were observed, and perhaps some CTLs, to one of the peptides contained in the vaccine, but there again was no detectable effect on CD4 or viral load (91). Hopes that the use of lipopeptide vaccines might improve immunogenicity remain to be realized (39, 107).

Recombinant Virus Vaccines

The prophylactic vaccine type that is next furthest in testing is recombinant virus, with poxviruses leading the list, often combined with recombinant protein vaccines. Canarypox, which undergoes abortive replication in mammalian cells, is currently being tested in a number of clinical trials. Canarypox expressing gp120, Gag, and protease followed by peptide vaccination induced weak neutralizing antibodies in only one-third of recipients, with an equivalent number demonstrating CTLs (99). A canarypox incorporating gp120, gp41, Gag, protease, and parts of Nef and Pol given with or followed by recombinant gp120 induced CTLs in 61% of recipients at some time during the trial, but the level of CTL responses was strikingly weak compared with the levels seen in infected persons (35). In addition, these vaccines have not induced responses to the dominant CTL epitopes such as an A2 Gag epitope targeted by most infected persons of this haplotype (24). Mouse experiments indicate that recombinant poxvirus followed by boosting with viruslike particles may enhance immune responses, and this needs to be tested in humans (80). Murine studies also suggest that mucosal immunization with vaccinia may circumvent prior vaccinia immunity in mice (10). These results may be important because they suggest independent compartmentalization of the mucosal and systemic immune systems. Combinations of vaccinia vectors, for example, with IL-12-expressing vectors, have increased cell-mediated immunity, but only in certain combinations and doses, so optimal immunization is likely to be a complex issue (43). Novel strains of vaccinia, such as modified vaccinia Ankara (MVA), may have enhanced immunogenicity and may be particularly immunogenic following DNA immunization (104).

Adenovirus vectors are another example of recombinant virus vector in vigorous development. In the past year, adenovirus prime followed by gp120 boost in an animal model resulted in partial protection of two of six animals even though only the Env protein was used as an immunogen. Replication-defective adenovirus can induce both CTL and humoral immune responses in mice (16), and the potential to use these in combination with other vaccines makes them attractive candidates. Recent safety concerns related to the use of adenovirus vectors can be expected to slow development of this very promising approach.

One of the more novel approaches to appear recently is the use of alpha virus vectors such as Venezuelan equine encephalomyelitis (VEE) (21). VEE replicon particles have been shown both to induce virus-specific immune responses and to protect challenged animals from disease progression. Four of four vaccinated animals were protected against disease for at least 16 months, and vaccination reduced peak viral load by 100-fold (31). In support of the protection being immunologically mediated, it was shown that the extent of reduction in viral load was directly correlated with the strength of the immune response induced by the vectors. The fact that these replicons preferentially target dendritic cells in the mucosa suggests that they may be particularly immunogenic (75). Other novel approaches for which there are as yet fewer data include poliovirus vectors and influenza, both of which deserve additional testing.

Whole Inactivated Virus

An approach that has been repeatedly successful in other viral infections has yet to be proven to be sufficiently immunogenic using HIV-1, namely, the use of whole inactivated virus. Because of safety concerns, it has been used exclusively as a therapeutic vaccine in persons already infected. In the pre-HAART era this approach was decidedly unsuccessful, since viremia could not be controlled during the time of potential immune activation by vaccine. With the advent of HAART this approach is deservedly receiving a second look, with a number of trials in progress. Results from one study presented only in abstract form indicate that it may be capable of significant boosts in T-helper-cell responses, and this is further supported by additional recent data (81, 90). This may be the vaccine most able to induce T-helper-cell responses of the currently available approaches. It is also one of the few approaches thus far to be tested in children, in whom preliminary studies show it to be safe and well tolerated (106).

Live Attenuated Virus

Of the various vaccine approaches attempted thus far, live attenuated vaccines have induced the broadest and most durable protection, although the exact mechanisms of protection remain somewhat unclear (83). However, safety concerns have only increased in recent years. Live attenuated viruses with deletions in Nef, Vpr, and the negative regulatory element induced AIDS in 6 of 8 infant macaques, and longer follow-up of adults showed resurgence of viremia in 4 of 16 animals (6). In vitro passage of delta 3 (long terminal repeat [LTR], Vpr, and Nef) in tissue culture resulted in enhanced viral replication after 2 months in culture, and this was associated with evolution to more rapidly replicating virus. These included a 39-nucleotide insertion in the LTR, with maintenance of deletions (12) and a duplicated Sp1 region that led to increased LTR promoter activity (12). Other studies have shown that live attenuated virus vaccine may be less protective against challenge with more highly pathogenic viruses (68) and that protection against heterologous challenge is likely to be difficult to achieve (121).

Despite safety concerns, the live attenuated vaccine approach has the potential in animal models to provide key insights into the components of protective immunity. Studies have shown that protected animals tend to have higher CD8 antiviral factor production including beta chemokines (2) but that this is present both before and after vaccination, suggesting a possible genetic influence on responsiveness. The relationship between immune responses and control of viremia is likely to be complex, since recent studies show no simple correlation between the breadth or strength of the CTL response and protection from challenge. (83). Studies with tetramers to visualize antigen-specific CD8 cells directly suggest an increase in CTLs after infection in the absence of detectable proviral DNA, suggesting that this may be helping to control viremia, along with other mechanisms. The extent to which CD4 T-helper-cell responses contribute to any observed control of viremia needs to be determined in animals infected with attenuated viruses. One study in macaques has shown production of beta chemokines and IFN gamma similar to that seen in HIV-infected controllers, with up to 2% of all CD4 cells specific for SIV (40, 41).

Whether there are modifications of attenuated vaccines that will render them sufficiently immunogenic and safe to permit human trials remains an open question. Most have been loss-of-function mutations, but these may not provide a sufficient margin of safety to proceed. Another approach is gain-of-function mutations. One such approach is the use of a proteolysis-resistant NFkB inhibitor in the Nef region (95). This downregulates viral expression and results in an attenuated virus in cell culture, but whether it would provide a sufficient margin of protection in vivo is not clear.

Bacterial Vectors

A number of recombinant bacterial vectors have been proposed as candidate HIV-1 vaccines. These include listeria, salmonella, and BCG. In particular, intracellular bacteria such as listeria may be more efficient at delivering recombinant proteins into the class I pathway within infected cells, thus facilitating presentation for CTLs (79). In usual listeria infection, one sees the generation of a strong cellular immune response to listeria virulence antigens. It has previously been shown that these recombinant bacterial vectors can generate class I restricted CTLs; now it has been shown that they can also generate T-helper-cell responses of the TH1 type (79). Other approaches such as the use of recombinant BCG and recombinant salmonella have been advocated for additional study, with results awaited (36, 110, 111). None has yet completed clinical trials in humans.

Pseudovirions and Viruslike Particles (VLPs)

Pseudovirions and viruslike particles are noninfectious virions that contain all the virion proteins required for assembly but do not contain viral RNA and thus are not replication incompetent. The use of these particles as immunogens has been explored in animal models and more recently in humans. Insect-derived Gag VLPs that were modified by inserting gp160-derived peptides or gp120 into the particle membrane were used to vaccinate macaques (85). All vaccinated monkeys became infected, but clearance of viremia was associated with accelerated appearance of neutralizing antibodies after challenge. Recent studies in humans include the demonstration that VLPs and AZT augment CTL responses in asymptomatic persons, but there was no clear evidence of functional immune enhancement, since this has no effect on viral load (11).

Polyepitope Vaccines

The in vitro and in vivo demonstrations of antiviral pressure exerted by CTLs have led to accelerated efforts to enhance these responses specifically. One approach is based on early studies of "string of beads" vaccines shown to be immunogenic in mice, in which multiple CTL epitopes are linked together in one construct (118). HIV-based polyepitope vaccines have been shown to be able to induce CTLs to nine of nine expressed epitopes in an animal model, and there is optimism that even more epitopes might be successfully presented on one vector (52). Immunogenicity appears to be enhanced if T-helper-cell responses are also included (52). Similarly, a polyepitope vaccine constructed with seven optimal A2 epitopes was recognized by cells from infected persons and able to induce CTLs in mice, again indicating that multiple epitopes can be simultaneously presented (120). A polyepitope vaccine that includes both macaque and human CTL epitopes has already been tested in monkeys in the form of a DNA vaccine and has shown immunogenicity in SIV (48). This vaccine, based on clade A epitopes, is expected to enter phase I human trials later this year in England and then be tested on-site in Africa. Induction of class II restricted T-helper-cell responses should also be feasible with this approach.

DNA Vaccines

The initial demonstration of protective efficacy of vaccine-induced immune responses with polynucleotide (DNA) vaccines was met with great optimism (114), but the robust responses seen in mice have been much more difficult to achieve in primates and humans. Numerous animal trials are in progress or have been completed, yet the striking results in mice have not been repeated with HIV or SIV thus far.

Interpretation of preclinical data showing immunogenicity in animal models is limited by the lack of challenge in some models (7). Intravaginal and intramuscular administration of DNA vaccines in chimpanzees can induce IgG and IgA, antibodies, CTLs, and T help (7), but the lack of challenge in this model prevents conclusions from being drawn as to the potential efficacy of these responses. Animal models have shown responses to both structural and regulatory proteins (4). *vif, vpu,* and *nef* regulatory genes are immunogenic in mice, which is not particularly surprising. Tat DNA vaccine elicits Ab and CTL responses, using transdominant mutants (25). However, the best targets to pursue remain unclear.

DNA vaccines have now been tried in a number of phase I human clinical trials. Immune responses including T-helper-cell responses have been induced but have been short lived (14). In another study, 15 HIV-1 seropositive persons were given a DNA vaccine expressing the *env* and *rev* gene products. Short-term follow-up limits conclusions that can be drawn in terms of persistence of what was likely induction of low-level immune responses (13). In another trial of seropositive persons, DNA immunization with *nef* or *tat* genes induced T-helper-cell responses and increased CTL precursors but had no effect on viral load (20). The combination of vaccine plus HAART appeared to augment induction of CTL responses; additional studies are in progress and should provide evidence as to the potential promise of this approach.

DNA vaccines may ultimately be more effective in combination with other approaches, such as DNA priming followed by boosting with live vector vaccines (48). Alternatively, there may be ways to augment immunogenicity of these vaccines. A number of trials in animal models are addressing potential ways to achieve enhanced immunogenicity. These include coexpression of adhesion molecules, growth factors, and CD40 ligand (8, 51, 57, 58, 59, 60, 62), as well as modifications in delivery systems (119). Modulation of antigen expression by modification of Gag sequences (94, 126) and enhancement of antigen secretion in vivo (112) also represent approaches that are being pursued at the present time.

Live HIV Vaccines

The advent of HAART has made it possible to use the equivalent of live HIV as a therapeutic vaccine. Structured interruption in therapy to allow a regulated amount of virus expression and then prompt reinstitution of therapy has been suggested from anecdotal cases to enhance immunity to HIV (71, 87). The best results have been observed in animals and humans who are treated in the acute stages of AIDS virus infection and then have treatment interrupted. In some cases this has led to sustained control of viremia (71, 87), but the extent to which the treatment interruptions have facilitated this and the precise immune enhancements that may be contributing to control remain poorly characterized. Additional studies in humans are currently under way, but results are not yet known. Animal data using this approach are needed; preliminary studies suggest that treatment in acute SIV infection may lead to augmented immune control once therapy has been stopped (70). Animals with acute SIV infection were treated with PMPA at defined times after infection, and then therapy was later stopped. Although postinoculation treatment did not prevent infection, it led to lower viral loads at steady state once therapy was stopped. In another study (97), early treatment of macaques followed by immunization suggested that viral load was lower at steady state once therapy was stopped, but limited follow-up hampers interpretation of these studies.

Trials on the Horizon

The HIV vaccine field remains without a clear front-runner, but there are multiple trials in progress or on the horizon that should at least provide evidence of the relative immunogenicity of different approaches and the potential to use different vaccines in combination to enhance immunogenicity. A large-scale trial of recombinant gp120 vaccine is in progress in the United States and abroad. Trials of a DNA vaccine produced by Merck have been initiated at a number of centers around the United States. In addition, there is growing enthusiasm for therapeutic vaccines, with numerous trials now in progress, using a variety of different vaccine candidates. New approaches to vaccination include the use of autologous dendritic cells, which have been shown to be highly immunogenic in humans using influenza peptides (32). Other approaches such as alloimmunization have also been proposed (108).

Summary and Conclusions

The most important conclusion that can be drawn from recent advances in HIV research is that this virus can be immunologically controlled in some individuals. However, since the virus does not appear to be eradicated under any naturally occurring conditions, the most promising results are likely to relate to vaccines that will be able to attenuate disease course in persons once they become infected. The finding that the lowering of virus load in the acute phase of infection is associated with enhanced immune control of infection suggests that even a partially effective vaccine may confer significant benefit. In addition, immunity is likely to be enhanced through the use of combinations of vaccines. At the same time, we need a better understanding of pathogenesis and immunity in persons infected with different clades and in persons of diverse ethnic groups. We also need to support the development of an international infrastructure to test the vaccine candidates. There is at this time no clear front-runner candidate, and thus it is prudent to move forward with all possible approaches using rigorous methods to assess immunogenicity and efficacy. With much improved assays to measure vaccine-induced responses, a thorough dissection of the responses induced by candidate vaccines is possible.

REFERENCES

1. Abbas, A. K. 1996. Die and let live: eliminating dangerous lymphocytes. Cell 84:655–657.
1a. Addo, M. M., M. Altfeld, E. S. Rosenberg, R. L. Eldridge, M. N. Philips, K. Habeeb, A. Khatri, C. Brander, G. K. Robbins, G. P. Mazzara, P. J. Goulder, B. D. Walker, and HIVCS Collaboration. 2001. The HIV-1 regulatory proteins Tat and Rev are frequently targeted by cytotoxic T lymphocytes derived from HIV-1-infected individuals. Proc. Natl. Acad. Sci. USA 98:1781.
2. Ahmed, R. K., C. Nilsson, Y. Wang, T. Lehner, G. Biberfeld, and R. Thorstensson, R. 1999. β-chemokine production in macaques vaccinated with live attenuated virus correlates with protection against simian immunodeficiency virus (SIVsm) challenge. J. Gen. Virol. 80:1569–1574.
3. Altman, J. D., P. A. H. Moss, P. J. R. Goulder, D. H. Barouch, M. G. McHeyzer-Williams, J. I. Bell, A. J. McMichael, and M. M. Davis. 1996. Phenotypic analysis of antigen-specific T lymphocytes. Science 274:94–96.

4. Ayyavoo, V., S. Kudchodkar, M. P. Ramanathan, P. Le, K. Muthumani, N. M. Megalai, T. Dentchev, L. Santiago-Barrios, C. Mrinalini, and D. B. Weiner. 2000. Immunogenicity of a novel DNA vaccine cassette expressing multiple human immunodeficiency virus (HIV-1) accessory genes. AIDS 14:1–9.

5. Baba, T. W., V. Liska, R. Hofmann-Lehmann, J. Vlasak, W. Xu, S. Ayehunie, L. A. Cavacini, M. R. Posner, H. Katinger, G. Stiegler, B. J. Bernacky, T. A. Rizvi, R. Schmidt, L. R. Hill, M. E. Keeling, Y. Lu, J. E. Wright, T. C. Chou, and R. M. Ruprecht. 2000. Human neutralizing monoclonal antibodies of the IgG1 subtype protect against mucosal simian-human immunodeficiency virus infection. Nature Med. 6:200–206.

6. Baba, T. W., V. Liska, A. H. Khimani, N. B. Ray, P. J. Dailey, D. Penninck, R. Bronson, M. F. Greene, H. M. McClure, L. N. Martin, and R. M. Ruprecht. 1999. Live attenuated, multiply deleted simian immunodeficiency virus causes AIDS in infant and adult macaques. Nature Med. 5:194–203.

7. Bagarazzi, M. L., J. D. Boyer, M. A. Javadian, M. A. Chattergoon, A. R. Shah, A. D. Cohen, M. K. Bennett, R. B. Ciccarelli, K. E. Ugen, and D. B. Weiner. 1999. Systemic and mucosal immunity is elicited after both intramuscular and intravaginal delivery of human immunodeficiency virus type 1 DNA plasmid vaccines to pregnant chimpanzees. J. Infect. Dis. 180:1351–1355.

8. Barouch, D. H., A. Craiu, M. J. Kuroda, J. E. Schmitz, X. X. Zheng, S. Santra, J. D. Frost, G. R. Krivulka, M. A. Lifton, C. L. Crabbs, G. Heidecker, H. C. Perry, M. E. Davies, H. Xie, C. E. Nickerson, T. D. Steenbeke, C. I. Lord, D. C. Montefiori, T. B. Strom, J. W. Shiver, M. G. Lewis, and N. L. Letvin. 2000. Augmentation of immune responses to HIV-1 and simian immunodeficiency virus DNA vaccines by IL-2/Ig plasmid administration in rhesus monkeys. Proc. Natl. Acad. Sci. USA 97:4192–4197.

9. Beddows, S., S. Lister, R. Cheingsong, C. Bruck, and J. Weber. 1999. Comparison of the antibody repertoire generated in healthy volunteers following immunization with a monomeric recombinant gp120 construct derived from a CCR5/CXCR4-using human immunodeficiency virus type 1 isolate with sera from naturally infected individuals. J. Virol. 73:1740–1745.

10. Belyakov, I. M., B. Moss, W. Strober, and J. A. Berzofsky. 1999. Mucosal vaccination overcomes the barrier to recombinant vaccinia immunization caused by preexisting poxvirus immunity. Proc. Natl. Acad. Sci. USA 96:4512–4517.

11. Benson, E. M., J. Clarkson, M. Law, P. Marshall, A. D. Kelleher, D. E. Smith, G. Patou, G. J. Stewart, D. A. Cooper, and R. A. French. 1999. Therapeutic vaccination with p24-VLP and zidovudine augments HIV-specific cytotoxic T lymphocyte activity in asymptomatic HIV-infected individuals. AIDS Res. Hum. Retroviruses 15:105–113.

12. Berkhout, B., K. Verhoef, J. L. van Wamel, and N. K. Back. 1999. Genetic instability of live, attenuated human immunodeficiency virus type 1 vaccine strains. J. Virol. 73:1138–1145.

13. Boyer, J. D., M. A. Chattergoon, K. E. Ugen, A. Shah, M. Bennett, A. Cohen, S. Nyland, K. E. Lacy, M. L. Bagarazzi, T. J. Higgins, Y. Baine, R. B. Ciccarelli, R. S. Ginsberg, R. R. MacGregor, and D. B. Weiner. 1999. Enhancement of cellular immune response in HIV-1 seropositive individuals: a DNA-based trial. Clin. Immunol. 90:100–107.

14. Boyer, J. D., A. D. Cohen, S. Vogt, K. Schumann, B. Nath, L. Ahn, K. Lacy, M. L. Bagarazzi, T. J. Higgins, Y. Baine, R. B. Ciccarelli, R. S. Ginsberg, R. R. Mac-Gregor, and D. B. Weiner. 2000. Vaccination of seronegative volunteers with a human immunodeficiency virus type 1 env/rev DNA vaccine induces antigen-specific proliferation and lymphocyte production of β-chemokines. J. Infect. Dis. 181:476–483.

15. Bratt, G., L. E. Eriksson, E. Sandstrom, G. Gilljam, J. Hinkula, J. Albert, R. Redfield, and B. Wahren. 1999. Long-term immunotherapy in HIV infection, combined with short-term antiretroviral treatment. Int. J. STD AIDS 10:514–521.

16. Bruce, C. B., A. Akrigg, S. A. Sharpe, T. Hanke, G. W. Wilkinson, and M. P. Cranage. 1999. Replication-deficient recombinant adenoviruses expressing the human immunodeficiency virus env antigen can induce both humoral and CTL immune responses in mice. J. Gen. Virol. 80:2621–2628.

17. Burton, D. R., and P. W. Parren. 2000. Vaccines and the induction of functional antibodies: time to look beyond the molecules of natural infection? Nature Med. 6:123–125.

18. Buseyne, F., M. McChesney, F. Porrot, S. Kovarik, B. Guy, and Y. Riviere. 1993. Gag-specific cytotoxic T lymphocytes from human immunodeficiency virus type 1-infected individuals: gag epitopes are clustered in three regions of the p24^{gag} protein. J. Virol. 67:694–702.

19. Cafaro, A., A. Caputo, C. Fracasso, M. T. Maggiorella, D. Goletti, S. Baroncelli, M. Pace, L. Sernicola, M. L. Koanga-Mogtomo, M. Betti, A. Borsetti, R. Belli, L. Akerblom, F. Corrias, S. Butto, J. Heeney, P. Verani, F. Titti, and B. Ensoli. 1999. Control of SHIV-89.6P-infection of cynomolgus monkeys by HIV-1 tat protein vaccine. Nature Med. 5:643–650.

20. Calarota, S. A., A. C. Leandersson, G. Bratt, J. Hinkula, D. M. Klinman, K. J. Weinhold, E. Sandstrom, and B. Wahren. 1999. Immune responses in asymptomatic HIV-1-infected patients after HIV-DNA immunization followed by highly active antiretroviral treatment. J. Immunol. 163:2330–2338.

21. Caley, I. J., M. R. Betts, N. L. Davis, R. Swanstrom, J. A. Frelinger, and R. E. Johnston. 1999. Venezuelan equine encephalitis virus vectors expressing HIV-1 proteins: vector design strategies for improved vaccine efficacy. Vaccine 17:3124–3135.

22. Cao, Y., L. Qin, L. Zhang, J. Safrit, and D. D. Ho. 1995. Virologic and immunologic characterization of long-term survivors of human immunodeficiency virus type 1 infection. N. Engl. J. Med. 332:201–208.

23. Carrington, M., G. W. Nelson, M. P. Martin, T. Kissner, D. Vlahov, J. J. Goedert, R. Kaslow, S. Buchbinder, K. Hoots, and S. J. O'Brien. 1999. HLA and HIV-1: heterozygote advantage and B*35-Cw*04 disadvantage. Science 283:1748–1752.

24. Carruth, L. M., T. F. Greten, C. E. Murray, M. G. Castro, S. N. Crone, W. Pavlat, J. P. Schneck, and R. F. Siliciano. 1999. An algorithm for evaluating human cytotoxic T lymphocyte responses to candidate AIDS vaccines. AIDS Res. Hum. Retroviruses 15:1021–1034.

25. Caselli, E., M. Betti, M. P. Grossi, P. G. Balboni, C. Rossi, C. Boarini, A. Cafaro, G. Barbanti-Brodano, B. Ensoli, and A. Caputo. 1999. DNA immunization with HIV-1 tat mutated in the trans activation domain induces hu-

moral and cellular immune responses against wild-type tat. J. Immunol. 162:5631–5638.

26. Clerici, M., N. I. Stocks, R. A. Zajac, R. N. Boswell, D. C. Bernstein, D. L. Mann, G. M. Shearer, and J. A. Berzofsky. 1989. Interleukin-2 production used to detect antigenic peptide recognition by T-helper lymphocytes from asymptomatic HIV-seropositive individuals. Nature 339:383–385.

27. Clerici, M., N. I. Stocks, R. A. Zajac, R. N. Boswell, C. S. Via, and G. M. Shearer. 1990. Circumvention of defective CD4 T helper cell function in HIV-infected individuals by stimulation with HLA alloantigens. J. Immunol. 144:3266–3271.

28. Collins, K. L., B. K. Chen, S. A. Kalams, B. D. Walker, and D. Baltimore. 1998. HIV-1 nef protein protects infected primary cells against killing by cytotoxic T lymphocytes. Nature 391:397–401.

29. Connor, R. I., B. T. Korber, B. S. Graham, B. H. Hahn, D. D. Ho, B. D. Walker, A. U. Neumann, S. H. Vermund, J. Mestecky, S. Jackson, E. Fenamore, Y. Cao, F. Gao, S. Kalams, K. J. Kunstman, D. McDonald, N. McWilliams, A. Trkola, J. P. Moore, and S. M. Wolinsky. 1998. Immunological and virological analyses of persons infected by human immunodeficiency virus type 1 while participating in trials of recombinant gp120 subunit vaccines. J. Virol. 72: 1552–1576.

30. Cox, J. H., R. P. Garner, R. R. Redfield, N. E. Aronson, C. Davis, N. Ruiz, and D. L. Birx. 1999. Antibody-dependent cellular cytotoxicity in HIV type 1-infected patients receiving VaxSyn, a recombinant gp160 envelope vaccine. AIDS Res. Hum. Retroviruses 15:847–854.

31. Davis, N. L., I. J. Caley, K. W. Brown, M. R. Betts, D. M. Irlbeck, K. M. Mc-Grath, M. J. Connell, D. C. Montefiori, J. A. Frelinger, R. Swanstrom, P. R. Johnson, and R. E. Johnston. 2000. Vaccination of macaques against pathogenic simian immunodeficiency virus with Venezuelan equine encephalitis virus replicon particles. J. Virol. 74:371–378.

32. Dhodapkar, M. V., R. M. Steinman, M. Sapp, H. Desai, C. F. Fossella, J. Krasovsky, S. M. Donahoe, P. R. Dunbar, V. Cerundolo, D. F. Nixon, and N. Bhardwaj. 1999. Rapid generation of broad T-cell immunity in humans after a single injection of mature dendritic cells. J. Clin. Invest. 104:173–180.

33. Dyer, W. B., G. S. Ogg, M. A. Demoitie, X. Jin, A. F. Geczy, S. L. Rowland-Jones, A. J. McMichael, D. F. Nixon, and J. S. Sullivan. 1999. Strong human immunodeficiency virus (HIV)-specific cytotoxic T-lymphocyte activity in Sydney blood bank cohort patients infected with nef-defective HIV type 1. J. Virol. 73:436–443.

34. Evans, D. T., D. H. O'Connor, P. Jing, J. L. Dzuris, J. Sidney, J. da Silva, T. M. Allen, H. Horton, J. E. Venham, R. A. Rudersdorf, T. Vogel, C. D. Pauza, R. E. Bontrop, R. DeMars, A. Sette, A. L. Hughes, and D. I. Watkins. 1999. Virus-specific cytotoxic T-lymphocyte responses select for amino-acid variation in simian immunodeficiency virus Env and Nef. Nature Med. 5:1270–1276.

35. Evans, T. G., M. C. Keefer, K. J. Weinhold, M. Wolff, D. Montefiori, G. J. Gorse, B. S. Graham, M. J. McElrath, M. L. Clements-Mann, M. J. Mulligan, P. Fast, M. C. Walker, J. L. Excler, A. M. Duliege, and J. Tartaglia. 1999. A canarypox vaccine expressing multiple human immunodeficiency virus type 1 genes

given alone or with Rgp120 elicits broad and durable CD8[+] cytotoxic T lymphocyte responses in seronegative volunteers. J. Infect. Dis. 180:290–298.

36. Falk, L. A., K. L. Goldenthal, J. Esparza, M. T. Aguado, S. Osmanov, W. R. Ballou, S. Beddows, N. Bhamarapravati, G. Biberfeld, G. Ferrari, D. Hoft, M. Honda, A. Jackson, Y. Lu, G. Marchal, J. McKinney, and S. Yamazaki. 2000. Recombinant bacillus Calmette-Guérin as a potential vector for preventive HIV type 1 vaccines. AIDS Res. Hum. Retroviruses 16:91–98.

37. Finzi, D., M. Hermankova, T. Pierson, L. M. Carruth, C. Buck, R. E. Chaisson, T. C. Quinn, K. Chadwick, et al. 1997. Identification of a reservoir for HIV-1 in patients on highly active antiretroviral therapy. Science 278:1295–1298.

38. Fuller, J. D., D. E. Craven, K. A. Steger, N. Cox, T. C. Heeren, and D. Chernoff. 1999. Influenza vaccination of human immunodeficiency virus (HIV)-infected adults: impact on plasma levels of HIV type 1 RNA and determinants of antibody response. Clin. Infect. Dis. 28:541–547.

39. Gahery-Segard, H., G. Pialoux, B. Charmeteau, S. Sermet, H. Poncelet, M. Raux, A. Tartar, J. P. Levy, H. Gras-Masse, and J. G. Guillet. 2000. Multiepitopic B- and T-cell responses induced in humans by a human immunodeficiency virus type 1 lipopeptide vaccine. J. Virol. 74:1694–1703.

40. Gauduin, M. C., R. L. Glickman, S. Ahmad, T. Yilma, and R. P. Johnson. 1999. Characterization of SIV-specific CD4[+] T-helper proliferative responses in macaques immunized with live-attenuated SIV. J. Med. Primatol. 28:233–241.

41. Gauduin, M. C., R. L. Glickman, S. Ahmad, T. Yilma, and R. P. Johnson. 1999. Immunization with live attenuated simian immunodeficiency virus induces strong type 1 T helper responses and β-chemokine production. Proc. Natl. Acad. Sci. USA 96:14031–14036.

42. Gerlach, J. T., H. M. Diepolder, M. C. Jung, N. H. Gruener, W. W. Schraut, R. Zachoval, R. Hoffmann, C. A. Schirren, T. Santantonio, and G. R. Pape. 1999. Recurrence of hepatitis C virus after loss of virus-specific CD4[+] T-cell response in acute hepatitis C. Gastroenterology 117:933–941.

43. Gherardi, M. M., J. C. Ramirez, D. Rodriguez, J. R. Rodriguez, G. Sano, F. Zavala, and M. Esteban. 1999. IL-12 delivery from recombinant vaccinia virus attenuates the vector and enhances the cellular immune response against HIV-1 env in a dose-dependent manner. J. Immunol. 162:6724–6733.

44. Goebel, F. D., J. W. Mannhalter, R. B. Belshe, M. M. Eibl, P. J. Grob, V. de Gruttola, P. D. Griffiths, V. Erfle, M. Kunschak, and W. Engl. 1999. Recombinant gp160 as a therapeutic vaccine for HIV-infection: results of a large randomized, controlled trial. AIDS 13:1461–1468.

45. Goulder, P. J., C. Brander, K. Annamalai, N. Mngqundaniso, U. Govender, Y. Tang, S. He, K. E. Hartman, C. A. O'Callaghan, G. S. Ogg, M. A. Altfeld, E. S. Rosenberg, H. Cao, S. A. Kalams, M. Hammond, M. Bunce, S. I. Pelton, S. A. Burchett, K. McIntosh, H. M. Coovadia, and B. D. Walker. 2000. Differential narrow focusing of immunodominant human immunodeficiency virus gag-specific cytotoxic T-lymphocyte responses in infected African and Caucasoid adults and children. J. Virol. 74:5679–5690.

46. Goulder, P. J. R., S. L. Rowland, A. J. McMichael, and B. D. Walker. 1999. Anti-HIV cellular immunity: recent advances towards vaccine design. AIDS 13:s121–136.

47. Guidotti, L. G., R. Rochford, J. Chung, M. Shapiro, R. Purcell, and F. V. Chisari. 1999. Viral clearance without destruction of infected cells during acute HBV infection. Science 284:825–829.

48. Hanke, T., R. V. Samuel, T. J. Blanchard, V. C. Neumann, T. M. Allen, J. E. Boyson, S. A. Sharpe, N. Cook, G. L. Smith, D. I. Watkins, M. P. Cranage, and A. J. McMichael. 1999. Effective induction of simian immunodeficiency virus-specific cytotoxic T lymphocytes in macaques by using a multiepitope gene and DNA prime-modified vaccinia virus Ankara boost vaccination regimen. J. Virol. 73:7524–7532.

49. Harrer, T., E. Harrer, S. A. Kalams, P. Barbosa, A. Trocha, R. P. Johnson, T. Elbeik, M. B. Feinberg, S. P. Buchbinder, and B. D. Walker. 1996. Cytotoxic T lymphocytes in asymptomatic long-term nonprogressing HIV-1 infection. Breadth and specificity of the response and relation to in vivo viral quasi-species in a person with prolonged infection and low viral load. J. Immunol. 156:2616–2623.

50. Harrer, T., E. Harrer, S. A. Kalams, T. Elbeik, S. I. Staprans, M. B. Feinberg, Y. Cao, D. D. Ho, T. Yilma, A. M. Caliendo, R. P. Johnson, S. P. Buchbinder, and B. D. Walker. 1996. Strong cytotoxic T cell and weak neutralizing antibody responses in a subset of persons with stable nonprogressing HIV type 1 infection. AIDS Res. Hum. Retroviruses 12:585–592.

51. Ihata, A., S. Watabe, S. Sasaki, A. Shirai, J. Fukushima, K. Hamajima, J. Inoue, and K. Okuda. 1999. Immunomodulatory effect of a plasmid expressing CD40 ligand on DNA vaccination against human immunodeficiency virus type-1. Immunology 98:436–442.

52. Ishioka, G. Y., J. Fikes, G. Hermanson, B. Livingston, C. Crimi, M. Qin, M. F. del Guercio, C. Oseroff, C. Dahlberg, J. Alexander, R. W. Chesnut, and A. Sette. 1999. Utilization of MHC class I transgenic mice for development of minigene DNA vaccines encoding multiple HLA-restricted CTL epitopes. J. Immunol. 162:3915–3925.

53. Jin, X., D. E. Bauer, S. E. Tuttleton, S. Lewin, A. Gettie, J. Blanchard, C. E. Irwin, J. T. Safrit, J. Mittler, L. Weinberger, L. G. Kostrikis, L. Zhang, A. S. Perelson, and D. D. Ho. 1999. Dramatic rise in plasma viremia after CD8$^+$ T cell depletion in simian immunodeficiency virus-infected macaques. J. Exp. Med. 189:991–998.

54. Johnson, R. P., R. L. Glickman, J. Q. Yang, A. Kaur, J. T. Dion, M. J. Mulligan, and R. C. Desrosiers. 1997. Induction of vigorous cytotoxic T-lymphocyte responses by live attenuated simian immunodeficiency virus. J. Virol. 71:7711–7718.

55. Kalams, S. A., S. P. Buchbinder, E. S. Rosenberg, J. M. Billingsley, D. S. Colbert, N. G. Jones, A. K. Shea, A. K. Trocha, and B. D. Walker. 1999. Association between virus-specific cytotoxic T-lymphocyte and helper responses in human immunodeficiency virus type 1 infection. J. Virol. 73:6715–6720.

55a. Kalams, S. A., and B. D. Walker. 1998. The critical need for CD4 help in maintaining effective cytotoxic T lymphocyte responses [comment]. J. Exp. Med. 188:2199.

56. Kaul, R., F. A. Plummer, J. Kimani, T. Dong, P. Kiama, T. Rostron, E. Njagi, K. S. MacDonald, J. J. Bwayo, A. J. McMichael, and S. L. Rowland-Jones. 2000.

HIV-1 specific mucosal CD8+ lymphocyte responses in the cervix of HIV-1-resistant prostitutes in Nairobi. J. Immunol. 164:1602–1611.

57. Kim, J. J., K. A. Simbiri, J. I. Sin, K. Dang, J. Oh, T. Dentchev, D. Lee, L. K. Nottingham, A. A. Chalian, D. McCallus, R. Ciccarelli, M. G. Agadjanyan, and D. B. Weiner. 1999. Cytokine molecular adjuvants modulate immune responses induced by DNA vaccine constructs for HIV-1 and SIV. J. Interferon Cytokine Res. 19:77–84.

58. Kim, J. J., N. N. Trivedi, L. K. Nottingham, L. Morrison, A. Tsai, Y. Hu, S. Mahalingam, K. Dang, L. Ahn, N. K. Doyle, D. M. Wilson, M. A. Chattergoon, A. A. Chalian, J. D. Boyer, M. G. Agadjanyan, and D. B. Weiner. 1998. Modulation of amplitude and direction of in vivo immune responses by co-administration of cytokine gene expression cassettes with DNA immunogens. Eur. J. Immunol. 28:1089–1103.

59. Kim, J. J., A. Tsai, L. K. Nottingham, L. Morrison, D. M. Cunning, J. Oh, D. J. Lee, K. Dang, T. Dentchev, A. A. Chalian, M. G. Agadjanyan, and D. B. Weiner. 1999. Intracellular adhesion molecule-1 modulates β-chemokines and directly costimulates T cells in vivo. J. Clin. Invest. 103:869–877.

60. Kim, J. J., J. S. Yang, D. J. Lee, D. M. Wilson, L. K. Nottingham, L. Morrison, A. Tsai, J. Oh, K. Dang, T. Dentchev, M. G. Agadjanyan, J. I. Sin, A. A. Chalian, and D. B. Weiner. 2000. Macrophage colony-stimulating factor can modulate immune responses and attract dendritic cells in vivo. Hum. Gene Ther. 11:305–321.

61. Koblin, B. A., B. H. van Benthem, S. P. Buchbinder, L. Ren, E. Vittinghoff, C. E. Stevens, R. A. Coutinho, and G. J. van Griensven. 1999. Long-term survival after infection with human immunodeficiency virus type 1 (HIV-1) among homosexual men in hepatitis B vaccine trial cohorts in Amsterdam, New York City, and San Francisco, 1978–1995. Am. J. Epidemiol. 150:1026–1030.

62. Kusakabe, K., K. Q. Xin, H. Katoh, K. Sumino, E. Hagiwara, S. Kawamoto, K. Okuda, Y. Miyagi, I. Aoki, K. Nishioka, and D. Klinman. 2000. The timing of GM-CSF expression plasmid administration influences the Th1/Th2 response induced by an HIV-1-specific DNA vaccine. J. Immunol. 164:3102–3111.

63. LaCasse, R. A., K. E. Follis, M. Trahey, J. D. Scarborough, D. R. Littman, and J. H. Nunberg. 1999. Fusion-competent vaccines: broad neutralization of primary isolates of HIV. Science 283:357–362.

64. Langlois, A. J., R. C. Desrosiers, M. G. Lewis, V. N. Kewal-Ramani, D. R. Littman, J. Y. Zhou, K. Manson, M. S. Wyand, D. P. Bolognesi, and D. C. Montefiori. 1998. Neutralizing antibodies in sera from macaques immunized with attenuated simian immunodeficiency virus. J. Virol. 72:6950–6955.

65. Lechner, F., D. K. Wong, P. R. Dunbar, R. Chapman, R. T. Chung, P. Dohrenwend, G. Robbins, R. Phillips, P. Klenerman, and B. D. Walker. 2000. Analysis of successful immune responses in persons infected with hepatitis C virus. J. Exp. Med. 191:1499.

66. Le Gall, S., L. Erdtmann, S. Benichou, C. Berlioz-Torrent, L. Liu, R. Benarous, J. M. Heard, and O. Schwartz. 1998. Nef interacts with the mu subunit of clathrin adaptor complexes and reveals a cryptic sorting signal in MHC I molecules. Immunity 8:483–495.

67. Leno, M., L. Carter, D. J. Venzon, J. Romano, P. D. Markham, K. Limbach, J. Tartaglia, E. Paoletti, J. Benson, G. Franchini, and M. Robert-Guroff. 1999. CD8+ lymphocyte antiviral activity in monkeys immunized with SIV recombinant poxvirus vaccines: potential role in vaccine efficacy. AIDS Res. Hum. Retroviruses 15:461–470.

68. Lewis, M. G., J. Yalley-Ogunro, J. J. Greenhouse, T. P. Brennan, J. B. Jiang, T. C. VanCott, Y. Lu, G. A. Eddy, and D. L. Birx. 1999. Limited protection from a pathogenic chimeric simian-human immunodeficiency virus challenge following immunization with attenuated simian immunodeficiency virus. J. Virol. 73:1262–1270.

69. Li, T. S., R. Tubiana, C. Katlama, V. Calvez, H. Ait Mohand, and B. Autran. 1998. Long-lasting recovery in CD4 T-cell function and viral-load reduction after highly active antiretroviral therapy in advanced HIV-1 disease. Lancet 351:1682–1686.

70. Lifson, J. D., J. L. Rossio, R. Arnaout, L. Li, T. L. Parks, D. K. Schneider, R. F. Kiser, V. J. Coalter, G. Walsh, R. J. Imming, B. Fisher, B. M. Flynn, N. Bischofberger, M. Piatak, Jr., V. M. Hirsch, M. A. Nowak, and D. Wodarz. 2000. Containment of simian immunodeficiency virus infection: cellular immune responses and protection from rechallenge following transient postinoculation antiretroviral treatment. J. Virol. 74:2584–2593.

71. Lisziewicz, J., E. Rosenberg, J. Lieberman, H. Jessen, L. Lopalco, R. Siliciano, B. Walker, and F. Lori. 1999. Control of HIV despite the discontinuation of antiretroviral therapy. N. Engl. J. Med. 340:1683–1684.

72. Little, S. J., A. R. McLean, C. A. Spina, D. D. Richman, and D. V. Havlir. 1999. Viral dynamics of acute HIV-1 infection. J. Exp. Med. 190:841–850.

73. Locher, C. P., R. M. Grant, E. A. Collisson, G. Reyes-Teran, T. Elbeik, J. O. Kahn, and J. A. Levy. 1999. Antibody and cellular immune responses in breakthrough infection subjects after HIV type 1 glycoprotein 120 vaccination. AIDS Res. Hum. Retroviruses 15:1685–1689.

74. Lyles, R. H., A. Munoz, T. E. Yamashita, H. Bazmi, R. Detels, C. R. Rinaldo, J. B. Margolick, J. P. Phair, and J. W. Mellors. 2000. Natural history of human immunodeficiency virus type 1 viremia after seroconversion and proximal to AIDS in a large cohort of homosexual men. J. Infect. Dis. 181:872–880.

75. MacDonald, G. H., and R. E. Johnston. 2000. Role of dendritic cell targeting in Venezuelan equine encephalitis virus pathogenesis. J. Virol. 74:914–922.

76. MacDonald, K. S., K. R. Fowke, J. Kimani, V. A. Dunand, N. J. Nagelkerke, T. B. Ball, J. Oyugi, E. Njagi, L. K. Gaur, R. C. Brunham, J. Wade, M. A. Luscher, P. Krausa, S. Rowland-Jones, E. Ngugi, J. J. Bwayo, and F. A. Plummer. 2000. Influence of HLA supertypes on susceptibility and resistance to human immunodeficiency virus type 1 infection. J. Infect. Dis. 181:1581–1589.

77. Malhotra, U., M. M. Berrey, Y. Huang, J. Markee, D. J. Brown, S. Ap, L. Musey, T. Schacker, L. Corey, and M. J. McElrath. 2000. Effect of combination antiretroviral therapy on T-cell immunity in acute human immunodeficiency virus type 1 infection. J. Infect. Dis. 181:121–131.

78. Mascola, J. R., M. G. Lewis, G. Stiegler, D. Harris, T. C. VanCott, D. Hayes, M. K. Louder, C. R. Brown, C. V. Sapan, S. S. Frankel, Y. Lu, M. L. Robb, H. Katinger, and D. L. Birx. 1999. Protection of macaques against pathogenic

simian/human immunodeficiency virus 89.6PD by passive transfer of neutralizing antibodies. J. Virol. 73:4009–4018.

79. Mata, M., and Y. Paterson. 1999. Th1 T cell responses to HIV-1 gag protein delivered by a Listeria monocytogenes vaccine are similar to those induced by endogenous listerial antigens. J. Immunol. 163:1449–1456.

80. Moldoveanu, Z., A. N. Vzorov, W. Q. Huang, J. Mestecky, and R. W. Compans. 1999. Induction of immune responses to SIV antigens by mucosally administered vaccines. AIDS Res. Hum. Retroviruses 15:1469–1476.

81. Moss, R. B., M. R. Wallace, W. K. Giermakowska, E. Webb, J. Savary, C. Chamberlin-Brandt, G. Theofan, R. Musil, S. P. Richieri, F. C. Jensen, and D. J. Carlo. 1999. Phenotype analysis of human immunodeficiency virus (HIV) type 1 cell-mediated immune responses after treatment with an HIV-1 immunogen. J. Infect. Dis. 180:641–648.

82. Musey, L., J. Hughes, T. Schacker, T. Shea, L. Corey, and M. McElrath. 1997. Cytotoxic-T-cell responses, viral load, and disease progression in early human immunodeficiency virus type 1 infection. N. Engl. J. Med. 337:1267–1308.

83. Nixon, D. F., S. M. Donahoe, W. M. Kakimoto, R. V. Samuel, K. J. Metzner, A. Gettie, T. Hanke, P. A. Marx, and R. I. Connor. 2000. Simian immunodeficiency virus-specific cytotoxic T lymphocytes and protection against challenge in rhesus macaques immunized with a live attenuated simian immunodeficiency virus vaccine. Virology 266:203–210.

84. Nixon, D. F., D. Douek, P. J. Kuebler, X. Jin, M. Vesanen, S. Bonhoeffer, Y. Cao, Y. Koup, D. D. Ho, and M. Markowitz. 1999. Molecular tracking of a human immunodeficiency virus nef specific cytotoxic T-cell clone shows persistence of clone-specific T-cell receptor DNA but not mRNA following early combination antiretroviral therapy. Immunol. Lett. 66:219–228.

85. Notka, F., C. Stahl-Hennig, U. Dittmer, H. Wolf, and R. Wagner. 1999. Accelerated clearance of SHIV in rhesus monkeys by virus-like particle vaccines is dependent on induction of neutralizing antibodies. Vaccine 18:291–301.

86. Ogg, G. S., X. Jin, S. Bonhoeffer, P. R. Dunbar, M. A. Nowak, S. Monard, J. P. Segal, Y. Cao, S. L. Rowland-Jones, V. Cerundolo, A. Hurley, M. Markowitz, D. D. Ho, D. F. Nixon, and A. J. McMichael. 1998. Quantitation of HIV-1-specific cytotoxic T lymphocytes and plasma load of viral RNA. Science 279:2103–2106.

87. Ortiz, G. M., D. F. Nixon, A. Trkola, J. Binley, X. Jin, S. Bonhoeffer, P. J. Kuebler, S. M. Donahoe, M. A. Demoitie, W. M. Kakimoto, T. Ketas, B. Clas, J. J. Heymann, L. Zhang, Y. Cao, A. Hurley, J. P. Moore, D. D. Ho, and M. Markowitz. 1999. HIV-1-specific immune responses in subjects who temporarily contain virus replication after discontinuation of highly active antiretroviral therapy [see comments]. J. Clin. Invest. 104:R13.

88. Oxenius, A., D. A. Price, P. J. Easterbrook, C. A. O'Callaghan, A. D. Kelleher, J. A. Whelan, G. Sontag, A. K. Sewell, and R. E. Phillips. 2000. Early highly active antiretroviral therapy for acute HIV-1 infection preserves immune function of $CD8^+$ and $CD4^+$ T lymphocytes. Proc. Natl. Acad. Sci. USA 97: 3382–3387.

89. Pantaleo, G., S. Menzo, M. Vaccarezza, C. Graziosi, O. J. Cohen, J. F. Demarest, D. Montefiori, J. M. Orenstein, C. Fox, L. K. Schrager, et. al. 1995.

Studies in subjects with long-term nonprogressive human immunodeficiency virus infection. N. Engl. J. Med. 332:209–216.

90. Patterson, B. K., D. J. Carlo, M. H. Kaplan, M. Marecki, S. Pawha, and R. B. Moss. 1999. Cell-associated HIV-1 messenger RNA and DNA in T-helper cell and monocytes in asymptomatic HIV-1-infected subjects on HAART plus an inactivated HIV-1 immunogen. AIDS 13:1607–1611.

91. Pinto, L. A., J. A. Berzofsky, K. R. Fowke, R. F. Little, F. Merced-Galindez, R. Humphrey, J. Ahlers, N. Dunlop, R. B. Cohen, S. M. Steinberg, P. Nara, G. M. Shearer, and R. Yarchoan. 1999. HIV-specific immunity following immunization with HIV synthetic envelope peptides in asymptomatic HIV-infected patients. AIDS 13:2003–2012.

92. Pitcher, C. J., C. Quittner, D. M. Peterson, M. Connors, R. A. Koup, V. C. Maino, and L. J. Picker. 1999. HIV-1-specific CD4+ T cells are detectable in most individuals with active HIV-1 infection, but decline with prolonged viral suppression. Nature Med. 5:518–525.

93. Polacino, P. S., V. Stallard, J. E. Klaniecki, S. Pennathur, D. C. Montefiori, A. J. Langlois, B. A. Richardson, W. R. Morton, R. E. Benveniste, and S. L. Hu. 1999. Role of immune responses against the envelope and the core antigens of simian immunodeficiency virus SIVmne in protection against homologous cloned and uncloned virus challenge in macaques. J. Virol. 73:8201–8215.

94. Qiu, J. T., R. Song, M. Dettenhofer, C. Tian, T. August, B. K. Felber, G. N. Pavlakis, and X. F. Yu. 1999. Evaluation of novel human immunodeficiency virus type 1 gag DNA vaccines for protein expression in mammalian cells and induction of immune responses. J. Virol. 73:9145–9152.

95. Quinto, I., M. Mallardo, F. Baldassarre, G. Scala, G. Englund, and K. T. Jeang. 1999. Potent and stable attenuation of live-HIV-1 by gain of a proteolysis-resistant inhibitor of NF-kappa B (I kappa B-alpha S32/36A) and the implications for vaccine development. J. Biol. Chem. 274:17567–17572.

96. Rosenberg, E. S., J. M. Billingsley, A. M. Caliendo, S. L. Boswell, P. E. Sax, S. A. Kalams, and B. D. Walker. 1997. Vigorous HIV-1-specific CD4+ T cell responses associated with control of viremia. Science 278:1447–1450.

97. Rosenwirth, B., W. M. Bogers, I. G. Nieuwenhuis, P. T. Haaft, H. Niphuis, E. M. Kuhn, N. Bischofberger, V. Erfle, G. Sutter, P. Berglund, P. Liljestrom, K. Uberla, and J. L. Heeney. 1999. An anti-HIV strategy combining chemotherapy and therapeutic vaccination. J. Med. Primatol. 28:195–205.

98. Rowland-Jones, S. L., T. Dong, L. Dorrell, G. Ogg, P. Hansasuta, P. Krausa, J. Kimani, S. Sabally, K. Ariyoshi, J. Oyugi, K. S. MacDonald, J. Bwayo, H. Whittle, F. A. Plummer, and A. J. McMichael. 1999. Broadly cross-reactive HIV-specific cytotoxic T-lymphocytes in highly-exposed persistently seronegative donors. Immunol. Lett. 66:9–14.

99. Salmon-Ceron, D., J. L. Excler, L. Finkielsztejn, B. Autran, J. C. Gluckman, D. Sicard, T. J. Matthews, B. Meignier, C. Valentin, R. El Habib, C. Blondeau, M. Raux, C. Moog, J. Tartaglia, P. Chong, M. Klein, B. Milcamps, F. Heshmati, and S. Plotkin. 1999. Safety and immunogenicity of a live recombinant canarypox virus expressing HIV type 1 gp120 MN tm/gag/protease LAI (ALVAC-HIV, vCP205) followed by a p24E-V3 MN synthetic peptide

(CLTB-36) administered in healthy volunteers at low risk for HIV infection. AIDS Res. Hum. Retroviruses 15:633–645.

100. Sandstrom, E., and B. Wahren. 1999. Therapeutic immunisation with recombinant gp160 in HIV-1 infection: a randomized double-blind placebo-controlled trial. Lancet 353:1735–1742.

101. Sarin, P. S., J. E. Talmadge, P. Heseltine, N. Murcar, H. E. Gendelman, R. Coleman, L. Kelsey, S. Beckner, D. Winship, and J. Kahn. 1999. Booster immunization of HIV-1 negative volunteers with HGP-30 vaccine induces protection against HIV-1 virus challenge in SCID mice. Vaccine 17:64–71.

102. Sattentau, Q. J., M. Moulard, B. Brivet, F. Botto, J. C. Guillemot, I. Mondor, P. Poignard, and S. Ugolini. 1999. Antibody neutralization of HIV-1 and the potential for vaccine design. Immunol. Lett. 66:143–149.

103. Schmitz, J. E., M. J. Kuroda, S. Santra, V. G. Sasseville, M. A. Simon, M. A. Lifton, P. Racz, K. Tenner-Racz, M. Dalesandro, B. J. Scallon, J. Ghrayeb, M. A. Forman, D. C. Montefiori, E. P. Rieber, N. L. Letvin, and K. A. Reimann. 1999. Control of viremia in simian immunodeficiency virus infection by CD8+ lymphocytes. Science 283:857–860.

104. Schneider, J., S. C. Gilbert, T. J. Blanchard, T. Hanke, K. J. Robson, C. M. Hannan, M. Becker, R. Sinden, G. L. Smith, and A. V. Hill. 1998. Enhanced immunogenicity for CD8+ cell induction and complete protective efficacy of malaria DNA vaccination by boosting with modified vaccinia virus Ankara. Nature Med. 4:397–402.

105. Schwartz, D., U. Sharma, M. Busch, K. Weinhold, T. Matthews, J. Lieberman, D. Birx, H. Farzedagen, J. Margolick, T. Quinn, B. Davis, O. Bagasra, R. Pomerantz, and R. Viscidi. 1994. Absence of recoverable infectious virus and unique immune responses in an asymptomatic HIV+ long-term survivor. AIDS Res. Hum. Retroviruses 10:1703–1711.

106. Sei, S., S. L. Sandelli, G. Theofan, S. Rato-Kim, M. Kumagai, L. D. Loomis-Price, J. H. Cox, P. Jarosinski, C. M. Walsek, P. Brouwers, D. J. Venzon, J. Xu, P. A. Pizzo, R. B. Moss, M. L. Robb, and L. V. Wood. 1999. Preliminary evaluation of human immunodeficiency virus type 1 (HIV-1) immunogen in children with HIV-1 infection. J. Infect. Dis. 180:626–640.

107. Seth, A., Y. Yasutomi, H. Jacoby, J. C. Callery, S. M. Kaminsky, W. C. Koff, D. F. Nixon, and N. L. Letvin. 2000. Evaluation of a lipopeptide immunogen as a therapeutic in HIV type 1-seropositive individuals. AIDS Res. Hum. Retroviruses 16:337–343.

108. Shearer, G. M., L. A. Pinto, and M. Clerici. 1999. Alloimmunization for immune-based therapy and vaccine design against HIV/AIDS. Immunol. Today 20:66–71.

109. Sitz, K. V., S. Ratto-Kim, A. S. Hodgkins, M. L. Robb, and D. L. Birx. 1999. Proliferative responses to human immunodeficiency virus type 1 (HIV-1) gp120 peptides in HIV-1-infected individuals immunized with HIV-1 rgp120 or rgp160 compared with nonimmunized and uninfected controls. J. Infect. Dis. 179:817–824.

110. Steger, K. K., P. J. Valentine, F. Heffron, M. So, and C. D. Pauza. 1999. Recombinant, attenuated, Salmonella typhimurium stimulate lymphoproliferative responses to SIV capsid antigen in rhesus macaques. Vaccine 17:923–932.

111. Steger, K. K., P. M. Waterman, and C. D. Pauza. 1999. Acute effects of pathogenic simian-human immunodeficiency virus challenge on vaccine-induced cellular and humoral immune responses to gag in rhesus macaques. J. Virol. 73:1853–1859.

112. Svanholm, C., L. Bandholtz, A. Lobell, and H. Wigzell. 1999. Enhancement of antibody responses by DNA immunization using expression vectors mediating efficient antigen secretion. J. Immunol. Methods 228:121–130.

113. Tasker, S. A., J. J. Treanor, W. B. Paxton, and M. R. Wallace. 1999. Efficacy of influenza vaccination in HIV-infected persons. A randomized, double-blind, placebo-controlled trial. Ann. Intern. Med. 131:430–433.

114. Ulmer, J., J. J. Donnelly, S. E. Parker, G. H. Rhodes, P. L. Felgner, V. J. Dwarki, S. H. Gromkowski, R. R. Deck, C. M. DeWitt, A. Friedman, L. A. Hawe, K. R. Leander, D. Martinez, H. C. Perry, J. W. Shiver, D. L. Montgomery, and M. A. Liu. 1993. Heterologous protection against influenza by injection of DNA encoding a viral protein. Science 259:1745–1749.

115. Wagner, L., O. O. Yang, E. A. Garcia-Zepeda, Y. Ge, S. A. Kalams, B. D. Walker, M. S. Pasternack, and A. D. Luster. 1998. β-chemokines are released from HIV-1-specific cytolytic T-cell granules complexed to proteoglycans. Nature 391:908–911.

116. Watson, A., J. McClure, J. Ranchalis, M. Scheibel, A. Schmidt, B. Kennedy, W. R. Morton, N. L. Haigwood, and S. L. Hu. 1997. Early postinfection antiviral treatment reduces viral load and prevents CD4+ cell decline in HIV type 2-infected macaques. AIDS Res. Hum. Retroviruses 13:1375–1381.

117. Watson, A., J. Ranchalis, B. Travis, J. McClure, W. Sutton, P. R. Johnson, S. L. Hu, and N. L. Haigwood. 1997. Plasma viremia in macaques infected with simian immunodeficiency virus: plasma viral load early in infection predicts survival. J. Virol. 71:284–290.

118. Whitton, J. L., N. Sheng, M. B. Oldstone, and T. A. McKee. 1993. A "string-of-beads" vaccine, comprising linked minigenes, confers protection from lethal-dose virus challenge. J. Virol. 67:348–352.

119. Widera, G., M. Austin, D. Rabussay, C. Goldbeck, S. W. Barnett, M. Chen, L. Leung, G. R. Otten, K. Thudium, M. J. Selby, and J. B. Ulmer. 2000. Increased DNA vaccine delivery and immunogenicity by electroporation in vivo. J. Immunol. 164:4635–4640.

120. Woodberry, T., J. Gardner, L. Mateo, D. Eisen, J. Medveczky, I. A. Ramshaw, S. A. Thomson, R. A. French, S. L. Elliott, H. Firat, F. A. Lemonnier, and A. Suhrbier. 1999. Immunogenicity of a human immunodeficiency virus (HIV) polytope vaccine containing multiple HLA A2 HIV CD8+ cytotoxic T-cell epitopes. J. Virol. 73:5320–5325.

121. Wyand, M. S., K. Manson, D. C. Montefiori, J. D. Lifson, R. P. Johnson, and R. C. Desrosiers. 1999. Protection by live, attenuated simian immunodeficiency virus against heterologous challenge. J. Virol. 73:8356–8363.

122. Wyatt, R., P. D. Kwong, E. Desjardins, R. W. Sweet, J. Robinson, W. A. Hendrickson, and J. C. Sodroski. 1998. The antigenic structure of the HIV gp120 envelope protein. Nature 393:705–711.

123. Yang, L. P., J. L. Riley, R. G. Carroll, C. H. June, J. Hoxie, B. K. Patterson, Y. Ohshima, R. J. Hodes, and G. Delespesse. 1998. Productive infection of neonatal CD8+ lymphocytes by HIV-1. J. Exp. Med. 187:1139–1144.

124. Yang, O. O., and B. D. Walker. 1997. CD8⁺ cells in human immunodeficiency virus type 1 pathogenesis: cytolytic and noncytolytic inhibition of viral replication. Advances in Immunol. 66:273–311.

125. Zajac, A. J., J. N. Blattman, K. Murali-Krishna, D. J. Sourdive, M. Suresh, J. D. Altman, and R. Ahmed. 1998. Viral immune evasion due to persistence of activated T cells without effector function. J. Exp. Med. 188:2205–2213.

126. zur Megede, J., M. C. Chen, B. Doe, M. Schaefer, C. E. Greer, M. Selby, G. R. Otten, and S. W. Barnett. 2000. Increased expression and immunogenicity of sequence-modified human immunodeficiency virus type 1 gag gene. J. Virol. 74:2628–2635.

INDEX

Page numbers followed by *t* and *f* indicate tables and figures, respectively. Those followed by *n* indicate notes, with the note number following the *n*.